Medical Speech–Language Pathology

A Practitioner's Guide

Second Edition

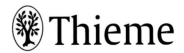

Medical Speech–Language Pathology

A Practitioner's Guide

Second Edition

Alex F. Johnson, Ph.D., C.C.C.-S.L.P.
Professor and Chair
Department of Communication Sciences and Disorders
Wayne State University
Detroit, Michigan

Barbara H. Jacobson, Ph.D., C.C.C.-S.L.P.
Assistant Professor
Voice Center
Vanderbilt University
Vanderbilt Medical Center
Nashville, Tennessee

Thieme
New York • Stuttgart

Thieme Medical Publishers, Inc.
333 Seventh Ave.
New York, NY 10001

Executive Editor: Timothy Hiscock
Editorial Assistant: David Price
Vice President, Production and Electronic Publishing: Anne T. Vinnicombe
Production Editor: Print Matters, Inc.
Sales Director: Ross Lumpkin
Associate Marketing Director: Verena Diem
Chief Financial Officer: Peter van Woerden
President: Brian D. Scanlan
Compositor: Compset, Inc.
Printer: Sheridan Books, Inc.

Library of Congress Cataloging-in-Publication Data

Medical speech-language pathology : a practitioner's guide/[edited by] Alex F. Johnson, Barbara H. Jacobson.
— 2nd ed.
    p.; cm.
  Includes bibliographical references and index.
  ISBN 1-58890-320-6 (US-HC) — ISBN 3-13-110532-1 (GTV-HC)
    1. Speech therapy. 2. Speech disorders. 3. Language disorders. I. Johnson, Alex F. II. Jacobson,
Barbara Holcomb.
  [DNLM: 1. Speech Disorders. 2. Deglutition Disorders. 3. Language Disorders. 4. Speech-Language
Pathology—methods. 5. Voice Disorders. WL 340.2 M489 2006]
RC423.M395 2006
616.85′5—dc22   2006044648

Important note: Medical knowledge is ever-changing. As new research and clinical experience broaden
our knowledge, changes in treatment and drug therapy may be required. The authors and editors of the
material herein have consulted sources believed to be reliable in their efforts to provide information that
is complete and in accord with the standards accepted at the time of publication. However, in view of the
possibility of human error by the authors, editors, or publisher of the work herein or changes in medical
knowledge, neither the authors, editors, or publisher, nor any other party who has been involved in the
preparation of this work, warrants that the information contained herein is in every respect accurate or
complete, and they are not responsible for any errors or omissions or for the results obtained from use of
such information. Readers are encouraged to confirm the information contained herein with other
sources. For example, readers are advised to check the product information sheet included in the package
of each drug they plan to administer to be certain that the information contained in this publication is
accurate and that changes have not been made in the recommended dose or in the contraindications for
administration. This recommendation is of particular importance in connection with new or infrequently
used drugs.

Some of the product names, patents, and registered designs referred to in this book are in fact registered
trademarks or proprietary names even though specific reference to this fact is not always made in the
text. Therefore, the appearance of a name without designation as proprietary is not to be construed as a
representation by the publisher that it is in the public domain.

Printed in the United States

5 4 3 2

TMP ISBN 1-58890-320-6
            978-1-58890-320-4
GTV ISBN 3-13-110532-1
            978-3-13-110532-5

This book is dedicated to the memory of Dr. Carol Frattali. She was a close friend,
a brilliant colleague, and a generous contributor to both editions of this book.
Her dedication to medical speech–language pathology was inspiring and motivating.

Contents

Preface ix

Acknowledgments xi

Contributors xiii

I. Medical Speech–Language Pathology: An Orientation 1

1. The Scope of Medical Speech–Language Pathology 3
   Alex F. Johnson and Barbara H. Jacobson

2. Medical Ethics and the Speech–Language Pathologist 8
   Edythe A. Strand, Kathryn M. Yorkston, and Robert M. Miller

II. Neurocognitive Communication Disorders 17

3. Brain Imaging in Aquired Language Disorders 19
   K. Paige George, Eric Vikingstad, Richard Silbergleit, and Yue Cao

4. Assessment of Aphasia 53
   Jacqueline J. Hinckley and Lori Bartels-Tobin

5. Aphasia Rehabilitation: Postacute Clinical Management 61
   Margaret Greenwald and Chad McCarney

6. Cognitive-Communication Rehabilitation Following Traumatic Brain Injury 71
   Carl Coelho and Kathleen M. Youse

7. Dementia: Diagnostic Approaches and Current Taxonomies 94
   Jennifer Horner, Michele L. Norman, and Danielle N. Ripich

8. Dementia: Communication Impairments and Management 110
   Michele L. Norman, Jennifer Horner, and Danielle N. Ripich

III. Disorders of Swallowing and Voice 129

9. Dysphagia: Basic Assessment and Management 131
   Jeri A. Logemann

10. The Use of Flexible Endoscopy to Evaluate and Manage Patients with Dyshagia 148
    Susan Langmore

11. Voice Disorders 158
    Barbara H. Jacobson, Joseph C. Stemple, Leslie E. Glaze, Bernice K. Klaben, and Michael Karnell

12. Rehabilitation of the Head and Neck Cancer Patients 182
    Michael S. Benninger, Cinthia Grywalski, and Debra Phyland

IV. Topics in Clinical Collaboration and Service Delivery **203**

13. Psychogenic Communication Disorders... 205
     Greg Mahr, Wendy Bertges Yost, and Barbara H. Jacobson

14. Current Trends and Issues in Health Care Delivery: What Speech–Language Pathologists Need to Know 213
     Janet E. Brown and Arlene Pietranton

15. Evidence-Based Practice and Outcomes-Oriented Approaches in Speech–Language Pathology................... 223
     Carol M. Frattali and Lee Ann Golper

16. Use of Data in Service Delivery... 236
     Nancy B. Swigert and Robert C. Mullen

17. Clinical Documentation in Medical Speech–Language Pathology 247
     Ann W. Kummer, Pete Johnson, and Katrina Zeit

18. Speech–Language Pathology in the Intensive Care Unit 260
     Alice K. Silbergleit and Michael A. Basha

19. Speech–Language Pathology Practice in the Acute Care Setting: A Consultative Approach 284
     Alex F. Johnson, Anne Marie Valachovic, and K. Paige George

V. Medical Perspectives **299**

20. Issues in Geriatric Medicine 301
     Thomas R. Palmer and Murray B. Hunter

21. Neurologic Disorders: An Orientation and Overview 315
     Nabih Ramadan and Daniel S. Newman

22. Medical and Surgical Management in Otolaryngology 337
     Glendon M. Gardner and Michael S. Benninger

23. Drug-Induced Communication and Swallowing Disorders 363
     Tami Remington and Susan C. Fagan

Index **379**

Preface

The interface of interdisciplinary knowledge, technological advances, and service delivery issues is realized in a remarkable way within the area of medical speech–language pathology. Since the publication of our last edition in 1998, the world of medical speech–language pathology has expanded, retracted, and expanded again. While reimbursement and policy issues affected the availability of services for some time immediately after the first edition was published, the demand for high quality services and the recognition of the vital role of speech–language pathology in helping patients medically and functionally has forced growth again. In this new edition of our book, we have tried to provide the basic information needed by clinicians committed to providing services in the medical setting and to also provide material of interest to those who need the most advanced information.

Each chapter is filled with important background information and with material that will hopefully guide and improve practice. The book is designed to be used as a text for medical speech–language pathology coursework, a reference book for those who work in health-care settings, and a compilation of up-to-date material focused on adult medical speech–language pathology areas. Additionally, it is hoped that researchers, physicians, and other rehabilitation professionals with an interest in the discipline of human communication disorders will find this text to be a window into the expanding world of medical speech–language pathology.

We have made a few changes in this edition of the text. We have redesigned the book to eliminate some redundancy, and hopefully readers will find this new organization to be more efficient and helpful for their purposes. Readers of the previous edition will note that we have removed the chapters that dealt with pediatric issues in medical speech–language pathology. This is an area of medical speech–language pathology that is rapidly expanding with regard to knowledge about swallowing and communication services to neonates, and about children with craniofacial deformities, developmental neurological and cognitive issues, respiratory issues, traumatic brain injury and so forth. Due to the need to limit the length of this text, the decision was made to eliminate the pediatric sections rather than provide cursory information that would not do justice to this specialty of medical speech–language pathology.

Our hope is that those who use this book will find that it provides information that improves their knowledge and skills, assists in the preparation of students and new professionals, and increases the opportunity for dialogue with colleagues across disciplines. We are convinced that the contributors to this text have kept these various purposes in mind as they have painstakingly put together such informative, interesting, current, and well-developed chapters. We believe that each chapter stands alone as an important information source for the discipline, that various chapters can combine as a significant review of a sub-area of speech–language pathology (acute patient care, neurologic disorders, voice, etc.), and that the entire work provides a comprehensive guide to patient care and best practice across the spectrum.

Acknowledgments

Every person who has authored or edited a book knows the work involved, the time expended, and the energy used. In our case, in this second edition, the work was complicated by "long distance" collaboration. Our first edition was completed while we were working together at Henry Ford Hospital. Our proximity provided daily communication, deliberation, and collaboration. This second edition was completed as we both moved to new positions in new states in new institutions. These changes have most certainly added to the complexity of completing this book. However, through this move we have developed new colleagues who have influenced our thinking about medical speech–language pathology. We have had the opportunity to invite some new contributors, and we have renewed our invitation to many of our chapter authors from the first edition. These relationships with new contributors, and certainly those from the previous edition, have been our sustenance in this work. We are indebted beyond comprehension to the talent and the patience of these contributors as we worked through this revision.

We also thank our editors at Thieme. They have been most helpful in providing support and leadership toward the completion of this project. We are grateful for the experience of working with Timothy Hiscock and David Price, who have guided us and have shared their expertise in this comprehensive and complex project.

We extend gratitude to those with whom we have worked and continue to work. The original impetus for the first edition grew from our collaborations with each other and with colleagues at Henry Ford Hospital in Detroit, Michigan. That remarkable experience in the 1990s shaped our understanding of medical speech–language pathology in a manner that continues to influence us in our own work and certainly in the development of this text. Our experience at Henry Ford with colleagues and students sharpened our view and engendered a love for this area of our field, and for that we will always be extremely grateful. Now we work in different institutions and express our gratitude also to those colleagues at Vanderbilt University and at Wayne State University who continue to guide our thinking. We are especially appreciative of our students, who are remarkable in asking questions that have yet to be answered.

Our families have been remarkably patient and offered true support over the years of development of the first and second edition. Our children (David, Jeffrey, Cristina), now into teens and young adulthood, have grown up over the years of our collaboration. Our spouses (Linda, Gary) have been enthusiastic in their support and interest and have offered encouragement at those moments when lethargy set in. Out of this collaboration, family friendships have grown and we know that they will endure.

Finally, we again thank each other! We have worked together now for almost twenty years, in one form or another. This book continues to represent those concepts and practices that we have embraced. We are so grateful for the opportunity to continue this collaboration, even when distance has changed our day-to-day interaction.

Contributors

EDITORS

Alex F. Johnson, Ph.D., C.C.C.-S.L.P.
Professor and Chair
Department of Communication Sciences and Disorders
Wayne State University
Detroit, Michigan

Barbara H. Jacobson, Ph.D., C.C.C.-S.L.P.
Assistant Professor
Voice Center
Vanderbilt University
Vanderbilt Medical Center
Nashville, Tennessee

CONTRIBUTORS

Lori Bartels-Tobin
Department of Communication
    Science and Disorders
University of South Florida
Tampa, Florida

Michael A. Basha, D.O., F.C.C.P.
Director of Critical Care Services
Division of Pulmonary and Critical Care Medicine
Physician HealthCare Network
Port Huron Hospital
Port Huron, Michigan

Michael S. Benninger, M.D.
Chair
Department of Otolaryngology—Head and Neck Surgery
Henry Ford Hospital
Henry Ford Health System
Detroit, Michigan

Janet E. Brown, M.A., C.C.C.-S.L.P.
Director, Healthcare Services in Speech
    Language Pathology
American Speech–Language-Hearing Association
Rockville, Maryland

Yue Cao, Ph.D.
Associate Professor
Departments of Radiation Oncology and Radiology
University of Michigan
Ann Arbor, Michigan

Carl Coelho, Ph.D., B.C.-N.C.D.
Professor and Head
Communication Sciences Department
University of Connecticut
Storrs, Connecticut

Susan C. Fagan, Pharm.D., B.C.P.S., F.C.C.P.
Professor
Clinical and Administrative Pharmacy
University of Georgia College of Pharmacy and
    Medical College of Georgia
Augusta, Georgia

Carol M. Frattali, Ph.D., B.C.-N.C.D.[†]
W.G. Magnuson Clinical Center, Speech–Language
    Pathology Section
National Institutes of Health
Bethesda, Maryland
Adjunct Professor
Department of Hearing and Speech Sciences
University of Maryland
College Park, Maryland
[†]Deceased

Glendon M. Gardner, M.D.
Department of Otolaryngology—Head and Neck Surgery
Henry Ford Hospital
Henry Ford Health System
Detroit, Michigan

K. Paige George, M.A.-C.C.C.-S.L.P.
Speech–Language Pathologist
Private Practice
Huntington Woods, Michigan

Leslie E. Glaze, Ph.D., C.C.C.-S.L.P.
Adjunct Assistant Professor
Department of Speech, Language and Hearing Sciences
University of Minnesota
Minneapolis, Minnesota

Lee Ann Golper, Ph.D., B.C.-N.C.D.
Associate Professor and Director, Speech–Language
    Pathology Division
Department of Hearing and Speech Sciences
Vanderbilt University
Vanderbilt Medical Center
Nashville, Tennessee

Margaret Greenwald, Ph.D.
Associate Professor
Department of Audiology and Speech–Language
    Pathology
Wayne State University
Detroit, Michigan

Cynthia Grywalski, M.A.
Speech–Language Pathologist
Division of Speech–Language Sciences and Disorders
Henry Ford Hospital
Henry Ford Health System
Detroit, Michigan

Jacqueline J. Hinckley, Ph.D.
Associate Professor
Department of Communication Science and Disorders
University of South Florida
Tampa, Florida

Jennifer Horner, Ph.D., J.D.
Associate Professor and Chair
Department of Rehabilitation Sciences
Medical University of South Carolina
College of Health Professions
Charleston, South Carolina

Murray B. Hunter, M.D.†
Senior Staff Physician
Department of Geriatrics
Henry Ford Center for Seniors
Henry Ford Health System
Detroit, Michigan
†Deceased

Pete Johnson, Ph.D.
Dysphagia Mentor
Coinvestigator/U.S. Site Coordinator—EMG/Dysphagia
    Study
Select Medical Rehabilitation Services
Clearwater, Florida

Michael Karnell, Ph.D.
Associate Professor
Department of Otolaryngology—Head and Neck Surgery
Department of Speech Pathology and Audiology
University of Iowa
Iowa City, Iowa

Bernice K. Klaben, Ph.D., C.C.C., S.L.P., B.R.S.-S.
Director of Clinical Practices
The Blaine Block Institute for Voice Analysis and
    Rehabilitation
Dayton, Ohio

Ann W. Kummer, Ph.D.
Professor
Department of Pediatrics
University of Cincinnati Medical Center
Director
Department of Speech Pathology
Cincinnati Children's Hospital Medical Center
Cincinnati, Ohio

Susan Langmore, Ph.D.
Associate Clinical Professor
Department of Otolaryngology—Head and Neck Surgery
Voice and Swallow Center
University of California–San Francisco
San Francisco, California

Jeri A. Logemann, Ph.D.
Professor
Department of Communication Sciences and Disorders
Northwestern University
Evanston, Illinois

Greg Mahr, M.D.
Medical Director
Henry Ford Kingswood Hospital
Ferndale, Michigan

Chad McCarney, M.S.
Research Assistant and Lecturer
Department of Audiology and Speech–Language Pathology
Wayne State University
Detroit, Michigan

Robert M. Miller, Ph.D., C.C.C.-S.L.P.
Senior Lecturer
Department of Speech and Hearing
University of Washington
Seattle, Washington

Robert C. Mullen, M.P.H.
Director, National Center for Treatment
    Effectiveness in Communication Disorders
American Speech–Language-Hearing Association
Rockville, Maryland

Daniel S. Newman, M.D.
Director, Department of Neurology
Harry J. Hoenselaar ALS Clinic
Henry Ford Hospital
Henry Ford Health System
Detroit, Michigan

Michele L. Norman, Ph.D.
Assistant Professor
Department of Gerontology
Virginia Commonwealth University Medical Center
School of Allied Health Professions
Richmond, Virginia

Thomas R. Palmer M.D.
Department of Family Medicine–Geriatrics
Henry Ford Hospital
Henry Ford Health System
Detroit, Michigan

Arlene Pietranton, Ph.D.
Executive Director
American Speech–Language-Hearing
    Association
Rockville, Maryland

Debra Phyland, M.App.Sc.
Lecturer
School of Human Communication Sciences
Latrobe University
Royal Victorian Eye and Ear Hospital
Melbourne, Victoria
Australia

Nabih Ramadan, M.D.
Professor and Chair
Departments of Neurology and Psychiatry and
   Behavioral Sciences
Rosalind Franklin University of Medicine
   and Science
North Chicago, Illinois

Tami Remington, Pharm.D.
Clinical Associate Professor and Clinical Pharmacist
College of Pharmacy
University of Michigan
Ann Arbor, Michigan

Danielle N. Ripich, Ph.D.
Professor and Dean
College of Health Professions
Medical University of South Carolina
Charleston, South Carolina

Alice K. Silbergleit, Ph.D., C.C.C.
Assistant Professor
Department of Neurology
Wayne State University
Director
Division of Speech–Language Sciences and
   Disorders
Henry Ford Hospital
Henry Ford Health System
Detroit, Michigan

Richard Silbergleit, M.D.
Director, Neuroimaging
Department of Diagnostic Radiology
William Beaumont Hospital
Royal Oak, Michigan

Joseph C. Stemple, Ph.D.
Professor, Department of Rehabilitation
   Sciences
College of Health Sciences
University of Kentucky
Lexington, Kentucky

Edythe A. Strand, Ph.D., C.C.C.-S.L.P.
Associate Professor and Consultant
Division of Speech Pathology
Department of Neurology
Mayo Clinic–Mayo College of Medicine
Rochester, Minnesota

Nancy B. Swigert, M.A.
President
Swigert & Associates, Inc.
Lexington, Kentucky

Anne Marie Valachovic, M.A.
Speech Pathologist
Division of Speech–Language Sciences
   and Disorders
Henry Ford Hospital
Henry Ford Health System
Detroit, Michigan

Eric Vikingstad, B.S.
Graduate Student
Department of Radiology
The University of Chicago
The University of Chicago Hospitals
Chicago, Illinois

Kathryn M. Yorkston, Ph.D.
Professor and Head
Division of Speech Pathology
Department of Rehabilitation Medicine
University of Washington
Seattle, Washington

Wendy Bertges Yost, Ph.D.
Clinical Psychologist
Henry Ford Hospital
Henry Ford Health System
Detroit, Michigan

Kathleen M. Youse, Ph.D., C.C.C.-S.L.P.
Assistant Professor
Division of Communication Disorders
College of Health Sciences
University of Kentucky
Lexington, Kentucky

Katrina Zeit, M.H.A., M.A.
Speech Pathologist and Project Manager
Department of Speech Pathology
Cincinnati Children's Hospital Medical Center
Cincinnati, Ohio

Section 1

**Medical Speech–Language Pathology:
An Orientation**

1

The Scope of Medical Speech–Language Pathology

Alex F. Johnson and Barbara H. Jacobson

✦ **Why Differentiate Medical from Nonmedical Speech–Language Pathology (SLP)?**
✦ **The Continuum of Care in Medical Speech–Language Pathology**
✦ **Subspecialization in Medical Speech–Language Pathology**
✦ **Procedures and Competencies in Medical Speech–Language Pathology**
✦ **Medical Speech–Language Pathology: Practice Trends**
✦ **Issues in Clinical Practice**
✦ **Issues in Service Delivery**

The field of speech–language pathology has a rich and long history of service to individuals who suffer from a variety of physical and psychological symptoms and diseases. The study of speech–language sciences and disorders includes attention to:

✦ The underlying anatomy and physiologic processes that are used in thinking about, understanding, formulating, and producing communication
✦ The psychological and social mechanisms that nurture communication or destroy it
✦ The physical processes that allow sound to be generated, transmitted, and perceived
✦ The conditions, both developmental and acquired, that impede the use of communication
✦ The environmental inputs and factors that encourage or discourage communication in all its forms
✦ The effects of communication and swallowing problems on individuals and on society

When such topics are studied from perspectives that emphasize the physical processes, causes, associated signs and symptoms, pathophysiology, and underlying disease processes, then we are using models and tools developed in the medical sciences. Over hundreds of years, those who have studied human medicine and disease have used a common model to expand the understanding of disease and approaches to its treatment. It should be no secret to those in our discipline that our processes and models have evolved from a similar framework, as have those in many other health disciplines (dentistry, optometry, veterinary medicine, psychology,

etc.). Although those who study medicine have developed and emphasized the use of surgery and pharmaceutical treatments, speech–language pathologists have provided distinctive behavioral and physiologic approaches to patient management.

✦ Why Differentiate Medical from Nonmedical Speech–Language Pathology?

There are few good reasons for differentiating medical and nonmedical speech–language pathology practice. Every clinician practicing in the field needs to know about the care of individuals with a variety of disorders. Regardless of the setting in which he or she practices, the speech–language pathologist must understand the causes and effects of communication disorders. This understanding can only come from in-depth knowledge of the physical, anatomic, psychological, and physiologic processes involved in communication, and from knowledge of the conditions producing the disorders that interrupt it. Thus, a medical (cause-effect scientifically based) perspective is useful to every speech–language pathologist.

Although this broad perspective on medical speech–language pathology holds true for most practitioners, it is important to highlight two general views regarding the categorization of speech–language pathology into components that are medical and those that are nonmedical. One school proposes that *a distinct* category of professional practice

3

within the field encompasses a body of information and a range of clinical activities that impact a patient's medical status or are impacted by a patient's medical condition. Proponents of this school of thought suggest that this aspect of speech–language pathology practice should be delimited and defined by the term *medical*. This approach serves to signal the key feature of the speech–language practice being discussed and also differentiate it from other aspects of the field (i.e., educational, developmental, etc.). This first view was highlighted in the 2000 revision of the Speech–Language Pathology (SLP) Scope of Practice of the American Speech–Language-Hearing Association (2001). In this document the concept of communication enhancement in the "absence of known diseases of impairments" was explicated.

A second perspective suggests that all speech–language pathology is medical. That is, the bases of our understanding of human communication and its disorders are found in the interplay among the physical, biologic, and behavioral sciences. This viewpoint emphasizes that, regardless of the setting in which we practice, the types of patients (or clients or students) whom we treat, or the nature of our clinical activities, the practice of the profession is based in clinical science and is therefore medical. This group would argue that there is no area of practice that could be considered nonmedical. Although this appears true when one focuses on understanding the underlying bases of human communication, it is a less precise description of the services that are delivered in non–health care environments. The professional activities of many speech–language pathologists concentrate on the use of language and communication for particular purposes in highly specific settings, such as the school or the workplace. Additionally, in the field there is an important continuing trend toward recognizing the needs of persons who experience communication challenges as a result of accent, stylistic differences, or other nonclinical situations. It is perhaps easier and more fruitful to consider these concerns in a social or educational context. An argument can be made for differentiating this particular set of practices from those directed to more immediate health concerns of the patient.

Our own position represents a compromise between these two perspectives. At the superordinate level, it is easy to recognize the interplay among the behavioral, physical, and life sciences in understanding the nature and treatment of speech, language, and swallowing disorders. At the more direct practice level, the benefit of discussing a "category" of practice within the field helps to align discussion for the important details of clinical diagnosis and treatment for the practitioner. Thus, we recognize the essential contribution of the scientific bases of the discipline, acknowledging that this foundation is shared with other health science professions. At the same time, we argue that there are speech-language pathologists who apply this information in nonmedical settings with persons who may or may not be ill, directed toward expected outcomes that are vocational or educational. Thus, for pragmatic reasons, we feel comfortable in utilizing the term *medical speech–language pathology* to categorize an aspect of speech–language professional practice that is not necessarily specific to a setting. Instead it represents a specific approach to patient care and a specific set of clinical processes and outcomes that are related to the medical, social, and psychological well-being of the patient.

The practice of medical speech–language pathology may be examined from three different viewpoints. These reflect the ways that we can characterize this area of specialization within the larger field of speech–language pathology. These viewpoints also guide how we regard our professional identity and how we plan for the future. Medical speech–language pathology may defined by (1) *where* it is practiced (the continuum of care); (2) *who* delivers speech–language services (the specialists and subspecialists); and (3) *how* and *what* types of services are performed (procedures and competencies). The contributors in this text reflect these various approaches to medical speech–language pathology in their chapters. As the reader progresses through this text, discussion of setting-specific (acute care, rehabilitation, outpatient) issues, skills and knowledge of practitioners, and skills and competencies will be found.

✦ The Continuum of Care in Medical Speech–Language Pathology

Medical speech–language pathology can be practiced in a variety of settings including academic facilities (university medical centers), community hospitals, outpatient clinics, subacute care facilities, rehabilitation settings, home care, nursing homes, and hospices. Medical speech–language pathologists can view themselves within the context of these physical environments.

The emphasis on various skills and knowledge shifts, depending on where services are delivered. For example, clinicians must be attuned to rapid changes in communication and swallowing as well as medical status when they practice in acute care settings. Their focus of management is primarily consultative. In chronic care environments, speech–language pathologists work to strengthen functional communication for patients whose disease processes are relatively stable. Interventions are rehabilitative or monitoring in nature. However, practice in both environments requires a strong base of knowledge in the pathophysiology of communication disorders (e.g., neurologic disease) as well as the effects of other diseases and conditions on patients.

✦ Subspecialization in Medical Speech–Language Pathology

Medical speech–language pathology may also be viewed in terms of areas of specialization. Clinicians often identify themselves by the type of disorders they treat or the kind of patients they see. Some of the areas that have become quite developed within the field include neurogenic communication disorders, voice disorders, swallowing disorders, tracheostomy/ventilator-dependent patients, and a host of pediatric areas. The extent and depth of knowledge necessary for comprehensive diagnosis and treatment in these areas have prompted the need for specialization. This focus by disorder in medical speech–language pathology follows the medical model. Many physicians train in a particular specialty (neurology or otolaryngology) and then seek further education in a subspecialty (laryngology or electrophysiology).

The move toward specialty recognition as a formal process of acknowledging a professional's area of concentration and expertise is emerging within the discipline of speech–language pathology. For example, several special-interest divisions within the American Speech–Language–Hearing Association (ASHA) have begun the process of setting standards for speech–language pathologists to obtain specialty recognition. Of particular interest to those in medical settings will be the evolution of the new specialty board and recognition process for those interested in swallowing and its disorders. This new specialty board has established criteria for recognition as part of ASHA's specialty recognition process. Additionally, the American Academy of Neurologic Communication Disorders and Sciences (ANCDS) has established and validated a program of specialty certification for practitioners who work with adults or children with neurologically based communication disorders. Information for this process can be found at www.ANCDS.edu.

✦ Procedures and Competencies in Medical Speech–Language Pathology

The practice of medical speech–language pathology may also be considered in the context of tasks, protocols, and competencies. This focus has become more common as diagnosis and treatment rely on technology (videofluoroscopy, endoscopy, augmentative communication technologies, etc.).

Because of the potential for risk to patients during various procedures, clearly defined competencies (skill and knowledge based) are required for ensuring the safety of patients and for the proper interpretation of results. This trend for instrumentally based practice is reflected in the development of several practice guidelines by ASHA. In addition, several groups, including the special interest divisions of ASHA, have developed competencies for a variety of areas of practice in medical speech–language pathology. Although these competencies are early in their development, it is probable that ASHA and other professional groups will be disseminating information about practice in this area.

✦ Medical Speech–Language Pathology: Practice Trends

Medical speech–language pathology is both dynamic and developing. The area is dynamic because constant changes in the state of knowledge in medicine, rehabilitation, and psychology, as well as political, economic, and competitive forces push for constant reconsideration and realignment in service delivery. It is developmental in the sense that new research-based evidence for diagnosis and treatment is emerging on a regular basis. Thus, the field continually needs to change to serve the profession, our patients, and the institutions where we practice speech–language pathology.

In 2002, ASHA published a report highlighting the state of SLP practice in health care settings. This report included foci on reimbursement issues and effects, caseload type and activities, and work setting issues. This is the first comprehensive report on the status of health care SLP practice and should be reviewed by every practitioner in our field. It is beyond the scope of this introductory chapter to review all of the dimensions of the report; however, some findings from the survey are as follows:

◆ Thirty-one percent of SLP practitioners' time was spent in treating dysphagia and over 50% of their time was spent in treating cognitive and language disabilities.

◆ A surprising number of SLP practitioners, 66%, received regular referrals for augmentative and alternative communication issues.

◆ Forty-five percent of respondents spent time in training and supervising clinical practicum students and clinical fellows, with most of this activity occurring in acute and rehabilitative settings rather than home care or skilled nursing programs.

◆ Less than 2% of respondents in health care reported using SLP assistants.

◆ Sixty-nine percent of respondents indicated that there was difficulty in hiring qualified SLPs for their setting. (Source: www.asha.org/members/slp/healthcare/work.htm.)

✦ Issues in Clinical Practice

Consultative Practice

In consultative practice, service delivery is characterized by intensive short-term interventions that may or may not include direct treatment with the patient. Chapter 18 contains a more extensive description of this practice modality. In medical speech–language pathology, consultation has evolved primarily in acute care settings as a means of effectively managing the care of patients with communication and swallowing disorders who are hospitalized for a relatively short stay. Instead of following standard evaluation and treatment protocols, practice emphasizes answering the referral question posed by the physician, monitoring communication and swallowing status, patient and family education, and discharge planning. This diversion from the strictly rehabilitative focus maintained in the past can be a difficult adjustment for medical speech–language pathologists. Many practitioners derive a great deal of satisfaction from developing therapeutic relationships with the patients they treat, and those connections may not be possible within the practice of consultation.

Technological Developments in Clinical Practice

New technologies that have been applied in speech–language pathology have developed within the past several years. Instrumentation for clinical practice in voice, swallowing, craniofacial anomalies, and other areas involving movement of the speech/swallowing musculature has allowed for new measures and observations of the physiologic aspects of speech. Communication aids and tools for the nonoral population also continue to expand options for enhancing interaction and productivity. New computer technologies have also had an effect on practice. General applications for use in business and home are being adapted for clinical settings. In addition, applications are being specifically developed for use by the SLP practitioner in clinical and administrative functions. Finally, the Internet is emerging as a source of information and tools for communication among professionals, interaction with resource centers focused on specific topics, and access to new information for incorporation into practice.

Ethical Issues

Ethical practice refers to the application of standards of service delivery. These standards include avoiding misrepresentation of services, performing only those activities for which one is qualified (i.e., certified, competent), adhering to preferred practice patterns, and providing service in the best interest of the patient, among others. Ethics also may be viewed from the perspective of its formal discipline (see Chapter 2). As the scope of practice expands in medical speech–language pathology, so do the number of situations in which ethical concerns may arise.

The specialty of swallowing has become the most visible area in which ethical issues emerge. The management of swallowing disorders is a high-volume activity for many medical speech–language pathologists. Dysphagia assessment and treatment, along with endoscopy, are service activities that carry the most risk for harm to the patient. Both ethical practice and ethics are important issues in this specialty. The question of competency, in the face of uneven graduate education in dysphagia in the past, continues to be at the forefront of discussion. Decision making in dysphagia practice requires an understanding of the principles of ethics and their application to questions of patient and family decisions regarding type of feeding, withdrawal of feeding, and oral feeding in the presence of aspiration risk. At this writing, most SLP practitioners understand and adhere to ethical standards of practice, but tend to be undereducated in the area of ethics.

Interprofessional Issues

A variety of disciplines and professions interact in medical speech–language pathology practice. Regardless of setting type or clinical specialization area, SLP practitioners come into contact with a myriad of physician specialists and generalists, rehabilitation professionals, nurses, psychologists, audiologists, and others as they go about the business of caring for their patients. As professionals attempt to work together there is sometimes a tendency for individual clinicians to engage in conflict over issues of turf, competence, or perceived power. These conflicts increase in frequency (and sometimes intensity) when the practice environment calls for reductions in resource utilization. Some organizations have developed new approaches to delivering services that attempt to avoid the "turf" competition by facilitating team approaches and product line approaches to avoid the traditional departmental structure. These models warrant careful study as vehicles for delivering improved care and quality. However, they do serve as a threat to some aspects of discipline-specific knowledge and skill development. A rush to develop new teams or product lines should not obviate the need for development of specialized skills in meeting the needs of patients with communication or swallowing disorders by the speech–language pathologist.

✦ Issues in Service Delivery

The health insurance industry has drastically changed its way of doing business and has caused havoc in the delivery of all health care services, including speech–language pathology. Major effects in all health settings include increased attention to costs and resources used, major attempts to control costs by reducing the length and variety of patient services, an emphasis on prevention over treatment, and measurement of performance from a variety of perspectives and clinical outcomes.

The careful observer of these issues recognizes that the entire process of serving patients via the health care system

has changed or is changing. Speech–language pathologists now must understand and appreciate the significance of a variety of new methodologies for funding their programs. These methods, which include capitation arrangements, extend beyond the traditional fee-for-service models. In addition to impacting the financial components of speech–language pathologists' practice, protocols have been and are being developed that determine who will get service and under what conditions. These factors have moved the speech–language pathologist into the role of needing to work to maintain relationships with referral sources, including insurance companies. The current market also requires that clinicians are continuously able to demonstrate the rationale for their services as well as all costs incurred on behalf of the patient.

✦ Conclusion

This chapter has highlighted some of the professional issues that may be consequential to speech–language pathologists who practice in medical settings. This discussion was not intended to be exhaustive, but to provide a framework and context for consideration of some of the subsequent chapters. Several of the concerns raised in this chapter are discussed in some detail in Chapters 14 and 15.

The following suggestions are offered as medical speech–language pathologists continue to adapt and grow during this time of change:

1. *Consider continuing education a professional mandate for survival.* The only way for the modern speech–language pathologist to maintain currency during this highly volatile and variable time is through ongoing acquisition of new information. Medical speech–language pathologists should concentrate on information specific to their area of subspecialty to maintain clinical expertise and currency. In addition, attention should be given to reading and attending conferences that address the various social, political, and financial trends impacting the health system.

2. *Know and maintain high standards of practice.* It is essential for practitioners entrusted with the care of their patients' communication and swallowing needs to know the standards of the profession and provide for safe, efficient, and timely care. Resources available include those from a variety of professional associations including ASHA and the various specialty interest divisions; the Standards Council and the Professional Services Board; related professional organizations (Academy of Neurological Communication Disorders and Sciences); and accrediting bodies [Commission of Accreditation of Rehabilitation Facilities (CARF) and the Joint Committee on Accreditation of Healthcare Organizations (JCAHO)]. Review of current journals addressing medical speech–language pathology topics can help professionals determine their currency and appropriateness in providing quality service that is consistent with the highest standards of practice.

3. *Establish familiarity with other professionals and practitioners.* Medical speech–language pathologists, experts in the communication process, need to have contact and familiarity with various other professionals in the health care system who interact in serving patients with communication disorders. The primary physicians, specialists, nurses, dietitians, pharmacists, and rehabilitation personnel influence

the care of the patient. Thus, as a manager of one aspect of care, the SLP practitioner needs to understand the implications and issues of other providers. Establishment of strong positive relationships among the various health care providers serves the interest of the patient.

4. *Consider roles and responsibilities beyond existing models.* Speech–language pathologists are sometimes classified as rehabilitation professionals. Although rehabilitation is a key activity in the chain of services provided, much of the expected growth in health care is anticipated in the areas of preventive care, consultation, collaboration in acute and primary care, and so forth. It is important for medical speech–language pathologists to participate in these other aspects of the health care delivery system.

5. *Professional involvement.* Another way to ensure currency and quality is through ongoing involvement by speech–language pathologists in speech–language–hearing associations, related professional organizations, and consumer support organizations. Involvement with such groups provides important vehicles for networking, exchange of information and ideas, and an ongoing source of new resources and data. These inputs to professional practice allow for continuous improvement of the program with attention to those issues that are shaping the current health care system environment.

Study Questions

1. What are the "medical" speech–language pathology skills and knowledge that you need for your particular work setting?

2. Describe the SLP continuum of care.

3. What are competencies?

4. What are the implications of specialty development in neurogenic communication disorders or dysphagia for you as a professional? Will you pursue one or both of these credentials? On what basis are you making this decision?

5. What are the important trends reflected in ASHA's 2002 health care survey that are consistent or inconsistent with your own observations?

References

American Speech–Language-Hearing Association. (2001). *Scope of Practice in Speech–Language Pathology.* Rockville, MD: ASHA.

American Speech–Language-Hearing Association. (2002). *Speech–Language Pathology Health Care Survey: Executive Summary.* www.asha.org/members/slp/healthcare/exec_sum.htm

2

Medical Ethics and the Speech–Language Pathologist

Edythe A. Strand, Kathryn M. Yorkston, and Robert M. Miller

- ✦ **Professional Ethics and Rules of Conduct**
- ✦ **Basic Principles of Medical Ethics**
- ✦ **Factors Contributing to Ethical Dilemmas, Barriers to Ethical Decision Making, and Techniques to Facilitate Resolution in Speech–Language Pathology**
- ✦ **Case Examples of Ethical Dilemmas in Speech–Language Pathology**

The field of biomedical ethics has seen a rapid expansion in recent years. Controversial and troubling issues related to health care, such as abortion, euthanasia, the patient's right to choose or refuse treatment, and the distribution of health care, have been the focus of numerous debates and publications. Scholars have used philosophical and theoretical foundations of biomedical ethics as a tool for deliberating many ethical dilemmas in medical practice (Engelhardt, 1986). Clinicians have looked for a way to systematically approach difficult moral decisions in clinical practice. Numerous publications have focused attention on a set of basic moral principles with which to guide clinical decisions (Ahronheim, Moreno, & Zuckerman, 1994; Beauchamp & Childress, 1983; Dunn, Gallagher, & Hodges, 1994; Elliott & Elliott, 1991; English, 1994; Gillon, 1994; Harron, Burnside, & Beauchamp, 1983; Jonsen, Siegler, & Winslade, 1992; Pellegrino, 1993). Beauchamp and Childress (1989) note that it is through examining moral principles and determining how these principles apply to individual cases that one is guided in the discussion and eventual resolution of these problems.

Principles of biomedical ethics are applicable to the speech–language pathologist (SLP) and other ancillary medical personnel who work closely with patients over a period of time, especially in the medical setting. Information about medical ethics in general is not yet routinely included in the curriculum of many speech pathology programs, yet those students who are choosing to practice in medical settings will be faced with many ethical decisions, either as an individual or as part of a rehabilitation team. SLPs are increasingly studying issues related to both clinical

ethics and professional ethics. These issues are extremely applicable to our clinical practice and our clinical relationship with patients. This chapter introduces the student or SLP to basic definitions of some of the principles of medical ethics and gives examples of how these principles might be relevant in the practice of speech–language pathology. (Because these descriptions are necessarily short, we have included a list of references in **Appendix 2–1** that may be of interest to SLPs who work in a medical setting.) Several cases are used to present difficult ethical problems. These cases involve moral decisions regarding maintenance or quality of life, the right of patients to make decisions about their own treatment; the responsibilities of the clinician to be truthful, loyal, and beneficent to the patient; and access to assessment and treatment in speech pathology.

✦ Professional Ethics and Rules of Conduct

Professionals are individuals who have specific training in an area of expertise. Professions often maintain organizations that specify credentials and qualifications for entry into the field, and certify that individuals in that group have the requisite knowledge and skills to provide that particular service to the consumer. Professions have also used their organizations to codify professional issues relating to morality, ethics, and rules of conduct. Professional organizations related to health care also specify obligations that relate to the patient-professional relationship. The Code of Ethics of the American Speech-Language-Hearing Association (ASHA) is focused toward "preserving the highest standards of integrity and ethical principles" (American Speech–Language–Hearing Association, 2003a, 2003b). ASHA's Code of Ethics delineates a set of guidelines that serve to protect patients and secure quality clinical service for them, as well as holds the clinician to a set of principled standards of conduct. The principles of ethics and rules of ethics, as described in ASHA's Code of Ethics, relate to the SLP's responsibilities to patients, to the public in general, and to the conduct of research (Strand, 2003). Standard III-F of the ASHA Speech–Language Pathology Standards for the Certificate of Clinical Competence indicates that the applicant must demonstrate knowledge of standards of ethical conduct. It is important that all SLPs review and discuss ASHA's Principles of Ethics and Rules of Ethics as well as have an understanding of the basic principles of medical ethics.

> **Question: *What if the patient and family are making the wrong decision? Do they still have the right to autonomy?***
>
> Consider the example of a 42-year-old woman who has a very severe verbal apraxia subsequent to an embolic ischemia (stroke) as a result of surgery. She has a very mild aphasia, and no cognitive deficits. She is educated, self-sufficient in activities of daily living, and well informed as to the options open to her. The speech–language pathologist has recommended a high-tech augmentative communication system to maximize her communication efficiency. She refuses, however, because, she says, the system "draws attention to my disability." Even though the speech–language pathologist may believe it is in the patient's best interest to use the augmentative system, the apraxic speaker has the right to autonomy—to decide not to invest the time, money, and effort to use a system that is unacceptable to her lifestyle.

✦ Basic Principles of Medical Ethics

The literature in medical ethics relies heavily on the use of ethical principles as a guide to moral decision making. Authors vary with respect to what principles are most important, how those principles relate to one another, and when one principle takes precedence over another. Several commonly discussed principles are autonomy, beneficence, nonmaleficence, and justice (Beauchamp & Childress, 1989; Horner, 2003; Strand, 2003). Three additional principles are important to the patient–professional relationship: veracity, confidentiality, and fidelity. A brief discussion of each of these major principles follows, to illustrate some of the issues involved in ethical dilemmas and how these principles can guide the clinician toward ethical action. We briefly discuss the meaning of each term, and then provide an example of how this principle addresses ethical dilemmas in speech pathology.

Autonomy

The principle of autonomy refers to the right of individuals to self-determination (Beauchamp & Childress, 1983). That is, individuals determine their own course of action and make decisions concerning their own fate. If people are autonomous, they are free to choose a self-formulated plan of action. They are free of control or influence by people or institutions and by personal limitations (such as lack of information or understanding that would prevent making a meaningful decision). Therefore, a person who is in some way influenced or controlled by others because of some diminished competency (e.g., dementia) is considered to have diminished autonomy. Autonomy, therefore, refers to people's self-contained ability to make informed decisions for themselves. In contrast, people with little or no autonomy are dependent on others, whether or not they are capable of deliberating or acting on their own. In recent years, those involved in the practice of clinical medicine have shifted away from a paternalistic attitude of making decisions for patients, and toward respecting the autonomy of patients to make decisions for themselves.

SLPs often provide assessment and treatment to patients who already experience diminished autonomy, not because it is imposed on them by government or the health care system, but because of diminished competence. As will be shown in one of the cases to follow, the degree to which such reduced competency (e.g., early stages of progressive dementia accompanying Parkinson's disease) impacts our respect for patient autonomy presents real ethical dilemmas.

Respect for autonomy is one of the most common principles involved in moral dilemmas that face SLPs who work with patients with degenerative neurologic disease, as well as other disorders that are encountered in the medical setting. Although respect for autonomy is one of the fundamental obligations in medical management, it is dependent in part on the maintenance of the patient's ability to communicate. Facilitating communicative efficiency and/or providing some means of augmentative communication may allow the patient to retain personal autonomy and the ability to make personal choices about medical care. However, even when communication is maintained and facilitated, the principle of patient autonomy still presents difficult moral dilemmas. This is especially true when one considers the sometimes-contrasting principle of beneficence.

Beneficence and Nonmaleficence

Autonomy and beneficence have been said to be the conflict at the roots of bioethics (Engelhardt, 1986). In medical practice, the principle of beneficence refers to furthering the optimal health interests of the patient (English, 1994). Beneficence, in its simplest form, implies being kind and merciful. Beneficence refers to "doing good," and includes any action that results in benefiting another. Beneficence implies that positive steps are taken to prevent harm, remove from harm, as well as contribute to another's welfare.

Beauchamp and Childress (1989) note that beneficence goes beyond being kind. They point out the importance of the obligation to balance the potential good against the potential harm that might result from an action or decision. They note that one cannot usually perform actions that are beneficial or that prevent harm without also creating risks. Therefore, the balance of potential good versus potential harm is an important aspect of this principle.

Question: *I have heard the word paternalism. How does that word fit in?*

Until recently, beneficence often took precedence over autonomy. The doctor or health care professional "knew best," and the beneficent decision was made for the patient. This has been known as "paternalism." In fact, paternalism is sometimes considered to occur whenever beneficence outweighs autonomy.

In clinical practice, it is common for autonomy to come in conflict with beneficence. For example, a patient with a progressive swallowing problem may be advised that a percutaneous endoscopic gastrostomy (PEG) is the most appropriate intervention at a particular time and is necessary for adequate nutrition and hydration. The speech–language pathologist (SLP) employs the principle of *beneficence* in the recommendation. The patient may be unwilling to accept the recommendation and choose to continue oral nutrition. In this case, autonomy takes precedence over beneficence.

Although the principle of beneficence includes acts to prevent harm or remove from harmful conditions, the principle of nonmaleficence refers to the noninfliction of harm on others. These two principles are not easily separable. Beauchamp and Childress (1989), however, consider nonmaleficence to be distinct from beneficence because of the conviction that our obligations not to injure patients are distinct from, and more stringent than, our responsibilities to benefit patients. Nonmaleficence encompasses both intentional harm as well as the risk of harm, and the line between them is not always clear. Using the example of the dysphagia patient described above, we see not only that the principles of autonomy may conflict with the principle of beneficence, but also that nonmaleficence comes into play because of the risk of harm. That is, deciding to continue oral feeding risks maleficence because of the risk of aspiration, dehydration, and malnutrition.

Justice

The formulation of a single unifying theory of justice has been an elusive problem (Beauchamp & Childress, 1989). There are different theories of justice described in the literature that attempt to simplify and give order to diverse rules and judgments. These theories have been used to determine how health care services should be distributed. For example, egalitarian theories emphasize equal access to goods (or health care). Libertarian theories emphasize invoking fair procedures over outcome. Utilitarian theories emphasize a variety of different criteria to maximize the public good. That is, there are trade-offs in balancing private and public benefit. Important questions concerning the right to equal access to health care, the right to a particular minimum of care, and how to establish priorities when allocating health care resources all involve the principle of justice. How one comes to answers in any particular situation will depend on the theoretical perspective taken.

Question: *Can you give me an example of how the principle of justice comes into play in the field of speech pathology?*

One example relates to the number of treatment sessions allowed for patients in the rehabilitation setting. Certain reimbursement systems are based on the principle of equal access to treatment, regardless of outcome (libertarian). That is, a given diagnosis allows a specified number of treatment sessions. This allowed number is the same for all patients with that diagnosis. Conversely, those who make decisions from a utilitarian perspective would say the number of sessions should be based on a variety of individualized factors (e.g., severity, prognosis) that relate to the potential outcome.

The principle of justice is often explained in terms of "fairness." In medical ethics, the discussion of justice often focuses on the distribution of services under a particular moral vision. The focus is on the comparative treatment of individuals given limited resources. The SLP, although not usually in the front lines of establishing systems of health care delivery, does struggle with problems related to patient access of assessment and treatment. We are faced with determining how much treatment is appropriate, what is the minimal treatment one can recommend given the financial resources available, and who to treat and not to treat given limited resources. These dilemmas facing SLPs in the medical setting keep getting worse because authorization limits the stays on rehabilitation units to shorter durations and allows fewer outpatient treatment visits.

Veracity, Confidentiality, and Fidelity

The principles of veracity, confidentiality, and fidelity are discussed together because they are all important to the patient–health care professional relationship. They also often overlap in practice as well as in principle, and together sometimes come in conflict with the necessity to be beneficent and obey the law. All three of these principles are often discussed as "obligations" to the patient by the health care professional.

Veracity refers to the obligation to be honest. When health care professionals are in a caregiving relationship with the patient, they promise to be truthful and not deceive. The obligation for veracity stems from the necessary relationship of trust between the health care professional and the patient. The patient expects the professional to be honest, and the professional expects patients to be truthful and open about concerns, attitudes, and information regarding their health and mental status. In addition to being truthful and open, however, there is the expectation that information about the patient's health care status will remain confidential.

The *principle of confidentiality* involves widespread rules and practices. These have always been considered to have grave importance. In general, the principle implies that professionals may not reveal the confidences entrusted to them in the course of their providing medical attention. In practice, confidentiality is often difficult to implement, given the number of people who have access to a patient's chart because they may be directly involved in the delivery of some health care service. Charts typically do not note what information the patient desires to keep confidential and what they have given permission to disclose. The SLP, for example, may often have much information about a patient's medical history and health care status. The principle implies that we adhere to rules of confidentiality and not disclose the information to which we have access. That, in fact, is essential to preserving fidelity.

The term *fidelity* implies the obligation of keeping promises or agreements inherent in the relationship with a patient. These promises include being beneficent, not doing harm, telling the truth, and maintaining confidentiality. The necessity to preserve fidelity (by telling the truth and maintaining confidentiality) sometimes comes in conflict, however, with the duty to obey the laws of country and be beneficent to all persons. Fidelity also refers to the clinician's implicit promise to maintain services even when the patient decides not to follow the clinician's advice or recommendations.

Question: *Can you give me an example of problems with confidentiality and fidelity with which a SLP may be faced?*

One SLP had been working for some time with a 12-year-old head-injured girl. The girl, who had come to trust the speech pathologist, confided to her that her father was abusing her. She implored her not to tell anyone. The speech pathologist knows that it is her obligation to inform the county social service department. What is the ethical course of action here? In this case, the speech pathologist decided to have many talks with the girl, until she was able to convince her that it was important to tell someone.

✦ Factors Contributing to Ethical Dilemmas, Barriers to Ethical Decision Making, and Techniques to Facilitate Resolution in Speech–Language Pathology

The two major areas of functional impairment encountered by SLPs in a medical setting are communication deficits and swallowing disorders. Inherent in these overlapping populations are factors that potentially contribute to the development of an ethical dilemma, as well as barriers to the resolution of those dilemmas. There are some factors, however, that if recognized, may be controlled to prevent the development of an ethical dilemma, or obviate the barriers to ethical decision making. These barriers may include failure to accede to the principles of medical ethics, developing strict and limiting policies or laws that affect patient care, team communication failures, and acting self-defensively because of a fear of blame.

Failure to understand or accede to the principles of medical ethics may occur for many reasons. Perhaps the most frequently encountered problem concerns the failure to accept a patient who invokes autonomy. For example, patients who are unable to express their wishes regarding alternative forms of nutritional management may have previously declared to a family member that they would never accept a feeding tube to sustain their life. A clinician who recognizes a high aspiration risk would be forced to grapple with the seeming conflict between the principles of beneficence and autonomy. The issues revolving around each of these principles must be openly discussed and weighed before a clinical course of action is determined. Failure to identify how the two principles are in conflict can be

a barrier to the process of decision making and can have dire consequences.

Strict and limiting policies or laws have been encountered that have either contributed to the development of an ethical dilemma or provided a barrier to the resolution of such a dilemma. For example, a patient was transferred into a skilled nursing facility (SNF) with a policy that prevented any form of syringe feeding. After admission, this patient was discovered to be rapidly losing weight and needing IVs to maintain hydration. The patient had been nutritionally maintained with syringe feeding at home, by the family, for 2 years prior to the SNF admission. There had been no instance of acute airway compromise and no evidence of insidious pulmonary decline related to aspiration. An experienced SLP diagnosed an oral-stage dysphagia and demonstrated on repeat clinical examinations and on a video fluoroscopic swallow study that the patient showed no evidence of aspiration when formula was placed in the mouth via syringe. Although in general syringe feeding should be discouraged, and utilized only with stringent guidelines and criteria, the unyielding policy of this SNF precipitated an ethical dilemma that escalated to involve the issues of feeding tube placement, surgical risk, and the loss of pleasure derived from eating. A more carefully worded policy could have prevented this dilemma.

Some states have laws that limit a clinician's authority to post patient care instructions at the bedside. This law prevents an SLP from affixing feeding recommendations to direct caregivers in safe swallowing techniques. Although this may be a well-intentioned law that protects the patient's right to confidentiality, it places some patients in jeopardy. These laws may be enforced even when the patient and family desire to have the information posted. Here, again, there is potential for conflict between "best clinical practice standards" and a benevolent principle designed to prevent disclosure of privileged information. The strictly stated policy in this case both precipitated an ethical dilemma and acted as a barrier to solving that dilemma.

Team communication failures also serve as barriers to the processes of ethical decision making. These may occur because the medium most often used for communication is the medical chart. The patient's chart is an artificial mode of communication and is not conducive to complex decision making. In particular, it does not facilitate the health care team's ability to come to consensus on important issues, because it is a serial log of communication where consensus cannot easily be developed. Such a method of communication does not then facilitate ethical decisions.

Consider, for example, the case of a terminally ill patient who is suffering from unremitting pain and desiring not to participate in medical procedures that are performed for purposes of diagnosis and assessment. All consultants involved with the case should be made aware of the patient's wishes, and intervention decisions should be driven by the desire to provide comfort and compassion. Unfortunately, the medical chart, a medical/legal document, frequently fails to communicate to all involved health professionals this essential information. Commonly, such patients are transported to radiology for nonessential x-rays, or are visited by laboratory technicians to draw blood for analysis. Face-to-face team meetings can facilitate communication for the purpose of coordinating care that is truly in the best interest of the patient. Clarity and access to information are essential elements in preventing ethical dilemmas.

Acting self-defensively because of fear of liability or blame has the potential not only to precipitate an ethical dilemma but also to compromise patient care. An SLP's decision to recommend a feeding tube in an acutely ill patient may be based on the clinician's subjective fear that the patient might develop complications as a result of oral feedings. Rather than using more objective measures, good clinical judgment, and considering all relevant factors in the individual case, a clinical decision can be unduly influenced by the clinician's anxiety, perhaps based on a previous, unfortunate experience. Recommendations regarding nutritional management have the inherent potential to result in a medical complication. They are rarely easy decisions, but they are determinations that must be based on the facts of the individual case and in consultation with the primary care team. By allowing fear and anxiety to guide recommendations, clinicians will experience an unresolved conflict between their desire to adhere to the principle of beneficence and their desire to avoid maleficence.

Despite one's best efforts, ethical dilemmas are inevitable in the context of a health care environment. The extreme complexity of modern medical care, technology, and the expanse of human relationships and emotions provide the ingredients to precipitate ethical dilemmas. When such conflicts arise, one should consider several techniques that can facilitate their resolution. For example, conflicts should be clearly defined, articulated, and broken down into their component parts; available options should be listed and objectively evaluated; and dialogue between all stakeholders should be encouraged whenever possible. Avoiding emotional attachment to a point of view, a major barrier to the resolution of a dilemma, should be avoided.

✦ Case Examples of Ethical Dilemmas in Speech–Language Pathology

So far in this chapter we have focused on professional ethics, the principles of medical ethics, and how to avoid some of the barriers to resolution of ethical dilemmas. Emphasis was given to describing what contributes to the dilemma. Now we discuss how ethical dilemmas are dealt with in a medical setting.

Clinical ethics is a term that has been used to describe the discipline that provides a structured approach to identifying, analyzing, and resolving ethical issues in clinical medicine (Jonsen et al, 1992). This structured approach to examining moral principles is a process, not a construct. It is the process by which principles of medical ethics can be applied to specific situations and cases (Pannbaker, Middleton, & Vekovius, 1995). In an effort to illustrate this process of communication and decision making, we present two case examples in which an ethical dilemma occurred. Following each case is a discussion by a small group of practicing SLPs. The cases presented come from the clinicians' experience, and the discussions demonstrate the process of applying the principles of medical ethics to difficult situations in which SLPs often find themselves. The discussions are similar to those that might occur in a patient staff meeting, a rehabilitation team meeting, or a discharge-planning meeting. They point out the principles of medical ethics as they are applied to real cases, and strategies for approaching difficult clinical problems. This type of forum is an important teaching mechanism for students in the medical professions, yet is somewhat neglected in the field of speech–language pathology.

Clinicians asked themselves the following questions to guide the discussion: What are the facts of this case? What other information do we need? What principles of medical ethics are important in this situation? How do the principles of autonomy, beneficence, and nonmaleficence come into conflict? How do the facts of this case help us resolve the conflict? Is there anything the team could or should have done to prevent this situation in the first place? Are there barriers to ethical decision making that the clinician or team should be aware of as they approach ethical dilemmas? What are the important issues relevant to our responsibility in this case? What are our options for action?

These questions are often structured so that one always begins by reviewing the facts of the case. From the facts, one can list issues that pertain to the medical ethics principles discussed earlier in this chapter. For example, in the first case to be discussed, listing the facts leads one to determine that the main issues involved are the patient's cognitive competency, the patient's request not to have a feeding tube, and the current risks to his well-being. This leads to a discussion of the principles of autonomy, beneficence, and maleficence. The principle of autonomy alone would lead to the decision to let him continue as he has, living alone and eating normally. The principle of beneficence (doing good and preventing harm) would dictate that any necessary steps be taken to prevent probably frequent aspiration. Some would even argue that allowing this patient oral nutrition so greatly risks his well-being that maleficence is at issue. The discussion is therefore guided by the questions, but the questions do not necessarily lead to one "right" answer.

The discussion that follows each of the cases presented is not scripted, nor was there any attempt to direct the discussion. Each bullet represents a turn by one of the three speech pathologists involved in the discussion. Although no specific directions were given to guide the discussion, there is an approach to the process of discussion that the three speech pathologists followed, and that may be helpful when approaching a similar discussion in your workplace. First, make sure there is not a lack of communication or failure to get the people together who are involved in the case. Make sure that all participants have all the facts and the answers to any questions they have. Second, make sure that possible barriers to the resolution of dilemmas, discussed earlier in this chapter, are not impeding the discussion. Then examine the principles involved in the case and how they might come into conflict. Finally, list alternative courses of action.

In the discussion following each of the cases presented, it will be clear that these are indeed ethical dilemmas because the principles do not fall into a hierarchy in terms of their importance. Clinical decisions are often made only after weighing the consequences of possible solutions.

Case 1

R.L. is a 76-year-old man with advanced Parkinson's disease. He has moderately severe dysarthria and a history of aspiration pneumonia and weight loss. On admission to the hospital, he denied episodes of choking or other difficulty with swallowing. He lives alone, and has a part-time assistant. Prior to admission, he signed an advance directive not to have a stomach tube placed at any stage in his disease. The primary physician feels that the patient is competent enough to make this decision. The speech pathologist, concerned about R.L.'s recent precipitous weight loss, along with the history of aspiration pneumonia, completed a bedside swallow evaluation. She found the patient had a great deal of difficulty swallowing both thin liquids and some solid food. Further, the patient appeared confused, and had difficulty following directions. This information was presented at rounds. Excerpts from the discussion of this case follow.

The participants begin by making sure they have all the facts they need.

◆ In reviewing the facts of this case, we have a case of a degenerative disease that we know is often accompanied by cognitive changes. We also see a clear risk of aspiration. We don't know when the advanced directive was signed. Do we know that this is still his wish?

◆ This also brings up another question. What is the physician using as a measure of the patient's competence? Is she basing it on current information, or basing it on her relationship with the patient 10 years ago? I would want to know a little more about the patient's competency.

◆ I'd also like to know a little more about how the family feels about the patient's decision and his competency to make this decision today. Does the family feel his advanced directives are in fact still current and correspond to his wishes? If so, then there are few options available at this point.

◆ This case reflects an interesting problem that advanced directive always raises. When patients are healthy they can write advanced directives, but when a life-threatening situation actually arises, predetermined directives may well undergo new scrutiny by the patients.

◆ Another problem this case illustrates is the role of knowledge or understanding of intervention strategies and the possible misconceptions about some techniques. Sometimes the connotations may be quite different from the reality (e.g., that a feeding tube is only used as a life-prolonging measure). The patient may make a decision based on misinformation.

◆ Also, when the ultimate decision gets closer and closer, something that has been unthinkable becomes more and more attractive.

◆ The decision about a feeding tube may also have been made prior to the advent of a PEG, which is an entirely different procedure than an open gastrostomy or nasogastric (NG) tube. If this were done over 10 years ago, we would have been talking about a whole different kind of procedure, and a different set of potential conflicts.

Now the discussion shifts to examination of the principles involved:

◆ A lot of what this case presents, too, is the obvious conflict between respect for the patient's autonomy and consideration of the clinician's recommendations, which are made in the spirit of "do no harm," and do what is in the best interest of the patient. On the surface, there is not really an ethical dilemma here. The speech pathologist, in spite of finding aspiration, could decide to respect the patient's autonomy and his right to make these decisions. In that case, the clinician would simply make certain management suggestions to minimize the risk without ever deciding that it was inappropriate for the patient to eat at all.

◆ But that leads to the flip side of autonomy, which brings into play the principle of beneficence, and doing good for the patient. These principles come into conflict here, because if therapists only respect patient autonomy, they run the risk of not upholding the principle of beneficence. In fact, they risk maleficence, or doing harm to the patient.

◆ In this case it is also possible that some of the barriers to ethical decision making would arise: Emotionality, for example, is probable. One person could get very strongly fixed on one side of advocating for the patient's right for autonomy, whereas a speech pathologist might become emotionally involved in the aspect of taking every measure possible in order for the patient not to aspirate at all, (perhaps because of fear of blame). A lot of that can be alleviated by very clear communication. The speech pathologist may say, yes we recognize the risk for aspiration here, but there are other considerations that we have to take into account before deciding on a course.

◆ Communication is a critical factor in this case. As the scenario reads I could interpret it to mean that all of the communication has been done via the medical chart. First there is the advanced directive at some previous date signed in the medical chart. There is the physician's note in the medical chart that the patient is cognitively competent. All of these issues could be communicated without any face-to-face communication. Perhaps one way to begin to solve the ethical dilemma is to bring all the players together for an online discussion.

Case 2

T.W. is a 30-year-old single woman with a diagnosis of Huntington's disease who was referred to the clinic by her family physician for evaluation of swallowing difficulty. The only information we had when we met her, other than her diagnosis, was the clinic nurse's note that she weighed 94 pounds and was 5'8" tall. The reason for her low body weight was clear when we met the patient. She exhibited severe chorea and was essentially in constant motion. The dietitian estimated that her daily calorie intake was approximately 1900 calories, but that her calorie needs were between 4000 and 5000 per day. Her swallow was characterized by lack of coordination, mild-to-moderate risk of aspiration, and difficulty in transport of the food to her mouth. She indicated that eating was a time-consuming activity that she did not particularly enjoy. When alternative means of feeding were discussed, she firmly refused. When risks to health of malnutrition, dehydration, and aspiration were presented, she said that she "didn't have much to live for anyway." When the patient left the clinic, a clinician who was just beginning her clinical fellowship year told her supervisor, "She's risking her own death through malnutrition or aspiration. Are we just going to let her do that? Isn't that condoning her suicide? That doesn't seem right. What should I do?" The supervisor motioned the clinician into her office and said, "Lets talk."

The supervisor begins by a review of the facts of the case.

◆ Let's start with a review of the facts in this case. That's a major problem here. There is a lot we don't know in this case. We don't know the degree of dementia. We don't know to what degree this woman presents conflicting wishes with respect to wanting to live. We don't know what the family situation is with regard to support. The first dilemma here is whether we can get all the information we need to facilitate decision making regarding this patient's care.

◆ We do know that she has calorie needs more than she can meet by her oral intake alone, given the degree of motor difficulty she has and given the fact she is already spending an inordinate amount of time per day trying to feed herself. Also, she has a risk of aspiration because of her incoordination and poor swallowing function. Finally, we have the fact that she is adamantly refusing a tube. Here again, we probably have the connotation of a feeding tube (prolonging life) coming into play. We probably have an obligation at least to educate the patient about what a feeding tube offers in terms of quality of life versus prolonging life. I think a lot of times we see patients shake their head "no" when the subject is brought up. After we explain what it is, how it is used, and what our experience with other patients has been, then they often agree to it, saying, "Oh, this is different from what I thought."

Now the discussion turns to a poignant issue related to autonomy.

◆ In a way this case brings up the most emotional and perhaps difficult ethical decision of all: the patient's right to choose to continue living. What is the role of the SLP in contributing to that decision? Do we have any role?

◆ The reason I remember this patient so vividly, and remember what she said to us, was that she was a very attractive young woman who was moving constantly. Someone asked her about her decision. As she was moving, she turned to them and said, "Would you want to live like this?" It just stopped the whole conversation.

◆ This case really emphasizes how, as clinicians, we can't completely divorce our own feelings about the worth of life, our own self-image and with what we would be willing to live and cope. It also illustrates how we might transfer our own personal feelings to patients when we help them cope with some very difficult personal decisions. One of the questions I have about this case is why did the patient come to the clinic, given that we are a speech and swallowing clinic? I see from the chart that she was referred by her family physician. What was she really hoping to get from the visit? It is important to make sure we ask why the patient chose to make the appointment, even if it was due to a physician referral. There would also be a tendency here, on the basis of the facts as presented, for abandonment by the clinic, with us throwing up our hands and saying we have nothing to offer; there's nothing we can do.

◆ Or, saying if you don't want what we have to offer, namely a PEG, don't come back because this is what is best.

◆ I hope what we did was to provide her with some management suggestions to minimize her risk of aspirating, educate her with regard to what her caloric needs were, and perhaps provide her with appropriate consultation with other people who might be able to provide her with adaptive aids for self-feeding. Then it would have been important to let her know that we would be there for her as consultants whenever she had questions or issues regarding feeding, swallowing, or communicating, making it clear we were available and willing to help.

◆ Which is promoting patient autonomy while still being beneficent.

◆ I remember her talking about how she wasn't married, would never be married or have children, and how no one depended on her. "Why do you insist I keep on living?" is what she said to us.

◆ We do come across patients, on a fairly regular basis, who are making that decision. Or at least who have a desire not to live with a degenerative disease any longer. Including this issue in a chapter such as this points out that our role as a clinician involves more than just assessment and treatment of communication and swallowing disorders. When these issues come up, we have to remember that there is no one right answer. We don't really have a role other than to keep in mind that the patient has a right to autonomy, and that our job is to provide information, be supportive, and do as much good for the patient as possible.

Now the discussion turns to our role as educators. How do we help students and CFY clinical fellows learn to deal with ethical dilemmas?

◆ This brings us to the final aspect of this case: the distraught clinician beginning her CFY and being unsure how to deal with intervention in this case. How does a young clinician acquire skills in these difficult situations? As an academic institution, how do we train students to approach a problem from an ethical perspective? How do we provide training for clinical decisions that involve ethical dilemmas?

◆ It's important to remember that clinicians who are well skilled and have no reservations about their fundamental clinical knowledge are still struggling with issues related to ethical management. How do we expect students or beginning clinicians to handle these issues when they are still learning how to do a physical exam or how to choose the appropriate test to give? How do we put them in a position where they can productively learn about issues that are less tangible and more tied to principle rather than accepted practice?

◆ It may be that the supervisor needs to guide the student in steps. One way to do that may be by going through the questions we've used to guide our discussion: What are the facts? What principles are presented in this case? What principles come into conflict? What barriers are there to coming to ethical decisions?

◆ Right from the start we have to recognize that students and beginning clinicians have little experience here and therefore are ill equipped to deal with this issue. It is likely they will react on a very different level from those of us who have been in these situations numerous times. They may first and foremost be absolutely overwhelmed by the devastation they see caused by the disease itself and its consequences related to speech and swallowing. I think they are going to be less well equipped to see the big picture and how all of this relates to, in this case, the woman's mortality. I think they will at first react at a very emotional level, and will not be able to rationally look at the facts of the case.

◆ One important aspect to remember when considering how to train clinicians with respect to clinical decision making involving ethical dilemmas is that one needs to develop a "fund of knowledge" on which to draw. One does that by honing observation skills, and learning how to clearly interpret what one sees. How does an experienced clinician, who has only recently been introduced to the principles of medical ethics, or a beginning clinician practicing in the medical setting for the first time, begin to establish an experience base from which to learn?

✦ There is no short cut to the experience. Every case that a beginning clinician has is a learning experience. It's important to keep in mind that each case is a new learning experience and that we shouldn't generalize too fast. There is a general tendency to take what we learned from the last case and apply it to the current case. Sometimes, even though there may be similarities that are apparent at first, there may be very different sets of circumstances that require very different approaches to the ethical dilemmas they present.

✦ It is a very important process to evaluate the cases according to the principles of medical ethics, so that you begin to establish a fund of experience in this area. Issues related to ethical dilemmas and techniques for resolving barriers pose particular challenges, because there are no textbooks that tell you the right answers. There are no checklists or guidelines for dealing with those clinical problems that involve ethical questions. That is why developing a fund of experience is so important. Clinicians have to learn from each case by talking about it honestly. If they present problems, discuss them, and talk about what worked and what didn't and why.

✦ Wisdom comes from a lot of experience, including the failures as well as the successes.

✦ Yes, it is important that we don't avoid the very uncomfortable process of critically evaluating how we have handled each patient. And it's important to lay the blame on ourselves if blame is appropriate. That is to say: "I didn't handle this case in the best possible way. How can I apply this experience in the future with other cases?" Because that is how we learn.

Study Questions

1. Principles of medical ethics
   A. are applicable to speech–language pathologists and other health professionals as well as to physicians.
   B. are not taught in medical schools.
   C. are applied to moral decision making in health care.
   D. A and C above.

2. ASHA's Code of Ethics
   A. is focused toward preserving the highest standards of integrity.
   B. delineates guidelines to serve and protect quality clinical service to the patient.
   C. holds the clinicians to a set of principled standards of conduct.
   D. All of the above.

3. ASHA's Standards for the Certificate of Clinical Competence
   A. does not include a statement regarding the necessity of knowledge of standards of ethical conduct.
   B. should include a statement regarding the necessity of knowledge of standards of ethical conduct.
   C. has a statement regarding the necessity of knowledge of standards of ethical conduct.
   D. None of the above.

4. Autonomy and beneficence
   A. have been said to be the conflict at the roots of bioethics.
   B. are sometimes in contradiction to each other.
   C. A and B.
   D. None of the above.

5. The principle of justice
   A. has much to do with the distribution of services in health care.
   B. focuses on the right of the individual to make decisions for herself.
   C. focuses on the duty of the professional to do good.
   D. focuses on the duty of the professional to prevent harm.

6. Clinical ethics
   A. describe a discipline that provides specific answers to ethical dilemmas.
   B. involve a structured approach to examining moral principles.
   C. refer to a process, not a construct.
   D. B and C above.

References

Ahronheim, J.C., Moreno, J. & Zuckerman, C. (1994). *Ethics in Clinical Practice.* Boston: Little, Brown

American Speech–Language-Hearing Association. (2003). Code of Ethics (revised). ASHA Supplement 23. Rockville, MD: American Speech–Language-Hearing Association

American Speech–Language-Hearing Association. (2003). Code of Ethics. Retrieved http://www.asha.org/NR/rdonlyres/F51E46C5-3D87-44AF-BFDA-46D32F85C60/0/18763_4.pdf). Retrieved July 11, 2004, from

Beauchamp, T.L. & Childress, J.F. (1983). *Principles of Biomedical Ethics.* New York: Oxford University Press

Beauchamp, T.L. & Childress, J.F. (1989). *Principles of Biomedical Ethics.* New York: Oxford University Press

Dunn, P.M., Gallagher, T.H. & Hodges, M.O. (1994). Medical Ethics: An Annotated Bibliography. *Annual of Internal Medicine, 121,* 627–632

Elliott, C. & Elliott, B. (1991). From the Patient's Point of View: Medical Ethics and the Moral Imagination. *Journal of Medical Ethics, 17,* 173–178

Engelhardt, H.T. (1986). *The Foundations of Bioethics.* New York: Oxford University Press

English, D.C. (1994). *Bioethics: A Clinical Guide for Medical Students.* New York: Norton Medical Books

Gillon, R. (1994). Medical Ethics: Four Principles Plus Attention to Scope. *British Medical Journal, 309,* 184–188

Harron, F., Burnside, J. & Beauchamp, T. (1983). *Health and Human Values: A Guide to Making Your Own Decisions.* New Haven, CT: Yale University Press

Horner, J. (2003). Morality, Ethics and the Law: Introductory Concepts. *Seminars in Speech and Language, 24,* 263–274

Jonsen, A.R., Siegler, M. & Winslade, W.J. (1992). *Clinical Ethics: A Practical Approach to Ethical Decisions in Clinical Medicine.* New York: McGraw-Hill

Pannbaker, M.H., Middleton, G.F. & Vekovius, G.T. (1995). *Ethical Practice in Speech–Language Pathology and Audiology: Case Studies.* San Diego: Singular Press

Pellegrino, E.D. (1993). The Metamorphosis of Medical Ethics: A 30-Year Retrospective. *Journal of the American Medical Association, 269,* 1158–1162

Strand, E. (2003). Clinical and Professional Ethics in the Management of Motor Speech Disorders. *Seminars in Speech and Language, 24,* 301–312

Appendix 2–1 Selected Resources for the SLP

Bach, J.R. & Barnett, V. (1994). Ethical Considerations in the Management of Individuals with Severe Neuromuscular Disorders. *American Journal of Physical and Medical Rehabilitation, 73,* 134–140

Banja, J.D., Bilsky, G.S. (1993). Discussing Cardiopulmonary Resuscitation with Elderly Rehabilitation Patients. *American Journal of Physical and Medical Rehabilitation, 72,* 168–171

Callahan, D. (1993). Allocating Health Care Resources. The Vexing Case of Rehabilitation. *American Journal of Physical and Medical Rehabilitation, 72,* 101–105

Dougherty, C.J. (1994). Quality-Adjusted Life Years and the Ethical Values of Health Care. *American Journal of Physical and Medical Rehabilitation, 73,* 61–65

Haas, J. (1993). Ethical Considerations of Goal Setting for Patient Care in Rehabilitation Medicine. *American Journal of Physical and Medical Rehabilitation, 72,* 228–232

Jennings, B. (1993). Healing the Self: The Moral Meaning of Relationships in Rehabilitation. *American Journal of Physical and Medical Rehabilitation, 72,* 401–404

Kottke, F.J. (1982). Philosophic Considerations of Quality of Life for the Disabled. *Archives of Physical and Medical Rehabilitation, 63,* 60–62

Meier, R.H. & Purtilo, R.B. (1994). Ethical Issues and the Patient-Provider Relationship. *American Journal of Physical and Medical Rehabilitation, 73,* 365–366

Pearlman, R.A. & Jonsen, A. (1985). The Use of Quality-of-Life Considerations in Medical Decision Making. *Journal of the American Geriatrics Society 33,* 344–352

Purtilo, R.B. (1986). Ethical Issues in the Treatment of Chronic Ventilator-Dependent Patients. *Archives of Physical and Medical Rehabilitation, 67,* 718–721

Purtilo, R.B. & Meier, R.H. (1993). Team Challenges: Regulatory Constraints and Patient Empowerment. *American Journal of Physical and Medical Rehabilitation, 72,* 327–330

Sivak, E.D., Gipson, W.T. & Hanson, M.R. (1982). Long-Term Management of Respiratory Failure in Amyotrophic Lateral Sclerosis. *Annals of Neurology, 12,* 18–23

Strax, T.E. (1994). Ethical Issues of Treating Patients with AIDS in a Rehabilitation Setting. *American Journal of Physical and Medical Rehabilitation, 73,* 293–295

Venesy, B.A. (1994). A Clinician's Guide to Decision Making Capacity and Ethically Sound Medical Decisions. *American Journal of Physical and Medical Rehabilitation, 73,* 219–226

Section 2

Neurocognitive Communication Disorders

3

Brain Imaging in Acquired Language Disorders

K. Paige George, Eric Vikingstad, Richard Silbergleit, and Yue Cao

✦ **Neuroimaging Techniques**
✦ **Neuroimaging of Acquired Language Disorders**

With the many advances in the field of neuroimaging, understanding of the neural organization of language and its associated disorders has greatly increased (Dronkers, Redfern, & Knight, 2000; Kertesz, 1979; Pizzamiglio, Galati, & Committeri, 2001; Small and Burton, 2002). Neuroimaging techniques provide a valuable means to study brain structure (i.e., anatomy) and function (i.e., blood flow and metabolism) in both neurologically intact and brain damaged individuals. The structural imaging modalities of computed tomography (CT) and magnetic resonance imaging (MRI) have enabled the first studies correlating living language behavior with precise lesion localization (Kertesz, 1979; Naeser & Hayward, 1978). Functional neuroimaging with single photon emission computed tomography (SPECT), positron emission tomography (PET), and perfusion-weighted and diffusion-weighted magnetic resonance imaging (PWI and DWI, respectively) has shown how focal damage disrupts blood flow and metabolism not only at the site of damage, but remotely from it with corresponding behavioral consequences (Hillis, Kane, Tuffiash, Ulatowski, Barker, Beauchamp, & Wityk, 2001c; Metter, 1987; Metter, Hanson, Jackson, Kempler, van Lancker, Mazziotta, & Phelps, 1990; Metter, Wasterlain, Kuhl, Hanson, & Phelps, 1981). Over the past 15 years, functional imaging with PET and functional magnetic resonance imaging (fMRI) has enabled the study of brain activity during task performance (e.g., reading single words or sentences) in neurologically intact and brain-damaged individuals. These studies have allowed researchers to see the brain "at work" during processing of language, attention, and memory. PET and fMRI have also been used to show how brain activity changes with aphasia recovery, both spontaneously and in response to drug or behavioral intervention (Cao, Vikingstad, George, Johnson, & Welch, 1999; Hillis, Wityk, Tuffiash, Beauchamp, Jacobs, Barker, & Selnes, 2001; Musso, Weiller, Kiebel, Muller, Bulau, & Rijntjes, 1999; Small, Flores, & Noll, 1998).

Speech–language pathologists can apply the wealth of information from the neuroimaging literature to enhance clinical practice (Kendall and Gonzalez Rothi, 2001; Raymer, 2001). Knowledge of the neural correlates of acquired language disorders can be used to predict potential deficits. As a result, initial evaluations can be targeted toward the expected impairments of language, which may lead to more timely diagnosis and development of treatment plans. Clinicians will also be better prepared to make evidence-based judgments of prognosis based on findings from neuroimaging studies of aphasia recovery. Finally, information from the imaging literature can provide a basis for counseling patients and their families about the neurophysiology of aphasia and neural mechanisms of recovery, in both the acute and chronic phases of injury.

We begin with a description of the primary neuroimaging techniques including CT, MRI, SPECT, PET, and fMRI, covering technical aspects as well as clinical and research applications. The second section reviews how structural and functional imaging has expanded understanding of the neural bases of acquired language disorders, predominantly aphasia. The chapter concludes with a brief discussion about the future directions for neuroimaging and its application to human communication disorders. To supplement this information, the reader is referred to Chapter 21 in this text.

✦ Neuroimaging Techniques

Computed Tomography

Computed tomography (CT), sometimes called a "CAT scan" (computed axial tomography), is an x-ray technique that provides more detailed images of soft tissue, bone, and body organs than do regular radiographs (plain x-ray films).

Table 3–1 Applications of CT in Clinical Brain Imaging and Neuroscience Research

	Imaging Technique	Application
Clinical central nervous system (CNS) applications	Anatomic imaging	Cerebrovascular disease
		Congenital malformation
		Infection
		Neoplasm
		Trauma
	Angiography	Aneurysm
		Arteriovenous malformation
		Vascular occlusive disease
Neuroscience applications	Anatomic imaging	Brain morphology studies
		Lesion localization studies
	Perfusion imaging	Activation studies
		Cerebrovascular disease

An x-ray is a beam of radiation that can penetrate a solid substance. With CT, sensitive x-ray equipment rotates around a patient's body to acquire multiple images from different angles, and then with the aid of a computer joins them together to show a cross-sectional image or "slice" of brain tissue and internal organs. Two- and three-dimensional renderings can be produced. CT's utility continues to grow as faster machines and higher resolution studies become more available and more affordable. CT of the head is commonly used to detect:

✦ Ischemic or hemorrhagic strokes

✦ Injuries from head and facial trauma, including bone fractures, soft tissue damage, and intracranial bleeds

✦ Intracranial mass lesions such as neoplasms or hematomas

✦ Central nervous system infections such as encephalitis or abscesses

✦ Intracranial calcifications suggestive of neurologic infections, disease, or neoplasm

✦ Enlarged brain ventricles in patients with hydrocephalus

✦ Focal cerebral atrophy in patients with suspected dementia

✦ Aneurysm or arteriovenous malformation details with a vascular imaging technique known as CT angiography

Table 3–1 highlights clinical and research applications of CT.

General Principles

In CT of the head, numerous tightly collimated x-ray beams are passed through the skull and brain at different angles. As x-ray beams pass through tissue, they are absorbed or attenuated (weakened) as some fraction of the x-ray beam interacts with electrons of the body's atoms that are in the beam's path. When the x-ray beam and the electrons interact, some of the x-ray energy is deflected from its course. This interaction results in a scattering of the x-ray. As a result, less energy exits the body along the path of the x-ray beam than entered the body. Special sensors detect how much the tissues in the beam's path attenuate the x-ray beam transmitted through the patient (**Fig. 3–1**). As a patient lies still during the study, the scanner gantry (or frame) rotates around the person, transmitting and recording x-ray beams at different angles. A special computer then records and analyzes the x-ray data to form a map of the degree of x-ray attenuation at each point in a slice of tissue. The CT image is this map presenting cross-sectional images or "slices" of the head and brain (**Fig. 3–2**).

Bone, cerebrospinal fluid (CSF), blood, and gray and white matter have different electron densities and as a result are distinguishable by CT. Bone, for example, has a high electron density and therefore maximally attenuates the x-ray beam. Bone appears hyperdense or white on CT. In contrast, air does not significantly attenuate the x-ray beam and is hypodense or black on the CT scan as typically viewed. CSF attenuates the beam less than brain but more than air and is dark, but not as

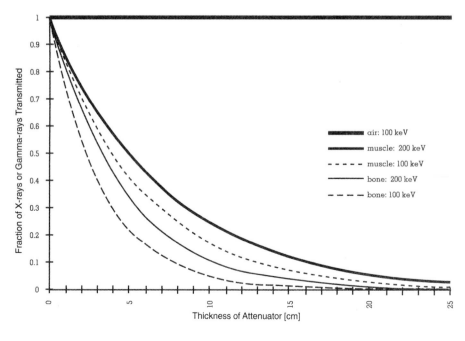

Figure 3–1 A demonstration of the effects of tissue type and photon energy on x-ray attenuation. Transmission of radiation decreases exponentially with attenuator thickness. The degree of attenuation increases as attenuator electron density increases and photon energy decreases.

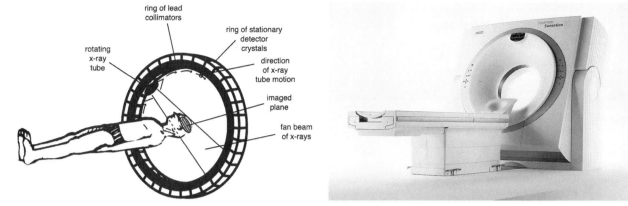

Figure 3–2 (A) A schematic drawing of a CT scanner. The ring of collimated detector crystals and the rotating x-ray tube are shown. **(B)** Photograph of a modern CT scanner. (Courtesy of Siemens Medical Corporation, New York, NY.)

black as air. The density of brain tissue and spinal cord is higher than CSF and these structures appear gray on CT images (**Fig. 3–3**). Pathologic conditions can change the expected attenuation of a tissue. For example, an infarct of brain parenchyma will appear hypodense (dark) on CT rather than its typical gray color.

At times, it may be helpful to enhance the contrast between different tissues to clearly resolve anatomic details and neuropathology. One method to enhance the CT images is to inject an iodinated contrast material into the bloodstream. As this radiopaque material flows through the vasculature, normal and compromised blood vessels can be discerned. Contrast

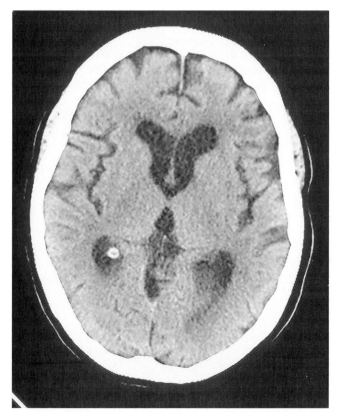

Figure 3–3 Axial CT image of a normal brain. Notice that cerebrospinal fluid (CSF) is dark, brain tissue is gray, and bone is white. (Photograph courtesy of Richard Silbergleit.)

enhancement improves the diagnosis of arteriovenous malformations, aneurysms, tumors, infarctions, certain infections, and demyelinating disease (Gray & Cummings, 1994). An area that has been contrast-enhanced appears whiter or denser on the CT. Iodinated contrast does not cross the blood–brain barrier. Many pathologic processes including most tumors and abscesses disrupt the blood–brain barrier and show enhancement with contrast.

CT scanner performance has improved significantly in the years since its inception. Modern spiral (helical) CT has greatly improved the accuracy of CT to image disease and injury. Spiral CT derives its name from the path the x-ray transmitter takes during scanning. Slices as thin as 0.5 mm can be taken in 0.37 seconds. The benefit of spiral CT is that higher-quality images are obtained with less radiation and in a very brief amount of time. A spiral scan can be achieved in one breath hold, which is especially beneficial for elderly, pediatric, or trauma patients who may not tolerate a longer scan. The speed of spiral CT contrasts with that of a conventional CT scan, which can take up to 45 minutes to obtain. Multislice spiral CT scanners, which can obtain several image slices at a time, are now becoming common. In 2004, 16-slice scanners were the state of the art, and 32-, 40-, and 64-slice scanners have been announced.

Strengths and Limitations of Computed Tomography

CT of the head is the most widely available imaging modality and the least expensive. A noncontrast CT is generally the first neuroimaging study for suspected stroke or head trauma. It is particularly useful for imaging bone, making it the test of choice for facial and skull fractures. The initial CT can rule out hemorrhages, brain tumors, and infections. It has some limitations, however. CT does not reliably detect ischemic (thrombotic or embolic) strokes within the first 24 to 48 hours of onset, and very small strokes are occasionally missed. Tissue contrast between gray and white matter is not as great as on MRI. Furthermore, CT exposes the patient to small amounts of ionizing radiation in the form of x-rays, which may be of particular concern for pregnant women and young children, especially those requiring multiple examinations. **Table 3–2** highlights the strengths and weaknesses of this modality.

Table 3–2   Summary of the Strengths and Weaknesses of CT, MRI, SPECT, and PET

Modality	Strengths	Weaknesses
CT	Excellent spatial resolution	Radiation exposure
	Excellent temporal resolution	Limited versatility
	Excellent geometric accuracy	
	Widely available	
MRI	Low risk	Cannot image patients with metallic implants, artificial valves, etc.
	Extremely versatile	Possible mild geometric distortion
	Excellent soft tissue contrast	
	Excellent spatial resolution	
	Moderate temporal resolution	
	Quantitative measurements possible	
SPECT	Extremely versatile	Radiation exposure
	Potential for coincidence detection	Poor spatial resolution
	Widely available	Very poor temporal resolution
	Pseudo- or nonquantitative measurements	
PET	Extremely versatile	Radiation exposure
	Moderate spatial resolution	Poor temporal resolution
	Quantitative measurements possible	Low availability
		High cost

Advanced Computed Tomography Imaging Techniques

Advanced CT imaging techniques include computed tomographic angiography (CTA) and CT perfusion imaging. CTA involves injection of an iodinated contrast agent into the bloodstream and the collection of thin axial slices. Workstations are then used to obtain three-dimensional (3D) images of the vascular system. This is often useful in identifying and better evaluating abnormalities of the cerebral vasculature including aneurysms, arteriovenous malformations (AVMs), and vascular occlusions. CT perfusion involves sequential measurements of an area of brain during iodinated contrast injection. Measurements of regional cerebral blood flow (rCBF), mean transit time (MTT), and regional cerebral blood volume (rCBV) are obtained. CT can also be used to visualize cerebral perfusion by having a patient inhale xenon contrast (Xe-CT CBF), rather than injecting contrast material. CT perfusion studies have the potential to reveal regions of functional activity and can show whether brain tissue is receiving adequate blood flow to maintain tissue viability. Areas that are hypoperfused can be targeted with thrombolytic therapy [e.g., tissue-type plasminogen activator (tPA)] to enhance blood

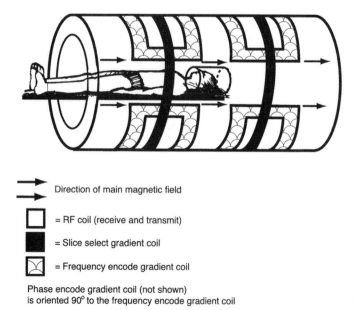

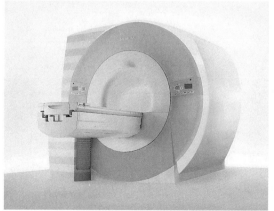

A   **B**

Figure 3–4 (A) Schematic of an MRI scanner showing patient positioning and the locations of the gradient and RF coils. **(B)** Photograph of a modern MRI scanner. (Courtesy of Siemens Medical Corporation, New York, NY.)

flow and restore function to that region. In emergency rooms, CT, CTA, and/or Xe-CT CBF are used increasingly for the evaluation of patients with acute stroke who may be candidates for thrombolytic therapy (Kilpatrick, Yonas, Goldstein, Kassam, Gebel, Wechsler, Jungreis, and Fukui, 2001; Schellinger, Fiebach, and Hacke, 2003).

Magnetic Resonance Imaging

Magnetic resonance imaging (MRI) uses radiofrequency (RF) waves and a strong magnetic field rather than x-rays to produce extremely high resolution images of internal organs and soft tissues, including brain. Since its development in the 1980s, MRI has been the preferred modality for diagnosing most diseases of the brain and spine. Superior anatomic detail can be obtained, with excellent delineation of gray and white matter. MRI is a powerful and versatile imaging technique that poses minimum risk to most patients (**Fig. 3–4**).

MRI is used to detect:

✦ Stroke, often within 6 hours of symptom onset
✦ Brain tumors, both primary and metastatic (**Fig. 3–5**)
✦ White matter disease (e.g., demyelinating lesions, lacunar infarcts, progressive multifocal leukoencephalopathy)

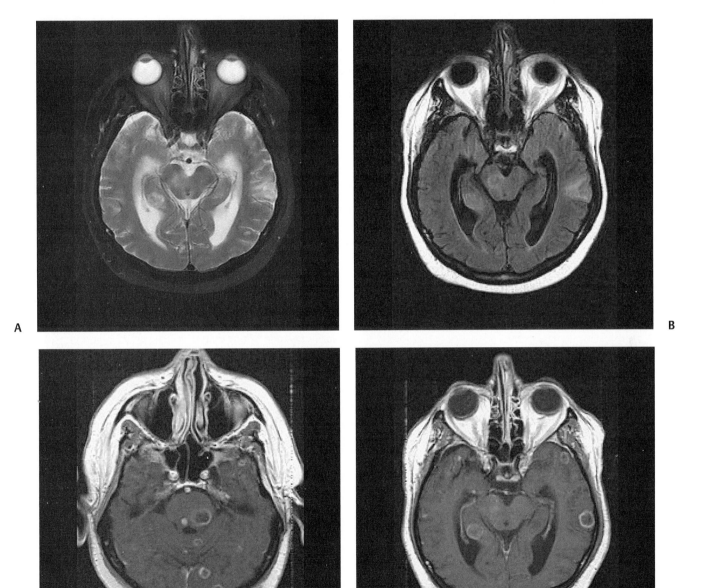

A   B

C   D

Figure 3–5 Axial magnetic resonance images of a patient with multiple metastases from lung cancer. **(A)** Axial T2–weighted image shows subtle high signal intensity in the left temporal lobe. **(B)** The signal abnormality is more pronounced on the fluid-attenuated inversion recovery (FLAIR) images. **(C)** Axial magnetization prepared rapid acquisition gradient echo (MPRAGE) image demonstrates several ring enhancing lesions in the left cerebellum, upper pons, and occipital lobe. **(D)** Axial MPRAGE image demonstrates several ring-enhancing lesions including two in the left temporal lobe (Images courtesy of Richard Silbergleit.)

Table 3–3 Applications of MR in Clinical Brain Imaging and Neuroscience Research

	Imaging Technique	Application
Clinical CNS applications	Anatomic imaging	Cerebrovascular disease
		Congenital malformation
		Infection
		Neoplasm
		Trauma
		White matter disease
	Angiography	Aneurysm
		Arteriovenous malformation
		Vascular occlusive disease
Neuroscience applications	Anatomic imaging	Brain morphology studies
		Lesion localization studies
	Angiography	CNS pulsatility
	Diffusion imaging	Cerebrovascular disease
		Epilepsy
		Neoplasm
	Blood oxygenation imaging	Activation studies
	Perfusion imaging	Activation studies
		Cerebrovascular disease
	Spectroscopic imaging	Activation studies
		Alzheimer's disease
		Huntington's disease
		Migraine
		Neoplasm
		Parkinson's disease
		Schizophrenia

+ Central nervous system infection (e.g., meningitis, encephalitis, and abscess)
+ Disease of the eye and ear
+ Focal cortical atrophy in a patient with possible dementia
+ Diffuse axonal injury and contusion following traumatic brain injury

Table 3–3 summarizes clinical and research applications of MRI.

General Principles

Magnetic resonance imaging takes advantage of the inherent magnetic properties of spinning hydrogen atoms in our bodies to generate a picture of a section of tissue. Hydrogen is the most abundant atom in the body, found in both water and fat. The nuclei of hydrogen atoms consist of a single proton that possesses an intrinsic magnetic moment. A magnetic moment can be best thought of as a tiny bar magnet within the nucleus of an atom. Under normal conditions, these biologic "magnets" are randomly oriented. When the body is placed within the strong external magnetic field of the MRI scanner, they tend to come into alignment with the field. Once the hydrogen atoms or "magnets" have aligned themselves with the magnetic field, a pulse of electromagnetic RF energy is applied that can move the protons out of alignment. After the pulse, the protons again align with the external magnetic field in a process called relaxation. Various tissues relax at different rates depending on their chemical nature, allowing the separation of gray matter, white matter, CSF, etc. During the relaxation process, RF energy is emitted from the tissue, and this is measured in RF coils or sensors surrounding the anatomy of interest. The duration, strength, and source location of the emitted energy are collected and translated by specialized equipment into the MR image. Two-dimensional (2D) sections in the axial, coronal, sagittal, and oblique planes, and 3D renderings of the brain can be displayed. A typical MRI scan takes anywhere from 30 to 90 minutes.

One of the greatest strengths of MRI is that it can produce tremendous variations in image contrast by utilizing the MR characteristics of different tissues. This is achieved by timing the application of RF and magnetic energy into tissue as well as by timing the collection of emitted RF energy. This is called a pulse sequence. Three tissue parameters commonly used to generate contrast in an MRI are proton density (PD), T1 (spin-lattice relaxation time), and T2 (spin-spin relaxation time). PD-weighted images show limited contrast between white and gray matter, but have high signal and good anatomic detail. Alternatively, white and gray matter can be discriminated by their T1 and T2 characteristics on T1-weighted and T2-weighted images. T1-weighted images are especially useful for distinguishing between gray and white matter. On T1-weighted images, CSF is black (hypointense), gray matter is dark gray, and white matter is light gray (hyperintense). T2-weighted images generally have poorer anatomic quality, but are better for detecting most pathologic lesions. Neurologic disease that increases the water content of brain tissue appears darker on T1-weighted images and lighter on T2-weighted images. Most lesions including tumors, infarct, and infection increase the water content of the affected tissue (**Fig. 3–6A–D**).

It is also possible to artificially enhance image contrast by introducing an exogenous contrast agent. Gadolinium has the property of altering the T1 and T2 in blood as well as blood vessel-rich tissue and in areas of blood–brain barrier disruption. Contrast enhancement of images results in striking signal intensity differences between these regions and the surrounding tissue (**Fig. 3–6E,F**). These differences are especially useful for imaging brain vasculature and cerebral perfusion, and in identifying compromises of the blood–brain barrier. This is important for detection of cerebrovascular disease, infection, and neoplasm.

Strengths and Limitations

For all its diagnostic and investigational power, MRI is a surprisingly low-risk procedure. Unlike most other medical imaging modalities, MRI does not use ionizing radiation and is free of the dangers associated with x-rays and gamma rays. The large magnetic field of the scanner does pose a risk to those patients with pacemakers or certain metallic implants

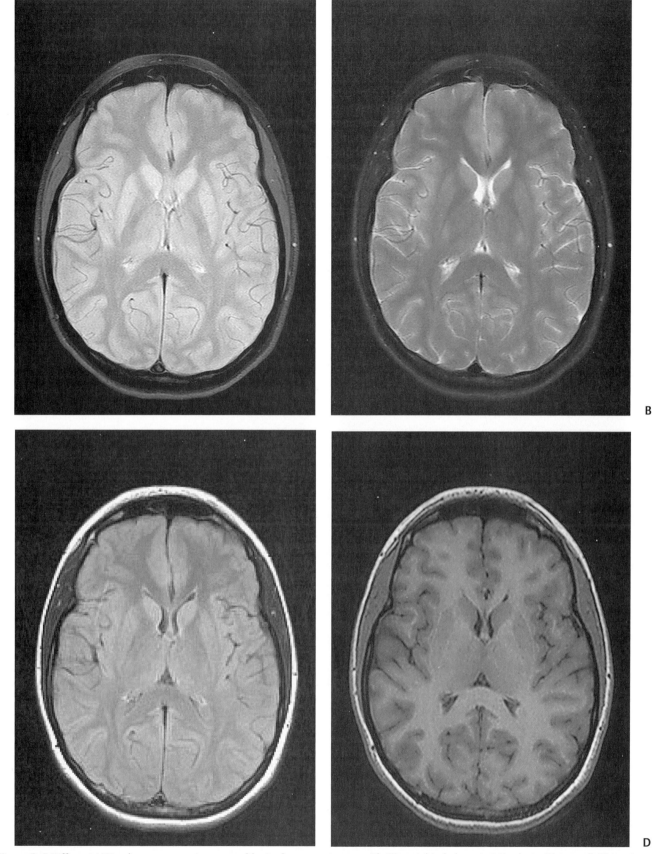

A

B

C

D

Figure 3–6 Different MRI pulse sequences in a normal brain demonstrate many of the different tissue contrast characteristics that can be obtained with MRI. **(A)** Axial proton density (PD) weighted image. Gray matter is brighter than white matter and CSF is gray. **(B)** Axial T2–weighted image. CSF is the brightest tissue. Gray matter is brighter than white matter. **(C)** FLAIR image. This sequence gives an image with T2–weighted characteristics but with pure fluid turning dark. It is ideal for evaluation of lesions that are bright on T2–weighted images that may be obscured by location near bright CSF. **(D)** Axial magnetization prepared rapid acquisition (MPR) image. This technique provides an image with mostly T1–weighted characteristics but with decreased signal in the fat compared to a traditional T1 image.

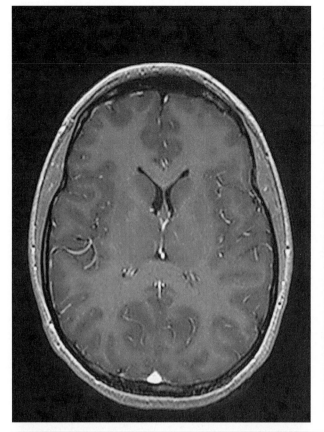

E

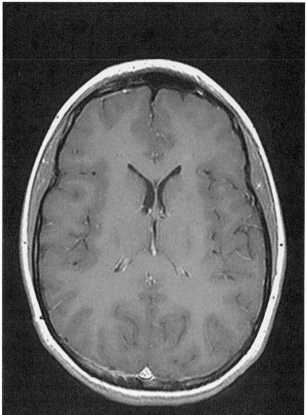

F

G

Figure 3–6 *(Continued)* **(E)** Axial-enhanced MPR image. Several normal blood vessels enhance and become visible after contrast administration. **(F)** Traditional T1–weighted enhanced image. Fat is the brightest tissue on the image. White matter is brighter than gray matter and CSF is black. **(G)** Coronal maximum intensity projection (MIP) view of 3D time-of-flight unenhanced MR angiogram of the intracranial circulation demonstrates the internal carotid, vertebral, and basilar arteries and their major branches. (Images courtesy of Richard Silbergleit.)

(including some heart valves, clips, and stents), and such individuals are not eligible for MR scanning. Most new implants are designed to be MRI compatible. Advantages of MRI include excellent spatial and temporal resolution, and its ability to be made sensitive to a diverse and widespread set of physical and physiologic parameters. MRI is superior to CT for the detection and localization of ischemic infarcts, aneurysms, and arteriovenous malformations. It can demonstrate an infarct within minutes to a few hours of onset, whereas commonly hours to days must pass before CT scanning detects infarction. CT, however, surpasses MRI in more reliably demonstrating an acute cerebral hemorrhage and in detecting bony pathology. MRI

tends to be the modality of choice for the diagnosis of vascular dementia (Gray and Cummings, 1994). It is also superior to CT in the later stages of traumatic brain injury for its ability to detect subtle structural changes such as atrophy, small chronic hemorrhages, and small infarcts.

MRI has its drawbacks as well. MRI may be unbearable for the claustrophobic patient, as the bore of a typical MRI scanner is rather narrow. In addition, the noise output of the scanner is considerable, and requires the use of hearing protection during scanning. General anesthesia is required for some patients. MRI is also susceptible to several artifacts, most notably patient motion, susceptibility effects, and metal artifact. For young, elderly, or trauma patients who cannot remain still, a satisfactory MRI may not be possible due to motion artifact. Susceptibility artifacts arise most frequently near bony or air-filled structures like the sinuses or the petrous part of the temporal bone, where the MR signal is often minimized. Metal artifact arises when some sort of metallic object is overlooked during patient screening and is brought into the scanner. **Table 3–2** lists strengths and weaknesses of MR imaging.

Advanced Magnetic Resonance Imaging Techniques

As well as being a technique to image anatomy, MR image contrast can be made sensitive to blood flow, blood oxygenation, functional activity, chemical composition, water diffusion, and tissue perfusion. These MR techniques include MR angiography (MRA), MR spectroscopy (MRS), diffusion-weighted MRI (DWI), perfusion-weighted MRI (PWI), and functional MRI (fMRI). Although structural MRI depicts brain anatomy, MRA images brain blood flow depicting vascular anatomy (arterial or venous) (**Fig. 3–6G**). MRA plays a central role in the evaluation of patients with diseases of the cerebral vasculature (e.g., arterial occlusive disease, sinus thrombosis, aneurysms, and arteriovenous malformations). MRS detects the chemical composition of diseased tissue. It is commonly used to study epilepsy, Alzheimer's disease, brain tumors, and the effects of drugs on brain metabolism. DWI and PWI are sensitive to changes in the diffusion of water in tissues and changes in tissue perfusion, respectively, that occur with ischemia. DWI has been used as an early indicator of dense ischemia or infarct, sometimes within minutes to hours of symptom onset (Gonzalez, Schafer, Buonanno, Schwamm, Budzik, Rordorf, Wang, Sorensen, & Koroshetz, 1999; Singer, Chong, Lu, Schonewille, Tuhrim, & Atlas, 1998) (**Fig. 3–7**). PWI reveals areas of brain tissue that are poorly perfused, and coupled with diffusion imaging, these techniques provide a powerful means for the early detection of stroke or stroke risk (Hillis, Wityk, Barker, and colleagues, 2002) (**Fig. 3–8**). Early detection of stroke is becoming increasingly important, as certain new therapies have a very narrow administration time window (e.g., thrombolytic therapy). Functional MRI (fMRI) was developed to study functional activity of the brain by detecting changes in blood oxygenation in brain regions during task performance. This latter MRI technique has many exciting applications in the research arena to study normal and disordered language processing.

Functional Magnetic Resonance Imaging

Functional MRI (fMRI) is a noninvasive imaging technique that produces high-resolution images of brain activity. Although conventional MRI uses ubiquitous hydrogen atoms to piece together a structural map of the brain, fMRI is tuned to detect the magnetic signatures of more specialized elements and molecules associated with certain brain activity and physiology. Most commonly, fMRI is used to detect changes in blood oxygenation levels during performance of motor, sensory, or cognitive tasks. Current fMRI studies use the BOLD (blood oxygenation level dependent) method, which takes advantage of the difference in magnetic properties of oxy- and deoxyhemoglobin to generate images that are sensitive to the oxygenation level of blood (Ogawa, Lee, Kay, & Tank, 1990; Ogawa, Menon, Tank, Kim, Merkle, Ellermann, & Ugurbil, 1993). Deoxyhemoglobin is a marker for oxygen-depleted blood. It is paramagnetic, and can act as an endogenous contrast agent or indicator of regional changes in blood oxygenation associated with neural activity. The BOLD signal change relies on the ratio of oxygenated and deoxygenated hemoglobin. In activated regions of the brain, this ratio changes as blood flow increases surpass oxygen use in brain tissue, decreasing the level of paramagnetic deoxyhemoglobin. This decrease in deoxyhemoglobin, or increase in the level of oxygenated blood, is the source of the BOLD signal (Ogawa et al., 1990, 1993). Functional signal changes can then be mapped onto a high-resolution MRI scan of the same subject to reveal changes in blood oxygenation, and assumed brain activity (McLaughlin, Rogers, & Shibata, 2003).

Functional MRI has been used primarily as a research tool to map human brain function. Functional MRI experiments have been used to identify regions of normal brain activity associated with a wide variety of functions, including human visual, auditory, sensory, and motor systems, as well as language comprehension and production (Belliveau, Kennedy, McKinstry, Buchbinder, Weisskoff, Cohen, Vevea, Brady, and Rosen, 1991; Binder, 2000; Binder, Frost, Hammeke, Cox, Rao, & Prieto, 1997; Friederici, Meyer, & von Cramon, 2000; Huang, Carr, & Cao, 2002). With fMRI, carefully controlled activation tasks are designed to isolate sensory, motor, or higher cognitive functions, such as language. During a scan, a large number of images are rapidly acquired [e.g., for echo-planar fMRI, the entire brain, typically in 4- or 5-mm contiguous slices, every 2 to 4 seconds (McLaughlin et al., 2003)], while a participant performs a task that is expected to change brain activity between two or more well-defined states—an experimental task and a control task (Matthews and Jezzard, 2004). Examples of language tasks might include naming pictures, generating a verb associated with a written noun (e.g., shown the written word *ball*, the participant says "kick"), making judgments about the semantic relatedness of two words (e.g., determining if the words *cat* and *dog* belong to the same semantic category), or making rhyme judgments about written words (e.g., determining if "kloj" and "plap" rhyme). A control task is also performed to remove the portion of the hemodynamic response not connected specifically with the task of interest. Control tasks in language experiments can be designed simply to remove early visual (e.g., passively viewing a cross-hair) or auditory processing (passively listening to a tone), or they may be designed to isolate specific components of language—phonologic (e.g., nonword rhyming task—*spag–klag*) vs. semantic processing (e.g., shirt-pants). Brain activity in the experimental state is then subtracted from or compared (via *t*-test or correlational type analysis) to activity in the control state. The result is a functional map of the location and intensity of the hemodynamic response associated with the process of interest. The functional image maps are then converted into maps of activated "voxels" or pixels using various computer algorithms, and the image is then overlaid onto a structural MRI of the individual participant's brain.

In addition to fMRI's widespread use in cognitive neuroscience research, there has been an interest in developing preoperative fMRI tasks that can be used clinically to identify language lateralization and eloquent cortex (i.e., essential for

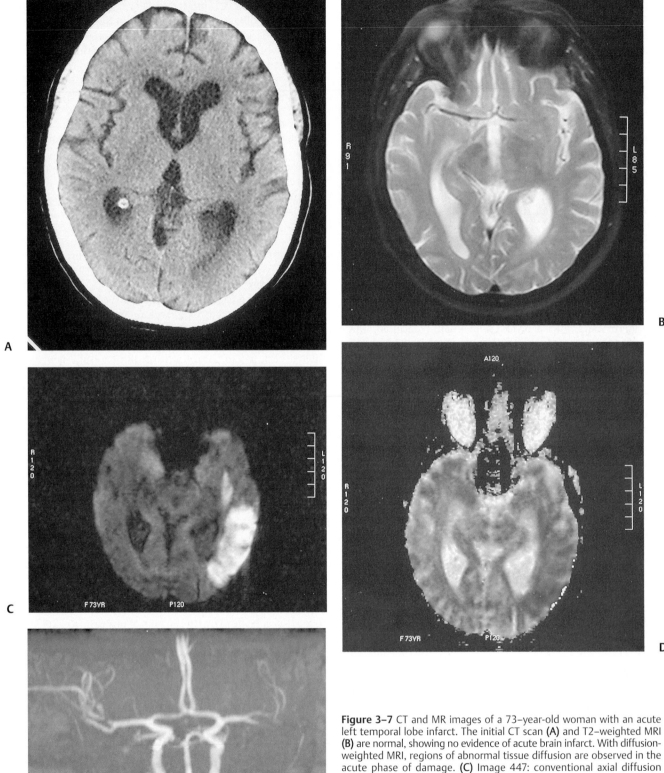

Figure 3–7 CT and MR images of a 73–year-old woman with an acute left temporal lobe infarct. The initial CT scan **(A)** and T2–weighted MRI **(B)** are normal, showing no evidence of acute brain infarct. With diffusion-weighted MRI, regions of abnormal tissue diffusion are observed in the acute phase of damage. **(C)** Image 447: conventional axial diffusion weighted image (b = 1000) demonstrates high signal intensity in the left temporal lobe. **(D)** Image 450: axial apparent diffusion coefficient (ADC) image shows low intensity in the same area, confirming that this represents restricted diffusion associated with an acute infarct. **(E)** Image 454: 3D time-of-flight magnetic resonance angiography (MRA) demonstrates occluded branches of the left middle cerebral arteries. (Courtesy of Richard Silbergleit.)

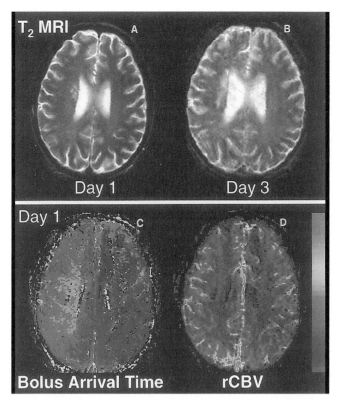

Figure 3–8 Axial T2–weighted MRI of a right-hemisphere periventricular stroke at day 1 **(A)** and day 3 **(B)**, and axial gadolinium injection perfusion-weighted MRI of the same patient at day 1 showing arrival time of the gadolinium bolus **(C)** and regional cerebral blood volume (rCBV) **(D)**. Note that at day 1 the perfusion images reveal a larger area of abnormal cerebral tissue than that detected by the T2–weighted MRI. By day 3, however, T2–weighted MRI demonstrates an enlarged lesion similar to that detected by perfusion imaging at day 1. (Courtesy of Peter Barker.)

Strengths and Limitations

The BOLD method has several advantages over other functional techniques, including a high signal-to-noise ratio, allowing the study of individual subjects, the capability of imaging the whole brain, temporal resolution of a few seconds [limited by the hemodynamic response itself (Matthews and Jezzard, 2004)], and good spatial resolution [the ability to detect the signal within 3 mm of where it was generated (Rugg, 1999)]. Because fMRI does not impose the risk of radiation exposure or use radioactive tracers, it is ideal for studying patients repeatedly over time. This is particularly exciting as a means of examining progressive neurologic diseases as well as neural mechanisms of recovery, both spontaneous and treatment-induced (Mayer, 2003). One of fMRI's major advantages is the ability to measure changes in the BOLD signal after perception or response to a single stimulus, a design known as event-related fMRI (Wise, 2003). This allows for experimental randomization and post-hoc analysis of single trials (e.g., comparing activation associated with correct vs. incorrect responses), which was not available previously with PET or fMRI.

The largest drawback of the BOLD fMRI scheme lies in questions about the true source of the BOLD effect. It has been shown that a fraction of the functional signal arises not from the brain capillaries and parenchyma (presumably at the site of activation), but rather from larger draining veins (Lai, Hopkins, Haake, and colleagues, 1993). Certain techniques are available to minimize signal contributions from these veins. In BOLD fMRI, however, this "brain–vein" dilemma somewhat limits the accuracy with which neural activity can be localized. Other limitations with fMRI are the same as those found with structural MRI, including the inability to scan patients with pacemakers or metallic implants (e.g., some heart valves, aneurysm clips), and difficultly imaging the basal temporal and orbitofrontal regions due to minimization of the MR signal by the temporal bone and frontal sinuses (susceptibility artifact). Motion artifact, from patient head movement and even of the brain intrinsically [for example, pulsations associated with respiratory or cardiac rhythms (Matthews and Jezzard, 2004)] can also be a problem. Statistical realignment procedures can be used to correct for motion artifact. Until recently, activation tasks involving spoken language production could not be performed with fMRI due to motion caused by vocalization. Rather, spoken language production tasks were done "silently" or covertly by thinking of a response instead of actually vocalizing. Several researchers have devised methods, however, to correct for signal distortion associated with overt speech production (Huang et al., 2002; Nelles, Lugar, Coalson, Miezin, Petersen, & Schlaggar, 2003) (**Fig. 3–9**).

Single Photon Emission Computed Tomography

Single photon emission computed tomography (SPECT) is a nuclear imaging technique that measures brain metabolism and rCBF through the use of radioactive tracers to produce 2D or 3D images of active brain regions. SPECT tracers have been developed to assess predominantly cerebral perfusion, but also blood–brain barrier integrity, neurotransmitter

motor, sensory, cognitive, or language function) for the purpose of surgical planning in epilepsy and lesion excision (e.g., tumor or arteriovenous malformation) (Binder, Swanson, Hammeke, Morris, Mueller, Fischer, Benbadis, Frost, Rao, & Haughton, 1996; Hirsch, Ruge, Kim, Correa, Victor, Relkin, Labar, Krol, Bilsky, Souweidane, DeAngelis, & Gutin, 2000). Currently there are more invasive techniques (e.g., the Wada test for language lateralization, and intraoperative brain mapping) that are standards of care, but given fMRI's strength as a non-invasive measure with high temporal and spatial resolution, there is a great desire to develop this application. There has also been considerable interest in using BOLD fMRI to study brain activity in several disease states. For instance, fMRI has been shown to detect early stages of neuropathology in Alzheimer's disease before clinical expression of cognitive decline (Bookheimer, Strojwas, Cohen, Sounders, Pericak-Vanc, Mazziotta, & Small, 2000). Functional recovery of motor and language ability in stroke patients has been examined, and these studies indicate that there are clear changes in functional organization following brain damage (Cao, D'Olhaberriague, Vikingstad, Levine, & Welch, 1998; Cao, Vikingstad, Huttenlocher, Towle, & Levin, 1994; Cao et al., 1999). We will discuss several studies using fMRI to study language reorganization following stroke-induced aphasia later in the chapter.

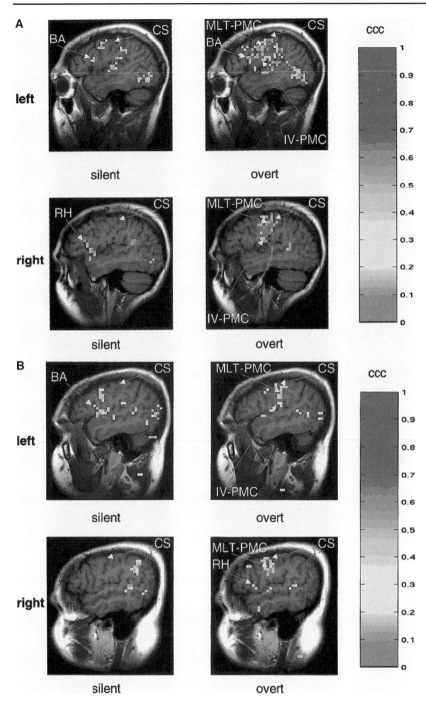

Figure 3–9 (A) Typical activation patterns obtained during silently speaking a letter name (two left panels). The Broca area was activated in both the silent and overt conditions, but to a large extent in the overt condition (right, top panel). The middle-inferior portion of the primary motor cortex (PMC) was activated bilaterally during overtly speaking a letter name, but not during silently speaking a letter name. **(B)** Typical activation patterns observed during silently generating an animal name (two left panels) and overtly generating an animal name (two right panels). Note that the Broca area was not activated during overt animal-name generation (right, top panel), but activated to a large extent during silent animal-name generation (left, top panel). The "mouth, lips, and tongue" region of the primary motor cortex was activated bilaterally during overt speech, but not during silent speech. In addition, overt speech activated the leftmost inferior portion of the primary motor cortex, and the activated cluster was disconnected from one in the middle portion of the primary motor cortex (right, top panel). MLT-PMC, the "mouth, lips, and tongue" region of the primary motor cortex; IV-PMC, the "inferior vocalization" region of the primary motor cortex; CS, central sulcus; BA, Broca area; RH, right homologue of Broca area; CCC, cross-correlation coefficient. See Color Plate 3–9B. [Reprinted with permission from Huang, J., Carr, T.H., and Cao, Y. (2001). Comparing Cortical Activations for Silent and Overt Speech Using Event-Related fMRI. *Human Brain Mapping, 15,* 39–53. Copyright 2001, John Wiley & Sons, Inc.]

uptake (e.g., receptor binding), and the presence of certain antibodies (e.g., indicative of tumor). SPECT has found a niche providing a measure of cerebral perfusion, and these maps of rCBF are of particular diagnostic value in acute stroke, dementia, traumatic brain injury, and epilepsy. SPECT is a relatively inexpensive imaging modality that is being used with increasing frequency to evaluate brain function in the clinical setting.

SPECT can be used in both the resting state (baseline blood flow and metabolism) as well as functional activation studies. SPECT scanning might be used to detect:

♦ Abnormal perfusion in a patient with a possible degenerative disease (e.g., Alzheimer's dementia vs. frontotemporal lobe degeneration)

♦ Abnormal perfusion in a patient with small cortical or subcortical lesion(s) not revealed by CT or MRI (e.g., mild traumatic brain injury)

♦ Cerebral ischemia in the hyperacute phases of stroke (i.e., within 3 hours of symptom onset)

♦ Seizure foci in a patient with epilepsy

♦ Dopamine uptake in a patient with Parkinson's disease

Table 3–4 highlights clinical and research applications of SPECT.

General Principles

Unlike CT and MRI, SPECT uses radioactive isotopes, called radionuclides (**Table 3–5**) to acquire images. Prior to scanning,

Table 3–4 Applications of SPECT in Clinical Brain Imaging and Neuroscience

	Radiopharmaceutical Class	Application
Clinical CNS applications	Blood–brain barrier (BBB) agents	Assessment of brain death
		Detect compromise of BBB
		Neoplasm
	Cerebral perfusion agents	Cerebrovascular disease
		Dementing illnesses
		Epilepsy
		Trauma
	Receptor binding agents	Glioma, pituitary tumor
Neuroscience applications	Cerebral perfusion agents	Activation studies
	Receptor binding agents	Cerebrovascular disease
		Dementing illnesses
		Depression
		Epilepsy
		Migraine
		Schizophrenia
	Labeled antibodies	Alzheimer's disease
		Neoplasm

These radiopharmaceuticals accumulate in different brain regions in different amounts proportional to the specificity rate of the pharmaceutical for the tissue of blood flow and the volume of tissue. The differential tracer uptake is the basis for SPECT imaging. The most common radiopharmaceuticals used in SPECT studies include the blood–brain barrier agents technetium-99m (^{99m}Tc)–hexamethylpropyleneamine oxime (HMPAO) and (^{99m}Tc)–ethyl cysteinate dimer (ECD), the cerebral perfusion agent xenon 133 (^{133}Xe), and the receptor binding agent iodine 123 (^{123}I). In SPECT, the radiopharmaceuticals contain a radionuclide that emits gamma rays as it decays. Surface detectors from the SPECT scanner measure the distribution of the gamma rays emitted by a radiopharmaceutical as it decays within a slice (or volume) of tissue (**Fig. 3–10**).

Data collection and image reconstruction in SPECT share some similarities with CT. In SPECT, a camera known as the Anger or gamma camera slowly rotates about the patient (reminiscent of an x-ray tube in motion with CT), collecting emission projections at many different angles. Although a CT scanner typically acquires data from one slice at a time (unless it is operating in spiral mode), the Anger camera collects projections from a volume of tissue. The image reconstruction algorithms used in CT and SPECT are based on the same theory, and both utilize sets of projection data to assemble the tomographs. Slices can be reformatted in any angle, including the axial, coronal, and sagittal planes (**Figs. 3–11, 3–12, and 3–13**). It is also possible to fuse SPECT images with those of CT and MRI to create a single image that combines anatomy and physiology. From these data, 3D surface and volume rendered images can be created facilitating sizing and localization of a lesion. Imaging times in SPECT are usually in the neighborhood of 15 to 30 minutes.

a radiopharmaceutical is introduced into the patient's body by either injection or inhalation and allowed to distribute within body and brain tissues. A radiopharmaceutical is a radioactive substance that can be selectively absorbed by certain cells in the brain or body and therefore can serve as a tracer of certain physiologic or biochemical processes.

Strengths and Weaknesses

SPECT imaging has several strengths and weaknesses (**Table 3–2**). Because the technique employs radioactive pharmaceuticals, the patient is exposed to ionizing radiation.

Table 3–5 Common SPECT and PET Radiopharmaceuticals

	Radiopharmaceutical Class	Radiopharmaceutical	Radionuclides
SPECT	Blood–brain barrier agents	DTPA, TlCl	^{99m}Tc, ^{201}Tl
	Cerebral perfusion agents	HMPAO, ECD, Xe	^{99m}Tc, ^{133}Xe
	Receptor binding agents	Acetylcholine, benzodiazepine, dopamine, and somatostatin receptor agents	^{111}In, ^{123}I
	Labeled antibodies	Antibody specific to neoplasm, amyloid, etc.	^{99m}Tc, ^{123}I, ^{131}I
PET	Blood–brain barrier agents	EDTA	^{68}Ga
	Cerebral perfusion agents	H_2O, CO, CO_2	^{15}O
	Receptor binding agents	Acetylcholine, benzodiazepine, dopamine, histamine, opium, and serotonin receptor agents	^{11}C, ^{18}F
	Metabolic tracers	Methionine, O_2, FDG	^{11}C, ^{15}O, ^{18}F
	Neurotransmitter tracers	L-Dopa	^{18}F
	Labeled antibodies	Antibody specific to glioma	^{124}I

DTPA, diethylenetriamine pentaacetic acid; ECD, ethyl cysteinate dimer; EDTA, ethylenediaminetetraacetic acid; FDG, fluorodeoxyglucose; HMPAO, hexamethylpropyleneamine oxime; TlCl, thallium chloride.

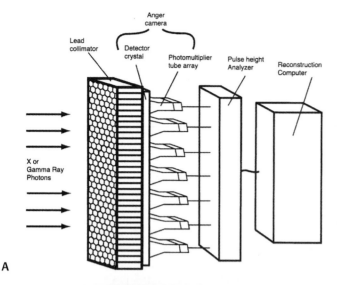

A

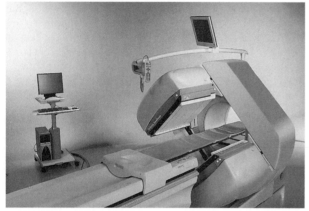

B

Figure 3–10 (A) Schematic of a SPECT gamma camera system showing the collimator, detector crystal, and photomultiplier tube array. **(B)** Photograph of a modern SPECT imaging system. (Infinia image courtesy of GE Healthcare, Buckinghamshire, UK. Copyright General Electric.)

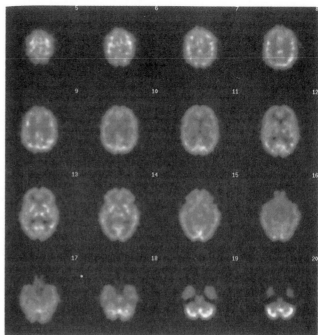

Figure 3–11 Axial SPECT images of cerebral perfusion in a healthy subject obtained using the radiopharmaceutical ^{99m}Tc-ECD. Notice that perfusion levels in the parietal cortex approach those of the occipital cortex and that the distribution of tracer appears rather smooth. (See Color Plate 3–11.) (Courtesy of David Wang.)

distribution of these radiopharmaceuticals throughout the brain and body.

PET scanning is the most costly of the imaging modalities in terms of labor and facilities, and requires a special machine called a cyclotron on site to produce nuclides. As a

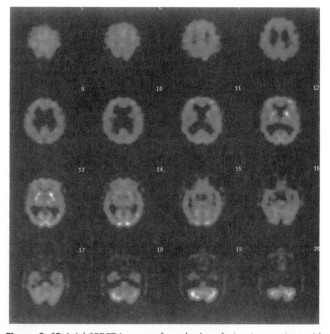

Figure 3–12 Axial SPECT images of cerebral perfusion in a patient with Alzheimer's dementia obtained using the radiopharmaceutical ^{99m}Tc-ECD. Perfusion in the parietal cortex is significantly reduced compared to that of the occipital cortex. This pattern of perfusion is typical in Alzheimer's type dementia, and is in clear contrast to that seen in healthy individuals (**Fig. 3–11**). (See Color Plate 3–12.) (Courtesy of David Wang.)

Furthermore, the radiation exposure is not limited to the imaged region, as the radiopharmaceutical distributes throughout the body. The use of radiation also prevents the rapid repetition of experiments because the radiation dose must be kept at an acceptable level and one must wait for the decay or elimination of radioactivity from previous scans before proceeding with the next. SPECT imaging does not possess the spatial or temporal resolution of MRI and CT; however, its ability to investigate a wide range of physiologic and biochemical processes not available to conventional radiologic techniques is a tremendous strength. SPECT scanning systems are also considerably less expensive and found in more clinical settings than PET.

Positron Emission Tomography

Positron emission tomography (PET) depicts rCBF, brain metabolism (e.g., oxygen and glucose), neurotransmitter metabolism, and drug concentrations in brain tissue through the use of injected radioactive isotopes or radionuclides. Like SPECT, PET measures emissions from radioactively labeled pharmaceuticals that have been injected into the body to create multicolored 2D and 3D images of the

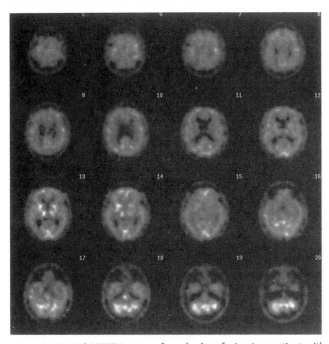

Figure 3–13 Axial SPECT images of cerebral perfusion in a patient with multiinfarct dementia (MID) obtained using the radiopharmaceutical ^{99m}Tc-ECD. Unlike the case of Alzheimer's type dementia (Fig. 3–12), perfusion levels in the parietal cortex approach those of the occipital cortex. The pattern of perfusion, however, appears mottled when compared to the healthy scan (**Fig. 3–11**), a trademark of MID. (See Color Plate 3–13.) (Courtesy of David Wang.)

result, the use of PET in clinical settings has been very slow to develop, and has been used primarily as a research tool. PET has seen widespread use in research for its ability to measure brain function both at rest and during activation studies where a subject performs a specific task during imaging. In these studies, abnormal brain function has been shown in patients with aphasia, Alzheimer's disease, primary progressive aphasia, Tourette's syndrome, stuttering, epilepsy, and Parkinson's disease (Jeffries, Schooler, Schoenbach, Herscovitch, Chase, Braun, 2002; Metter and Hanson, 1994; Nestor, Graham, Fryer, Williams, Patterson, & Hodges, 2003; Small, Ercoli, Silverman, Huang, Komo, Bookheimer, Lavretsky, Miller, Siddarth, Rasgon, Mazziotta, Saxena, Wu, Mega, Cummings, Saunders, Pericak-Vance, Roses, Barrio, Phelps, 2000). PET has also been used extensively to study normal motor, sensory, and cognitive processing, including language (Petersen, Fox, Posner, Mintun, and Raichle, 1988; Petersen, Fox, Snyder, & Raichle, 1990; Wise, Hadar, Howard, & Patterson, 1991). See **Table 3–6** for clinical and research applications of PET.

General Principles

Unlike SPECT in which the administered radiopharmaceutical emits gamma rays, PET radiopharmaceuticals are positron (positively charged electrons) emitters. These positron emitting isotopes are chemically incorporated into biologically active radiopharmaceuticals, enabling examination of a number of physiologic and biochemical processes. The positrons emitted by the radioisotopes are measured noninvasively by detectors

Table 3–6   Applications of PET in Clinical Brain Imaging and Neuroscience Research

	Radiopharmaceutical Class	**Application**
Clinical CNS applications	Metabolic tracers	Differentiation of recurrent tumor from radiation necrosis
Neuroscience applications	Cerebral perfusion agents	Alzheimer's disease
		Cerebrovascular disease
		Functional imaging
	Receptor binding agents	Alcoholism
		Alzheimer's disease
		Epilepsy
		Mood disorder
		Schizophrenia
		Parkinson's disease
	Metabolic tracers	Activation studies
		AIDS
		Alzheimer's disease
		Cerebrovascular disease
		Depression
		Epilepsy
		Neoplasm
		Parkinson's disease
	Neurotransmitter tracers	Parkinson's disease
		Schizophrenia
	Labeled antibodies	Glioma

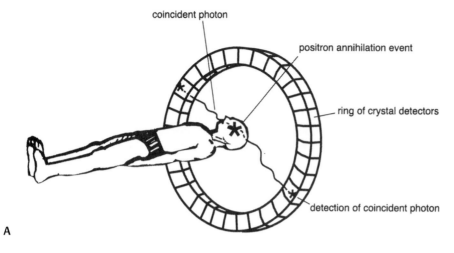

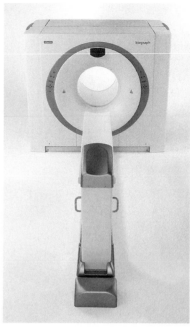

Figure 3–14 (A) Schematic of a PET scanner showing the ring of crystal detectors, and an annihilation even with subsequent coincidence detection. **(B)** Photograph of a modern PET/CT scanner. (Courtesy of Siemens Medical Corporation, New York, NY.)

arranged outside the body, and tomographic images are reconstructed. PET images accurately reveal the distribution of the administered radiopharmaceutical in the region of the body being studied (**Fig. 3–14**). Radionuclides commonly found in PET radiopharmaceuticals include fluorine 18 [^{18}F] fluorodeoxyglucose (FDG), which is used to measure glucose metabolism, [^{15}O] O_2, which is used to measure oxygen metabolism, and [^{15}O] water, which is used to measure cerebral blood flow (CBF) (Metter and Hanson, 1994). In general, PET radiopharmaceuticals used in brain imaging fall into one of six categories: blood–brain barrier agents, cerebral perfusion agents, tracers of metabolism, neurotransmitter tracers, agents that bind to specific central nervous system (CNS) receptors, and labeled antibodies (**Table 3–5**).

PET scanners in general perform better than SPECT systems in terms of resolution and scanning times. Modern PET scanners can attain in-plane spatial resolution on the order of 3 to 5 mm, and slice thicknesses of approximately 1 cm. Scan times are still rather long, especially when compared to the faster functional MRI techniques, and a typical scan may require from 1 to 20 minutes to complete. This limits somewhat the ability of PET to examine rapidly changing processes.

Strengths and Limitations

PET scanning is a tremendously versatile technique as it can image brain function at rest and during task performance (**Fig. 3–15**). Radiopharmaceuticals have been developed that allow PET to trace physiologic processes ranging from blood flow to energy and neurotransmitter metabolism. Other strengths of this technique include the ability to make quantitative physiologic measurements. Such measurements can be made of the entire brain, including the orbital region of the frontal lobe and the basal region of the temporal region; fMRI is generally poor at imaging these regions.

PET does have several drawbacks, however. As with SPECT imaging, PET scanning exposes the subject to a radioactive

tracer, which limits PET's desirability for repetitive or lengthy studies. Also, PET scanning is easily the most expensive of the imaging modalities discussed in this chapter. There are also some limitations in using PET during functional imaging studies. PET has a poor signal-to-noise ratio, and frequently PET data must be averaged over several subjects or several repetitions to attain adequate signal and to reduce noise. Definitive individual studies are therefore difficult to obtain. With improving

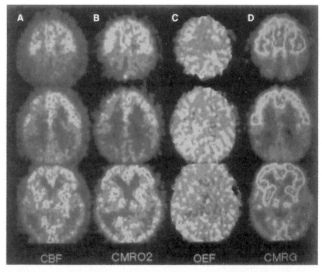

Figure 3–15 Axial PET images of **(A)** cerebral blood flow (CBF), **(B)** cerebral metabolism rate of oxygen ($CMRO_2$), **(C)** oxygen extraction fraction (OEF), and **(D)** cerebral metabolism rate of glucose (CMRG) in a patient with Alzheimer's disease. Significant reductions of CBF and CMRG and moderate reduction of $CMRO_2$ were noted in the parietotemporal region. A slight increase in OEF was observed in the same region. (See Color Plate 3–15.) [From Fukuyama, H., Ogawa, M., Yamauchi, H., Yamaguchi, S., Kimur, J., Yonekura, Y., Konishi, J. (1994). Altered Cerebral Metabolism in Alzheimer's Disease: A PET Study. *Journal of Nuclear Medicine, 35,* 1–6. Copyright 1994, Society of Nuclear Medicine, Inc., with permission.]

Table 3–7 Summary of the Applications of CT, MRI, SPECT, and PET

Modality		Primary Applications
CT	Clinical	Cerebrovascular disease, congenital malformation, neoplasm, trauma, angiography
	Neuroscience	Lesion studies, brain morphology studies
MRI	Clinical	Cerebrovascular disease, congenital malformation, infection, neoplasm, white matter disease, angiography
	Neuroscience	Activation studies, cerebral perfusion studies, in vivo spectroscopy, diffusion imaging, lesion studies, brain morphology studies
SPECT	Clinical	Dementing illnesses, neoplasm, cerebrovascular disease, epilepsy
	Neuroscience	Activation studies, cerebral perfusion studies, receptor mapping studies
PET	Clinical	Differentiation of recurrent tumor from radiation necrosis
	Neuroscience	Activation studies, cerebral perfusion studies, baseline metabolic studies (glucose, oxygen, and amino acids), receptor mapping studies

technologies, newer PET scanners, however, are approaching the point where individual data may be considered reliable. PET also suffers from rather poor temporal resolution when compared to rapid fMRI techniques. One PET CBF measurement can be obtained over 1 to 2 minutes, whereas the whole brain can be imaged in 2 to 3 seconds with echoplanar fMRI. See **Table 3–2** for a summary of strengths and weaknesses of PET.

Table 3–7 summarizes the clinical and research applications of CT, MRI, SPECT, and PET. The remainder of the chapter focuses on the application of these technologies to the study of acquired language disorders.

✦ Neuroimaging of Acquired Language Disorders

This section highlights key findings from structural and functional neuroimaging studies of patients with acquired language disorders, predominantly patients with aphasia. From these investigations, insights into the localization of aphasia, the neural basis of language deficits, and mechanisms of recovery have been gained. Three methods used in neuroimaging research are reviewed: (1) the lesion-deficit or clinical-anatomic approach, (2) baseline CBF and metabolism studies, and (3) functional brain activation studies. The overall aim of the lesion-deficit approach is to correlate a specific

language deficit or aphasia syndrome with precise lesion localization identified on structural CT or conventional MRI. The logic behind this method is that if an individual can no longer perform a certain language function, then the damaged area must be critical or essential for that function (Binder and colleagues, 1997). Lesion-deficit studies have been the central means to establish the neural correlates of aphasia and associated language disorders. The second type of study uses the functional neuroimaging technologies of SPECT, PET, or DWI and PWI to examine CBF and metabolism while an individual is at "rest" during imaging. These studies have been referred to as baseline CBF and metabolism, steady-state, or resting studies. They have advanced understanding of the relationship between abnormal neurophysiology and clinical deficits as well as the neurophysiologic mechanisms of aphasia recovery. The final type of study uses functional neuroimaging (e.g., FDG-PET and fMRI-BOLD techniques) to show brain regions that are active in both brain-damaged and neurologically intact individuals during performance of specific language tasks, such as reading words, naming pictures, or comprehending sentences. Unlike lesion-deficit studies, which identify brain areas that are critical for language performance, activation studies enable researchers to visualize all brain regions that participate in a specific language task (Binder and colleagues, 1997). Some brain regions may be critical for efficient language performance, whereas others may serve a more supportive or secondary role. These studies have been particularly exciting for advancing neurologic models of normal language processing and investigating neural mechanisms of aphasia recovery, both spontaneous and treatment-induced. The information from this broad literature base can be applied to inform many aspects of the clinical decision-making process, from differential diagnosis to determining prognosis (Kendall and Gonzalez-Rothi, 2001; Raymer, 2001).

Lesion-Deficit Studies

Historical Perspective

The study of the anatomic localization of aphasia began in the 19th century with the work of Paul Broca, Carl Wernicke, and Ludwig Lichtheim, who made the first clinical-anatomic correlations from the postmortem study of patients with aphasia (Broca, 1861; Wernicke, 1874; Lichtheim, 1885). From these efforts the classical model of language and the brain was developed, which posits the existence of cerebral language centers in the left perisylvian region that support speaking, listening, reading, and writing. In its simplest version, Wernicke's area in the left posterior-superior temporal gyrus [Brodmann area (BA) 22] encompasses the center for receptive aspects of language, namely decoding of auditory word forms. Broca's area in the left posterior end of the inferior frontal lobe (BA 44–45) is the center for expressive aspects of language, namely motor planning of speech. These two areas are connected by a white matter fiber tract, the arcuate fasciculus. A third brain area, the angular gyrus in the inferior parietal lobe (area 39), is the critical center for word reading. It enables the translation of visual input into an auditory code, with subsequent access of meaning through Wernicke's area (**Fig. 3–16**) for a depiction of the left lateral surface of the brain including Brodmann areas.

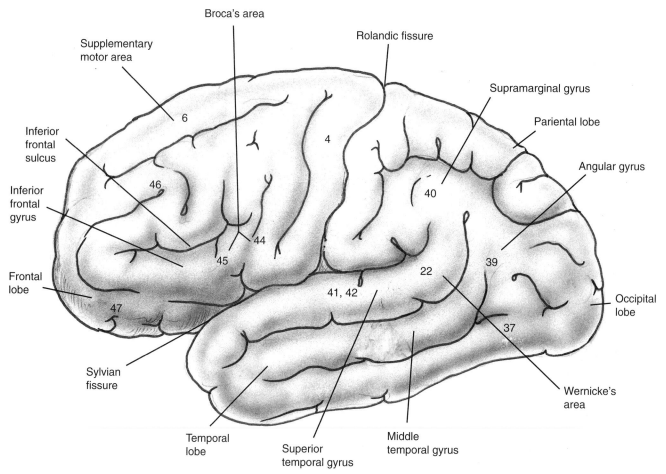

Broca's area
Rolandic fissure
Supplementary motor area
Supramarginal gyrus
Pariental lobe
Inferior frontal sulcus
Angular gyrus
Inferior frontal gyrus
Frontal lobe
Occipital lobe
Sylvian fissure
Wernicke's area
Temporal lobe
Superior temporal gyrus
Middle temporal gyrus

6   4   46   40   44   45   47   41, 42   22   39   37

Figure 3–16 Diagrammatic representation of the lateral surface of the left cerebral hemisphere. Brodmann's areas 44 and 45 correspond to Broca's area, and area 22 to Wernicke's area. Areas 41 and 42 correspond to the primary auditory cortex; these areas are deep in the sylvian fissure and cannot be visualized in a lateral view of the brain. Area 40 is the supramarginal gyrus and area 39 is the angular gyrus. The names of gyri and corresponding Brodmann numbers discussed in the text are also listed.

According to the classical model, focal brain damage to the language areas or connections between them results in different aphasia syndromes. Damage to Wernicke's area (BA 22) causes Wernicke's aphasia, a syndrome characterized by fluent but paraphasic speech output, auditory comprehension impairment, and poor repetition. Damage to Broca's area (BA 44–45) causes Broca's aphasia, a syndrome characterized by nonfluent speech output, relatively intact auditory comprehension, and poor repetition. Damage to the fiber tract that connects Broca's and Wernicke's areas, the arcuate fasciculus, causes conduction aphasia. This syndrome is characterized by fluent speech output, intact comprehension, and poor repetition. The classical model lost favor in the first half of the 20th century, but was revitalized by the late Norman Geschwind and still undergoes revision today (Geschwind, 1965, 1970; Mesulam, 1990, 1998). Debate continues as to the exact brain regions that support receptive and expressive language, as well as to the specific linguistic function of Broca's and Wernicke's areas (Grodzinsky, 2000; Hickok and Poeppel, 2004; Mohr, 1976; Wise, Scott, Blank, Mummery, Murphy, and Warburton, 2001). Despite these shortcomings, the classical model is still widely applied to interpret the behavioral consequences of brain injury and disease upon language function (Damasio, 2001).

Neuroanatomic Correlates of Aphasia

With the advent of CT in the 1970s and the development of MRI in the 1980s, the precise characterization of structural lesions in living patients has been realized. As a result, the anatomic correlates of aphasia and associated disorders have been described in much greater detail than permitted with postmortem studies (Naeser and Hayward, 1978; see Damasio, H., 1991 for a review). Clinicians regularly use lesion localization data to predict behavioral consequences of damage in a given brain region. Initial testing can then be targeted toward the most probable deficits, which is particularly important in the acute setting where the patient's testing tolerance may be poor. If the pattern of observed language deficits is not consistent with lesion data, it may prompt a request for further neurologic workup. It is important to recognize, however, that there is variation in the presentation of aphasia. This variation results from differences in the exact placement of a lesion as well as differences in normal neural and vascular anatomy. Variation also arises because of differences in organization of neural networks that support normal language processing (A. Damasio, 1991).

Numerous imaging studies have been conducted to more definitively describe the neuroanatomic correlates of aphasia (H. Damasio, 1991; Damasio & Geschwind, 1984; Naeser and

Table 3–8   Lesion Location and Clinical Manifestations of the Classic Aphasia Syndromes

Aphasia Syndrome	Clinical Manifestation	Classical Lesion Location
Broca's aphasia	Major deficit of speech production with nonfluent, sparse, halting, hesitating speech, often misarticulated, frequently missing function words	Posterior aspects of left third frontal convolution—Broca's area (areas 44 and 45), adjacent premotor and motor regions, with extension into underlying white matter, basal ganglia, and insula
Wernicke's aphasia	Major deficit of auditory comprehension with fluent paraphasic output (phonemic, morphological, and semantic paraphasias)	Posterior region of left superior temporal gyrus and possibly adjacent parietal cortex (lower segment of supramarginal and angular gyri)
Anomic aphasia	Deficit of single word production, typically for common nouns, with variable auditory comprehension problems	Inferior parietal lobe (angular gyrus) or the connections between parietal and temporal lobes; damage to left anterior temporal cortex
Global aphasia	Major deficits affecting both language comprehension and production	Large left perisylvian region, extending deep into underlying white matter, lenticular and caudate nuclei
Conduction aphasia	Deficits of repetition and spontaneous speech (phonemic paraphasias)	Left perisylvian damage to primary auditory cortex (areas 41 and 42), surrounding association cortex (area 22), and variable damage to the insula, its subcortical white matter, and the supramarginal gyrus (area 40); sparing of superior temporal gyrus (Wernicke's area)
Transcortical motor aphasia	Deficit of speech production similar to Broca's aphasia with relatively spared repetition	Anterior and superior to Broca's area (Watershed zone); or white matter tracts deep to Broca's area
Transcortical sensory aphasia	Deficit of auditory comprehension, with relatively spared repetition	Posterior parietotemporal lesions; posterior section of middle temporal gyrus (area 37) and in the angular gyrus (area 39) or in underlying white matter with relative sparing of Wernicke's area (area 22 in the superior temporal gyrus (watershed zone)

Adapted from Caplan, D. (1994). Language and the Brain. In M.A. Gernsbacher (Ed.), *Handbook of Psycholinguistics*. San Diego, CA: Academic Press, Inc.; Damasio, H. Neuroanatomical Correlates of the Aphasias. (1991). In M.T. Sarno (Ed). *Acquired Aphasia, 2nd ed.* (pp. 27–43). San Diego: Academic Press; Damasio, A. Signs of Aphasia. (1991). In M.T. Sarno (Ed) *Acquired Aphasia, 2nd ed.* (pp. 27–43). San Diego: Academic Press.

Hayward, 1978). **Tables 3–8** and **3–9** summarize the lesion localization data for the classic aphasia syndromes and related disorders. These efforts have shown that lesions anterior to the rolandic fissure in the left frontal lobe result in the nonfluent aphasias, Broca's and transcortical motor. Lesions posterior to the rolandic fissure in the left parietal and temporal lobes result in the fluent aphasias, Wernicke's, conduction and transcortical sensory. Lesions that encompass the sylvian fissure produce repetition impairments. These neuroanatomic correlations have been found to be fairly reliable, but some exceptions have been found.

Several investigations have identified atypical lesion sites for the different aphasia syndromes (Basso, Lecours, Moraschini, & Vanier, 1985; Vignolo, Boccardi, & Caverni, 1986; Kertesz, 1979; see Dronkers et al., 2000 for a review). Patients have been found who have fluent aphasia with anterior lesions, nonfluent aphasia with posterior lesions, and global aphasia with only partial lesions in the perisylvian cortex (Basso and colleagues, 1985; Cappa and Vignolo, 1983). Additionally, the lesions that cause chronic Broca's, Wernicke's, and conduction aphasia have been found to be different from what classic theory predicts. Isolated damage to Broca's area does not cause chronic Broca's aphasia but instead a transient impairment of articulation and language (Dronkers, 1992; Mohr, 1976; Mohr, Pessin Finkelstein, Funkenstein, Duncan, & Davis, 1978). For classic Broca's aphasia, the lesion may include Broca's area, but must extend beyond into other frontal and subcortical regions. Broca's area can even be spared in Broca's aphasia (Dronkers, Shapiro, Redfern, & Knight, 1992). It has also been shown that damage to classic Wernicke's area does not cause Wernicke's aphasia. Instead, isolated damage to Wernicke's area causes chronic conduction aphasia with a lasting impairment of repetition (Dronkers, Redfern, Ludy, & Baldo, 1998). For chronic Wernicke's aphasia, the lesion may include Wernicke's area (left posterior-superior temporal gyrus), but must also extend into the middle temporal gyrus or inferior parietal lobe. Wernicke's aphasia may even be caused by damage outside of Wernicke's area (Dronkers, Redfern, & Ludy 1995). The classic lesion localization of conduction aphasia, a disconnection of the anterior and posterior language regions from damage to the arcuate fasciculus, has also been challenged (Anderson, Gilmore, Roper, Crosson, Bauer, Nadeau, Beversdorf, Cibula, Rogish, Kortencamp, Hughes, Gonzalez Rothi, & Heilman, 1999; Damasio & Damasio, 1989; Dronkers et al., 2000). Damage that severs the left arcuate fasciculus has been shown to result in deficits more characteristic of severe Broca's aphasia, with speech output limited to the production of recurring stereotypic utterances (e.g., "No, no"; "Yeah, yeah"; "Yes, I know"; "I know") (Dronkers et al., 2000). The exact locus is at the point where the fibers of the arcuate fasciculus join together and ascend out of the temporal lobe and over the ventricles. Deep parietal lesions and even small subcortical strokes can cause this damage, which disrupts

Table 3–9 Related Syndromes

Syndrome	Clinical Manifestations	Lesion Location
Mutism	Minimal or absent speech output; a spontaneous speech and motor output; normal comprehension of oral and written language	Mesial aspect of frontal lobe involving the supplementary motor area (mesial portion of area 6), its connections, and anterior cingulate (area 24)
Alexia without agraphia (pure alexia)	Inability to read, with preserved ability to write spontaneously or to dictation; speech, auditory comprehension, and repetition are intact	Left occipital lobe damage; primary visual cortex (area 17), part of visual association cortices (areas 18 and 19), with extension into mesial occipitotemporal regions (mesial area 37) and posterior parahippocampal gyrus; lesion disrupts connections between right and left hemispheres coursing through splenium of corpus callosum
Pure word deafness	Profound loss of auditory comprehension and inability to repeat, with normal fluent speech and occasional paraphasia	Bilateral damage to the superior temporal gyri
Alexia with agraphia	Inability to read and write	Left posterior parietal damage between Wernicke's area and the visual association cortices

communication between posterior and anterior language regions. Conduction aphasia is now more commonly thought to be caused by *cortical* damage in the left perisylvian region. The specific regions include, but not necessarily all in combination, the primary auditory cortex (areas 41 and 42), the superior temporal gyrus (Wernicke's area), the supramarginal gyrus, the insula, and the underlying white matter (H. Damasio, 1991). Two different types of conduction aphasia have been described as well, each with a different lesion locus (Shallice, 1988). In repetition conduction aphasia, patients have an underlying verbal short-term memory disorder. The associated lesion is in the left inferior supramarginal gyrus (Sakurai, Takeuchi, Kojima, Yazawa, Murayama, Kaga, Momose, Nakase, Sakuta, & Kanazawa, 1998). In the second type, reproduction conduction aphasia, patients have a more generalized phonologic impairment, resulting in the production of phonemic paraphasias. The lesion involves the periventricular white matter, which connects the auditory cortex to the supramarginal gyrus (Sakurai and colleagues, 1998). These studies demonstrate that the neuroanatomic correlates of aphasia are much more complex than initially assumed.

Other neuroimaging studies have sought to make more detailed clinical-anatomic correlations by localizing specific impairments of language rather than an entire aphasia syndrome. Alexander, Naeser, and Palumbo (1990) examined the influence of locus of lesion in patients with nonfluent aphasia following damage in and around Broca's area. They grouped patients by lesion site: (1) the left frontal operculum (Broca's area), (2) lower motor cortex, or (3) immediately subjacent subcortical white matter. They then identified the associated language symptoms. Damage restricted to the frontal operculum resulted in deficits similar to transcortical motor aphasia: nonfluent, sparse grammatical output, with intact repetition. Damage to the lower motor cortex or its efferent subcortical projections caused dysarthria with disrupted articulation and prosody. Damage to the lower motor cortex and subcortical white matter caused dysarthria and phonemic errors. Studies such as this one can be applied clinically to predict not only the presence of nonfluent aphasia, but also how the pattern of speech and language production might differ based on the site and extent of lesion.

Dronkers (1996) studied another disorder commonly associated with nonfluent aphasia: speech apraxia. Apraxia of speech is a motor speech disorder that affects the planning and programming of speech. Dronkers overlapped the lesions of 25 patients with this disorder and found that all of them had damage to the superior tip of the precentral gyrus of the insula. Nineteen other patients were examined who did not have apraxia of speech, and interestingly their lesions did not encompass the insula. Damage to the anterior insula has been shown by others to result in speech apraxia (Taubner, Raymer, & Heilman, 1999).

The neuroanatomic correlates of auditory comprehension deficits have been investigated. The reason for comprehension failure can stem from a number of sources: (1) an inability to perceive or discriminate phonemes, (2) an inability to decode syntactic relationships within a sentence, or (3) an inability to understand the semantic meaning of words (Kirshner, 1995a). It is not surprising that a single locus for comprehension failure has not been found. Dronkers, Wilkins, Van Valin, Redfern, and Jaeger (2004) recently used more advanced data analysis techniques to identify the critical brain regions associated with performance on a test of auditory sentence length comprehension. They examined 64 chronic left hemisphere stroke patients, eight right hemisphere patients, and 15 neurologically intact older adults. They found that damage in the following brain regions corresponded with poorer language performance: (1) the posterior middle temporal gyrus (MTG) and underlying white matter, (2) the anterior superior temporal gyrus, (3) the superior temporal sulcus (STS) and angular gyrus, and (4) two regions in the midfrontal cortex in Brodmann's areas 46 and 47. Interestingly, damage to Broca's and Wernicke's areas did not affect performance on this measure. Further study showed that damage to the MTG corresponded with the poorest performance of word level comprehension, whereas the other regions contributed to deficits of sentence level comprehension. Based on converging evidence from the results of this study and others, the following roles for each of these regions in the left hemisphere were proposed: (1) the posterior middle temporal gyrus and underlying white matter (posterior BA 21 and superior BA 37) in single-word comprehension; (2) the anterior temporal gyrus (anterior BA 22) in morphosyntactic aspects of sentence length comprehension; (3) the STS and angular gyrus (BA 39) in auditory short-term memory processes engaged during sentence comprehension; and (4) the left frontal cortex (BA 46–47) in working memory processes that facilitate the selection and manipulation of

Table 3–10 Proposed Contributions of Different Brain Areas to Language Comprehension

Components of Language Comprehension	Contributing Brain Areas
Word-level comprehension: linking concepts to words	Left posterior middle temporal gyrus and underlying white matter (posterior BA 21 and superior BA 37)
Sentence-level comprehension	
Processing of *basic* morphosyntactic structures	Left anterior temporal gyrus (BA 22)
Auditory short-term verbal memory necessary when comprehension requires auditory rehearsal of sentence	Left superior temporal sulcus and angular gyrus (BA 39)
Working memory processes for processing of *complex* morphosyntactic structures	Left frontal cortex (BA 46–47)

Adapted from Dronkers, N.F., Wilkins, D.P., Van Valin, R.D., Redfern, B.B., Jaeger, J.J. (2004). Lesion Analysis of the Brain Areas Involved in Language Comprehension. *Cognition, 92,* 145–177

semantic and syntactic information during sentence comprehension (**Table 3–10**). The results from this study can be used not only to anticipate patients who might have sentence length comprehension impairments, but also to provide greater insight into the possible underlying cause of the failure to understand spoken language.

In conclusion, lesion-deficit studies using modern structural neuroimaging have been invaluable for characterizing the neuroanatomic correlates of aphasia and associated disorders. Not only has the localization of the classic aphasia syndromes been more accurately described, but the localization of more focal deficits affecting language production and comprehension has been identified. This information can be used to guide differential diagnosis and to make general predictions about the potential for certain language deficits to persist. It is important to recognize, however, that some exceptions to typical lesion-deficit correlations will be found.

Neuroanatomic Correlates of Aphasia Recovery

There is increasing pressure in the clinical setting to make evidence-based decisions of prognosis for recovery of language function. Fortunately, the lesion localization data just discussed can be used to inform such decisions. The role of lesion size and location has also been examined in aphasia recovery research.

Demeurisse and Capon (1987) found that lesion volume had a significant relationship to ultimate aphasia severity when damage affected *both* cortical and subcortical regions. Patients with large cortical/subcortical strokes had poorer outcomes. When damage was restricted to subcortex, however, aphasia outcome could not be predicted based on lesion volume. Others have had similar findings (Kertesz, Harlock, & Coates, 1979; Naeser, Helm-Estabrooks, Haas, Auerbach, & Srinivasan, 1987; Yarnell, Monroe, & Sobel, 1976;).

Overall, lesion location, not lesion size, has been shown to be a better predictor of aphasia recovery (Naeser and Palumbo, 1994). A number of critical lesion sites have been

identified that result in limited recovery of spontaneous speech. Knopman, Selnes, Nicccum, Rubens, Yock, and Larson (1983) discovered that persistent nonfluency was associated with damage to the left precentral gyrus and underlying white matter. Naeser, Palumbo, Helm-Estabrooks, Stiassny-Eder, and Albert (1989) examined the lesions of patients with either severely limited verbal output or those with nonfluent Broca's aphasia and agrammatic utterances. The patients with the most severe speech fluency deficit had lesions extending into two critical subcortical white matter pathways. The first is the medial subcallosal fasciculus (MSF), which is located in the lateral angle of the frontal horn deep to Broca's area. The MSF contains a pathway whereby fibers pass from the supplementary motor area (SMA) and the cingulate gyrus (BA 24) to the caudate nucleus. The second is the middle one third of the periventricular white matter (M 1/3 PVWM) near the body of the left lateral ventricle. The M 1/3 PVWM is found deep to the lower motor and sensory cortex areas of the mouth (**Fig. 3–17**). Damage to both regions in *combination* resulted in severe nonfluency due to disruption of pathways that facilitate speech initiation, motor execution, and sensory feedback (Naeser and Palumbo, 1994). Dronkers, Redfern, and Shapiro (1993) found that lesions severing the arcuate fasciculus dramatically reduced speech output to the level of recurrent stereotypies (e.g., "Well, well"; "You know, you know"). These studies and others show the importance of preserving specific subcortical white matter pathways for recovery of speech fluency (Ludlow, Rosenberg, Fair, Buck, Schesselman, & Salazar, 1986; Dronkers and colleagues, 2000).

The relationship between lesion site and recovery of auditory comprehension has been examined. Naeser et al. (1987) found that patients with Wernicke's aphasia had poor recovery of auditory comprehension when damage involved more than one half of Wernicke's area. It was also poor when damage extended beyond Wernicke's area into the middle temporal gyrus. A similar pattern was found in patients with global aphasia who had large cortical/subcortical lesions involving Wernicke's area (Naeser, Gaddie, Palumbo, and Stiassny-Eder, 1990). Dronkers, Wilkins, Van Valin, Redfern, and Jaeger (2004) found too that damage to the temporal lobe, specifically the middle temporal gyrus, greatly reduced recovery of auditory comprehension ability in patients with chronic aphasia.

Neuroanatomic Correlates and Prediction of Treatment Candidacy

Lesion localization data have been used to identify candidates for different treatment approaches. The lesion loci of patients with Broca's aphasia who make a good versus poor response to melodic intonation therapy (MIT) have been explored (Naeser, 1994; Naeser and Helm-Estabrooks, 1985). MIT is a program designed to improve verbal expression in patients with severe limitations of speech fluency by teaching them to produce phrases and sentences using continuous voicing and exaggerated intonation (Helm-Estabrooks & Albert, 1991). Patients found to benefit from MIT had lesions that spared critical white matter pathways (e.g., medial subcallosal fasciculus area and the middle third of the periventricular white matter), as well as more than half of Wernicke's area and the subcortical temporal isthmus (Naeser, 1994). The lesion locus of patients with global aphasia who make a good versus poor response to computed visual communication (C-VIC) has been

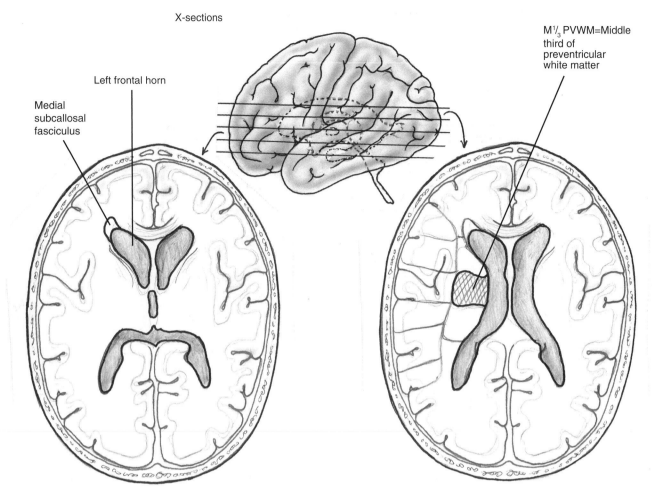

Figure 3–17 A diagrammatic representation of the two critical white matter areas for recovery of spontaneous speech (Naeser, 1994). The lesion must damage these two areas in *combination* for recovery to be poor: (1) The medial subcallosal fasciculus (MSF), which is located in the lateral angle of the frontal horn deep to Broca's area. It contains a pathway through which fibers pass from the supplementary motor area (SMA) and the cingulate gyrus (BA 24) to the caudate nucleus. (2) The middle one-third of the periventricular white matter (PVWM), which is near the body of the left lateral ventricle. It contains part of the motor/sensory pathways for the mouth. As a result of damage to these two specific areas, pathways are no longer available for speech initiation, motor execution, or sensory feedback.

examined. With C-VIC, patients who have no spontaneous speech or the ability to read or write or use pictures and icons on the computer to communicate. Patients who make a good response to this treatment approach had left hemisphere lesions that spared the SMA and cingulate gyrus, as well as Wernicke's area in the posterior temporal lobe or the subcortical temporal isthmus.

Lesion-Deficit Studies: Conclusions

The results from lesion-deficit studies combined with clinical expertise can inform the clinical decision-making process in terms of evaluation planning, determining candidacy for certain treatment approaches, and counseling patients and their families about the potential for language recovery. The challenge for clinicians is to obtain structural imaging information that demonstrates the true locus and extent of damage. Unfortunately, CT and MRI data are often obtained in the hyperacute phase of illness to rule out the presence of brain hemorrhage for the purposes of medical management. At this time point, the true lesion margins causing the language symptoms cannot be fully appreciated, and later

scans are not routinely obtained. With developments in MRI technology, specifically perfusion and diffusion weighted imaging, this problem is being resolved to some degree. The application of these techniques is discussed later. An additional challenge for clinicians is to have radiologists read imaging studies to the level of detail necessary to make accurate predictions. A better alternative is for speech–language pathologists to read brain scans with physicians for the purpose of identifying critical structures that might affect language as well as the potential for recovery (Kendall and Gonzalez-Rothi, 2001).

Cerebral Blood Flow and Metabolism: Baseline Studies

Functional imaging with SPECT, PET, DWI, or PWI has been used to examine abnormalities of CBF (perfusion) or metabolism while a patient is in a passive or "resting" state during imaging. These studies have shown that acquired language disorders result not only from direct structural damage, but also indirectly from loss of tissue integrity in regions where blood flow and brain metabolism have been compromised.

It is also clear that recovery of language occurs in part when brain function in undamaged regions is restored. This section reviews results from studies that show these findings.

Remote Effects of Structural Lesions

A major focus of resting studies has been to examine the consequences of a radiologically identifiable structural lesion on areas *not* seen to be directly damaged by neurologic insult. These studies have shown that structural damage causes abnormalities of brain metabolism and blood flow that extend beyond the site of lesion into distant *undamaged* regions of the brain (Kuhl, Phelps, Kowell, Metter, Selin, Winter, 1980). There are two primary mechanisms that explain how a region remote from direct damage may function abnormally.

The first occurs when structural damage in one brain region impairs the nerve impulses to a distant, but neuronally connected brain region(s). The undamaged region may no longer receive excitatory or inhibitory input from or through the area of damage and therefore no longer functions appropriately. This phenomenon is referred to as diaschisis (Feeney and Baron, 1986). Regression or reversal of diaschisis is thought to account for some early signs of recovery in aphasia (Pizzamiglio et al., 2001).

The second mechanism is when tissue or cellular functionality of a remote region is compromised by a reduction in blood flow. Studies have shown that similar structural lesions among patients can cause different behavioral consequences. For example, a solitary basal ganglion lesion seen in one patient may be associated with one cluster of language symptoms, whereas the same basal ganglion lesion in another patient may result in a different cluster of deficits. The theory of diaschisis does not explain this phenomenon well (Hillis, Barker, Wityk, Aldrich, Restrepo, Breese, & Work, 2004a). Functional imaging, however, has demonstrated that there are differences in blood flow and metabolism patterns in other areas of the brain among these patients. Brain tissue remote from the lesion may receive adequate blood flow to survive and avoid structural change, but may or may not receive enough to support behavioral function (Mies, Auer, Ebhardt, Traupe, & Heiss, 1983; Metter & Hanson, 1994; Barber, Darby, Desmond, Yang, Gerraty, Jolley, Donnan, Tress, & Davis, 1998; Hillis and colleagues, 2004a).

Blood flow and metabolism alterations in brain regions separate from the structural lesion may occur in distant sites as a result of a global or regional ischemia or may occur in areas adjacent to the structural lesion where there is enough blood flow from other vessels to prevent infarction or structural change. A major thrust of research has been to develop drug therapies and surgical or vascular interventions to treat the hypoperfused regions surrounding the lesion core, the so-called ischemic penumbra (Wise, 2003). Neurologic sequelae are reduced when perfusion can be restored promptly to these salvageable areas.

Neurophysiology of Aphasia: Positron Emission Tomography Studies

Metter and colleagues (Metter, 1987; Metter et al., 1981; Metter, Riege, Hanson, Kuhl, Phelps, Squire, Wasterlain, & Benson, 1983; Metter, Kempler, Jackson, Hanson, Mazziotta, & Phelps, 1989) have conducted a number of resting PET studies to explore the neuropathophysiology of aphasia. They have had several important findings:

1. Metabolic depression extends beyond the site of damage, suggesting that structurally undamaged tissue may be abnormal.

2. Hypometabolism occurs in the left temporoparietal cortex in essentially all adults with aphasia regardless of the locus of structural lesion.

3. The degree of hypometabolism in the left prefrontal cortex differentiates patients with Broca's, Wernicke's, and conduction aphasia. Patients with Broca's aphasia have the greatest abnormality, followed by patients with Wernicke's aphasia. No prefrontal abnormality occurs in patients with conduction aphasia.

4. Damage to subcortical regions including the internal capsule, basal ganglia, thalamus, and/or insula causes functional disruption to subcortical-cortical networks that support language processing.

5. The type of aphasia is more closely associated with the locus of physiologic abnormality than the locus of structural lesion.

Based on their studies, Metter and colleagues have argued for a two-compartment brain model of the neuropathophysiology of aphasia (see Metter and Hanson, 1994). Dysfunction in the temporoparietal cortex is essential for the development of language abnormalities in all aphasia types. What ultimately distinguishes the classic aphasia syndromes, however, is subcortical-frontal dysfunction. Damage to these language pathways causes different levels of impairment to speech fluency and other aspects of language expression.

Neurophysiology of Aphasia: Perfusion-Weighted and Diffusion-Weighted Imaging Studies

Hillis and colleagues (Hillis et al., 2001c; Hillis, Wityk, Barker, & Caramazza, 2003) have used the advanced MRI techniques of PWI and DWI to investigate the relationship between regions of dysfunctional tissue and language deficits in patients with acute (within 24 hours of onset) left hemisphere stroke. Very early after insult, PWI shows poorly perfused brain regions, whereas DWI shows densely ischemic brain regions that are likely to infarct. In combination, these techniques reveal structural damage as well as associated physiologic abnormality. Hillis and colleagues have used this information to make lesion-deficit correlations in the acute phase before any major brain reorganization or rehabilitation has taken place. This is in contrast to lesion-deficit studies, which make such correlations in patients with chronic damage. In these patients, lesions have stabilized, and the brain has likely undergone some form of structural and functional modification in response to injury.

Using PWI and DWI, Hillis et al. (2001c) examined the relationship between hypoperfusion, but not infarct, in Wernicke's area and single-word comprehension deficits. They studied 80 patients within 24 hours of onset of left hemisphere stroke. They found a significant relationship between the magnitude of delay in perfusion to Wernicke's area (left BA 22) and the rate of errors on a word comprehension test. In another study, Hillis, Kane, Tuffiash, Ulatowski, Barker, Beauchamp, and Wityk (2001b) used PWI and DWI to examine the relationship between neural dysfunction in Wernicke's area and the left inferior temporal lobe (BA 37), and performance on tests of single-word comprehension and naming. They studied six acute left hemisphere stroke patients with hypoperfusion in Wernicke's area, and one patient with additional hypoperfusion in BA 37. They hypothesized that reperfusion of dysfunctional brain tissue would lead to recovery of language. To restore perfusion, they administered an experimental medical therapy (e.g., medically induced blood pressure elevation), which successfully increased blood flow to Wernicke's area (BA 22) in five of the patients. As a result, their naming and comprehension deficits resolved. In the one patient with dysfunction in both Wernicke's area and BA 37, medical therapy restored blood flow to BA 37 but not Wernicke's area. As a result, she continued to have impaired single-word comprehension, but not naming deficits. Based on the pattern of results, the authors argued that Wernicke's area was critical for both single-word comprehension and production: specifically linking word forms with meaning or a lexical-semantic interface. They proposed that BA 37 was critical for word form retrieval during language production (e.g., phonologic output lexicon), but not for normal single-word comprehension. Though speculative, these results show the exciting applications of PWI and DWI to study brain–language relationships in patients with acute brain damage.

Hillis et al. (2002) studied the neural basis of aphasia following subcortical stroke. They proposed that subcortical aphasia results (1) directly by damaging subcortical structures that support language, (2) indirectly through disruption of subcortical-cortical networks (diaschisis), or (3) through associated cortical hypoperfusion. They examined 115 patients within 24 hours of symptom onset with DWI, PWI, and comprehensive language testing. Of those patients studied, 37 had damage restricted to the subcortical white matter, basal ganglia, or thalamus. Twenty-five (68%) had aphasia, and of those patients, all had associated cortical hypoperfusion in the perisylvian region of the left middle cerebral artery (MCA). Six patients with subcortical infarct and cortical hypoperfusion went on to receive medical therapy to restore cortical perfusion. As a result, they all had marked language gains with full recovery in most patients. Hillis and colleagues attributed the subcortical aphasia to associated cortical hypoperfusion, although disrupted cortical-subcortical connections or diaschisis may also have been the underlying cause of aphasia. This study did not rule out this latter possibility.

In a subsequent study, Hillis and colleagues (2004a) used PWI and DWI to examine a group of patients with a variety of fluent and nonfluent aphasias following acute left basal ganglia stroke. They argued that if diaschisis was the mechanism of aphasia, they should observe consistent language symptoms for similar lesions. For patients with lesions involving the basal ganglia, this was not found. In fact, a wide variety of language deficits or none at all were documented. Hillis and colleagues used this evidence to argue for the important role of cortical hypoperfusion in aphasia following left basal ganglia stroke. In support of this hypothesis, they found different degrees of cortical hypoperfusion measured with PWI in specific regions of the perisylvian cortex. They also demonstrated a strong relationship between the type of aphasia (e.g., Broca's, Wernicke's, conduction) and region of cortical hypoperfusion. Interestingly, regions of hypoperfusion and associated aphasia type were similar to those from lesion-deficit studies of classic aphasia syndromes.

Cerebral Blood Flow and Metabolism and Recovery of Aphasia: Baseline Studies

Baseline or resting studies of CBF and metabolism have advanced understanding of the neural mechanisms of language recovery. Two primary issues have been investigated. The first has been to determine whether early measurements of CBF and metabolism can be used to predict language outcome in patients with aphasia. The results have been mixed. The second has been to better understand the relationship between change in CBF or metabolism in brain regions ipsilateral or contralateral to a lesion and the level of aphasia recovery. In general, patients with a good recovery regain the functional integrity of the left hemisphere.

Karbe, Kessler, Herholz, Fink, and Heiss (1995) studied 22 patients with aphasia following left hemisphere stroke to determine if the degree of metabolic disturbance in language-relevant brain regions in the acute phase (3 weeks post-onset) could predict outcome of aphasia in the chronic phase of recovery (2 years post-onset) All patients underwent resting PET studies of regional cerebral metabolic rates of glucose (CMRGl) and had comprehensive neuropsychological testing, including the Token Test and a word fluency test (e.g., generating words beginning with the letters /f/, /a/, /s/) at the two time points. The authors found a significant relationship between acute measurements of metabolic abnormality in the left hemisphere and later performance on these specific language tests. Those with acute (3 weeks post-onset) metabolic abnormality in the left temporal lobe had a poorer performance on the Token Test at 2-years poststroke. Similarly, those with acute metabolic abnormality in the left prefrontal cortex had poorer performance on the test of word fluency 2 years poststroke. Therefore, early measurements of CMRGl predicted later recovery potential.

Not all studies have found that early measurements of brain function predict later recovery of language ability. Mimura, Kato, Kato, Sano, Kojima, Naeser, and Kashima (1998) conducted two different studies examining the relationship between aphasia recovery and CBF measured with SPECT early (within the first year) and late in the recovery process (approximately 7 years poststroke). In the first study, they examined 20 patients with aphasia following left hemisphere stroke at 3 and 9 months post-onset. At each time point, patients were administered the Japanese Standard Language Test of Aphasia (SLTA) and had SPECT scans. The most significant findings were that initial CBF measurements, left or right, did not predict level of language performance 9 months poststroke. However, language improvement was associated with increased perfusion (CBF) in the left hemisphere over time. Change in perfusion in the right hemisphere did not correspond with change in language performance over time. In the second study, they examined 16 aphasic patients with SPECT and the SLTA approximately 7 years poststroke. All patients had undergone prior language testing approximately 6 months post-onset. The authors found that patients with both good and poor recoveries had decreased perfusion levels in the damaged left hemisphere in this late recovery period. Patients with good recovery, however, had reestablished normal perfusion in the right hemisphere, particularly in the right frontal and thalamic areas, whereas patients in the poor recovery group had diminished right hemisphere CBF. The results confirm the importance of restoring left hemisphere brain function in tissue adjacent to the lesion for a good language recovery in the first year post-onset. Much later in the recovery process, good recovery was associated with restoration of perfusion in the right hemisphere.

Other studies have shown the importance of restoring brain function in the damaged left hemisphere, but restoring function in the right hemisphere earlier in the recovery period is important as well. Cappa, Perani, Grassi, Bressi, Alberoni, Franceschi, Bettinardi, Todde, and Fazio (1997) studied eight aphasic patients with resting PET and a battery of language tests at 2 weeks and 6 months post-onset of left hemisphere stroke. During the acute stage, they found hypometabolism in structurally undamaged regions of both the left and right hemispheres. At 6-month follow-up, regional glucose metabolism had increased in both hemispheres, with a particularly strong relationship between improved language performance and changes in glucose metabolism in the right hemisphere. They concluded that in the acute phase, patients with aphasia have bilateral depression of metabolism. With recovery, regression of metabolic depression or reversal of diaschisis in undamaged regions leads to restoration of language ability.

In summary, it is unclear whether early measurements of CBF and metabolism can be used to reliably predict language outcome. Further longitudinal study is needed. It is possible that a critical time period exists when early measurements have some predictive value (e.g., 3 weeks versus 3 months post-onset). The findings discussed, however, highlight the importance of restoring blood flow and metabolism in tissue adjacent to the lesion and remote from it to maximize recovery of language.

Cerebral Blood Flow and Metabolism: Conclusions

Many valuable insights into the nature of language deficits and mechanisms of recovery have been gained from baseline CBF and metabolisms studies. Unfortunately, in the clinical setting, patients with aphasia commonly do not undergo functional imaging to show the true extent of a structural lesion or the associated functional defect. Therefore, clinicians must make predictions about potential deficits and prognosis based on structural imaging data often gathered in the acute phase before the true extent of a lesion can be visualized. As PWI and DWI become more readily used in acute assessment of stroke, clinicians will be able to better appreciate the true locus and extent of brain damage. What can be gleaned from these studies is that in the acute phase, the language impairment seems much greater due to temporary disruption of cellular function and abnormalities of blood flow and metabolism. With recovery, there will be some reversal of diaschisis, reperfusion of ischemic tissue, and reactivation of viable neurons leading to less severe clinical deficits (Raymer, 2001). It is important to consider these variables when evaluating a patient in the acute phase and determining potential for aphasia recovery.

Functional Brain Activation Studies

This section highlights key findings from functional activation studies using PET and fMRI to show the utility of these techniques for developing new models of normal language processing, as well as for understanding neural mechanisms of language deficits and mechanisms of aphasia recovery.

Functional Imaging Studies of Normal Language Processing

Functional imaging studies of neurologically intact adults have focused on isolating and localizing specific subcomponents of language including phonetics, phonology, orthography, semantics, and syntax (Binder et al., 1997; Demonet, Chollet, Ramsay, Cardebat, Nespoulous, Wise, Rascol, Frackowiak, 1992; Kuperberg, Holcomb, Sitnikova, Greve, Dale, & Caplan, 2003; Petersen et al., 1988, 1990). From these efforts new models of the neural correlates of language and its subcomponents have been developed, which are much more detailed linguistically and anatomically than the classical model. These studies have shown that language is subserved by *networks* made up of many brain regions or "modules" that may include, but extend beyond, Broca's and Wernicke's areas into other sylvian and extrasylvian regions (Binder et al., 1997; Mesulam, 1990, 1998; Petersen et al., 1988). These neural regions are widely dispersed and each module "acts as a partial contributor rather than the purveyor of a whole complicated process" (A. Damasio, 1991, p. 27). Therefore, although Wernicke's area may participate in some aspect of language comprehension (e.g., decoding the speech signal), it is not the center for all of comprehension. Instead, the joint activation of multiple brain regions with relative specialization (e.g., orthographic, phonologic, semantic, syntactic) enables normal comprehension (Keller, Carpenter, & Just, 2001). It has also been shown that regions that support other cognitive processes, such as executive function and working memory, may be recruited depending on the complexity of the language task to be performed. The neural models developed from functional activation studies can be used to anticipate potential language deficits given a known lesion site. Additionally, because of their greater detail both linguistically and anatomically, they can be used to better delineate the locus of breakdown in the language-processing network (Kendall & Gonzalez Rothi, 2001; Raymer, 2001).

The neural correlates of normal single-word comprehension have been examined with functional imaging (Binder and colleagues, 1997, Demonet and colleagues, 1992). These studies have identified the functional anatomy of the component cognitive processes involved in comprehension of single words. These include extracting phonetic cues from the speech signal (phonetic processing), mapping that percept onto a lexical-phonologic representation (e.g., phonologic input lexicon), and then accessing an associated semantic representation (meaning or comprehension). Martin (2003), in a review of neuroimaging studies, identified the following neural correlates for single-word comprehension: (1) phonetic analysis to the *bilateral* superior temporal lobes; (2) lexical-phonologic representations to the left superior temporal lobe or superior temporal sulcus; and (3) semantic representations to widely distributed regions across the left middle and inferior temporal gyri, with some degree of right hemisphere participation. These three different systems have been referred to as the auditory "what" pathway that enables comprehension of words (e.g., mapping of speech onto meaning) (Hickok and Poeppel, 2004). For comprehension tasks that demand greater analysis or manipulation of semantic information, left inferior frontal and prefrontal regions were shown to participate. From a clinical perspective, this neural model of normal single-word comprehension can be used to make more specific predictions of the component processes disrupted in auditory

Table 3–11 Tasks Used in Functional Activation Studies of Single-Word Production

Tasks	Example
Picture naming (silent or overt)	Name color or black-and-white objects
Noun generation (silent or overt)	Name as many animals OR tools
Verb generation (silent or overt)	See or hear *ball* → "kick OR throw OR hit"
Word generation from a letter cue (silent or overt)	See or hear the letter *A* → "apple, ant, ark"
Word repetition (silent or overt)	Repeating a heard word
Word reading (silent or overt)	Reading words: strategy may vary from phonologically decoding word to using a whole word route

See Indefrey, P. & Levelt, W.J.M. (2000). The Neural Correlates of Language Production. In M.S. Gazzaniga (Ed.), *The New Cognitive Neurosciences*. Cambridge, MA: MIT Press.

comprehension. For example, patients with damage in the superior temporal gyrus may have a deficiency accessing phonologic word forms associated with a concept, whereas those with damage in the middle or inferior temporal gyrus may have impairment at the level of semantics. The ability of this model to inform diagnosis and treatment is obviously much greater than the classical model.

The neural correlates of single-word production have also been investigated with functional neuroimaging. Indefrey and Levelt (2003) completed a meta-analysis of 58 word production experiments that used different tasks and functional imaging techniques to create a model of single-word production. The benefit of doing a meta-analysis is that brain activation, which relates more to the specific task used or to some other aspect of experimental design (e.g., task difficulty or how long a subject was able to look at a stimulus), can be distinguished from brain activation related specifically to the component processes involved in single-word production. In these studies, a wide variety of tasks were used including verb generation, noun generation, picture naming, word reading, and word repetition (**Table 3–11**). Some of the production tasks were performed with overt vocalization, whereas others were performed covertly (e.g., thinking a response versus speaking it). Each task was analyzed for its component cognitive processes according to a psycholinguistic theory of single-word production (Levelt, Roelofs, and Meyer, 1999). The core processes identified were (1) activation of conceptual information (e.g., lexical-semantics), (2) phonologic word form retrieval (e.g., phonologic output lexicon), (3) phonologic encoding (e.g., delineation of appropriate syllabification and stress), and (4) phonetic encoding and articulation. Localization of these production processes was left lateralized and included (1) lexical-semantics to the left midsegment of the middle temporal gyrus; (2) phonologic word form retrieval to the left posterior superior and middle temporal gyri (Wernicke's area) and left thalamus; (3) phonologic encoding to the left posterior inferior frontal gyrus (Broca's area) and the midsuperior temporal gyrus (both these regions came close to criteria in the meta-analysis for acceptable levels of activation, but did not actually meet the criteria); and (4) overt articulation to the

primary motor and sensory areas bilaterally. Other regions activated during overt articulation included the left anterior superior temporal gyrus, the right SMA, and the left and medial cerebellum. Supplementary motor activation (left and right) was thought to reflect motor planning and imagination of articulation. This left-lateralized word production network was found to span across both posterior and frontal language regions and had some overlap with brain regions involved in single-word comprehension (e.g., middle temporal gyrus in lexical-semantics, superior temporal gyrus in phonologic word form retrieval). Again the clinical utility of this model can be appreciated when trying to determine the potential cause(s) of word production failure in a patient during naming or spontaneous output.

In summary, functional activation studies have advanced our understanding of the neural correlates of normal comprehension and production of single words. Unlike the classical model, brain–language correlations are based on neuroimaging of normal brain activity. Additionally, the analysis of language is based on cognitive processing models rather than behavioral descriptions of language such as auditory comprehension, speech fluency, or repetition. The neural correlates of normal language processing are especially helpful for predicting potential deficits in the subcomponents of language (e.g., phonologic input/output vs. semantics), which may facilitate planning for diagnostic evaluations and development of a treatment plan. As will be discussed later, knowledge of normal neural networks can help us to better understand how the brain reorganizes following injury both spontaneously and following treatment. The reader is referred to Martin (2003), Gernsbacher and Kaschek (2003), Small and Burton (2002), Wise (2003), and Indefrey and Levelt (2000) for more thorough discussions of neuroimaging of normal language processing.

Functional Activation Studies of Aphasia

Functional activation studies have been important for the investigation of not only normal language processing but also the neurophysiology of language deficits and mechanisms of aphasia recovery (Mayer, 2003). With PET and fMRI, it has become possible to visualize the neural networks that subserve language processing in the intact brain and then to compare how these networks change following brain damage (Buckner and Petersen, 2000). Functional MRI has been particularly well suited for single-case studies of patients with aphasia, given its high anatomic resolution in individual subjects and ability to image patients repeatedly over time.

Neural Bases of Language Deficits

An interesting avenue of study using activation paradigms has been to demonstrate abnormal patterns of brain activity in patients who make persistent language errors. Warburton, Price, Swinburn, and Wise (1999) studied six patients with chronic aphasia during a verb generation task (e.g., producing verbs associated with auditory noun cues, such as "apple"—"slice, eat, peel, wash"). Brain activity of the patient group was measured with PET and compared to activity in a normal control group. Both groups showed a pattern of left lateralized activation in the inferior temporal, frontal, and prefrontal cortices. A smaller degree of right hemisphere activation in these regions was also found. A slightly different pattern was noted, however, in one patient who performed more poorly on the task. He activated the same regions as the normal control group, with one exception. He failed to activate the left prefrontal cortex, a region that was structurally intact. Poorer performance on the task was thought to reflect the combined effect of structural damage in the parietotemporal region as well as the lack of activation in left prefrontal cortex attributed to diaschisis. The authors went on to hypothesize that behavioral therapy could focus on reestablishing brain activity in the undamaged prefrontal region, which in turn might foster recovery of potentially viable neurons surrounding the site of damage. Obviously, further investigation is needed to test their hypothesis.

Price, Warburton, Moore, Frackowiak, and Friston (2001) in a PET study also found evidence of abnormal brain activity in undamaged regions suggestive of diaschisis. They compared patterns of brain activation in four patients with aphasia who had damage in classic Broca's area to the normal pattern. All participants performed a "feature detection" task on visually presented letter strings or words. They indicated with a key-press if letters contained a vertical feature that ascended above the main body of the letter ("b, d, f, h" would get a "yes" response, whereas "n, o, p, q" would get a "no" response). The feature detection task stayed constant, but the target stimulus was either a string of consonants or a word. Normal participants activated a left lateralized network that included the posterior inferior frontal (pIFG), posterior middle temporal (pMTG), and the posterior inferior temporal gyri (pITG). In contrast, patients with aphasia activated the left middle temporal gyrus, but did not, as might be expected, activate the damaged left IFG. Of further interest was that they failed to activate the undamaged pITG. Instead, there was a decrease in activation of the pITG during decisions made on words. The authors concluded the aberrant response in the left pITG occurred when the demands on the damaged left IFG increased. As a result, the pITG did not receive adequate input from the damaged IFG, and the function of that region was compromised. This phenomenon was termed *dynamic diaschisis* to explain how a usually viable cortical region responds abnormally due to dependence on and interaction with a damaged region. The authors went on to hypothesize that the same undamaged region might respond normally under another cognitive or sensorimotor condition, if interaction with the damaged region was not required.

The context-sensitive nature of diaschisis was demonstrated in a follow-up study with one patient who performed a subsequent semantic similarity task on words (e.g., determining which of two words were semantically related to a target word). It was hypothesized the left pITG would activate normally during the semantic task, but not the feature detection task. The findings supported this hypothesis. The single patient activated the left pITG during the semantic task like the normal participants, but not during the feature detection task. The authors went on to highlight the potential importance of developing specific strategies to reactivate undamaged regions affected by dynamic diaschisis during speech–language therapy. A reversal of diaschisis or the reestablishment of connections between brain regions that support language processing has been hypothesized before as an important mechanism of aphasia recovery (Zahn, Drews, Specht, Kemeny, Reith, Willmes, Schwarz, & Huber, 2004). As models of the neural anatomy and connectivity of language processes become better established through PET and fMRI activation studies and other techniques to map human cortex, such therapeutic approaches will be an exciting avenue to investigate.

Functional Activation Studies of Aphasia Recovery

Over time, most patients with aphasia experience some degree of recovery of language function despite persistent damage to left hemisphere language regions (Thompson, 2000a,b). In the early phase of recovery, language improvement has been attributed to a regression of diaschisis or the reestablishment of connections between undamaged regions that have been temporarily deactivated following injury (Pizzamiglio et al., 2001). Functional imaging studies at rest and during task performance have both demonstrated the importance of restoring brain function in undamaged regions in both the left and right hemispheres (Cappa et al., 1997). In the later or more chronic phases of recovery, language improvement is thought to result from a reorganization of the large-scale neural networks that support language function. (Thompson, 2000a,b; Zahn, Huber, Drews, Specht, Kemeny, Reith, Willmes, & Schwarz, 2002; Zahn et al., 2004.) With reorganization, undamaged regions of the brain compensate for damaged regions to foster language recovery. Three primary mechanisms have been proposed (Wise, 2003). The first is that there is a restitution of undamaged regions in the left hemisphere, particularly at the edge of a lesion. According to this hypothesis, recovery occurs because of redundancy within the neural system, whereby, unimpaired neurons that can normally support the behavior are recruited. The second mechanism of recovery assumes that there is a shift of language function to homologous regions in the right hemisphere that have latent language function. The third mechanism of recovery is that patients adopt a different cognitive strategy to bypass the damaged language network. The use of the alternative strategy enables patients with aphasia to achieve similar language performance as normal individuals simply by a different means (Marshall, 1984). There is evidence from functional activation studies to demonstrate that one or all three of the mechanisms occur during aphasia recovery.

The importance of restoring left hemisphere language regions has been demonstrated in a number of studies (Calvert, Brammer, Morris, Williams, King &, Matthews, 2000; Cao et al., 1999; Heiss, Kessler, Thiel, Ghaemi, & Karbe, 1999; Knopman, Rubens, Selnes, Klassen, & Meyer, 1984; Rosen, Petersen, Linenweber, Snyder, White, Chapman, Dromerick, Fiez, & Corbetta, 2000; Warburton and colleagues, 1999). Heiss et al. (1999) found in a PET activation study that restitution of left temporal regions corresponded with a good recovery. They studied 23 patients with anterior lesions (frontal and subcortical) and temporal lesions during rest and a word repetition task (repeating nouns) at 2 weeks and 8 weeks poststroke. Neurologically intact adults had increased activation in left frontal regions and bilateral activation in posterior superior temporal regions. The patients with anterior damage who had a good recovery (as measured by Token Test performance), had activation in the right IFG and right superior temporal gyrus (STG) at 2 weeks. By 8 weeks these patients no longer had significant right IFG activation, but had regained activation in the left STG. The temporal group who had a poorer recovery activated left Broca's area and the SMA at 2 weeks. By 8 weeks, the patients with temporal lobe damage activated

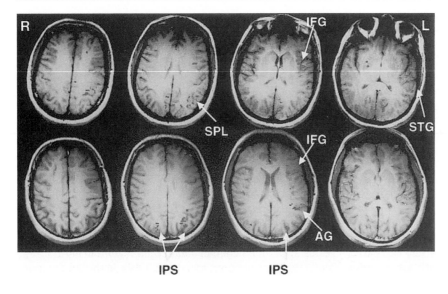

Figure 3–18 Functional MRI activation patterns observed in normal subjects during silent picture naming (top row images) and silent verb generation (bottom row images). Two cortical regions in the left hemisphere: inferior frontal lobe (IFL) and inferior parietal-superior temporal lobes (IPS) were markedly activated during picture naming. Activation was also observed in the left insula, bilateral occipital lobe, and left primary sensorimotor cortex. During verb generation, three cortical regions in the left hemisphere (IFL, IPS, and the banks of the intraparietal sulcus-IPS) were activated to a large degree. To a smaller extent, the right hemisphere homologues activated. [From Cao, Y., Vikingstad, E.M., George, K.P., Johnson, A.F., & Welch, K.M.A. (1999). Cortical Language Activation in Stroke Patients Recovering from Aphasia with Functional MRI. *Stroke, 30,* 2331–2340, with permission.]

the precentral gyrus bilaterally and the right STG. They did not regain activation of the left STG. It was concluded that the right hemisphere was recruited when the homologous left hemisphere regions were damaged; however, good recovery occurred when left hemisphere temporal regions could be reintegrated into the language network.

A number of investigations have shown that activation of both undamaged regions in the left hemisphere as well as the right contribute to aphasia recovery (Cao and colleagues, 1999; Heiss and colleagues, 1999; Karbe, Thiel, Weber-Luxenburger, Herholz, Kessler, & Weiss, 1998; Perani, Cappa, Tettamanti, Rosa, Scifo, Miozzo, Basso, & Fazio, 2003; Weiller, Isensee, Rijntjes, Huber, Muller, Bier, Dutschka, Woods, Noth, & Diener, 1995; Zahn et al., 2004). Weiller and colleagues (1995) in a PET activation study examined rCBF in six patients with a partial recovery from Wernicke's aphasia and six normal controls during nonword repetition and verb generation. The primary finding was that patients with aphasia had increased rCBF in right hemisphere homologues of Broca's and Wernicke's areas, whereas normal participants had prominent left lateralized rCBF in these areas. The patients also had greater rCBF volumes in left frontal and prefrontal regions compared to normal controls. The authors concluded that partial recovery of Wernicke's aphasia resulted from a redistribution of language function to a preexisting network that involved both the left and right hemispheres.

Cao and colleagues (1999) in an fMRI-BOLD study demonstrated that *combined* activation of undamaged regions in

the left hemisphere and compensatory activation of regions in the right hemisphere contributed to aphasia recovery. They studied seven patients with relatively good recovery of aphasia and normal controls during performance of covert picture naming and verb generation (e.g., thinking *"kick"* when shown the word *ball*). Normal controls activated a left dominant network in the inferior frontal lobe (IFL) (i.e., inferior frontal gyrus, middle frontal gyrus), and the inferior parietal-superior temporal lobes (IPSTL). A smaller extent of activation in right hemisphere homologues was also found (**Fig. 3–18**). In comparison, patients with aphasia activated a bilateral network with significant increases in right hemisphere activation (IFL and IPSTL), and associated nonsignificant decreases in left hemisphere activation (IFL and IPSTL) for both paradigms. For picture naming, right frontal and posterior activation increased, whereas for verb generation only right posterior activation increased. Patients with better naming performance (as measured outside the scanner) had bilateral activation in the IFL, whereas those with poorer performance (but still relatively good recovery of naming) had right dominant IFL activation. This study is of particular importance because it demonstrates that patients who experienced better recovery of language, specifically naming ability, engaged a bilateral network of brain regions rather than a right dominant network. Although a right dominant network was capable of supporting recovery of naming ability, recovery was not as great as when a bilateral network was engaged (**Figs. 3–19** and **3–20**).

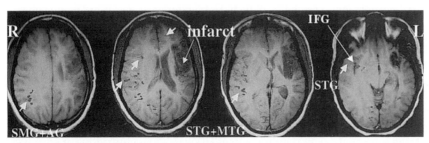

Figure 3–19 Functional MRI activation obtained from a single patient with poorer recovery of naming ability during picture naming. The patient had a large left frontotemporoparietal infarct with extension to the basal ganglia resulting in global aphasia. With recovery, the patient's aphasia evolved to an anomic profile, but she continued to have naming deficits. Activation was almost exclusively in the right hemisphere (comprising 92% of all cortical activity). Right hemisphere activation was observed in the supramarginal gyrus (SMG), angular gyrus (AG), inferior frontal gyrus (IFG) and middle frontal gyrus (MFG), the insula, and the superior temporal gyrus (STG). The left hemisphere was markedly void of activity; activation was found only in the left MFG and left STG. [From Cao, Y., Vikingstad, E.M., George, K.P., Johnson, A.F., & Welch, K.M.A. (1999). Cortical Language Activation in Stroke Patients Recovering from Aphasia with Functional MRI. *Stroke, 30,* 2331–2340, with permission.]

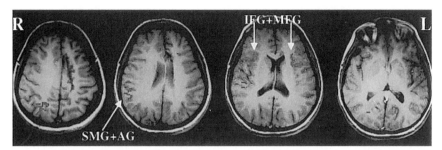

Figure 3–20 Functional MRI activation obtained from a single patient with a good recovery of naming ability during verb generation. The patient had a left anterior superior frontal infarct resulting in an acute transcortical motor aphasia. With recovery, the patient's aphasia evolved to an anomic profile. Activation was bilaterally represented in the frontal lobe (inferior and middle frontal gyri), and right dominant in the supramarginal gyrus (SMG) and angular gyrus (AG), superior temporal gyrus (STG), and the intraparietal sulcus. These right hemisphere regions mirrored left hemisphere activation found in normal controls. The patient also exhibited left hemisphere activation in the superior temporal gyrus. Bilateral activation in the right hemisphere corresponded with a better recovery of naming ability. Of further interest was that the left SMG, a structurally intact region commonly activated in normal subjects, failed to activate. This lack of activation may reflect diastases. [From Cao, Y., Vikingstad, E.M., George, K.P., Johnson, A.F., & Welch, K.M.A. (1999). Cortical Language Activation in Stroke Patients Recovering from Aphasia with Functional MRI. *Stroke, 30*, 2331–2340, with permission.]

The compensatory potential of the right hemisphere to support language recovery has been shown in other studies. Thulborn, Carpenter, and Just (1999) in a longitudinal fMRI study examined brain activation in two patients with good recovery of aphasia and six normal controls during sentence comprehension. Normal controls activated a left lateralized network predominantly in Broca's and Wernicke's areas. In contrast, the patients showed a shift in activation away from the areas of damage in the left hemisphere to their right hemisphere homologues. This left-to-right shift increased over the recovery time period. The first patient had a dense expressive aphasia, which resolved in the acute phase following medical therapy. Functional MRI at 3 days and 6 months post-onset showed strong right dominance in Broca's area, with left dominance in Wernicke's area during the sentence comprehension task. The second patient had chronic epilepsy and had a stroke immediately following surgery to resect the epileptic focus. He developed a dense Wernicke's aphasia that improved over time to enable his return to work. As a patient being surgically treated for epilepsy, prestroke fMRI data were fortuitously available for comparison. From the time of the pre-event fMRI, lateralization during sentence comprehension shifted from strong left dominance in Wernicke's area to weak right dominance after 3 months and right dominance by 9 months. Lateralization in Broca's area shifted from weak right dominance in Broca's area before the stroke, to weak left dominance by 9 months. The authors argued that language recovery was associated with a redistribution of workload over an existing large-scale language network, which continued to change over many months following injury. The finding that normal controls had activation in both the left and right hemispheres suggests that new areas were not adopted, but rather redundant neurons in the language network were activated to maintain language function.

A shift in activation from the left to the right hemisphere has not always been found to correspond with a favorable recovery of language, however. Rosen et al. (2000) used fMRI and PET to study the reorganization of neural networks in patients with chronic left inferior frontal infarcts. They used a word stem completion task (e.g., shown *COU*, patient generates "COUple"), which is known to place demands on the left IFG. The authors found an absence of activation in the left IFG and increased activation in the right IFG. The increased right IFG activation, however, did not correspond with greater accuracy on the word-stem completion task. The authors entertained the possibility that right hemisphere activation may indicate participants adopted a different processing strategy to perform the task (e.g., generating words based on their spelling versus how they sound). The finding that right IFG activation and word stem completion did not correlate, however, implies that another strategy was not adopted. Rather, the authors interpreted increased right IFG activation as a maladaptive response due to abnormal loss of inhibitory control of the left IFG over the right IFG. Of further interest was that patients with the best performance on the word-stem completion task and the best recovery of aphasia had increased activation in perilesional tissue in the left IFG. As found in many of the other studies, extension of language function into perilesional tissue or reactivation of still viable neurons in the left hemisphere has been the most effective mechanism of recovery.

Another possible neurologic mechanism of recovery is that an individual with aphasia adopts a different cognitive strategy to maintain language performance and thereby bypasses a damaged language network. The use of a different strategy was demonstrated in a fMRI study of a 28-year-old woman with partial recovery of aphasia following a left frontal ischemic stroke (Calvert et al., 2000). Brain activation was measured during performance of a verbal semantic decision task (e.g., determining if a word belonged to the category of living or nonliving things) and a nonword rhyme decision task (e.g., "flait and klate"). Of significance during the semantic decision task, the patient showed much greater activation of extrastriate visual cortex bilaterally than the control group. This increased activation was attributed to the patient's placing greater demands on visual processing to make semantic decisions, rather than a transfer of linguistic function to visual processing areas. Activation during the rhyming task was left lateralized in posterior and frontal brain regions in the control group. In contrast, the patient activated the right inferior frontal gyrus, the region homologous to the infarct, as well as perilesional tissue in the left hemisphere inferior to Broca's area. This study confirms the presence of all three mechanisms of recovery: (1) recruitment of perilesional tissue in the left hemisphere; (2) compensation by the right inferior frontal lobe, the region homologous to the site of injury; and (3) adoption of a novel processing strategy to perform the task.

Functional Activation Studies of Speech–Language Therapy

Another exciting application of functional neuroimaging is to identify how patterns of language reorganization can be influenced by treatment (Thompson, 2000). Belin, Van Eeckhout, Zilbovicius, Remy, Francoois, Guillaume, Chain, Rancurel, and

Samson (1996) measured relative CBF with PET to examine changes in brain activation in seven nonfluent aphasic patients following successful treatment with melodic intonation therapy (MIT). MIT is a well-established treatment program used to facilitate speech production in patients with persistent nonfluency (Albert, Sparks, and Helm, 1973). With MIT, patients learn to speak with simplified and exaggerated prosody that emphasizes both the melody (two notes, high and low) and rhythm (two durations, long and short) of words and phrases. The authors contrasted patterns of brain activity in patients with chronic, severe nonfluent aphasia during four different tasks: (1) rest, (2) hearing words read with natural intonation, (3) repetition of single words with natural intonation, and (4) repetition of single words with MIT-like intonation. Unfortunately, a normal control group was not used for comparison. It was hypothesized that different patterns of brain activation would be seen during normal production, which would reflect a residual deficit-related state, whereas activation during MIT-like production would reflect a recovery-related state. Aphasic patients' performance on both repetition tasks was variable, but more MIT words were produced accurately than without MIT. The authors found that passive listening to words (hearing words) and word repetition without MIT resulted in abnormal activation of *right* hemisphere regions homologous to normal left hemisphere language regions. Additionally, during the word repetition task without MIT, a decrease in activation in left Broca's area was also observed compared to passively listening to words. A different pattern of brain activation was found for MIT repeated words compared to repetition without MIT. MIT-like word repetition resulted in *left* hemisphere activation in Broca's area and the adjacent left prefrontal cortex, and a decrease in activation in the right homologue of Wernicke's area. The authors argued that right hemisphere activation was related to persistence of aphasia and not to functional recovery of aphasia. This study also shows how language therapy can be used to reactivate disrupted left-hemisphere language regions.

Small et al. (1998) demonstrated how retraining letter to sound correspondences in a patient with phonologic dyslexia resulted in a reorganization of the network that supports sentence level reading. Patients with phonologic dyslexia have an inability to phonologically decode words and therefore rely on a whole-word route when reading. Treatment for this patient involved learning letter-to-sound correspondences to facilitate reading of words and nonwords. Brain activation was measured during performance of a sentence level reading task (e.g., modified version of the Token Test; De Renzi & Vignolo, 1962; McNeil & Prescott, 1978). Prior to treatment, the primary locus of activation was in the left angular gyrus (BA 39), a region known to support recognition of word forms. Following treatment, activation decreased in the left angular gyrus and there was an increase in activation in the left lingual gyrus (BA 18). The lingual gyrus overlaps with visual processing regions that support the decomposition of written words (e.g., phonologic decoding) (Petersen, et al., 1988, 1990). The results from this study provide clear evidence of a change in brain activity through the adoption of a different cognitive strategy (reading by letter-to-sound correspondences, not a whole-word route) to restore sentence level reading.

Thompson, Gitleman, and Fix (see Thompson, 2000b) used fMRI to measure and observe changes in functional anatomy in a 52-year-old right-handed man with chronic agrammatic aphasia. The patient participated in an intensive 32-week course of linguistic-specific therapy to improve syntactic comprehension. Prior to treatment, fMRI activation studies of auditory sentence comprehension (i.e., sentence picture matching) compared to a control task of single-word reading showed significant activation in the right homologue of Wernicke's area (BA 22) and the dorsolateral prefrontal cortex (BA 46). Following treatment, increased activation was observed in right hemisphere homologous areas in and around Wernicke's area (BA 22, 21, and 37), as well as in Broca's area (BA 44 and 45). These changes in functional anatomy corresponded with improvements in sentence comprehension. This study provides support for the compensatory role of the right hemisphere to enhance language performance.

Functional activation studies can be applied in a number of ways to test the benefits of speech–language therapy. One important avenue of investigation will be to examine the potential of therapy to reactivate remote brain regions that have been functionally disconnected by distant structural damage. Another will be to understand whether therapy to stimulate a behavior enhances neurologic reorganization better than therapy that teaches the use of strategies to circumvent a damaged network (Thompson, 2000a). It will also be critical to study how combined drug and behavioral interventions affect neural reorganization.

✦ Conclusion

Neuroimaging has been invaluable to the study of acquired language disorders. Lesion-deficit studies using CT and conventional MRI have been used to localize lesions in aphasia and to identify brain regions that are critical for performance of particular language functions. Resting studies with PET, SPECT, DWI, and PWI have been instrumental in showing the remote effects of structural damage and given insights into the neurophysiologic mechanisms of aphasia recovery. Of great interest in recent years have been PET and fMRI activation studies, which have led to new insights into the organization of normal language processing. From these investigations, neural models of language processing have been developed that are much more detailed, both linguistically and anatomically, than the classical model of Broca, Wernicke, Lichtheim, and Geschwind. More than ever before, functional neuroimaging has helped to elucidate the neural mechanisms of aphasia recovery. We have now been able to see that regression of diaschisis, reperfusion of ischemic tissue, and reactivation of viable neurons all lead to improved language function. The importance of restoring function in the left hemisphere is clear, whereas the exact role of the right hemisphere in recovery remains to be elucidated. It is also evident that speech–language intervention fosters visible change at the neural level. This information has many applications to clinical care of patients with aphasia from diagnosis to prediction of recovery.

In the future, it will be exciting to use functional activation studies to examine brain plasticity and test the effectiveness of different speech–language interventions. The neurologic mechanisms of learning and restitution of language function have yet to be fully understood. Although activation studies hold promise, it is still a challenge to develop activation paradigms to isolate the processes of interest and make accurate interpretations of the significance of brain activity. There is still much work to be done both with behavioral and neuroimaging studies.

Study Questions

1. Mr. S. is a 60-year-old man with new onset of fluent paraphasic speech output and poor comprehension. MRI results show a large left temporoparietal stroke. What other information from MRI would be helpful? What are the potential speech and language deficits? What decisions about prognosis can be made? What information can be shared with the family about the neural mechanisms of recovery in the acute compared to the chronic phase of stroke?

2. Mrs. T. is a 75-year-old woman with nonfluent aphasia following a large frontal-subcortical stroke 6 months ago.

What potential deficits does this patient have? What information do you want to gain from structural neuroimaging? What is the prognosis for recovery of speech fluency? What information can be shared with the family to develop realistic expectations and goals for Mrs. T?

3. Mr. V. is a 65-year-old man with a 1-year history of progressive word-finding difficulty. You notice a number of phonologic errors in his spontaneous speech during the initial interview. CT and MRI are normal. What other neuroimaging studies would be beneficial? Where do you predict the locus of neural dysfunction might be?

References

Albert, M.L., Bachman, D.L., Morgan, A., & Helm-Estabrooks, N. (1988). Pharmacotherapy for Aphasia. *Neurology, 38,* 877–879

Albert M.L., Sparks, R.W., & Helm, N.A. (1973). Melodic Intonation Therapy for Aphasia. *Archives of Neurology, 29,* 130–131

Alexander, M.P., Naeser, M.A., & Palumbo, C. (1990). Broca's Area Aphasias: Aphasia After Lesions Including the Frontal Operculum. *Neurology, 40,* 353–362

Anderson, J.M., Gilmore, R., Roper S., Crosson B., Bauer, R.M., Nadeau S., Beversdorf D.Q., Cibula J., Rogish M. 3rd, Kortencamp S., Hughes J.D., Gonzalez Rothi, L.J., & Heilman, K.M. (1999). Conduction Aphasia and the Arcuate Fasciculus: A Reexamination of the Wernicke' Geschwind Model. *Brain and Language, 70,* 1–12

Barber, P.A., Darby, D.G., Desmond, PM., Yang, Q., Gerraty, R.P., Jolley, D., Donnan, G.A., Tress, B.M., & Davis, S.M. (1998). Prediction of Stroke Outcome with Echoplanar Perfusion- and Diffusion-Weighted MRI. *Neurology, 51,* 418–426

Basso, A., Lecours, A., Moraschini, S., & Vanier, M. (1985). Anatomoclinical Correlations of the Aphasias as Defined Through Computerized Tomography: Exceptions. *Brain and Language, 26,* 201–229

Belin, P., Van Eeckhout, P, Zilbovicius, M., Remy P., Francoois, C., Guillaume, S., Chain F., Rancurel, G., & Samson Y. (1996). Recovery from Nonfluent Aphasia after Melodic Intonation Therapy: A PET Study. *Neurology, 47,* 1504–1511

Belliveau J.W., Kennedy D.N., McKinstry C., Buchbinder, B.R., Weisskoff, R.M., Cohen, M.S., Vevea, J.M., Brady, T.J., & Rosen, B.R. (1991). Functional Mapping of the Human Visual Cortex by Magnetic Resonance Imaging. *Science, 254,* 716–719

Benton, A. (1991). Aphasia: Historical Perspectives. In: M.T. Sarno (Ed.), *Acquired Aphasia,* 2nd ed. (pp. 1–26). San Diego: Academic Press

Binder, J.R. (2000). The New Neuroanatomy of Speech Perception. *Brain, 123, (12),* 2371–2372

Binder, J.R., Frost, J.A., Hammeke, T.A., Cox, R.W., Rao, S.M., & Prieto, T. (1997). Human Brain Language Areas Identified by Functional Magnetic Resonance Imaging. *Journal of Neuroscience, 17,* 353–362

Binder, J.R., Swanson, S.J., Hammeke, T.A., Morris, G.L., Mueller, W.M., Fischer, M., Benbadis, S., Frost, J.A., Rao, S.M., & Haughton, V.M. (1996). Determination of Language Dominance Using Functional MRI: A Comparison with the WADA Test. *Neurology, 46,* 978–984

Blumstein, S.E., Baker, E., & Goodglass, H. (1977). Phonological Factors in Auditory Comprehension in Aphasia. *Neuropsychologia, 15,* 19–30

Boatman, D., Gordon, B., Hart, J., Selnes, O., Miglioretti, D., & Lenz, F. (2000). Transcortical Sensory Aphasia: Revisited and Revised, *Brain, 123,* 1634–1642

Bonne, O., Gilboa, A., Louzoun, Y., Kempf-Sherf, O., Katz, M., Fishman, Y., Ben-Nahum Z., Drausz, Y., Bocher, M., Lester, H., Chisin, R., & Lerer, B. (2003). Cerebral Blood Flow in Chronic Symptomatic Mild Traumatic Brain Injury. *Psychiatry Research, 124,* 141–152

Bookheimer, S.Y., Strojwas, M.H., Cohen, M.S., Saunders, A.M., Pericak-Vanc, M.A., Mazziotta, J.C., & Small, G.W. (2000). Patterns of Brain Activation in People at Risk for Alzheimer's Disease. *New England Journal of Medicine, 343,* 450–456

Broca, P. (1861). Remarques sur le siege de la faculte du langage articule, suivies d'une observation d'aphemie. *Bulletin de la Societe d'Anatomie (Paris), 2,* 330–357

Broca, P. (1863). Localisation des Functions Cerebrales: Siege du Langage Articule. *Bulletin de la Societe d'Anthropologie, 4,* 200–203

Broca, P. (1865). Du Siege de la Faculte du Langage Articule. *Bulleltin de la Societe d'Anthropologie, 6,* 337–393

Buckner, R.L. & Petersen, S.E. (2000). *Neuroimaging of Functional Recovery.* In H.S. Levin & J. Grafman (Eds.), Cerebral Reorganization of Function After Brain Damage (pp. 318–329). New York: Oxford University Press

Calvert, G.A., Brammer, M.J., Morris, R.G., Williams, S.C.R., King, N., & Matthews, P.M. (2000). Using fMRI to Study Recovery from Acquired Dysphasia. *Brain and Language, 71,* 391–399

Cao, Y., D'Olhaberriague, L., Vikingstad, E.M., Levine, S.R., & Welch, K.M. (1998). Pilot Study of Functional MRI to Assess Cerebral Activation of Motor Function after Poststroke Hemiparesis. *Stroke, 29,* 112–22

Cao Y., Vikingstad E.M., George K.P., Johnson, A.J., & Welch K.M.A. (1999). Cortical Language Activation in Stroke Patients Recovering from Aphasia with Functional MRI. *Stroke, 30,* 2331–2340

Cao, Y., Vikingstad, E.M., Huttenlocher, P.R., Towle, V.L., & Levin, D.N. (1994). Functional Magnetic Resonance Studies of the Reorganization of the Human Hand Sensorimotor Area After Unilateral Brain Injury in the Perinatal Period. *Proceedings of the National Academy of Sciences U.S.A., 91,* 9612–9616

Cappa, S.F., Perani, D., Grassi, F., Bressi, S., Alberoni, M., Franceschi, M., Bettinardi, V., Todde, S., & Fazio, F. (1997). A PET Follow-Up Study of Recovery After Stroke in Acute Aphasics. *Brain and Language, 56,* 55–67

Cappa S.F., & Vignolo, L.A. (1983). CT Scan Studies of Aphasia. *Human Neurobiology, 2(3),* 129–134

Damasio, A. (1991). Neuroanatomical Correlates of the Aphasias. In M.T. Sarno (Ed.), *Acquired Aphasia,* 2nd ed. (pp. 27–43). San Diego: Academic Press

Damasio, A.R., Damasio, H., Rizzo, M., Varney, N., & Gersh, F. (1982). Aphasia with Nonhemorrhagic Lesions in the Basal Ganglia and Internal Capsule. *Archives of Neurology, 39,* 15–24

Damasio, A.R. & Geschwind N. (1984). The Neural Basis of Language. *Annual Review of Neuroscience, 7,* 127–147

Damasio, H. (1991). Neuroanatomical Correlates of the Aphasias. In M.T. Sarno (Ed.), *Acquired Aphasia,* 2nd ed. (pp. 45–71). San Diego: Academic Press

Damasio, H., & Damasio, A.R. (1989). *Lesion Analysis in Neuropsychology.* New York: Oxford University Press

Damasio, H., Tranel, D., Grabowski, T., Adolphs, R., & Damasio, A. (2004). Neural Systems Behind Word and Concept Retrieval. *Cognition, 92,* 179–229

Demeurisse, G., & Capon, A. (1987). Language Recovery in Aphasic Stroke Patients: Clinical, CT and CBF Studies. *Aphasiology, 1,* 301–315

Demonet, J.F., Chollet, F., Ramsay, S., Cardebat, D., Nespoulous, J.L., Wise, R. Rascol, A., & Frackowiak, R. (1992). The anatomy of phonological and semantic processing in normal subjects. *Brain, 115,* 1753–1768

De Renzi, E., & Vignolo, L.A. (1962). The token test: a sensitive test to detect receptive disturbances in aphasics. *Brain, 85,* 665–678

Dronkers, N.F. (1996). A New Brain Region for Coordinating Speech Articulation. *Nature, 384,* 159–161

Dronkers, N.F. (2000). The Pursuit of Brain-Language Relationships. *Brain and Language, 71,* 59–61

Dronkers, N.F., Redfern, B.B., & Knight, R.T. (2000). The Neural Architecture of Language Disorders. In M.S. Gazzaniga (Ed.), *The New Cognitive Neurosciences* (pp. 949–958). Cambridge, MA: MIT Press

Dronkers, N.F., Redfern, B.B., & Ludy, C. (1995). Lesion Localization in Chronic Wernicke's Aphasia. *Brain and Language, 51,* 62–65

Dronkers, N.F., Redfern, B.B., Ludy, C., & Baldo, J. (1998). Brain Regions Associated with Conduction Aphasia and Echoic Rehearsal. *Journal of the International Neuropsychological Society, 4,* 23–24

Dronkers, N.F., Redfern, B., & Shapiro, J.K. (1993). Neuroanatomic correlates of production deficits in severe Broca's aphasia. *Journal of Clinical and Experimental Neuropsychology, 15(1),* 59–60

Dronkers, N.F., Shapiro, J.K., Redfern B., & Knight, R.T. (1992). The role of Broca's area in Broca's Aphasia. *Journal of Clinical and Experimental Neuropsychology, 14,* 52–53

Dronkers, N.F., Wilkins, D.P., Van Valin, R.D., Redfern, B.B., & Jaeger, J.J. (1994). A Reconsideration of the Brain Areas involved in the Disruption of Morphosyntactic Comprehension. *Brain and Language, 47,* 461–463

Dronkers, N.F., Wilkins, D.P., Van Valin, R.D., Redfern, B.B., Jaeger, J.J. (2004). Lesion Analysis of the Brain Areas Involved in Language Comprehension. *Cognition, 92,* 145–177

Feeney, D.M. & Baron, J.C. (1986). Diaschisis. *Stroke, 17,* 817–830

Freedman, M., Alexander M.P., & Naeser, M.A. (1984). Anatomic Basis of Transcortical Motor Aphasia. *Neurology, 34,* 409–417

Friederici, A.D., Meyer, M., & von Cramon, D.Y. (2000). Auditory Language Comprehension; An Event-Related fMRI Study on the Processing of Syntactic and Lexical Information. *Brain and Language, 74,* 289–300

Gernsbacher, M.A. & Kaschek, M.P. (2003). Neuroimaging studies of language production and comprehension. *Annual Review of Psychology, 54,* 91–114

Geschwind, N. (1965). Disconnexion Syndromes in Animals and Man. *Brain, 88,* 237–294, 585–644

Geschwind, N. (1970). The Organization of Language in the Brain. *Science, 170,* 940–944

Gold, B.T. & Kertesz, A. (2000). Right Hemisphere Semantic Processing of Visual Words in an Aphasic Patient: An fMRI Study. *Brain and Language, 73,* 456–465

Gonzalez R., Schaefer P., Buonanno F.S., Schwamm, L.H., Budzik, R.F., Rordorf, G., Wang, B., Sorensen, A.G., & Koroshetz, W.J. (1999). Diffusion-Weighted MR Imaging: Diagnostic Accuracy in Patients Imaged within 6 Hours of Stroke Symptom. *Radiology, 210,* 155–162

Gorelick, P.B., Hier, D.B., Benevento, L., Levitt, S., & Tan, W. (1984). Aphasia after left thalamic infarction. *Archives of Neurology, 41,* 1296–1298

Grafman, J. (2000). Conceptualizing Functional Neuroplasticity. *Journal of Communication Disorders, 33,* 345–356

Gray, K.F. & Cummings, J.L. (1994). Neuroimaging in Dementia. In A. Kertesz (Ed.), *Localization and Neuroimaging in Neuropsychology* (pp. 621–651). San Diego: Academic Press

Grodzinsky, Y. (2000). The Neurology of Syntax: Language Use without Broca's Area. *Behavioral Brain Sciences, 23,* 1–21

Hart, J., & Gordon, B. (1990). Delineation of Single-Word Semantic Comprehension Deficits in Aphasia, with Anatomical Correlation. *Annals of Neurology, 27,* 226–231

Heiss, W.D., Emunds, H.G., & Herholz, K. (1993). Cerebral Glucose Metabolism as a Predictor of Rehabilitation after Ischaemic Stroke. *Stroke, 24,* 1784–1788

Heiss, W.D., Karbe, H., & Weber, L.G., Herholz, K., Kessler, J., Pietrzyk, U., & Pawlik, G. (1997). Speech-induced cerebral metabolic activation reflects recovery from aphasia. *Journal of the Neurological Sciences, 145,* 213–217

Heiss, W.D., Kessler, J., Thiel, A., Ghaemi, M., & Karbe, H. (1999). Differential Capacity of Left and Right Hemispheric Areas for Compensation of Poststroke Aphasia. *Annals of Neurology, 45,* 430–438

Heiss W.D., Thiel, A., Winhuisen, L., Muhlberger, B., Kessler, J., & Herholz K. (2003). Functional Imaging in the Assessment of Capability for Recovery after Stroke. *Journal of Rehabilitation Medicine, 41, (suppl),* 27–33

Helm-Estabrooks, N.E., & Albert, M.L. (1991). *Manual of Aphasia Therapy.* Austin, TX: Pro-Ed

Hickok, G. & Poeppel, D. (2004). Dorsal and Ventral Streams: A Framework for Understanding Aspects of the Functional Anatomy of Language. *Cognition, 92,* 67–99

Hillis, A.E., Barker, P.B., Beauchamp, N.J., Winters, B.D., Mirski, M., & Wityk, R.J. (2001a). Restoring Blood Pressure Reperfused Wernicke's Area and Improved Language. *Neurology, 56,* 670–672

Hillis, A.E., Barker, P.B., Wityk, R.J., Aldrich, E.M., Restrepo, L., Breese, E.L., & Work, M. (2004a). Variability in Subcortical Aphasia is Due to Variable Sites of Cortical Hypoperfusion. *Brain and Language, 38,* 524–530

Hillis, A.E., Kane, A., Tuffiash,E., Ulatowski, J.A., Barker, P.B., Beauchamp, N.J., & Wityk R.J. (2001b). Reperfusion of Specific Brain Regions by Raising Blood Pressure Restores Selective Language Functions in Subacute Stroke. *Brain and Language, 79,* 495–510

Hillis, E.E., Wityk, R.J., Barker, P.B., Beauchamp, N.J., Gailloud P., Murphy, K., Cooper, O., & Metter, E.J. (2002). Subcortical Aphasia and Neglect in Acute Stroke: The Role of Cortical Hypoperfusion. *Brain, 125,* 1094–1104

Hillis, A.E., Wityk, R.J., Barker, P.B., & Caramazza, A. (2003). Neural Regions Essential for Writing Verbs. *Nature Neuroscience, 6,* 19–20

Hillis, A.E., Wityk, R.J., Tuffiash, E., Beauchamp, N.J., Jacobs, M.A., Barker, P.B., & Selnes, O.A. (2001c). Hypoperfusion of Wernicke's Area Predicts Severity of Semantic Deficit in Acute Stroke. *Annals of Neurology, 50,* 561–566

Hillis, A.E., Work, M., Barker, P.B., Jacobs, M.A., Breese, E.L., & Maurer K. (2004b). Re-examining the Brain Regions Crucial for Orchestrating Speech Articulation. *Brain, 127,* 1479–1487

Hirsch, J., Ruge, M.I., Kim, K.H., Correa, D.D., Victor, J.D., Relkin, N.R., Labar, D.R., Krol, G., Bilsky, M.H., Souweidane, M.M., DeAngelis, L.M., & Gutin, P.H. (2000). An Integrated Functional Magnetic Resonance Imaging Procedure for Preoperative Mapping of Cortical Areas Associated with Tactile, Motor, Language, and Visual Functions. *Neurosurgery, 47,* 711–721

Ho, S.S., Berkovic, S.F., Newton, M.R., Austin, M.C., McKay, W.J., & Bladin, P.F. (1994). Parietal Lobe Epilepsy: Clinical Features and Seizure Localization by Ictal SPECT. *Neurology, 44,* 2277–2284

Holland, A.L., Fromm, V., DeRuyter, F., & Stein, M. (1996). Treatment Efficacy for Aphasia. *Journal of Speech and Hearing Research, 39,* S27–S36

Huang J., Carr, T.H., & Cao, Y. (2002). Comparing Cortical Activations for Silent and Overt Speech Using Event-Related fMRI. *Human Brain Mapping, 15,* 39–53

Indefrey, P. & Levelt, W.J.M. (2000). The Neural Correlates of Language Production. In M.S. Gazzaniga (Ed.), *The New Cognitive Neurosciences.* Cambridge, MA: MIT Press

Jeffries, K.J., Schooler, C., Schoenbach, C., Herscovitch, P., Chase, T.N., & Braun, A.R. (2002). The functional neuroanatomy of Tourette's syndrome: An FDG PET study III: Functional coupling of regional cerebral metabolic rates. Neuropsychopharmacology, 27, 92–104

Just, M.A., Carpenter, P.A., Keller, T.A., Eddy, W.F., & Thulborn, K.R. (1996). Brain Activation Modulated by Sentence Comprehension. *Science, 274,* 114–116

Karbe, H., Kessler, J., Herholz, K., Fink, G.R., & Heiss, W.D. (1995). Long-term Prognosis of Post stroke Aphasia Studied with Positron Emission Tomography. *Archives of Neurology, 52,* 186–190

Karbe, H., Thiel, A., Weber-Luxenburger, G., Herholz, K., Kessler, J., & Heiss, W.D. (1998). Brain Plasticity in Poststroke Aphasia: What is the Contribution of the Right Hemisphere? *Brain and Language, 64,* 215–230

Keller, T.A., Carpenter, P.A., & Just, M.A. (2001). The Neural Bases of Sentence Comprehension: An fMRI Examination of Syntactic and Lexical Processing. *Cerebral Cortex, 11,* 223–237

Kempler, D., Metter, E.J., Jackson, C.A., Hanson, W.R., Riege, W.H., Mazziotta, J.C., & Phelps, M.E. (1988). Disconnection and Cerebral Metabolism. The Case of Conduction Aphasia. *Archives of Neurology, 45,* 275–279

Kendall, D.L. & Gonzalez Rothi, L.J. (2001). Epilogue: Neuroimaging with A View To Prediction and Prognosis. *Topics in Language Disorders, 21,* 75–80

Kertesz, A. (1979). *Aphasia and Associated Disorders: Taxonomy, Localization and Recovery.* New York: Grune & Stratton

Kertesz, A. (1988). Recovery of Language Disorders—Homologous Contralateral or Connected Ipsilateral Compensation? In S. Finger (Ed.), *Brain Injury and Recovery: Theoretical and Controversial Issues* (pp. 307–321) New York: Plenum

Kertesz, A. (1994). Localization and Function: Old Issue Revisited and New Developments. In A. Kertesz (Ed.), *Localization and Neuroimaging in Neuropsychology* (pp. 1–33). San Diego: Academic Press

Kertesz, A., Harlock, W., Coates, R. (1979). Computer Tomographic Localization, Lesion Size and Prognosis in Aphasia and Nonverbal Impairment. *Brain and Language, 8,* 34–50

Kertesz A., Lau, WK., & Polk, M. (1993). The Structural Determinants of Recovery in Wernicke's Aphasia. *Brain and Language, 44,* 153–164

Kilpatrick, M.M., Yonas, H., Goldstein, S., Kassam, A.B., Gebel, J.M. Jr., Wechsler, L.R., Jungreis, C.A., & Fukui, M.B. (2001). CT-based Assessment of Acute Stroke: CT, CT angiography, and Xenon-Enhanced CT Cerebral Blood Flow. *Stroke, 32,* 2543–2549

Kinsbourne, M. (1998). The Right Hemisphere and Recovery from Aphasia. In: B. Stemmer & H.A. Whitaker (Eds.), *Handbook of Neurolinguistics* (pp. 386–394). San Diego: Academic Press

Kirshner, H.S. (1995a). Classical Aphasia Syndromes. In H.S. Kirshner (Ed.), *Handbook of Neurological Speech and Language Disorders* (pp. 57–89). New York: Marcel Dekker

Kirshner, H.S. (1995b). Introduction to Aphasia. In H.S. Kirshner (Ed.), *Handbook of Neurological Speech and Language Disorders* (pp. 1–21). New York: Marcel Dekker

Knopman D.S., Rubens A.B., Selnes O.A., Klassen, A.C., & Meyer, M.W. (1984). Mechanisms of Recovery from Aphasia: Evidence for Serial Xenon 133 Blood Flow Studies. *Annals of Neurology, 15,* 530–535

Knopman D.S., Selnes O.A., Niccum N., & Rubens, A.B., (1984). Recovery of Naming in Aphasia: Relationship to Fluency, Comprehension and CT findings. *Neurology, 34,* 1461–1471

Knopman, D.S., Selnes, O.A., Niccum, N., Rubens, A.B., Yock, D., & Larson, D. (1983). Longitudinal Study of Speech Fluency in Aphasia. CT Correlates of Recovery and Persistent Non-Fluency. *Neurology, 33,* 1170–1178

Kuhl, D.E., Phelps, M.E., Kowell, A.P., Metter, E.J., Selin, C., & Winter, J. (1980). Effects of Stroke on Local Cerebral Metabolism and Perfusion: Mapping by Emission Computed Tomography of 18FDG and 13NH3. *Annals of Neurology, 8,* 47–60

Kuperberg, G.R., Holcomb, P.J., Sitnikova, T., Greve, D., Dale, A.M., & Caplan, D. (2003). Distinct Patterns of Neural Modulation during the Processing of Conceptual and Syntactic Anomalies. *Journal of Cognitive Neuroscience, 15,* 272–293

Lai, S., Hopkins, A.L., & Haake, E.M., et al. (1993). Identification of Vascular Structures as a Major Source of Signal Contrast in High Resolution 2D and 3D Functional Activation Imaging of the Motor Cortex at 1.5T. *Magnetic Resonance Medicine, 30,* 387–392

Levelt, W.J., Roelofs, A., & Meyer, A.S. (1999). A theory of lexical access in speech production. *Behavioral Brain Science, 22,* 1–38; discussion 38–75

Lichtheim, L. (1885). [On Aphasia.] *Brain, 7,* 433–485 (Originally published in *Deutsches Archiv fuer Klinische Medizin,* 1885, *36,* 204–268

Ludlow, C.L., Rosenberg, J., Fair, C., Buck, D., Schesselman, S., & Salazar, A. (1986). Brain Lesions Associated with Non-Fluent Aphasia Fifteen Years Following Penetrating Head Injury. *Brain, 109,* 55–80

Martin, R.C. (2003). Language Processing: Functional Organization and Neuroanatomical Basis. *Annual Review of Psychology, 54,* 55–89

Marshall, J.F. (1984). Brain Function: Neural Adaptations and Recovery from Injury. *Annual Review of Psychology, 35,* 277–308

Matthews, P.M. & Jezzard, P. (2004). Functional Magnetic Resonance Imaging. *Journal of Neurology, Neurosurgery and Psychiatry, 75,* 6–12

Mayer, J. (2003). The Role of fMRI in Aphasiology: Interface Between Technology, Theory and Clinical Care. In Perspectives on Neurophysiology and Neurogenic Speech and Language Disorders. American Speech–language-Hearing Association Division 2 Newsletter (pp. 4–7)

McLaughlin, S.A., Rogers, M.A., & Shibata, D.A. (2003). A Primer on Functional Magnetic Resonance Imaging (fMRI). In Perspectives on Neurophysiology and Neurogenic Speech and Language Disorders. American Speech-language-Hearing Association Division 2 Newsletter (pp. 25–32)

McNeil, M.R., & Prescott, T.E. (1978). *Revised Token Test.* Baltimore: University Park Press

Mesulam, M.-M. (1990). Large Scale Neurocognitive Networks and Distributed Processing for Attention, Language, and Memory. *Annals of Neurology; 28:*597–613

Mesulam, M.-M. (1998). From Sensation to Cognition. *Brain, 121,* 1013–1052

Metter, E.J. (1991). Brain-Behavior Relationships in Aphasia Studied by Positron Emission Tomography. *Annals of the New York Academy of Science, 620,* 153–164

Metter, E.J., & Hanson, W.R. (1994). Use of Positron Emission Tomography to Study Aphasia. In A. Kertesz (Ed.), Localization and Neuroimaging in Neuropsychology (pp. 123–149). Academic Press: San Diego

Metter, E.J., Hanson, W.R., Jackson, C.A., Kempler, D., van Lancker, D., Mazziotta, J.C., & Phelps, M.E. (1990). Temporoparietal Cortex in Aphasia: Evidence from Positron Emission Tomography, *Archives of Neurology, 47,* 1235–1238

Metter, E.J., Jackson, C.A., & Kempler, D. (1992). Temporoparietal Cortex and the Recovery of Language Comprehension in Aphasia. *Aphasiology, 6,* 349–358

Metter, E.J., Kempler, D., Jackson,C., Hanson, W.R., Mazziotta, J.C., & Phelps, M.E. (1989). Cerebral Glucose Metabolism in Wernicke's, Broca's, and Conduction Aphasias. *Archives of Neurology, 46,* 27–34

Metter, E.J., Riege, W.H., Hanson, W.R., Jackson, C.A., Kempler, D., & van Lancker, D. (1988). Subcortical Structures in Aphasias. An Analysis Based on (F-18)-Fluorodeoxy-Glucose Positron Emission Tomography, and Computed Tomography. *Archives of Neurology, 45,* 1229–1234

Metter, E.J., Riege, W.H., Hanson, W.R., Kuhl, D.E., Phelps, M.E., Squire, L.R., Wasterlain, C.G., & Benson, D.F. (1983). Comparisons of Metabolic Rates, Language and Memory in Subcortical Aphasia. *Brain and Language, 19,* 33–47

Metter, E.J., Wasterlain, C.G., Kuhl, D.E., Hanson, W.R., & Phelps, M.E. (1981). 18FDG Positron Emission Computed Tomography in a Study of Aphasia. *Annals of Neurology, 10,* 173–183

Mies, G., Auer, L.M., Ebhardt, G., Traupe, H., & Heiss, W.D. (1983). Flow and Neuronal Density in Tissue Surrounding Chronic Infarction. *Stroke, 14,* 22–27

Mimura, M., Kato, M., Kato, M., Sano, Y., Kojima, T., Naeser, M., & Kashima, H. (1998). Prospective and Retrospective Studies of Recovery in Aphasia: Changes in Cerebral Blood Flow and Language Functions. *Brain, 121,* 2083–2094

Mohr, J.P. (1976). Broca's Area and Broca's Aphasia. In H. Whitaker & H.A. Whitaker (Eds.), *Studies in Neurolinguistics* (vol. 1, pp. 201–235). New York: Academic Press

Mohr, J., Pessin, M., Finkelstein, S., Funkenstein, H.H., Duncan, G.W., & Davis, K.R., (1978). Broca Aphasia: Pathologic and Clinical. *Neurology, 28,* 311–324

Musso, M., Weiller C., Kiebel, S., Muller, S.P., Bulau, P., & Rijntjes, M. (1999). Training Induced Brain Plasticity in Aphasia. *Brain, 122(pt 9),* 1781–1790

Naeser, M.A. (1994). Neuroimaging and Recovery of Auditory Comprehension and Spontaneous Speech in Aphasia with Some Implications for Treatment in Severe Aphasia. In A. Kertesz (Ed.), *Localization and Neuroimaging in Neuropsychology* (pp. 245–295). San Diego, CA: Academic Press

Naeser, M.A., Gaddie, A., Palumbo, C.L., & Stiassny-Eder, D. (1990). Late Recovery of Auditory Comprehension in Global Aphasia. Improved Recovery Observed with Subcortical Temporal Isthmus Lesion vs. Wernicke's Cortical Area Lesion. *Archives of Neurology, 47,* 425–432

Naeser, M.A. & Helm-Estabrooks, N. (1985). CT Scan Lesion Localization and Response to Melodic Intonation Therapy with Nonfluent Aphasia Cases. *Cortex, 21,* 203–223

Naeser, M.A., Helm-Estabrooks, N., Haas, G., Auerbach, S., Srinivasan, M. (1987). Relationship between Lesion Extend in 'Wernicke's Area' on Computed Tomographic Scan and Predicting Recovery of Comprehension in Wernicke's Aphasia. *Archives of Neurology, 44,* 73–82

Naeser, M.A., & Hayward, R.W. (1978) Lesion Localization in Aphasia with Cranial Computed Tomography and the Boston Diagnostic Aphasia Exam. *Neurology, 28,* 545–551

Naeser, M.A., & Palumbo, C.L. (1994). Neuroimaging and Language Recovery in Stroke. *Journal of Clinical Neurophysiology, 11,* 150–174

Naeser, M.A. & Palumbo, C.L. (1995). How to Analyze CT / MRI Scan Lesion Sites to Predict Potential for Long-Term Recovery in Aphasia. In H.S. Kirshner (Ed.), *Handbook of Neurological Speech and Language Disorders* (pp. 91–148). New York: Marcel Dekker

Naeser, M.A., Palumbo C.L., Helm-Estabrooks, N., Stiassny-Eder, D. & Albert, M.S. (1989). Severe Non-fluency in Aphasia: Role of the Medial Subcallosal Fasciculus Plus Other White Matter Pathways in Recovery of Spontaneous Speech. *Brain, 112,* 1–38

Nelles, J.L., Lugar, H.M., Coalson, R.S., Miezin, F.M., Petersen, S.E., & Schlaggar, B.L. (2003). Automated Method for Extracting Response Latencies of Subject Vocalizations in Event-Related fMRI Experiments. *Neuroimage, 20,* 1865–1871

Nestor, P.J., Graham, N.L., Fryer, T.D., Williams, G.B., Patterson, K., & Hodges, J.R. (2003). Progressive non-fluent aphasia is associated with hypometabolism centered on the left anterior insula. *Brain, 126,* 2406–2418

Ogawa, S., Lee, T.M., Kay, A.R., & Tank, D.W. (1990). Brain Magnetic Resonance Imaging with Contrast Dependent on Blood Oxygenation. *Proceedings of the National Academy of Sciences U.S.A., 87,* 9868–9872

Ogawa S., Menon R.S., Tank D.W., Kim, S.G., Merkle, H., Ellermann, J.M., & Ugurbil, K. (1993). Functional Brain Mapping by Blood Oxygenation Level-Dependent Contrast Magnetic Resonance Imaging. A Comparison of Signal Characteristics with a Biophysical Model. *Biophysical Journal, 64,* 803–812

Perani, D., Cappa, S.F., Tettamanti, M., Rosa, M., Scifo, P., Miozzo, A., Basso, A. & Fazio, F. (2003). A fMRI Study of Word Retrieval in Aphasia. *Brain and Language, 85,* 357–368

Petersen, S.E., Fox, P.T., Posner, M.I., Mintun, M., & Raichle, M.E. (1988). Positron Emission Tomographic Studies of the Cortical Anatomy of Single-Word Processing. *Nature, 331,* 585–589

Petersen, S.E., Fox, P.T., Posner, M.I., Mintun, M., & Raichle, M.E. (1989). Positron Emission Tomographic Studies of the Cortical Anatomy of Single-Word Processing. *Nature, Feb 18;331(6157),* 585–589

Petersen, S.E., Fox, P.T., Snyder, A.Z., & Raichle, M.E. (1990). Activation of Extrastriate and Frontal Cortical Areas by Visual Words and Word-Like Stimuli. *Science, 249,* 1041–1044

Pizzamiglio, L., Galati, G., & Committeri, G. (2001). The Contribution of Functional Neuroimaging to Recovery After Brain Damage: A Review. *Cortex, 37,* 11–31

Poeppel, D. & Hickok, G. (2004). Towards a New Functional Anatomy of Language. *Cognition, 92,* 1–12

Price, C.J., Warburton, E.A., Moore, C.J., Frackowiak, R.S. & Friston, K.J. (2001). Dynamic diaschisis: Anatomically remote and context-sensitive human brain lesions. *Journal of Cognitive Neuroscience, 13(4),* 419–429

Raymer, A.M. (2001). Acquired Language Disorders. *Topics in Language Disorders, 21,* 42–59

Raymer, A.M., Foundas, A.L., Maher, L.M., Greenwald, M.L., Morris, M., Rothi, L.J., & Heilman, K.M. (1997). Cognitive Neuropsychological Analysis and Neuroanatomic Correlates in a Case of Acute Anomia. *Brain and Language, 58,* 137–156

Roeltgen, D., & Heilman, K.M. (1984). Lexical Agraphia: Further support for the Two System Hypothesis of Linguistic Agraphia. *Brain, 107,* 811–827

Rosen, H.J., Petersen, S.E., Linenweber, M.R., Snyder, A.Z., White, D.A., Chapman, L., Dromerick, A.W., Fiez, J.A., & Corbetta, M. (2000). Neural Correlates of Recovery from Aphasia after Damage to Left Inferior Frontal Cortex. *Neurology, 55,* 1883–1894

Roskies, A.L., Fiez, J.A., Balota, D.A., Raichle, M.E., & Petersen, S.E. (2001). Task-Dependent Modulation of Regions in the Left Inferior Frontal Cortex during Semantic Processing. *Journal of Cognitive Neuroscience, 13,* 829–843

Rugg, M.D. (1999). Functional Neuroimaging in Cognitive Neuroscience. In. C.M. Brown & P. Hagoort (Eds.), *The neurocognition of language* (pp. 15–36). Oxford: Oxford University Press

Sakurai, Y., Takeuchi, S., Kojima,E., Yazawa, I., Murayama, S., Kaga, K,. Momose, T., Nakase, H., Sakuta, M., & Kanazaw, I., (1998). Mechanism of Short-Term Memory and Repetition in Conduction Aphasia and Related Cognitive Disorders: A Neuropsychological, Audiological and Neuroimaging Study. *Journal of the Neurological Sciences, 154,* 182–193

Schellinger, P.D., Fiebach, J.B., & Hacke, W. (2003). Imaging-based Decision Making in Thrombolytic Therapy for Ischemic Stroke: Present Status. *Stroke, 34,* 575–583

Selnes, O.A., Knopman, D.S., Niccum, N., Rubens, A.B., & Larson, D. (1983). Computed Tomographic Scan Correlates of Auditory Comprehension Deficits in Aphasia: A Prospective Recovery Study. *Annals of Neurology, 13,* 558–566

Selnes, O.A., Knopman, D.S., Niccum, N., & Rubens, A.B. (1985). The Critical Role of Wernicke's Area in Sentence Repetition. *Annals of Neurology, 17,* 549–557

Selnes, O.A., Niccum, N., Knopman, D.S., & Rubens, A.B. (1984). Recovery of Single Word Comprehension: CT-Scan Correlates. *Brain and Language, 21,* 72–84

Shallice T. (1988). From Neuropsychology to Mental Structure. Cambridge: Cambridge University Press

Singer M., Chong J., Lu, D., Schonewille, W.J., Tuhrim, S., & Atlas, S.W. (1998). Diffusion-Weighted MRI in Acute Subcortical Infarction. *Stroke, 29,* 133–136

Small, G.W., Ercoli, L.M., Silverman, D.H., Huang, S.C., Komo, S., Bookheimer, S.Y., Lavretsky, H., Miller, K., Siddarth, P., Rasgon, N.L., Mazziotta, J.C., Saxena, S., Wu H.M., Mega. M.S., Cummings, J.L., Saunders, A.M., Pericak-Vance, M.A., Roses, A.D., Barrio, J.R., & Phelps, M.E. (2000). Cerebral Metabolic and Cognitive Decline in Persons at Genetic Risk for Alzheimer's Disease. *Proceedings of the National Academy of Sciences U.S.A., 97,* 6037–6042

Small, S.L., & Burton, M.W. (2002). Functional Magnetic Resonance Imaging Studies of Language. *Current Neurology and Neuroscience Report, 2,* 505–510

Small, S.L., Flores, D. K., & Noll, D.C. (1998). Different Neural Circuits Subserve Reading Before and After Therapy for Acquired Dyslexia. *Brain and Language, 62,* 298–308

Taubner, R.W., Raymer, A.M., & Heilman, K.M. (1999). Frontal-opercular Aphasia. *Brain and Language, 70,* 240–261

Thompson, C.K. (2000a). Neurobiology of Language Recovery in Aphasia. *Brain and Language, 71,* 245–248

Thompson, C.K. (2000b). Neuroplasticity. Evidence from Aphasia. *Journal of Communication Disorders, 33,* 357–366

Thulborn, K.R., Carpenter, P.A., & Just, M.A. (1999). Plasticity of Language-Related Brain Function During Recovery from Stroke. *Stroke, 30,* 749–754

Vignolo, L.A., Boccardi, E., & Caverni L. (1986). Unexpected CT-Scan Findings in Global Aphasia. *Cortex, 22,* 55–69

Warburton, E.A., Price, C.J., Swinburn, K. & Wise, R.J. (1999). Mechanisms of Recovery from Aphasia: Evidence from Positron Emission Tomography Studies. *Journal of Neurology, Neurosurgery, and Psychiatry, 66(2),* 155–161

Weiller C, Isensee C, Rijntjes M, Huber W, Muller S, Bier D, Dutschka, K., Woods, R.P., Noth, J., & Diener, H.C. (1995) Recovery from Wernicke's Aphasia: A Positron Emission Tomographic Study. *Annals of Neurology, 37,* 723–732

Wernicke, C. (1874). Der aphasische Symptomenkomplex. Breslau: Cohn & Weigert

Wise, R.J.S. (2003). Language Systems in Normal and Aphasic Human Subjects: Functional Imaging Studies and Inferences from Animal Studies. *British Medical Bulletin, 65,* 95–119

Wise, R., Chollet, F., Hadar, U., Friston, K., Hoffner, E., & Frackowiak R. (1991). Distribution of Cortical Neural Networks Involved in Word Comprehension and Word Retrieval. *Brain, 114,* 1803–1817

Wise, R., Hadar, U., Howard, D., & Patterson, K. (1991). Language activation studies with positron emission tomography. Ciba Foundation Symposium, 163, 218–228; discussion 228–234

Wise, R.J.S., Scott, S.K., Blank, C., Mummery, C.J., Murphy, K., & Warburton, E.A. (2001). Separate Neural Subsystems within 'Wernicke's Area.' *Brain, 124,* 83–95

Yarnell, P., Monroe, P., & Sobel, L. (1976). Aphasia Outcome in Stroke: A Clinical Neuroradiological Correlation. *Stroke, 7,* 516–522

Zahn, R., Drews, E., Specht, K., Kemeny, S., Reith, W., Willmes, K., Schwarz, M., & Huber, W. (2004). Recovery of Semantic Word Processing in Global Aphasia: A Functional MRI Study. *Cognitive Brain Research, 18,* 322–336

Zahn R., Huber, W., Drews, E., Specht, K., Kemeny, S., Reith, W., Willmes K., Schwarz, M. (2002). Recovery of Semantic Word Processing in Transcortical Sensory Aphasia: A Functional Magnetic Resonance Imaging Study. *Neurocase, 8(5),* 376–386

4

Assessment of Aphasia

Jacqueline J. Hinckley and Lori Bartels-Tobin

◆ Clinical Competencies
◆ Concepts and Principles Underlying the Assessment of Aphasia
◆ Goals and Methods for the Assessment of Aphasia

◆ Clinical Competencies

This chapter addresses some of the competencies described in Standard III-E of the Standards and Implementation for the Certificate of Clinical Competence in Speech-Language Pathology (ASHA, 2000):

> The applicant must possess knowledge of the principles and methods of prevention and assessment, and intervention for people with communication and swallowing disorders, including consideration of anatomical/physiological, developmental, and linguistic and cultural correlates of the disorders.

Specifically, the chapter describes the principles and methods of assessment for people with aphasia, including consideration of anatomic/physiologic, developmental, and linguistic and cultural correlates of aphasia.

◆ Concepts and Principles Underlying the Assessment of Aphasia

Theoretical and Conceptual Issues

The theoretical orientation of the clinician, as well as the purpose of the assessment, will drive the selection of certain assessment tools over others. Similarly, the underlying theoretical foundation of any given assessment tool relates to the type of information it can yield, and how it can inform the clinical process.

A structuralist view of aphasia emphasizes the neuroanatomic and neurophysiologic origins of the disorder, and links assessment techniques and results to the neurologic etiology (Gagnon & Martin, 2002; Lum, 2002). When guided by this theoretical view, the clinician is more likely to select assessment tools that will generate information about aphasic syndromes that are consistent with typical lesion site patterns, particularly those aphasia assessments that provide classical aphasia type and severity profiles.

A functionalist view of aphasia foregrounds the psycholinguistic and cognitive components and processes. An assessment driven by this theoretical view attempts to isolate the functional locus of the lesion within a particular model of the language system (Hillis, 2001). For example, performances on particular tasks may serve to isolate a breakdown in a particular language component. Adhering to a particular language model during an assessment may aid the clinician in determining more specifically the cognitive and linguistic characteristics of any given aphasia.

A newer theoretical orientation stems from ethnographic approaches and emphasizes the social implications of living with aphasia (Simmons-Mackie, 2001). Assessment occurs within the context of the social milieu, including family, friends, job, and hobbies. Conversational abilities and strategies are emphasized along with the social strategies that result in improved participation in various life activities. In this view, the emphasis is beyond the internal cognitive, linguistic, or neuroanatomic mechanisms of the individual. Rather, a seamless extension of the internal linguistic system with the external social environment is posited.

A framework that can accommodate the applications of all of these theoretical orientations is the World Health Organization's (WHO) (2001) International Classification of Functioning, Disability, and Health (ICF). This classification system is designed to accommodate theory as well as operational definitions and descriptions of illness and disability. It is intended to be context-inclusive and to be applicable to many cultures, not just based on Western concepts. In this framework, disability is an impairment of a body structure or body function, which may lead to limitations in activities or restrictions to participation in typical social roles. This framework also takes environmental factors and personal factors into account. Thus, the multiple factors that relate to social functioning can be accommodated in the framework.

An important characteristic of the WHO ICF framework is the interactivity between impairment, activity limitations, and participation restrictions. Observations of 20 adults with aphasia during the first year poststroke supports the notion that

Table 4–1   Application of Three Theoretical Models to the Case of Mr. A.

Mr. A., a 55-year-old, right-handed man, is referred for outpatient speech–language treatment 3 weeks after his single left hemispheric cardiovascular accident. He has a mild right hemiparesis of the right upper extremity. His auditory comprehension is relatively good in conversation. His language production is characterized by one- to three-word phrases, comprised mostly of content words. Prior to his stroke, Mr. A. had a successful, 20-year career in marketing and sales for a large company. He lives with his wife and has no children. He participated in golf and softball and enjoyed traveling with his wife.

	Structuralist Approach	Functionalist Approach	Social Approach
Assessment goals	Determine type and severity of aphasia; consider consistency of the diagnosis with the neurologic status.	Determine the language components and processes that are affected.	Determine Mr. A.'s previous and current social roles and functions.
Assessment tools	Standardized aphasia batteries, such as Boston Diagnostic Aphasia Examination, Western Aphasia Battery, Aphasia Language Profiles	Administer an in-depth battery to assess specific language skills. Selected tools from the Psycholinguistic Assessment of Language Processing in Aphasia (PALPA) might be selected to achieve this goal.	Conduct an interview of Mr. A. and his wife. Observe Mr. A.'s functional ability to communicate in several different contexts, including typical contexts that are personally relevant. This might involve the use of published assessment tools like the Communication Activities of Daily Living-2 (CADL-2), checklists, or other qualitative measures.
Clinical outcomes	Mr. A. would most likely be diagnosed with a Broca's type aphasia, consistent with his lesion in the left frontoparietal region.	In the case of Mr. A., specific difficulties in lexical access including the phonologic output lexicon might be identified.	Assessment information would indicate to the clinician the extent of the patient's ability and inability to communicate in daily settings with his wife, friends, or neighbors, as well as his ability to communicate in vocational and avocational settings, and his overall ability to participate in typical social roles.
ICF	Most consistent with the impairment level of the ICF framework	Most consistent with the impairment level of the ICF framework	Most consistent with the activity/participation levels of the ICF framework
Treatment planning	Treatments that are specifically intended for Broca's-type aphasia, such as syntax-focused treatments, would most likely be selected.	Treatments that specifically address the components identified in the assessment as impaired would be selected for treatment. An individualized cuing hierarchy might be developed based on his assessment performance and error patterns.	Intervention would focus on training Mr. A.'s wife, friends, or other communication partners with appropriate strategies. Mr. A. would also be trained to use effective communication strategies. Intervention would focus on personally relevant contexts such as golfing, work, or softball league.
Prognosis generation	Prognosis would be focused on the typical recovery patterns of individuals with Broca's aphasia.	Prognosis would be focused on initial response to treatment and the nature and extent of the damage to the language system.	Prognosis would emphasize Mr. A.'s motivation and his adaptation to disability, as well as his level of social support.

ICF, International Classification of Functioning, Disability, and Health.

either one of these categories may change more than the others, without a direct correlation (Irwin, Wertz & Avent, 2002).

It is important to select an appropriate theoretical and conceptual basis for an assessment that is consistent with clinical constraints and goals. An example of a case handled in the three theoretical orientations described is provided in **Table 4–1**.

Principles of Measurement

The validity, reliability, and standardization of our assessment tools are critical to our ability to arrive at appropriate conclusions from our assessments (Murray & Chapey, 2001; Spreen & Risser, 1998). Validity is the evidence that a test measures what it says it measures. Reliability is the demonstration that a test will consistently measure what it claims to measure. Conditions should be standardized so that they are similar across test administrations. The problems that are associated with poor reliability and validity of tests and measures are listed in **Table 4–2**.

Clinical time must be used effectively, and as a result, the appropriate tool for the assessment goal must be chosen and administered correctly. Conducting a longer than needed assessment may result in misuse of clinical resources, whereas too little assessment information may lead to incorrect diagnoses. We must also be concerned with using selected pieces of various tests to create an institution-specific protocol that may not be a reliable tool (Davis, 2000).

Table 4–2 Problems Associated with Poor Reliability and Validity of Testing and Observation Tools

Limitations in interpretation of data

Generation of conflicting data among instruments or observers

Establishment of inaccurate or incomplete diagnosis

Establishment of inappropriate or ineffective treatments

Miscommunication of results to patient, family, referral sources

Inaccurate prediction of the course of the disorder

Inaccurate prognosis for recovery

From Johnson, George, & Hinckley, 1998.

Disorder-Specific Considerations

To effectively conduct assessments in aphasia, we must be familiar with neurophysiologic underpinnings and correlates, cognitive-linguistic foundations, life-span issues, and sociocultural concerns.

Neuroanatomic/Neurophysiologic Considerations

Aphasia is the result of a stroke, head injury, or degenerative condition of the brain. The etiology of the aphasia may affect the prognosis and may also create other important assessment considerations owing to comorbidities or related disabilities.

When aphasia is the result of stroke or head injury, there is an expectation that continuous improvement will characterize the course over time. Approximately one third of all adults who have had a stroke experience aphasia (Laska, Hellblom, Murray, Kahan, & Von Arbin, 2001). Only 20% of adults with head injury have a language disorder that fits the classic criteria of aphasia (Sarno, Buonaguro & Levita, 1987). Primary progressive aphasia or aphasia due to other degenerative disease results in deterioration over time.

For the traumatic aphasias, time post-onset is an important factor in prognosis and in the determination of the type and nature of the intervention. It is generally accepted that the acute period of recovery extends from the time of the event to about 3 months post-onset. During this period, communication improvement is rapid, even without treatment, but is even greater when treatment is provided (Robey, 1998). During the postacute phase, or from 3 to 12 months post-onset, spontaneous recovery slows down, but important outcomes result from treatment. Finally, during the chronic phase, or beyond 12 months post-onset, communication performance tends to be stabilized without treatment or specific self-study or practice.

In contrast, aphasia due to degenerative disease can be expected to worsen over time. Assessment and intervention focus on maintenance of communication, environmental assistance, and compensatory strategies used by the person with aphasia and by his or her communication partners.

Determination of the type of aphasia is highly reliant on the site and the extent of the lesion (Godefroy, Dubois, Debachy, Leclerc, & Kreisler, 2002), although cerebral perfusion may be more accurately associated with the severity of aphasia than lesion volume alone (Fridriksson, Holland, Coull, Plante, Trouard, & Beeson, 2002). Anterior lesions are generally associated with poorer expressive abilities and relatively stronger comprehension, whereas the opposite pattern is generally observed with posterior lesions. Furthermore, the transcortical

aphasias have been associated with lesions outside of the perisylvian region.

Each of these etiologies is also associated with other characteristic health or psychosocial issues. Adults with aphasia due to stroke or degenerative diseases are more likely to be older adults (Bonita, 1992). Older individuals are more likely to be experiencing other health challenges besides those related to the stroke. They are also more likely to be dealing with issues of retirement, and their adult children may be managing their care. Aphasia due to head injury, however, is more likely to occur among adolescents and younger adults between the ages of 15 and 24 years. In this group, individuals may be grappling with substance abuse, issues of independent living, and decisions about how to manage a long life after the onset of aphasia.

Cognitive-Linguistic Considerations

The linguistic system breaks down in systematic ways in aphasia. The difference in processing verbs and nouns is a classic distinction between the nonfluent and fluent types of aphasia, with verbs more impaired in nonfluent aphasia and nouns more impaired in fluent aphasia (Druks, 2002). The production of nouns can also systematically break down based on particular linguistic characteristics, like word frequency, age of acquisition, familiarity, and imageability. There are grammatical distinctions between fluent and nonfluent aphasias as well. In some adults with nonfluent aphasia, agrammatism occurs and is characterized by a difficulty with closed-class words and a reliance on nouns (Thompson, 2001). Paragrammatism may occur in fluent aphasia and is characterized by substitutions of closed-class words (Chatterjee & Maher, 2000). Written language shows parallel linguistic disruptions, which are most obvious in writing and spelling production. Errors occur based on word frequency, regularity of spelling, and phonologic forms.

Although aphasia is typically considered a language disorder, there are certain cognitive changes that can be associated with the onset of aphasia. Attention may be compromised, and the allocation of cognitive resources to single or multiple tasks may be faulty (Fischler, 2000). Working memory, particularly for verbal material, is also typically reduced (Crosson, 2000). Although visual-spatial skills are not often impaired, high-level reasoning and problem solving may be compromised by an inability to rely on linguistic processing for completion of internal computation (Helm-Estabrooks, 2002). For example, adults with aphasia vary considerably in their ability to complete tasks such as Raven's Colored Progressive Matrices (David & Skilbeck, 1984) or the Wisconsin Card Sort (Purdy, 2002), in which nonverbal stimuli are manipulated, suggesting that these tasks might be most efficiently performed with intact language capacity.

It is critical to assess both the linguistic and cognitive abilities of the adult with aphasia. The linguistic profile contributes to understanding how the individual's strengths and weaknesses can affect communication, and the cognitive profile may be important for determining the most appropriate intervention strategy.

Life-Span Considerations

The age of onset of aphasia is important, because expectations for health and life activity change over the course of the life span. Younger individuals with aphasia have special needs that often go overlooked and underserved. Adults in their twenties who have aphasia will need to grapple with the development of gainful employment options, independent living, and the establishment of important social bonds. During the middle adult years, there are issues of returning to work and parenting, as well as marital relations. Older individuals may have more expectations for illness and decline of functioning than younger adults, although this decline in biologic functioning can be compensated for through cultural mechanisms (Baltes, 1993). Around the age of retirement or after, the maintenance of active social connections including family interactions and development of avocational activities take priority.

Assessment of lifestyle needs and desires can take place in the context of the WHO ICF (2001). This framework provides the impetus for identifying activities and social roles appropriate for the individual with aphasia as a goal in rehabilitation. To achieve this goal, appropriate assessment information must be collected about typical activities, family relationships, employment, civic activities, and hobbies. Qualitative approaches including interviews and questionnaires are probably the best techniques for collecting these data.

Sociocultural Considerations

As in any area of clinical practice, we must be alert to the individual's cultural background. A majority of individuals in the United States are bilingual or multilingual, with various cultural backgrounds. This background is critical to the appropriate assessment of aphasia.

Among bilingual (or multilingual) persons, aphasia onset may differentially affect their languages, or both (or all) their languages may be affected similarly (Fabbro, 2001). Similarly, the degree of improvement over time may differ among their languages. Thus, the language background of an individual, including the proficiency and typical patterns of usage of the languages, are important considerations in the assessment and management of aphasia. **Table 4–3** lists selected assessment

Table 4–3 Assessment Tools Appropriate for Use with Bilingual or Multilingual Adults with Aphasia

Tool	Description
Bilingual Aphasia Test (Paradis, 1987)	Subtests and stimuli provided for assessing all language modalities; designed to be translated
Multilingual Aphasia Examination (Benton, Hampsher, & Sivian, 1994)	Designed to be usable for a variety of languages; 11 subtests, pass/fail rating, multiple forms for repeat testing; oral spelling, visual naming, sentence repetition
Aachen Aphasia Test (Orgass & Poeck, 1969)	A standardized aphasia battery available in German, English, and Italian
Boston Diagnostic Aphasia Examination (Goodglass, Kaplan, & Barresi, 2000)	Available in English, Spanish, and Portuguese
Western Aphasia Battery (Kertesz, 1982)	Available in English and Cantonese
Communicative Abilities in Daily Living (Holland, Frattali, & Fromm, 1999)	A functional communication assessment based on role-playing available in English and Spanish

tools in the context of aphasia among bilingual/bicultural individuals.

✦ Goals and Methods for the Assessment of Aphasia

There are four basic purposes for which a clinician conducts an assessment. First, we must differentiate between aphasia and other possible speech, language, or cognitive disorders. Second, we must determine whether intervention is indicated, and if so, what the appropriate type and amount of intervention will be. Third, we must determine a prognosis or what is expected to occur over time for an individual with that particular communication diagnosis. Fourth, we must assess performance on specific measures to determine the outcomes of our intervention efforts.

Differential Diagnosis

Differential diagnosis is the determination of a particular communication diagnosis, to the exclusion of others. The clinician uses interview, case history, and formal and informal tests in a hypothesis-driven, process approach that will lead to a communication diagnosis.

The process approach to assessment (Helm-Estabrooks & Albert, 1991) involves generating a testable hypothesis about a possible communication diagnosis, and then testing that hypothesis against collected behavioral data. This begins with the case history, including review of medical records and interview data. Initial conversation with the person with aphasia and support persons will aid in lending support to our hypothesis.

Once we have gathered diagnosis-relevant information from the case history and initial interview, we move on to making our own observations about the patient's communication. The presence of word-finding difficulties does not exclude communication diagnoses other than aphasia, but all patients with aphasia have word-finding difficulties. We need to determine whether the patient is oriented to person, place, and time; if the patient does indeed have aphasia, we may need to use alternative response modalities (such as pointing to written choices) to help assess this. Finally, we compare the patient's language abilities relative to their cognitive abilities. If language is predominantly impaired, rather than cognition, we have support for our hypothesis of a diagnosis of aphasia. **Table 4–4** lists the tools with which to perform differential diagnosis in aphasia. In this case we are most likely to rely on a structuralist and functionalist theoretical approach, because our clinical questions revolve around the nature of the brain disorder and a details of the cognitive-linguistic performances.

Determining type of aphasia can most consistently be done through the analysis of performances on a standardized aphasia battery (**Table 4–4**). The classical syndromes of aphasia (Broca's, Wernicke's, transcortical aphasias, conduction, anomic, and global) are determined by the relative abilities of the individual on fluency in conversation, repetition abilities, and comprehension. These diagnostic categories are convenient ways to describe the general characteristics of an individual's aphasia, and can be used in intervention planning. Some specific treatment approaches are oriented to particular types of aphasia (Helm-Estabrooks & Albert, 1991).

Table 4–4 A Summary of Tools that Can Be Used for the Differential Diagnosis of Aphasia

Assessment Tool	Description	Examples of Tasks
Boston Diagnostic Aphasia Examination (Goodglass, Kaplan, & Barresi, 2000)	Expressive and receptive language skills, percentile ranking, 35 subtests	Speech output rating scale, oral word reading, oral automatized sequences
Western Aphasia Battery (Kertesz, 1982)	17 subscores, 7 major scores; expressive and receptive language skills, optional constructional section	Written word-picture matching, verbal and written picture description, reading comprehension
Aphasia Diagnostic Profiles (Helm-Estabrooks, 1992)	Nine subtests, behavior profile, expressive and receptive language	Oral story comprehension, picture naming, fluency
Minnesota Test for the Differential Diagnosis of Aphasia (Schuell, 1965)	Five sections, no composite scores, assume aphasia plus other deficits present	Aphasia with sensorimotor involvement, dysarthria, visual impairment
Examining for Aphasia (Eisenson, 1994)	Evaluates expressive and receptive language skills, 5 different composites, ranks aphasia severity	Oral reading, writing numerals and letters, computations
Bedside Evaluation and Screening Test of Aphasia (Fitch-West & Sands, 1987)	Screening tool, fill-in-the-blank results for type, degree, and bilateral involvement of aphasia	Conversational expression, object naming, reading
Aphasia Language Performance Scales (Keenan & Brassell, 1975)		
Sklar Aphasia Scale (Sklar, 1983)	Rating scales of informal interview and five 25-item subtests	Auditory decoding, oral and graphic encoding

Intervention Planning

Once we have determined the diagnosis of aphasia, we need to decide whether treatment is indicated. A summary of the decision-making process once the diagnosis is established is given in **Table 4–5**. We also want to consider the time post-onset of the aphasia. Treatment in the acute stage can maximize recovery potential, but treatment beyond the

Table 4–5 Hierarchy of Client Management Questions for Use After the Diagnosis Is Established

1. Is the client medically stable?

    YES: Proceed to Question 2.

    NO: Will ongoing assessment contribute to the medical management of the client?

    (1) If no, recheck after an appropriate interval.

    (2) If yes, continue with periodic reassessments.

2. Is the client entering a period of rapid recovery?

    YES: Initiate treatment to facilitate improvement.

    NO: Proceed to Question 3.

3. Is the client at the peak of communication abilities with expected future decrease in function?

    YES: Initiate appropriate education or intervention program.

    NO: Proceed to Question 4.

4. Is the client experiencing psychiatric or psychological complications?

    YES: Refer to appropriate services.

    NO: Proceed to Question 5.

5. Could a course of intervention significantly alter the person's level of productivity?

    YES: Initiate appropriate treatment.

    NO: No direct treatment indicated; consider support or maintenance program.

From Johnson, George & Hinckley, 1998.

spontaneous recovery period can also have important effects (Robey, 1998).

Once we have determined that treatment is indicated, we consider the factors that determine the type and frequency of treatment. Some aphasia treatment approaches are based on determination of the initial aphasia assessment. For example, some treatments are particularly designed for Wernicke's aphasia, or the syntactic deficits observed in Broca's agrammatic aphasia (Helm-Estabrooks & Albert, 1991). The theoretical orientation driving this approach to assessment and treatment is most consistent with the structuralist view.

In a functionalist approach, the clinician emphasizes the psycholinguistic and cognitive characteristics of the individual as some of the most important aspects for determining the nature of the intervention. In this approach, a detailed assessment of the cognitive-linguistic system helps to pinpoint the specific breakdowns in the language system. The Psycholinguistic Assessment of Language Processing in Aphasia (PAL:PA; Kay, Lesser, & Coltheart, 1992) is an example of a set of tasks designed for this purpose.

In a social approach to aphasia, the clinician emphasizes the functional and social consequences of the aphasia. Therefore, additional assessment tools that can provide a profile of typical communication activities or social activities would be utilized. Examples of assessment tools that might be used for further informing choices about the type of intervention are listed in **Table 4–6**.

Unfortunately, none of these theoretical approaches addresses the amount or frequency of therapy that would be maximally beneficial. For individuals with severe aphasia, more treatment will likely be provided. However, we need to consider the functional changes that come with the intervention. Individuals with mild aphasia may be able to communicate sufficiently for basic survival, but additional intervention may make the difference between a nonproductive lifestyle in the future and return to gainful employment or other productive activities.

Table 4–6 Assessment Tools Appropriate for Intervention Planning in Aphasia

Assessment Tool	Description	Examples of Tasks
Psycholinguistic Assessment of Language Processing in Aphasia (PALPA) (Kay, Lesser, & Coltheart, 1992)	Series of 60 individual subtests, recommends other subtests based on subtest performance, pinpoints loci of communication breakdown	Pointing Span for Noun-Verb Sequences (60); Spelling-Sound Regularity Reading Task (35); Nonword Spelling (45)
Revised Token Test (McNeil & Prescott, 1978)	Assesses auditory comprehension; 10 subtest mean scores, measures performance changes	Shapes of various colors and sizes are manipulated according to series of verbal commands
Boston Naming Test (Kaplan, Goodglass, & Weintraub, 1983)	Present 60 drawn pictures of items, uses various error codes and cuing	Labeling 60 pictured items
Boston Assessment of Severe Aphasia (Helm-Estabrooks, Ramsberger, Morgan, & Nicholas, 1989)	Assesses comprehension and expression, rating scale for verbal or gestural responses	Praxis, reading comprehension, auditory comprehension
Discourse Comprehension Test (Brookshire & Nicholas, 1993)	Reading or auditory comprehension of narratives	Patient answers yes/no questions about the narratives
Raven Colored Progressive Matrices (Raven, 1976)	Three sets of 12 responses; does not require verbal responses, assesses cognitive functioning	Each colored stimuli is patterned with a missing block, patient points to choices that complete the pattern
Cognitive-Linguistic Quick Test (Helm-Estabrooks, 2001)	Assesses five cognitive domains and gives composite severity score, verbal and nonverbal portions	Symbol cancellation, story retelling, clock generation

Frequency of treatment is generally dictated by reimbursement schedules; however, many individuals decide to pay privately for additional treatment by attending private practice clinics, university clinics, or aphasia centers. More treatment is associated with greater improvement. Furthermore, some subset of individuals with aphasia (about 20–25%) may be appropriate for intensive aphasia treatment, such as individual or group speech–language therapy a few hours a day. Individuals who are appropriate for intensive treatment are medically stable, have the cognitive and psychological stamina to participate in such a regimen, and have the social support that will aid them in completing the treatment course (Legh-Smith, Denis, Enderby, Wade, & Langton-Hewer, 1987).

Determining Prognosis

Prognosis is based on several demographic factors, as well as characteristics of the nature of the injury, the aphasia type and severity, and the general cognitive status of the patient. Some of this information may come from the case history and interview, and other information is derived from the clinician's initial assessment. An example of a checklist that aids in determining prognosis is given in **Table 4–7**. This checklist

Table 4–7 Prognostic Factors in Aphasia

Factor	Better Prognosis	Poorer Prognosis
Time post-onset	Less than 6 months	More than 6 months
Lesion type	Smaller, single, unilateral	Larger, multiple, bilateral
Type of aphasia	Anomic, conduction, transcortical	Global
Overall severity	Mild	Severe
Overall cognitive abilities	Relatively preserved	Relatively impaired
Initiation of treatment	Early post-onset	Later post-onset
Amount of treatment	More	Less

includes several critical factors that have been determined to contribute to prognosis.

Measuring Outcomes

Any course of intervention should end with the measurement of appropriate outcomes. Outcomes are changes in performance over a period of time that might be associated with treatment. Outcomes can be categorized by the time period that they reflect: intermediate, instrumental, and ultimate (Frattali, 1998). Intermediate outcomes are those that occur at the end of a session and help us to determine whether treatment should continue. Instrumental outcomes are those that help the client continue to learn even after treatment has ended. Ultimate outcomes relate to the social validity of the intervention, and might include measures such as return to gainful employment or community reintegration.

Outcomes can be measured on standardized aphasia batteries; however, there may not be a close relationship between performance on these measures and change in functional abilities (Irwin et al, 2002). As a result, it is important to consider functional outcomes, and to attend to the ultimate outcomes of our treatment. Functional assessment tools, including measures of community reintegration, return to employment, or other measures of ultimate outcome (Hinckley, 2002), are important ways for us to assess the value of our intervention services. **Table 4–8** gives examples of functional assessment tools.

✦ Conclusion

This chapter has presented the theoretical and conceptual foundations of assessment in aphasia. Principles and techniques for accomplishing the goals of assessment, including differential diagnosis, intervention planning, determining prognosis, and measuring outcomes, have been outlined.

Table 4–8   Examples of Functional Communication Assessment Tools in Aphasia

Assessment Tool	Description	Examples of Tasks
Communication Abilities in Daily Living (Holland, Frattali, & Fromm, 1999)	Measures functional, everyday communication skills, 3-point scale for each item	Role-playing a doctor's office visit, filling out forms, writing a grocery list
Communicative Effectiveness Index (Lomas et al, 1989)	16 statements regarding patient abilities in daily activities as ranked by caregiver	16 questions with scale lines, caregiver marks "X" on line, rating patient abilities
Discourse Abilities Profile (Terrell & Ripich, 1989)	Videotape session, rate discourse performance overall, checklist of absent or present feature	Examines spontaneous speech output for narrative, procedural, and conversational tasks
ASHA Functional Assessment of Communication Skills (FACS) (Frattali, Thompson, Holland, Wohl, & Ferketic, 1995)	Rates impairment effect on everyday activities of living	Examines four domains: reading, social communication, daily planning
Discourse Comprehension Test (Brookshire & Nicholas, 1993)		
Pragmatic protocol (Prutting & Kirchner, 1983)	Examines three different areas, judge behaviors appropriate/inappropriate	Utterance acts, propositional acts, illocutionary acts
Quantitative Production Analysis (Saffran, Berndt, & Schwartz, 1989)	Analysis of narrative production from taped session	Structural analysis, lexical content, total sentences
Correct Information Unit analysis (Nicholas & Brookshire, 1993)	Analysis of narrative production from taped session, concerned with content units and accuracy	Rules for counting content units, with examples, and for counting total words
Content unit analysis (Craig et al, 1992; Yorkston & Beukelman, 1980)	Obtain language sample using "cookie theft" picture, analyze content and efficiency of speech	Assign content units, syllables per minute, content units per minute

Study Questions

1. Compare and contrast the three theoretical orientations to aphasia, and state one diagnostic tool that belongs to that orientation.

2. List and define the three classifications of the World Health Organization.

3. How do reliability, validity, and standardization of assessment tools affect our diagnoses?

4. What considerations should the speech–language pathologist make to effectively conduct assessments of aphasia?

5. How do the three theoretical orientations to aphasia relate to treatment approaches?

6. What are the three types of outcomes that can be measured? Why is it important to measure outcomes?

7. List prognostic indicators used in aphasia to determine prognosis.

References

American Speech–Language-Hearing Association (2005) Background Information and Implementation for the Certificate of Clinical Competence in SLP. Rockville, MD

Baltes, P.B. (1993). The Aging Mind: Potential and Limits. *Gerontologist, 33,* 5, 580–594

Benton, A., deS. Hampsher, K., Sivian, A. (1994). *Multilingual Aphasia Examination* (3rd ed.) Lutz, FL: Psychological Assessment Resources, Inc

Bonita, R. (1992). The Epidemiology of Stroke. *Lancet, 339,* 342–344

Brookshire, R., & Nicholas, L. (1993) *Discourse Comprehension Test.* Tucson, AZ: Communication Skills Builders

Chatterjee, A. & Maher, L. (2000). Grammar and Agrammatism. In: S.E. Nadeau, L.J. Gonzalez Rothi & B. Crosson (Eds.), *Aphasia and Language: Theory to Practice.* New York: Guilford Press

Craig, H.K., Hinckley, J. J., Winkelseth, M., Carry, L., Walley, J., Bardach, L., Higman, B., Hilfinger, P., Schall, C. and Sheimo, D. (1993). Quantifying connected speech sample of adults with chronic severe aphasia. *Aphasiology, 7,* pp. 155–163

Crosson, B. (2000). Systems that support language processes: Attention. In: S.E. Nadeau, L.J. Gonzalez Rothi & B. Crosson (Eds.), *Aphasia and Language: Theory to Practice.* New York: Guilford Press

David, R.M. & Skilbeck, C.E. (1984). Raven IQ and Language Recovery Following Stroke. *Journal of Clinical Neuropsychology, 6,* 302–308

Davis, G.A. (2000). *Aphasiology.* Boston: Allyn & Bacon

Druks, J. (2002). Verbs and Nouns—A Review of the Literature. *Journal of Neurolinguistics, 15,* 289–319

Eisenson, J. (1994). *Examining for aphasia* (3rd ed) Austin, TX: Pro-Ed, Inc.

Fabbro, F. (2001). The Bilingual Brain: Bilingual Aphasia. *Brain & Language, 79,* 201–210

Fischler, I. (2000). Attention, Resource Allocation, and Language. In: S.E. Nadeau, L.J. Gonzalez Rothi & B. Crosson (Eds.), *Aphasia and Language: Theory to Practice.* New York: Guilford Press

Fitch-West, J., & Sands, E. (1998). *Bedside Evaluation and Screening Test of Aphasia* (2nd ed.). Austin, TX: Pro-Ed, Inc.

Frattali, C.M. (1998). Outcomes Measurement: Definitions, Dimensions, and Perspectives. In: Frattali, C.M. (Ed.), *Measuring Outcomes in Speech-Language Pathology.* New York: Thieme

Frattali, C, Thompson, C., Holland, A., Wohl, C, & Ferketic, M. (1995). *American Speech–Language-Hearing Association. Functional assessment of communication skills for adults.* Rockville, MD: ASHA

Fridriksson, J., Holland, A. L., Coull, B. M., Plante, E., Trouard, T. P., & Beeson, P. (2002). Aphasia Severity: Association with Cerebral Perfusion and Diffusion. *Aphasiology, 16,* 859–871

Gagnon, D.A. & Martin, N. (2002). Diagnosis, Prognosis, and Remediation of Acquired Naming Disorders from a Connectionist Perspective. In: Daniloff, R.G. (Ed.), *Connectionist Approaches to Clinical Problems in Speech and Language* (pp. 147–188). Mahwah, NJ: Lawrence Erlbaum

Godefroy, O., Dubois, C. Debachy, B., Leclerc, M., Kreisler, A. (2002). Vascular Aphasias: Main Characteristics of Patients Hospitalized in Acute Stroke Units. *Stroke, 33,* 702–705

Goodglass, H., Kaplan, E., & Barresi, B. (2000). *Boston Diagnostic Aphasia Examination* (3rd ed.). Philadelphia: Lea & Febinger

Helm-Estabrooks, N. (1992). *Aphasia Diagnostic Profiles.* Austin, TX: Pro-Ed, Inc.

Helm-Estabrooks, N. (2001). *Cognitive Linguistic Quick Test.* San Antonio, TX: The Psychological Corporation

Helm-Estabrooks, N. (2002). Cognition and Aphasia: A Discussion and a Study. *Journal of Communication Disorders, 35,* 171–186

Helm-Estabrooks, N. & Albert, M.L. (1991). *Manual of Aphasia Therapy.* Austin, TX: Pro-Ed

Helm-Estabrooks, N., Remsberger, G., Morgan, A., & Nicholas, M. (1989). *Boston assessment of severe aphasia.* Austin, TX: Pro-Ed, Inc.

Hillis, A.E. (2001). Cognitive Neuropsychological Approaches to Rehabilitation of Language Disorders: Introduction. In: Chapey, R. (Ed.), *Language Intervention Strategies in Aphasia and Related Neurogenic Communication Disorders* (pp. 513–523). Philadelphia: Lippincott Williams & Wilkins

Hinckley, J.J. (2002). Vocational and Social Outcomes of Adults with Chronic Aphasia. *Journal of Communication Disorders, 35,* 543–560

Holland, A., Frattali, C., & Fromm, D. (1999). *Communicative Activities of Daily Living-2.* Austin, TX: Pro-Ed, Inc.

Irwin, W.H., Wertz, R.T., & Avent, J.R. (2002). Relationships Among Language Impairment, Functional Communication, and Pragmatic Performance in Aphasia. *Aphasiology, 16,* 823–835

Johnson A.F., George K.P., Hinckley, J. Assessment (1998). In A.F. Johnson & B.H. Jacobson (Eds.) Medical Speech–Language Pathology: A Practitioner's Guide (1st ed.) New York: Thieme

Kalplan, E., Goodglass, H., & Weintraub, S. (1983). *Boston Naming Test* (2nd ed.). Philadelphia: Lea & Febinger

Kay, J., Lesser, R., & Coltheart, M. (1992). *Psycholinguistic Assessments of Language Processing in Aphasia.* East Sussex, UK: Psychology Press

Keenan, J., & Brassell, E. (1975). *Aphasia Language Performance Scales.* Murfressboro, TN: Pinnacle Press

Kertesz, A. (1982). *Western Aphasia Battery.* San Antonio, TX: Psychological Corporation

Laska, A.C., Hellblom, A., Murray, V., Kahan, T., & Von Arbin, M. (2001). Aphasia in Acute Stroke and Relation to Outcome. *Journal of Internal Medicine, 249,* 413–422

Legh-Smith, J.A., Denis, R., Enderby, P.M., Wade, D.T. & Langton-Hewer, R. (1987). Selection of Aphasic Stroke Patients for Intensive Speech Therapy. *Journal of Neurology, Neurosurgery, and Psychiatry, 50,* 1488–1492

Lomas, J., Pickard, L, Bester, S., Elbard, H., Finlayson, A., & Zoghaib, C. (1989). The communicative effectiveness index: Development and psychometric evaluation of a functional communication measure for adult aphasia. *Journal of Speech and Hearing Disorders, 54,* 113–124

Lum, C. (2002). *Scientific Thinking in Speech and Language Therapy.* Mahwah, NJ: Lawrence Erlbaum

McNeil, M. R., & Prescott, T.E. (1978). *Revised Token Test.* Austin, TX: Pro-Ed, Inc.

Murray, L.L. & Chapey, R. (2001. Assessment of Language Disorders in Adults. In: Chapey, R. (Ed.), *Language Intervention Strategies in Aphasia and Related Neurogenic Communication Disorders* (pp. 55–126). Philadelphia: Lippincott Williams & Wilkins

Nicholas, L., & Brookshire, R. (1993). A system for quantifying the informativeness and efficiency of connected speech in adults with aphasia. *Journal of Speech and Hearing Research, 36,* 338–350

Orgass, B., & Poeck, K. (1969). Assessment of aphasia by psychometric methods. *Cortex 5* (4), 317–330

Paradis, M. (1987). *The assessment of bilingual aphasia.* Hillsdale, NJ: Lawrence Erlbaum Associates

Prutting, C., & Kirchner, D. (1983). Applied pragmatics. In T. Gallagher and C. Prutting (Eds.), *Pragmatic assessment and intervention issues in language* (pp. 28–64). San Diego, CA: College-Hills Press, Inc.

Purdy, M. (2002). Executive Function Ability in Persons with Aphasia. *Aphasiology, 16,* 4–6, 549–557

Raven, J. (1976). *Coloured Progressive Matrices.* Los Angeles, CA: Western Psychological Services

Robey, R.R. (1998). A Meta-Analysis of Clinical Outcomes in the Treatment of Aphasia. *Journal of Speech, Language, and Hearing Research, 41,* 172–187

Saffran, E., Berndt, R., & Schwartz, M. (1989). The quantitative analysis of agrammatic production: Procedure and data. *Brain and Language, 37,* 440–479

Sarno, M.T., Buonaguro, A. & Levita, E. (1967). Characteristics of verbal impairment in closed head injury. *Arch of physical medicine & Rehab.* (67b) year 4. Aphasia in Closed Head Injury and Stroke. *Aphasiology, 1,* 331–338

Schuell, H. (1965). *The Minnesota Test for Differential Diagnosis of Aphasia.* Minneapolis, MN: University of Minnesota Press

Simmons-Mackie, N. (2001). Social Approaches to Aphasia Intervention. In: Chapey, R. (Ed.), *Language Intervention Strategies in Aphasia and Related Neurogenic Communication Disorders* (pp. 246–266). Philadelphia: Lippincott Williams & Wilkins

Sklar, M. (1983). *Sklar Aphasia Scale Revised.* Los Angeles, CA: Western Psychological Services

Spreen, O. & Risser, A.H. (1998). Assessment of Aphasia. In: M.T. Sarno (Ed.), *Acquired Aphasia,* 3rd ed. (pp. 71–156). New York: Academic Press

Terrell, B., & Ripich, D. (1989). Discourse competence as a variable in intervention. *Seminars in Speech and Language, 10* (4), 282–297

Thompson, C.K. (2001). Treatment of Underlying Forms: A Linguistic Specific Approach for Sentence Production Deficits in Agrammatic Aphasia. In: Chapey, R. (Ed.), *Language Intervention Strategies in Aphasia and Related Neurogenic Communication Disorders* (pp. 605–628). Philadelphia: Lippincott Williams & Wilkins

World Health Organization. (2001). International Classification of Functioning, Disability, and Health: ICF. Geneva: WHO

Yorkston, K., & Beukelman, D. (1980). An analysis of connected speech samples of asphasic and normal speakers. *Journal of Speech and Hearing Disorders, 45,* 27–36

5

Aphasia Rehabilitation: Postacute Clinical Management

Margaret Greenwald and Chad McCarney

✦ **Perspectives on Aphasia Rehabilitation**
✦ **Aphasia Rehabilitation for Individuals: Evidence-Based Practice**
✦ **Planning Aphasia Rehabilitation for Stroke Survivor Groups**

Note: This chapter addresses several areas of knowledge and skill identified by the American Speech–Language–Hearing Association as standard competencies for the Certificate of Clinical Competence in Speech–Language Pathology (ASHA, 2000). Specifically, this chapter relays knowledge in the areas of normal language processes (Standard III-B), acquired language disorders (Standard III-C), and principles and methods of assessment and treatment of individuals with acquired language disorders (Standard III-D).

This chapter is an overview of current principles and methods for rehabilitation of adult patients with acquired aphasia. The focus of this chapter is on management of aphasia in postacute clinical settings (for a discussion of rehabilitation in acute care settings, see Chapter 19). Current evidence-based approaches to aphasia treatment and management are emphasized, with illustrations of patient examples and the practical clinical decisions involved in designing treatment for individuals and patient groups.

✦ Perspectives on Aphasia Rehabilitation

Adults with acquired aphasia have impaired language skills secondary to neurologic injury or disease affecting the central nervous system (CNS), for example, cerebrovascular accident (CVA) or traumatic brain injury (TBI). Normal language can break down in varied and complex ways, yet patterns of similarity do emerge among aphasia patients that provide clues to the underlying source of impairment and to promising treatment approaches. The goal of aphasia rehabilitation is to assist patients, within the context of their environment and the type and extent of CNS damage, to reach their full potential in communication. Toward this end, the speech-language pathologist tailors treatment approaches to the

unique communication needs and concerns of each aphasia patient.

Classifications of "Functioning" and "Disability"

The World Health Organization's International Classification of Functioning, Disability, and Health (ICF; World Health Organization, 2001) is a framework for defining patient needs that may be addressed specifically in rehabilitation. The ICF includes codes defining language abilities and activity and participation codes that allow the clinician to report the range of effects that aphasia has on a patient's life, and potential improvements in life participation following aphasia treatment. These life participation concepts have been included in the American Speech–Language–Hearing Association (ASHA) revised Scope of Practice for Speech–language Pathology (ASHA, 2001). Aphasia rehabilitation focuses on one or more of the following interrelated aspects of aphasia: (1) cognitive-linguistic impairment; (2) resulting decline in skill areas of language (e.g., reading, comprehension, naming); and (3) the real-life effects of reduced language skill.

The Role of the Speech–Language Pathologist

Ideally, the speech–language pathologist (SLP) is prepared to assume the following roles in providing optimal patient care:

1. Communication partner. Knowledge of the patient's underlying aphasia allows the clinician to listen and to respond to the patient with particular sensitivity to communication cues and strategies that may be beneficial. Additionally, the clinician is attentive to spoken and unspoken cues that may indicate the patient's emotional state during communication attempts, and his/her goals and expectations for the therapy process.

Table 5–1 Evolution of Aphasia Subtypes: General Pattern of Improved Auditory Comprehension

	Nonfluent Aphasias: Auditory Comprehension		Fluent Aphasias: Auditory Comprehension	
	Poor	Good	Poor	Good
Repetition				
Poor	Global	Broca's	Wernicke's	Conduction
Good	Transcortical (TC) mixed	TC motor	TC sensory	Anomic

2. Diagnostician. An accurate diagnosis of the cognitive-linguistic deficits that characterize different forms of aphasia is the basis for treatment planning, and is important for educating stroke survivors, family members, and clinical staff about the communication strengths and weaknesses of the individual.

3. Therapist. Use of evidence-based or theory-driven treatments may increase the likelihood of treatment effectiveness in any given patient. When appropriate, the clinician may include other stroke survivors, family members, and clinical staff in the therapy process.

4. Researcher. Every clinician must evaluate the effectiveness of one treatment approach over another and document the treatment results; thus, there is no necessary division between clinician and researcher. Much will be gained from increased reporting of treatment results by clinicians in professional forums.

5. Educator/advocate. A variety of situations may arise in which the clinician can act in the role of advocate for the individual with aphasia. For example, the SLP plays an important role in educating clinical staff about the individual's aphasia and in advocating proper discharge planning. The clinician can also be an advocate for the stroke survivor in the community, for example, supporting the efforts of an individual to return to paid or volunteer work if appropriate, or assisting aphasia support groups. The SLP is able to offer ongoing patient and family education about ways to manage the effects of aphasia in many aspects of life participation.

The Continuum of Care and Aphasia Evolution

The approach to aphasia rehabilitation necessarily varies with the stroke survivor's stage of recovery and the setting in which intervention occurs. The SLP may be involved in providing care for individuals with aphasia at one or more of the following stages of recovery: acute care (acute hospital); subacute care (extended care facility); inpatient rehabilitation (rehabilitation hospital or unit); home care (patient's home); and outpatient rehabilitation (rehabilitation center). The aphasia rehabilitation methods we discuss in this chapter can apply to one or more of the postacute stages of recovery. In postacute settings, rehabilitation services often are implemented by multidisciplinary teams in which the SLP interacts closely with professionals in rehabilitation medicine, neurology, occupational therapy, physical therapy, nursing, neuropsychology, and social work in coordinating patient care.

In the early stages of aphasia recovery, treatment tasks aimed at facilitating restoration of language function (i.e., restitutive approaches) may maximize neurophysiologic recovery of normal language processes (Rothi, 1995). Compensatory (i.e., substitutive) communication strategies such as the use of a pointing board also may be employed in these early stages to maximize functional communication and to alleviate frustration on the part of the patient. These substitutive strategies typically become the focus of aphasia treatment in late stages of recovery, when the potential for neurophysiologic recovery is reduced.

In postacute aphasia rehabilitation and recovery, an individual's aphasia often evolves from one traditional subtype to another (Kertesz, 1979). This evolution of classification is based on relative improvement in fluency, auditory comprehension, and/or repetition ability. Of these three areas, improved auditory comprehension is likely to have the most functional benefit in daily life, as it increases patients' ability not only to comprehend the spoken messages of others but also possibly to detect and self-correct their own verbal errors (Duffy & Coelho, 2001; Schuell, 1953; but see Maher, Rothi & Heilman, 1994) (**Table 5–1**). Anomia is a feature of all aphasia subtypes, and anomic aphasia may persist despite the evolution of other aphasia symptoms (Kertesz, 1979) (**Table 5–1**).

The significance of aphasia evolution from a rehabilitation perspective is that the clinician must be flexible in modifying treatment goals and in systematically altering the difficulty level of treatment tasks to meet the current needs of the individual. As a patient's aphasia evolves, new therapy issues and concerns arise. For example, although improving auditory comprehension is a positive sign of evolution from Wernicke's aphasia to conduction aphasia, patients at this stage of recovery are likely to experience increased frustration as they begin to notice their own speech errors and to attempt self-correction. It is also important to note that the underlying aphasia subtype may remain the same even when the individual's functional communication improves significantly as a result of treatment. For example, a patient with anomic aphasia may remain anomic, but may learn effective strategies to compensate for the anomia.

✦ Aphasia Rehabilitation for Individuals: Evidence-Based Practice

Cognitive-linguistic impairments that underlie reduced language skill in aphasia can be linked to specific sources of disruption within the normal language system. Normal language is generally thought to involve interactive subcomponents that support comprehension via multiple input modalities (e.g., spoken words, pictures, gestures, written words, tactile input, environmental sounds), and that support expression through various output modes (e.g., speaking, drawing, gesturing, writing) (Caramazza, Hillis, Rapp, & Romani, 1990). Detailed discussion of models of single-word processing is beyond the scope of this chapter. Sample evidence-based approaches to treatment for impairments of language comprehension and expression are discussed below.

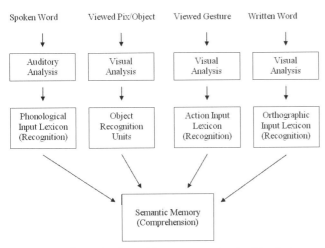

Spoken Word   Viewed Pix/Object   Viewed Gesture   Written Word

| Auditory Analysis | Visual Analysis | Visual Analysis | Visual Analysis |

| Phonological Input Lexicon (Recognition) | Object Recognition Units | Action Input Lexicon (Recognition) | Orthographic Input Lexicon (Recognition) |

Semantic Memory (Comprehension)

Figure 5–1 Schematic of cognitive processes involved in single-word comprehension (Adapted from Caramazza et al., 1990).

Table 5–2 Manipulating Difficulty of Sample Comprehension Tasks: Array Size and Semantic Relatedness

Category sorting (listed in increasing task difficulty)

Sort stimuli into distant semantic categories (e.g., transportation versus food)

Sort stimuli into close semantic categories (e.g., fruits versus vegetables)

Sort stimuli within semantic category (e.g., winter versus summer clothing)

Matching tasks (listed in increasing task difficulty)

Direct match of word to its picture (e.g., match "horse" to HORSE)

    Given 2 choices: target and 1 unrelated foil

    Given 3 or more choices: target and 2 or more unrelated foils

    Given 2 choices: target and 1 semantically related foil

    Given 3 or more choices: target and 2 or more semantically related foils

Match word to its semantic associate (e.g., match "horse" to SADDLE)

Rehabilitation of Single-Word Comprehension

Rehabilitation of comprehension impairment can be targeted to the general skill area affected (e.g., reading comprehension), or to the more detailed cognitive-linguistic component(s) affected (reference). **Figure 5–1** is a schematic of cognitive processes thought to be involved in comprehension of single words through various input modalities. Within this framework, normal comprehension occurs following perception of a stimulus, recognition of the stimulus as familiar (at the level of the input lexicon or object recognition units), and activation of its meaning within semantic memory (Riddoch, Humphreys, Coltheart, & Funnell, 1988). When semantic memory is disrupted, comprehension from all input modalities is impaired. Alternatively, comprehension can be disrupted from only one input modality in the context of normal comprehension via other modalities (Franklin, Turner, Ralph, Morris, & Bailey, 1996) (**Fig. 5–1**).

Rehabilitation of Impaired Semantic Memory

Poor comprehension due to impaired semantic memory is generally thought to result from poor activation of the semantic features that differentiate one single word concept from another (Rapp & Goldrick, 2000). Individuals with semantic memory impairment may be able to comprehend the general semantic category of a word (e.g., *animal*) though they are unable to comprehend more specific details of meaning that distinguish the target word (e.g., *zebra*) from a semantically related word (e.g., *giraffe*). The individual with semantic memory deficit may benefit from a variety of treatment tasks that require activation of semantic features (Behrmann & Lieberthal, 1989; Byng, Kay, Edmundson, & Scott, 1990; Grayson, Hilton, & Franklin, 1997; Ochipa, Maher, & Raymer, 1998). In general, the difficulty of a semantic task increases with the semantic relatedness of choices presented and with increasing number of choices (**Table 5–2**).

Semantic treatment tasks have included matching to definition, making yes/no judgments about the semantic features of target words, category sorting, and matching tasks (**Table 5–2**). Matching tasks can incorporate various combinations of stimuli across modality (e.g., spoken word-to-picture, spoken word-to-written word, picture-to-written word, gesture-to-picture). Comprehension treatment may begin with the least demanding semantic distinctions and may build to include closely related semantic distractors (e.g., the target *RABBIT* versus *mouse*) or matching of semantic associates (e.g., match the target *RABBIT* to choice of *CARROT, butter*, or *bread*) (Howard & Patterson, 1992).

An individual with a profound comprehension deficit may be unable to perform even the least difficult of the semantic tasks above, despite extensive modeling. In this case, the clinician can probe the patient's ability to perform the more basic task of matching two identical objects presented with one unrelated distractor (e.g., two cups and a pencil). If patients are unable to work at this more basic level when assessed across several sessions, they may not be ready to participate in language treatment. However, with aphasia evolution, this task is a possible starting point for comprehension treatment during the following weeks or months.

Rehabilitation of Modality-Specific Comprehension Deficits

Modality-specific comprehension impairment requires specific focus on tasks that facilitate semantic activation from the impaired modality. Treatment focusing on phonemic processing tasks led to improved comprehension via phonologic input in a patient with impaired auditory comprehension arising from prelexical phonologic disruption (Morris, Franklin, Ellis, Turner, & Bailey, 1996). Treatment aimed at encouraging analysis of characteristic visual features of objects may facilitate comprehension in individuals with impaired visual word recognition (Greenwald, Raymer, Richardson, & Rothi, 1995; Zihl, 2000). Gesture comprehension may be facilitated by having the patient match the clinician's gesture to a choice of objects or pictures (e.g., match the gesture denoting *DRINK* to a cup). Patients with poor comprehension in general may benefit from visual action therapy (VAT; Helm-Estabrooks, Fitzpatrick, & Barresi, 1982), a systematic nonverbal program aimed at facilitating gesture comprehension and production. Treatment focusing on access to semantic features via written word stimuli would be appropriate for individuals with modality-specific comprehension impairment from written words (e.g., Greenwald & Berndt, 1999). A variety of treatment approaches for acquired reading impairment are discussed below.

Compensatory Strategies for Improved Comprehension

Compensatory techniques can be introduced at various stages in recovery to meet the immediate needs of the person with aphasia. For example, an individual with poor comprehension in the auditory modality may be assisted with a communication board containing pictures or written words to aid comprehension. Gesture comprehension is often a useful treatment goal for a person whose comprehension is impaired through other input modalities. In this case, the clinician would incorporate gesture into all communicative interactions with the patient, train family members and clinical staff in the use of the same gestures, and facilitate the patient's comprehension of gestures through structured therapy tasks, as described above.

Patients with right hemisphere lesions may not exhibit the lexical-semantic deficits described above, but nevertheless may have difficulty with many forms of comprehension. Right hemisphere damage can disrupt comprehension of the central themes of discourse, connotative word meanings, figurative language, inferences, humor, and emotional and linguistic prosody (Myers & Brookshire, 1996). Specific suggestions for treatment of right hemisphere comprehension deficits are provided by Myers (1998).

Rehabilitation of Single-Word Expression

As depicted in a theoretical language model (**Fig. 5–2**), the ability to express a written or spoken name requires activation of the concept within semantic memory, and subsequent activation of the output lexicon wherein abstract word forms are retrieved for spoken or written language. In addition to this activation of whole-word forms at the lexical level, reading or spelling can be accomplished via sublexical conversion from grapheme to phoneme (reading) or from phoneme to grapheme (spelling). Irregularly spelled words (e.g., *yacht*) can be processed correctly only via lexical activation, whereas nonsense words (e.g., *flig*) are processed sublexically. Lexical or sublexical information presumably is held in working

memory during subsequent motor programming for expression (e.g., Martin & Freedman, 2001). Semantic concepts can also be expressed through gesture and drawing, which may become critical modes of expression for aphasia patients who have expressive impairments in the verbal and written modes (**Fig. 5–2**).

Rehabilitation of Impaired Naming

Disruption of word retrieval can affect oral naming, written naming, or both. A brief summary of treatment approaches for anomia is provided in **Table 5–3**. Individuals who produce semantically related errors in naming tasks (e.g., "chair" for TABLE) have imprecise activation of semantic features within semantic memory, disrupted egress of semantic information to the output lexicon(s), or possible damage to the output lexicon itself (Caramazza & Hillis, 1990). When written naming and verbal naming are similarly impaired, it is likely that the source of impairment is within semantic memory or in egress from semantic memory (**Table 5–3**).

Many studies of naming treatment have paired semantic treatment with activation of the output mode (i.e., phonologic or graphemic) through tasks of oral or written naming (Nickels & Best, 1996). Studies of patients with both semantic and phonologic impairment suggest that semantic comprehension tasks may be most effective when combined with phonologic output tasks in these patients (Drew & Thompson, 1999; LeDorze, Boulay, Gaudreau, & Brassard, 1994).

Anomia stemming from impaired retrieval of phonologic lexical forms for output (i.e., the phonologic output lexicon) has been addressed through treatments focusing on phonologic training, through phonologic cuing hierarchies (Greenwald et al., 1995; Hillis, 1993; Raymer, Thompson, Jacobs, & LeGrand, 1993), judgments about the phonologic information for words (e.g., initial phoneme, number of syllables) (Robson, Marshall, Pring, Chiat, 1998), or phonologic rehearsal (Mitchum & Berndt, 1994). A combination of semantic and phonologic tasks may facilitate improved naming in some patients (Marshall, Pring, & Chiat, 1998). Patients with good repetition ability may be

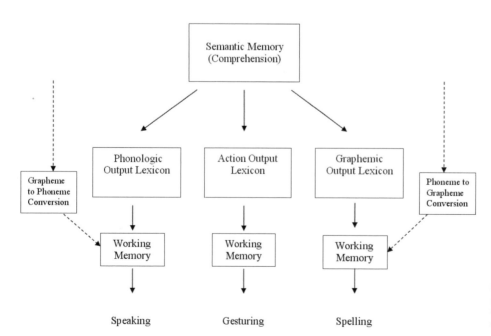

Figure 5–2 Schematic of cognitive processes involved in single-word expression (Adapted from Caramazza et al., 1990).

Table 5–3 Treatment for Impaired Word Retrieval (i.e., Anomia)

Role of the Speech–Language Pathologist (SLP)	Clinical Issues
Communication partner	How does the patient attempt to communicate when unable to name verbally? What is the patient's level of frustration when s/he is unable to retrieve a word?
Diagnostician	Compare oral naming versus written naming.
	1. If both are impaired in similar fashion, and comprehension is also impaired, a central semantic deficit is likely.
	2. If both are impaired in similar fashion, and comprehension is NOT impaired, a semantic "egress" deficit is likely.
	3. Or, only one naming mode may be impaired.
Therapist	*Patient A:* central semantic impairment; or *Patient B:* semantic egress deficit
	Both patients are likely to benefit from semantic treatment aimed at facilitating the ability to distinguish among increasingly close semantic features. Adding tasks of oral or written naming may increase the effectiveness of semantic tasks.
	Patient C: Oral naming deficit
	Patient may benefit from phonologic rehearsal, the use of phonologic cuing hierarchies, or combined semantic-phonologic treatment.
	Patient D: Written naming deficit
	Direct training of whole-word graphemic forms can be provided via item-specific practice, anagram and copy treatment, or homophone spelling.

candidates for treatment programs incorporating repetition (Greenwald et al., 1995), whereas patients with poor repetition ability may be better served through treatment programs that train phonologic awareness or semantic self-cuing strategies without requiring the patient to repeat. Treatment aimed at improving repetition ability alone would have no functional justification, because repetition is not a functional means of everyday communication.

When written naming is impaired relative to oral naming, treatment focusing on retrieval of lexical graphemic forms for output may be needed (i.e., treatment of the graphemic output lexicon). Unlike regularly spelled words, irregularly spelled words can only be spelled correctly via this lexical-semantic route; therefore, treatments of lexical graphemic output have focused on training of irregular word spelling (Hillis & Caramazza, 1987). Several effective treatment approaches for lexical graphemic impairment have been reported, including those focusing on item-specific training (Hillis & Caramazza, 1987), anagram and copy treatment (ACT; Beeson, 1999), copy and recall treatment (CART; Beeson, 1999), and spelling of homophones (Behrmann, 1987). Because spelling of regularly spelled words also can be accomplished via an alternate route of phoneme-to-grapheme conversion (**Fig. 5–2**), additional treatment approaches to writing and spelling are outlined briefly below.

Frustration commonly accompanies anomia even in its milder forms, and can be reduced in many cases when the clinician provides an alternative means of expression to the patient. For the patient with severely impaired oral naming, the most obvious compensatory strategies may be use of writing, a pointing board, or a notebook containing pictures, letters, or written words. Individuals who are unable to indicate a "yes" or "no" response verbally or through head movements may be able to respond consistently through yes/no practice using gesture or a pointing board. Patients with oral or written anomia of all severity levels may benefit from systematic practice in using alternative means to communicate their intent, as outlined in the therapy approach called "promoting aphasic communicative effectiveness" (PACE; Davis & Wilcox, 1981).

Establishing functional gesture as a viable alternative to naming may require systematic practice using a set of gestures such as Amer-Ind codes, which are easily recognized gestures based on Native American hand talk (Rao, 2001; Skelly, 1979). As noted above, individuals with severe comprehension impairment may be able to learn functional gestures through training with the VAT program (Helm-Estabrooks et al., 1982). When an underlying limb apraxia is present, it is still possible to improve the quality of gesture production through repetitive gesture production and systematic feedback (e.g., Ochipa, Maher, & Rothi, 1995).

Rehabilitation of Impaired Oral Reading

There are many different types of reading disorder that may accompany aphasia, distinguishable by observed error patterns and proficiency in reading regular words, irregular words, and nonsense words (e.g., *jisp*; Rothi, Coslett, & Heilman, 1984). These acquired dyslexias require distinct forms of treatment (**Table 5–4**), and a variety of studies provide evidence for the effectiveness of restitutive and compensatory treatments for specific forms of dyslexia. It is noteworthy, however, that in one study of 55 aphasic patients with acquired dyslexia who were not categorized by dyslexia subtype, computerized reading treatment appeared to improve reading and to facilitate recovery in other areas of language function (Katz & Wertz, 1997).

Letter-by-letter reading is a typical strategy used by patients with pure alexia (i.e., alexia without agraphia). This disorder reflects a more peripheral disorder in accessing lexical word forms in visual word recognition. These patients typically are able to read all types of reading stimuli (regularly spelled, irregularly spelled, high image, low image, nonsense words) with equal performance levels once they spell the stimulus aloud to themselves. A word length effect (predictably longer response times in reading long words versus short words) indicates letter-by-letter reading even when the patient does not name the letters overtly. Treatment of letter-by-letter reading has generally taken two forms: (1) encouraging letter-by-letter reading to make this a more efficient process in patients who have impaired

Table 5–4   Treatment for Impaired Reading

Role of the SLP	Clinical Issues
Communication partner	What is patient's desire/motivation to read? Does patient attempt to read?
Diagnostician	Is silent reading better than oral reading? In oral reading, are particular types of stimuli read better or worse than others (regular/irregular; real words/nonsense words; nouns/verbs/functors; concrete/abstract; long/short words; single words/sentences)?
Therapist	*Patient E:* Letter-by-letter reading: (1) facilitate improved letter-by-letter reading if it is poor; or (2) encourage whole-word residual reading by presenting written word stimuli at rapid speeds.
	Patient F: Deep dyslexia: (1) semantic treatment aimed at facilitating comprehension of written words; or (2) grapheme-to-phoneme conversion training to facilitate reading of regular words and reduce semantic errors by assisting the patient in sounding out the first letter.
	Patient G: Surface dyslexia: train whole-word reading of irregularly spelled words.

letter naming or are slow in letter-by-letter reading (Lott, Friedman, & Linebaugh, 1994); or (2) discouraging letter-by-letter reading as a strategy and assisting the patient in using residual whole-word recognition abilities by requiring the patient to read words presented at rapid exposure durations (speeds at which letter-by-letter reading is not possible) (Gonzalez Rothi & Moss, 1992), or through multiple oral rereading of a text passage (Beeson & Insalaco, 1998) (**Table 5–4**).

Deep dyslexia is characterized by frequent semantic errors in oral reading, as well as poor performance in reading nonsense words. These patients are thought to have one of three general problems involving the semantic system, thus giving rise to many semantic errors: difficulty accessing semantic information from print, degraded semantic memory itself, or difficulty using semantic information to access lexical phonology during oral reading (Coltheart, 1980). Treatment for deep dyslexia has focused on semantic memory, or on facilitation of grapheme-to-phoneme conversion. Treatment focusing directly on impaired semantic memory has incorporated comprehension tasks, such as pointing to the picture corresponding to the written word (Hillis, 1991). Treatment focusing on training grapheme-to-phoneme conversion has facilitated oral reading of regularly spelled words (de Partz, 1986), and reduced the number of semantic errors produced in oral reading (Mitchum & Berndt, 1991).

Surface dyslexia involves relatively good reading of regular words and nonsense words via the sublexical grapheme-to-phoneme route, but poor reading of whole words via the lexical route. Patients with this type of dyslexia have benefited from whole-word lexical treatment, wherein they receive practice in reading irregularly spelled words (Byng & Coltheart, 1986; Friedman & Robinson, 1991; Weekes & Coltheart, 1996).

Cross-cuing strategies may be highly successful with some dyslexic patients. For example, a patient who was completely unable to read from print, but who retained the ability to pronounce words spelled aloud to her, received a successful treatment in which she was taught to name printed letters aloud to self-cue oral reading (Greenwald & Rothi, 1998). A second patient who was unable to read from print demonstrated the retained ability to read if she traced the letters with her finger; this patient doubled her pretreatment reading speed through treatment aimed at maximizing this self-cuing strategy (Maher, Clayton, Barrett, Schober-Peterson, & Rothi, 1998). These are examples of treatment programs based on careful diagnosis by the SLP.

Rehabilitation of Impaired Spelling and Writing

Many patients who have aphasia also have spelling or writing impairments. These may co-occur with reading deficits or in patients with good reading ability. Patients often wish to regain the ability to sign their signature for functional purposes, and writing or spelling can be used as part of a strategy to circumvent verbal anomia or to self-cue verbal naming.

Impaired spelling should be distinguished from impaired writing. Patients may be unable to write correctly for a variety of reasons, including motoric weakness or deficits in motor programming for writing (i.e., apraxic agraphia); however, these patients may have intact linguistic spelling abilities when tested using an alternate modality such as oral spelling, typing, or spelling with anagram letters (Rapcsak & Beeson, 2000). Patients with deficient writing may benefit from assistance in letter formation, particularly in relearning to sign their name. When a spelling disorder is present, the particular form of spelling treatment must be matched to the subtype of spelling impairment.

Spelling disorders generally are measured by tasks of written naming and tasks of spelling to dictation (i.e., the clinician dictates spelling stimuli for the patient to spell). Similar to acquired dyslexia, there are several subtypes of acquired spelling impairment. Patients with "deep agraphia" produce many semantic errors in spelling (e.g., spelling BOAT for the target "car") and perform poorly in spelling nonsense words to dictation via the sublexical phoneme-to-grapheme route (Rapcsak & Beeson, 2000). Similar to treatment for deep dyslexia, described earlier, treatment for deep agraphia can focus on treatment of semantic memory (Hillis, 1991) or on treatment of the sublexical phoneme-to-grapheme route (Hillis Trupe, 1986). In contrast, patients with "surface agraphia" (i.e., lexical agraphia) have difficulty with whole-word spelling of irregular words, but are able to spell many regular words and nonsense words via the sublexical phoneme-to-grapheme route. Treatment for these patients has centered on maximizing optimal use of the sublexical route (Hillis & Caramazza, 1994), or on strengthening the graphemic output lexicon through whole-word spelling practice (as described earlier in regard to written naming). Greenwald (2004) incorporated lexical and sublexical spelling treatment into functional sentence spelling tasks for e-mail exchange.

Rehabilitation of Impaired Sentence Processing

Individuals with various types of aphasia can have impaired sentence processing, affecting comprehension and/or production. A variety of successful treatments have been devised to address these deficits. Detailed consideration of these complex disorders and their treatments is beyond the scope of this chapter (see Mitchum & Berndt, 2001). However, **Table 5–5**

Table 5–5 Treatment for Impaired Sentence Processing

Role of the SLP	Clinical Issues
Communication partner	What is the patient's impression of the deficit level/severity? A patient who was a talkative salesperson premorbidly may experience even a relatively mild sentence production deficit as extremely frustrating.
Diagnostician	Assess comprehension and production of specific types of sentences using appropriate materials. It is imperative to test difficult sentence processing abilities so that patients with milder forms of aphasia are not missed.
	Is the range of sentence types available for production reduced? Does the patient show worse word retrieval in sentences versus single word naming?
	Can the patient formulate difficult sentence constructions when constrained to begin a sentence with the agent vs. object?
	Do oral and written forms of sentence production differ?
Therapist	*Patient H:* Sentence comprehension deficit. One type of comprehension deficit involves not understanding who is doing the action in a passive sentence. Patient may benefit from sentence query therapy, in which clinician provides color-coded markings to identify the grammatical elements of a written sentence and asks questions about thematic roles.
	Patient I: Sentence production deficit. One type of production deficit is limitation to producing sentences only in subject-verb-object construction. The use of anagrams may be beneficial in showing the patient how an active sentence can become a passive sentence and still retain the same meaning (e.g., Mitchum & Berndt, 2001)

includes suggested questions and approaches that apply to treatment of sentence processing disorders.

Sentence comprehension skills of the individual aphasia patient can be misunderstood by family and caregivers of the patient, making education and advocacy in this area imperative for the SLP. Individuals with generally intact comprehension at the single-word level or for simple syntactic constructions may nevertheless have severely impaired comprehension of more complex sentence constructions. When these patients do not respond appropriately to a spoken complex sentence, this response may be interpreted inaccurately as resistance or lack of cooperation. The clinician must provide ongoing education about the patient's sentence processing abilities to caregivers and clinical staff, and demonstrate the most effective way of communicating with the patient to maximize sentence comprehension and production.

Special Technologies and Aphasia Treatment

Augmentative-alternative communication (AAC) strategies can enhance functional communication in persons with aphasia. AAC may replace, support, or supplement residual natural speech during communication interactions (Hux, Manasse, Weiss, & Beukelman, 2001). At the elementary level, basic communication of needs, wants, and feelings (e.g., pain) is targeted using single-word communication cards, gestures, picture/photo dictionary, communication book, alphabet board, or eye gaze. Drawing may be a viable form of expression for those individuals who report having a background or interest in drawing (Beeson & Ramage, 2000). At the intermediate level, daily communication in the home or other life participation contexts is targeted, using options such as drawing, electronic devices, generic and personalized communication booklets, gestures, and written choice communication (Garrett & Beukelman, 1992). Writing, drawing, and computerized (Katz, 2001) or electronic devices may be used at the advanced level to promote independent communication.

Multiple factors must be considered in evaluating AAC options for a person with aphasia, including communication needs, life participation goals, skill level, cost, and motivation. Successful AAC strategies allow patients with aphasia to maximize residual communicative strengths and individualism

(Hux et al., 2001), and to communicate their maximal level of functional information, communicative participation, and message meaning and intent (e.g., humor).

Despite the usefulness of AAC in the treatment of comprehension or expression impairments, many individuals who have learned to use AAC in individual sessions do not use it in social situations. Thus, there may be a need for acceptance models in the application of AAC in adult-acquired communication disorders (Lasker & Bedrosian, 2001). Numerous factors contribute to the success or failure of AAC approaches. Perhaps many persons with aphasia who are elderly find AAC unappealing because they have had a lifetime of natural communication and have difficulty adapting to AAC (Hux et al., 2001). Possibly preferences for more natural speech by the individual's family members and clinicians also influence poor AAC acceptance in aphasia (Lasker, 1997). AAC can improve important communications among family and friends. In the roles of educator/advocate as well as therapist, the SLP clinician may help to reduce the stigma of AAC during the individual's transition from natural communication to augmented communication.

Addressing the Real-Life Consequences of Aphasia

In recent years, many researchers and clinicians have placed increased emphasis on psychosocial aspects of rehabilitation directly related to life participation skills (Frattali, 1998; Simmons-Mackie, 2001). Clearly, aphasia rehabilitation focused only at the impairment level would be insufficient to meet the individual needs of the person with aphasia, because psychosocial factors are integral to communication in real-life contexts (Bouchard-Lamothe, Bopurassa, Laflamme, Garcia, Gailey, & Stiell, 1999). As noted above, the SLP fulfills the roles of communication partner and educator/advocate, and as therapist individualizes treatment tasks to address the goals and concerns of the person with aphasia. The psychosocial and life-participation approaches to aphasia rehabilitation emphasize communicative strengths of the individual that can be used to meet the daily and chronic challenges of aphasia, and focus on strengthening the individual's daily participation in activities of choice (Chapey, 2001).

The clinical methods used in psychosocial and life-participation approaches to aphasia rehabilitation vary widely to correspond with the abilities and interests of each person with aphasia. Space limitations allow only a sample of methods here. Overall, therapy tasks are conducted within dynamic communication interactions that represent natural adult social exchanges rather than artificial contexts (Leiwo, 1994). Qualitative as well as quantitative measures of communication ability are used to document treatment outcome (Damico, Simmons-Mackie, Oelschlaeger, Elman, & Armstrong, 1999).

In general, remediation of chronic aphasia is likely to be most effective when the individual's significant others are included in the real-life aspects of the rehabilitation process (Ryff & Singer, 2000). There is evidence that training communication partners can be effective in improving the communication and social participation of the person with aphasia (Boles, 1997). Attempts to assist the individual in overcoming chronic barriers in the environment that inhibit participation in daily activities can facilitate naturalistic communication (Lyon & Shadden, 2001). Social group therapy has been found to have a positive impact on both linguistic and psychosocial aspects of aphasia (Elman & Bernstein Ellis, 1999). Direct conversation therapy (Simmons-Mackie, 2000) and conversational coaching are methods for facilitating the individual's skill and confidence in conversation. Promising techniques for assisting conversational skills include scaffolded and supported conversation approaches, in which the listener provides cues and verbal models within the natural flow of conversation (Damico, 1992; Duchan, 1997). Collaborative drawing (Lyon, 1995) or pantomime (Demchuk, 1996) techniques are examples of enhanced compensatory strategy training that can facilitate generalization of compensatory strategies to real-life communicative contexts (Simmons-Mackie, 2001).

✦ Planning Aphasia Rehabilitation for Stroke Survivor Groups

At any stage in the continuum of aphasia rehabilitation, group intervention is an adaptable venue for treatment. Aphasia treatment groups serve a variety of functions: (1) providing education seminars for patients and families, (2) addressing specific language deficits and life participation goals, and (3) giving patients a comfortable environment to share the distressing elements of life with disrupted language skills. At the subacute stage of recovery, group sessions may include attempts to stimulate language skills such as auditory comprehension, and to facilitate early adjustment to abrupt changes in life participation. At the outpatient stage, greater emphasis may be placed on compensatory strategies and overall communicative function, as well as on psychosocial adjustment to aphasia across a wider range of life-participation contexts. For individuals with chronic aphasia, group sessions typically focus on each patient's objectives for transfer and maintenance of communication skills. Individuals most likely to benefit from group treatment at the chronic stage are those with identified personal goals and the ability to take the communication risks to increase the potential for further communication success. At any of these stages, group members may benefit from sharing communication hardships and communicatively isolating experiences with other group members to reduce loneliness, facilitate personal coping, and elevate confidence and desire for social contact.

Successful aphasia group formation depends on two primary membership characteristics. First, because every group member is encouraged to actively participate, group size should be limited to four or five members. Groups with more than five members generally produce unequal communication opportunities, thereby reducing sociocommunicative practice. Second, aphasia groups are best formed with aphasia severity in mind. When aphasia severity is not controlled, the vitality of the group can suffer as members with mild aphasia may become bored and members with severe aphasia may lose initiative in attempting to participate. Care in aphasia group formation and proper candidacy increase the likelihood of reliable attendance, active participation, moments of communicative spontaneity and social closeness.

As noted earlier, there is evidence that group rehabilitation for aphasia can facilitate improved linguistic skills and psychosocial adjustment (Elman & Bernstein Ellis, 1999). A summary of group therapy by Kearns and Elman (2001) included five types of aphasia groups (**Table 5–6**), and a wide range of approaches to group intervention and to measurement of group treatment outcomes.

Ongoing research is needed to further define models of aphasia group intervention that may be most effective in facilitating communication skills in real-life social contexts (Avent, 1997; Marshall, 1998). Clinical and research interest in group treatment is likely to increase, because it is a promising component of rehabilitation and follow-up care for individuals with aphasia and their families.

Table 5–6   Aphasia Group Types

Aphasia Group Type	Purpose
Direct language treatment	Highly structured stimulus-response training approach, often viewed as adjunct to individual treatment (e.g., Brookshire, 1997; Holland, 1970)
Indirect language treatment	Unstructured (general conversation, social groups, role playing, field trips) (e.g., Davis, 1992; Kearns & Simmons, 1985)
Sociolinguistic treatment	Interaction among patients is emphasized; role-playing in real-life situations; PACE activities (Avent, 1997; Wilcox & Davis, 1977)
Transition	Role-playing to prepare for new environment after dismissal from hospital (i.e., communicative demands, psychological adjustment, and development of alternative strategies) (Aten et al., 1981)
Maintenance	Regular stimulation of language skills; practice in using residual language skills; social interaction, social communication and entertainment; a source of information, support and referral for families (Brookshire, 1997; Hunt, 1976)

From Kearns & Elman, 2001.

Study Questions

1. What are the various roles of the speech–language pathologist in clinical practice? Give an example of each.

2. What distinguishes a central semantic impairment from a modality-specific semantic impairment?

3. What are some techniques for reducing frustration during communication breakdowns between aphasia patients and their family members?

4. Give specific examples of how knowledge of the general categories of acquired dyslexia can guide treatment decisions.

5. How would you explain sentence comprehension impairments to hospital staff attempting to communicate with a person with aphasia?

6. Discuss the value of a flexible approach to providing education and therapy services as part of aphasia rehabilitation.

7. Why is it important to consider group size, aphasia severity level, and patient prognosis when forming an aphasia group?

References

American Speech–Language-Hearing Association (ASHA) (2005). *Membership and Certification Handbook of ASHA* Rockville, MD.

American Speech–Language-Hearing Association (ASHA) (2001). *Scope of Practice* in *Speech–Language* Pathology, Rockville, MD.

Aten, J., Kushner-Vogel, D., Haire, A., West, J.F., O'Connor, S. & Bennett, L. (1981). Group Treatment for Aphasia Panel Discussion. In: R.H. Brookshire (Ed.), *Clinical Aphasiology Conference Proceedings* (pp. 141–154). Minneapolis, MN: BRK

Avent, J.R. (1997). Group Treatment in Aphasia Using Cooperative Learning Methods. *Journal of Medical Speech–language Pathology, 5,* 9–26

Beeson, P.M. (1999). Treating Acquired Writing Impairment. *Aphasiology, 13,* 767–785

Beeson, P.M. & Insalaco, D. (1998). Acquired Alexia: Lesions from Successful Treatment. *Journal of the International Neuropsychological Society, 4,* 621–635

Beeson, P.M. & Ramage, A.E. (2000). Drawing from Experience: The Development of Alternative Communication Strategies. *Topics in Stroke Rehabilitation, 7,* 10–20

Behrmann, M. (1987). The Rites of Righting Writing: Homophone Remediation in Acquired Dysgraphia. *Cognitive Neuropsychology, 4,* 365–384

Behrmann, M. & Lieberthal, T. (1989). Category-Specific Treatment of a Lexical-Semantic Deficit: A Single Case Study of Global Aphasia. *British Journal of Disorders of Communication, 24,* 281–299

Boles, L. (1997). Conversation Analysis as a Dependent Measure in Communication Therapy with Four Individuals with Aphasia. *Asia Pacific Journal of Speech, Language and Hearing, 2,* 43–61

Bouchard-Lamothe, D. Bourassa, S., Laflamme, B., Garcia, L.J., Gailey, G. & Stiell, K. (1999). Perceptions of Three Groups of Interlocutors of the Effects of Aphasia on Communication: An Exploratory Study. *Aphasiology, 13,* 839–856

Brookshire, R.H. (1997). *An Introduction to Neurogenic Communication Disorders,* 5th ed. St. Louis: Mosby Year Book

Byng, S. & Coltheart, M. (1986). Aphasia Therapy Research: Methodological Requirements and Illustrative Results. In: E. Hjelmquist & L.B. Nilsson (Eds.), *Communication and Handicap* (pp. 191–213). Amsterdam: North-Holland

Byng, S., Kay, J., Edmundson, A. & Scott, C. (1990). Aphasia Tests Reconsidered. *Aphasiology, 4,* 67–91

Caramazza, A. & Hillis, A.E. (1990). Where Do Semantic Errors Come From? *Cortex, 26,* 95–122

Caramazza, A., Hillis, A.E., Rapp, B.C. & Romani, C. (1990). The Multiple Semantics Hypothesis: Multiple Confusions? *Cognitive Neuropsychology, 7,* 161–189

Chapey, R. (2001). *Language Intervention Strategies in Aphasia and Related Neurogenic Communication Disorders,* 4th ed. Baltimore: Lippincott Williams & Wilkins

Coltheart, M. (1980). Deep Dyslexia: A Right Hemisphere Hypothesis. In: M. Coltheart, K.E. Patterson & J.C. Marshall (Eds.), *Deep Dyslexia* (pp. 326–380). London: Routledge & Kegan Paul

Damico, J. (1992). *Whole Language for Special Needs Children.* Buffalo, NY: Educom Associates

Damico, J., Simmons-Mackie, N., Oelschlaeger, M., Elman, R. & Armstrong, E. (1999). Qualitative Methods in Aphasia Research: Basic Issues. *Aphasiology, 13,* 651–666

Davis, G.A. (1992). *A Survey of Adult Aphasia.* Englewood Cliffs, NJ: Prentice Hall

Davis, G.A. & Wilcox, M.J. (1981). Incorporating Parameters of Natural Conversation in Aphasia Treatment. In R. Chapey (Ed.), *Language Intervention Strategies in Adult Aphasia.* Baltimore: Williams & Wilkins

de Partz, M. (1986). Reeducation of a Deep Dyslexic Patient: Rationale of the Method and Results. *Cognitive Neuropsychology, 3,* 149–177

Demchuk, M. (1996). Creative Communication in Aphasia. Paper presented to the annual meeting of the American Speech–language-Hearing Association, Seattle

Drew, R.L. & Thompson, C.K. (1999). Model-Based Semantic Treatment for Naming Deficits in Aphasia. *Journal of Speech, Language and Hearing Research, 42,* 972–989

Duchan, J. (1997). A Situated Pragmatics Approach to Supporting Children with Severe Communication Disorders. *Topics in Language Disorders, 17,* 1–18

Duffy, J. & Coelho, C. (2001). Schuell's Stimulation Approach to Rehabilitation. In: R. Chapey (Ed.), *Language Intervention Strategies in Aphasia and Related Neurogenic Communication Disorders,* 4th ed. (pp. 341–382). Baltimore: Lippincott Williams & Wilkins

Elman, R.J. & Bernstein Ellis, E. (1999). The Efficacy of Group Communication Treatment in Adults with Chronic Aphasia. *Journal of Speech, Language and Hearing Research, 42,* 411–419

Franklin, S., Turner, J., Ralph, M, Morris, J. & Bailey, P. (1996). A Distinctive Case of Word Meaning Deafness. *Cognitive Neuropsychology, 13,* 1139–1162

Frattali, C. (1998). Assessing Functional Outcomes: An Overview. *Seminars in Speech and Language, 19,* 209–221

Friedman, R.B. & Robinson, S.R. (1991). Whole-Word Training Therapy in a Stable Surface Alexic Patient: It Works. *Aphasiology, 5,* 521–528

Garrett, K.L. & Beukelman, D.R. (1992). Augmentative Communication Approaches for Persons with Severe Aphasia. In: K. Yorkston (Ed.), *Augmentative Communication in the Medical Setting* (pp. 245–321). Tucson, AZ: Communication Skill Builders

Gonzalez Rothi, L.J. & Moss, S. (1992). Alexia Without Agraphia: Potential for Model Assisted Therapy. *Clinics in Communication Disorders, 2,* 11–18

Grayson, E., Hilton, R. & Franklin, S. (1997). Early Intervention in a Case of Jargon Aphasia: Efficacy of Language Comprehension Therapy. *European Journal of Disorders of Communication, 32,* 257–276

Greenwald, M.L. (2004). "Blocking" Lexical Competitors in Severe Global Agraphia: A Treatment of Reading and Spelling. Neurocase, 10 (2), 156–174

Greenwald, M.L. & Berndt, R.S. (1999). Impairment of Abstract Letter Order Knowledge: Severe Alexia in a Mildly Aphasic Patient. *Cognitive Neuropsychology, 16,* 513–556

Greenwald, M.L., Raymer, A.M., Richardson, M.E. & Rothi, L.J.G. (1995). Contrasting Treatments for Severe Impairments of Picture Naming. *Neuropsychological Rehabilitation, 5,* 17–49

Greenwald, M.L. & Rothi, L.J.G. (1998). Lexical Access via Letter Naming in a Profoundly Alexic and Anomic Patient: A Treatment Study. *Journal of the International Neuropsychological Society, 4,* 595–607

Helm-Estabrooks, N., Fitzpatrick, P. & Barresi, B. (1982). Visual Action Therapy for Global Aphasia. *Journal of Speech and Hearing Disorders, 47,* 385–389

Hillis, A.E. (1991). Effects of Separate Treatments for Distinct Impairments Within the Naming Process. In: T. Prescott (Ed.), *Clinical Aphasiology,* vol. 19 (pp. 255–265). Austin, TX: Pro-Ed

Hillis, A.E. (1993). The Role of Models of Language Processing in Rehabilitation of Language Impairments. *Aphasiology, 7,* 5–26

Hillis, A.E. & Caramazza, A. (1987). Model-Driven Treatment of Dysgraphia. In: R.H. Brookshire (Ed.), *Clinical Aphasiology* (pp. 84–105). Minneapolis, MN: BRK

Hillis, A.E. & Caramazza, A. (1994). Theories of Lexical Processing and Rehabilitation of Lexical Deficits. In: M.J. Riddoch & G.W. Humpheys (Eds.), *Cognitive Neuropsychology and Cognitive Rehabilitation* (pp. 449–484). Hillsdale, NJ: Erlbaum

Hillis Trupe, A.E. (1986). Effectiveness of Retraining Phoneme to Grapheme Conversion. In R.H. Brookshire (Ed.), *Clinical Aphasiology* (pp. 163–171). Minneapolis, MN: BRK

Holland, A.L. (1970). Case Studies in Aphasia Rehabilitation Using Programmed Instruction. *American Speech and Hearing Association, 35,* 377–390

Howard, D. & Patterson, K. (1992). *Pyramids and Palm Trees.* Bury St. Edmunds, UK: Thames Valley Publishing

Hunt, M.I. (1976). Language Maintenance Group for Aphasics. Paper presented at the annual meeting of the American Speech and Hearing Association, Houston

Hux, K., Manasse, N., Weiss, A., & Beukelman, D.R. (2001). Augmentative and Alternative Communication for Persons with Aphasia. In: R. Chapey (Ed.), *Language Intervention Strategies in Aphasia and Related Neurogenic Communication Disorders,* 4th ed. (pp. 675–687). Baltimore: Lippincott Williams & Wilkins

Katz, R.C. (2001). Computer Applications in Aphasia Treatment. In: R. Chapey (Ed.), *Language Intervention Strategies in Aphasia and Related Neurogenic Communication Disorders,* 4th ed. (pp. 718–741). Baltimore: Lippincott Williams & Wilkins

Katz, R.C. & Wertz, R.T. (1997). The Efficacy of Computer-Provided Reading Treatment for Chronic Aphasic Adults. *Journal of Speech, Language and Hearing Research, 40,* 493–507

Kearns, K.P. & Elman, R.J. (2001). Group Therapy for Aphasia: Theoretical and Practical Considerations. In: R. Chapey (Ed.), *Language Intervention Strategies in Aphasia and Related Neurogenic Communication Disorders,* 4th ed. (pp. 316–337). Baltimore: Lippincott Williams & Wilkins

Kearns, K.P. & Simmons, N. (1985). Group Therapy for Aphasia: A Survey of Veterans Administration Medical Centers. In: R.H Brookshire (Ed.), *Clinical Aphasiology Conference Proceedings* (pp. 176–183). Minneapolis, MN: BRK

Kertesz, A. (1979). *Aphasia and Associated Disorders.* Orlando: Grune & Stratton

Lasker, J. (1997). Effects of Storytelling Mode on Partner's Communicative Ratings of an Adult with Aphasia (doctoral dissertation, University of Nebraska-Lincoln, 1997). *Dissertation Abstracts International, 59–02B,* 0627

Lasker, J.P. & Bedrosian, J.L. (2001). Promoting Acceptance of Augmentative and Alternative Communication by Adults with Acquired Communication Disorders. *Augmentative and Alternative Communication, 17,* 141–153

Le Dorze, G., Boulay, N., Gaudreau, J. & Brassard, C. (1994). The Contrasting Effects of A Semantic Versus a Formal-Semantic Technique for the Facilitation of Naming in a Case of Anomia. *Aphasiology, 8,* 127–141

Leiwo, M. (1994). Aphasia and Communicative Speech Therapy. *Aphasiology, 8,* 467–482

Lott, S.N., Friedman, R.B. & Linebaugh, C.W. (1994). Rationale and Efficacy of a Tactile-Kinaesthetic Treatment for Alexia. *Aphasiology, 8,* 181–195

Lyon, J. (1995). Drawing: Its Value as a Communication Aid for Adults with Aphasia. *Aphasiology, 9,* 33–50

Lyon, J. & Shadden, B. (2001). Treating Life Consequences of Aphasia's Chronicity. In: R. Chapey (Ed.), *Language Intervention Strategies in Aphasia and Related Neurogenic Communication Disorders,* 4th ed. (pp. 297–315). Baltimore: Lippincott Williams & Wilkins

Maher, L.M., Clayton, M.C., Barrett, A.M., Schober-Peterson, D. & Rothi, L.J.G. (1998). Rehabilitation of a Case of Pure Alexia: Exploiting Residual Abilities. *Journal of the International Neuropsychological Society, 4,* 636–647

Maher, L.M., Rothi, L.J.G. & Heilman, K.M. (1994). Lack of Error Awareness in an Aphasic Patient with Relatively Preserved Auditory Comprehension. *Brain and Language, 46,* 402–418

Marshall, R. (1998). *Introduction to Group Treatment for Aphasia: Design and Management.* Boston: Butterworth-Heinemann

Marshall, J., Pring, T. & Chiat, S. (1998). Verb Retrieval and Sentence Production in Aphasia. *Brain and Language, 63,* 159–183

Martin, R.C. & Freedman, M.L. (2001). Relations Between Language and Memory Deficits. In: R.S. Berndt (Ed.), *Handbook of Neuropsychology,* 2nd ed., Vol. 3 (pp. 239–256). Amsterdam: Elsevier

Mitchum, C. & Berndt, R.S. (1991). Diagnosis and Treatment of the Non-Lexical Route in Acquired Dyslexia: An Illustration of the Cognitive Neuropsychological Approach. *Journal of Neurolinguistics, 6,* 103–137

Mitchum, C. & Berndt, R.S. (1994). Verb Retrieval and Sentence Construction: Effects of Targeted Intervention. In: M.J. Riddoch & G. Humpreys (Eds.), *Cognitive Neuropsychology and Cognitive Rehabilitation* (pp. 317–348). Hillsdale, NJ: Erlbaum

Mitchum, C. & Berndt, R.S. (2001). Cognitive Neuropsychological Approaches to Diagnosing And Treating Language Disorders: Production and Comprehension of Sentences. In: R. Chapey (Ed.), *Language Intervention Strategies*

in Aphasia and Related Neurogenic Communication Disorders, 4th ed. (pp. 551–571). Baltimore: Lippincott Williams & Wilkins

Morris, J., Franklin, S., Ellis, A.W., Turner, J.E. & Bailey, P.J. (1996). Remediating a Speech Perception Deficit in an Aphasic Patient. *Aphasiology, 10,* 137–158

Myers, P.S. (1998). *Right Hemisphere Damage: Disorders of Communication and Cognition.* San Diego, CA: Singular Publishing Group

Myers, P.S. & Brookshire, R.H. (1996). Effect of Visual and Inferential Variables on Scene Descriptions by Right-Hemisphere-Damaged and Non-Brain-Damaged Adults. *Journal of Speech and Hearing Research, 39,* 870–880

Nickels, L. & Best, W. (1996). Therapy for Naming Disorders (Part II): Specifics, Surprises and Suggestions. *Aphasiology, 10,* 109–136

Ochipa, C, Maher, L.M. & Raymer, A.M. (1998). One Approach to the Treatment of Anomia. *ASHA Special Interest Division 2: Neurophysiology and Neurogenic Speech and Language Disorders, 15,* 18–23

Ochipa, C., Maher, L.M., & Rothi, L.J.G. (1995). Treatment of Ideomotor Apraxia. *Journal of the International Neuropsychological Society, 2,* 149

Rao, P. (2001). Use of Amer-Ind Code by Persons with Severe Aphasia. In: R. Chapey (Ed.), *Language Intervention Strategies in Aphasia and Related Neurogenic Communication Disorders,* 4th ed. (pp. 688–702). Baltimore: Lippincott Williams & Wilkins

Rapcsak, S. & Beeson, P.M. (2000). Agraphia. In: Nadeau, S., Rothi, L.J.G. & Crosson, B. (Eds.), *Aphasia and Language* (pp. 184–220). New York: Guilford Press

Rapp, B. & Goldrick, M. (2000). Discreteness and Interactivity in Spoken Word Production. *Psychological Review, 107,* 460–499

Raymer, A.M. & Rothi, L.J.G. (2001). Cognitive Approaches to Impairments of Word Comprehension and Production. In R. Chapey (Ed.), *Language Intervention Strategies in Aphasia and Related Neurogenic Communication Disorders,* 4th ed. (pp. 524–550), Baltimore: Lippincott, Williams & Wilkins.

Raymer, A.M., Thompson, C.K., Jacobs, B. & LeGrand, H.R. (1993). Phonologic Treatment of Naming Deficits in Aphasia: Model-Based Generalization Analysis. *Aphasiology, 7,* 27–53

Riddoch, M.J., Humphreys, G.W., Coltheart, M. & Funnell, E. (1988). Semantic Systems or System? Neuropsychological Evidence Re-examined. *Cognitive Neuropsychology, 5,* 3–25

Robson, J., Marshall, J., Pring, T. & Chiat, S. (1998). Phonologic Naming Therapy in Jargon Aphasia: Positive but Paradoxical Effects. *Journal of the International Neuropsychological Society, 4,* 675–686

Rothi, L.J.G. (1995). Behavioral Compensation in the Case of Treatment of Acquired Language Disorders Resulting from Brain Damage. In: R.A. Dixon & L. Backman (Eds.), *Compensating for Psychological Deficits and Declines: Managing Losses and Promoting Gains* (pp. 219–230). Mahwah, NJ: Lawrence Erlbaum

Rothi, L.J.G., Coslett, H.B. & Heilman, K.M. (1984). *Battery of Adult Reading Function.* Unpublished manuscript

Ryff, C.D. & Singer, B. (2000). Interpersonal Flourishing: A Positive Health Agenda for the New Millennium. *Personality and Social Psychology Review, 4,* 30–44

Schuell, H. (1953). Auditory Impairment in Aphasia: Significance and Retraining Techniques. *Journal of Speech and Hearing Disorders, 18,* 14–21

Simmons-Mackie, N. (2000). Social Approaches to the Management of Aphasia. In L. Worrall, L. & C. Frattali (Eds.), *Neurogenic Communication Disorders: A Functional Approach* (pp. 162–187). New York: Thieme

Simmons-Mackie, N. (2001). Social Approaches to Aphasia Intervention. In: R. Chapey (Ed.), *Language Intervention Strategies in Aphasia and Related Neurogenic Communication Disorders,* 4th ed. (pp. 246–268). Baltimore: Lippincott Williams & Wilkins

Skelly, M. (1979). *Amer-Ind Gestural Code Based on Universal American Indian Hand Talk.* New York: Elsevier

Weekes, B. & Coltheart, M. (1996). Surface Dyslexia and Surface Dysgraphia: Treatment Studies and Their Theoretical Implications. *Cognitive Neuropsychology, 13,* 277–315

Wilcox, M.H. & Davis, G. (1977). Speech Act Analysis of Aphasic Communication in Individual and Group Settings. In: R.H. Brookshire (Ed.), *Clinical Aphasiology Conference Proceedings* (pp. 166–174). Minneapolis, MN: BRK

World Health Organization (2001). *International Classification of Functioning, Disability and Health.* Geneva: WHO

Zihl, J. (2000). Visual Agnosia. In: J. Zihl (Ed.), *Rehabilitation of Visual Disorders After Brain Injury* (pp. 133–174). East Sussex, UK: Psychology Press

6

Cognitive-Communicative Rehabilitation Following Traumatic Brain Injury

Carl Coelho and Kathleen M. Youse

✦ Scope of Chapter
✦ Definitions and Mode of Injury
✦ Incidence
✦ Severity of Injury
✦ Cognitive and Communicative Sequelae Following Traumatic Brain Injury
✦ Rehabilitation of Traumatic Brain Injury
✦ Stages of Recovery Following Traumatic Brain Injury

✦ Scope of Chapter

This chapter provides an overview of the role of the speech–language pathologist in the management of individuals with traumatic brain injury (TBI). Although this discussion includes specific reference to cognitive rehabilitation, it is not intended to be a comprehensive presentation of that topic. Such an undertaking is beyond the scope of a single chapter. The reader is referred to texts on cognitive rehabilitation that cover the topic in greater depth (Finlayson & Garner, 1994; Mills, Cassidy, & Katz, 1997; Ponsford, Sloan, & Snow, 1995; Rosenthal, Griffith, Kreutzer, & Pentland, 1999; Sohlberg & Mateer, 2001; Stuss, Winocur, & Robinson, 1999; Ylvisaker & Feeney, 1998). Rather, the emphasis of this chapter is on an overview of intervention practices of speech–language pathologists in medical settings for individuals with TBI.

The chapter reviews the neuropathology and incidence of TBI, and describes the rehabilitation continuum in which individuals with TBI are assessed and treated. The practice patterns utilized in each setting are discussed and illustrated with case examples.

✦ Definitions and Mode of Injury

TBI may be thought of as a subset of acquired brain injury (ABI), which includes not only TBI but stroke, hypoxic-hypotensive injury, infectious disorders such as encephalitis, and brain tumors (Sohlberg & Mateer, 2001). This chapter focuses specifically on the management of TBI; however,

many of the interventions described are applicable to other categories of ABI as well. TBI may be classified into two broad categories— open and closed—based on whether or not the meninges remain intact. *Open* head injuries result when the scalp, skull, and meninges are penetrated, as in a gunshot wound. *Closed* head injuries typically result from mechanical forces. For example, if a moving head comes in contact with a stationary surface (e.g., automobile dash board or windshield) or if the head is struck with a moving object (e.g., with a baseball bat or pipe), resulting in skull fractures and tissue damage to the underlying brain surface. Another common mode of injury is referred to as *acceleration-deceleration*, in which the moving head suddenly stops but the brain continues to move in the original direction and then suddenly reverses its path. Once the brain collides with the inside surface of the skull, areas of contusion result. The point of initial impact is referred to as *coup,* and when the brain rebounds in the opposite direction and impacts another surface of the skull, *contrecoup.* Injury may also occur when the brain is scraped across the rough inner surfaces of the skull, particularly at the base of the skull. The orbital and lateral surfaces of the frontal and temporal lobes are vulnerable to this type of injury (Oder, Podreka, Spatt, & Goldenberg, 1996; Sohlberg & Mateer, 2001). These contusions and abrasions result in a variety of focal lesions. A different type of brain damage that often occurs during the acceleration-deceleration process is microscopic, that is, at the level of the brain cell axons and in particular, the long nerve fiber tracts. The jerking and/or twisting motion of the brain during the acceleration and deceleration may result in axonal stretching, shearing, and tearing. This type of injury results in widespread but irregular damage and is termed *diffuse axonal injury* (DAI). This damage results in disrupted neuronal communication among various brain regions (Sohlberg & Mateer, 2001). TBI is characterized not only by the *primary damage* (i.e., focal and diffuse lesions) just described, but also by a variety of *secondary factors* such as infection, oxygen deprivation, brain swelling, and elevation of intracranial pressure.

✦ Incidence

There are approximately 500,000 new cases of TBI each year in the United States, or roughly 200 cases per 100,000 persons. Adolescents and young adults ages 15 to 24 have the highest incidence of TBI, typically associated with motor vehicle accidents. Older adults over the age of 65 and children under the age of 5 have the next highest incidence of TBI, most commonly resulting from falls. Males are twice as likely to experience a TBI as females, and individuals with a previous TBI are three times more likely to suffer a subsequent TBI (Youse, Le, Cannizzaro, & Coelho, 2002).

✦ Severity of Injury

The seriousness of a TBI is determined by a variety of factors including the distribution of the injury (i.e., focal or multifocal lesions, and/or DAI), severity (i.e., size, location, and depth of lesions), and type of underlying pathology. There are several

Table 6–1 Indices of Traumatic Brain Injury (TBI) Severity

Classification	Glasgow Coma Scale (GCS) Score	Duration of Coma	Length of PTA
Severe	3–8	Over 6 hours	Over 24 hours
Moderate	9–12	Less than 6 hours	1–24 hours
Mild	13–15	20 minutes or less	60 minutes or less

From Sohlberg, M. M, & Mateer, C. A. (2001). *Cognitive Rehabilitation: An Integrative Neuropsychological Approach.* New York: Guilford Press, with permission.

indices of TBI severity (**Table 6–1**). Some of the more commonly applied measures are the Glasgow Coma Scale (GCS) (Jennett & Bond, 1975), duration of coma, and length of posttraumatic amnesia (**Table 6–2**). The GCS assesses severity of injury by rating the degree of eye opening, the best verbal response, and the best motor response. Coma is a prolonged period of unconsciousness, and in most instances a longer duration of coma is associated with greater severity of injury (see next section for more information pertaining to coma). Posttraumatic amnesia (PTA) refers to the length of time during which memories are not stored and thus new learning cannot occur. Severity of PTA is often measured by the Galveston Orientation and Amnesia Test (GOAT) (Levin, O'Donnell, & Grossman, 1979) (**Table 6–3**).

Table 6–2 Glasgow Coma Scale

Eye Opening		
None	1	Not attributable to ocular swelling
To pain	2	Pain stimulus is applied to chest or limbs
To speech	3	Nonspecific response to speech or shout, does not imply the patient obeys command to open eyes
Spontaneous	4	Eyes are open, but does not imply intact awareness
Motor Response		
No response	1	Flaccid
Extension	2	"Decerebrate"; adduction, internal rotation of shoulder, and pronation of the forearm
Abnormal flexion	3	"Decorticate"; abnormal flexion, adduction of the shoulder
Withdrawal	4	Normal flexor response; withdraws from pain stimulus with abduction of the shoulder
Localizes pain	5	Pain stimulus applied to supraocular region or fingertip causes limb to move in an attempt to remove it
Obeys commands	6	Follows simple commands
Verbal Response		
No response	1	(Self-explanatory)
Incomprehensible	2	Moaning and groaning, but no recognizable words
Inappropriate	3	Intelligible speech (e.g., shouting or swearing), but no sustained or coherent conversation
Confused	4	Patient responds to questions in a conversational manner, but the responses indicate varying degrees of disorientation and confusion
Oriented	5	Normal orientation to time, place, and person
Summed Glasgow Coma Scale score = E + M + V (3 to 15)		

From Jennett, B., & Bond, M. (1975). Assessment of Outcome After Severe Brain Damage. *Lancet, 1,* 480–487.

Table 6–3   Questions from the Galveston Orientation and Amnesia Test (GOAT)

1. What is your name?

   When were you born?

   Where do you live?

2. Where are you now?

   City?

   Hospital?

3. On what date were you admitted to this hospital?

   How did you get here?

4. What is the first event you can remember *after* the injury?

   Can you describe in detail (e.g., date, time, companions) the first event you can recall *after* injury?

5. Can you describe the last event you recall *before* the accident?

   Can you describe in detail (e.g., date, time, companions) the first event you can recall *before* the injury?

6. What time is it now?

7. What day of the week is it?

8. What day of the month is it?

9. What is the month?

10. What is the year?

From Levin, H.S., O'Donnell, V.M., and Grossman, R.G. (1979). The Galveston Orientation and Amnesia Test: A Practical Scale to Assess Cognition After Head Injury. *Journal of Nervous and Mental Disease, 167,* 675–684

✦ Cognitive and Communicative Sequelae Following Traumatic Brain Injury

No two injuries are the same; consequently, TBI results in a diverse, idiosyncratic constellation of cognitive-communicative, physical, and psychosocial deficits. The most common sequela of TBI is a reduced capacity to pursue premorbid interests and daily activities at a comparable functional level. Such difficulties exist along a broad continuum ranging from the need for additional time to complete tasks to total dependence on others for all basic needs. It has been estimated that 75% of all cases of TBI can be characterized as mild (defined in **Table 6–4**). The most characteristic features of TBI are the resulting cognitive disturbances that are often present

Table 6–4   Definition of Mild Traumatic Brain Injury

Trauma induced physiologic disruption of brain function as evidenced by at least one of the following:

A period of loss of consciousness not greater than 30 minutes

GCS score of at least 13 by 30 minutes following injury

Loss of memory for events before or after injury [posttraumatic amnesia (PTA) less than 24 hours]

Any alteration in mental state

Focal neurologic deficits which may or may not be transient

If standard radiologic studies (e.g., CT scan or MRI) are done, they must be interpreted as normal

From Mild Traumatic Brain Injury Committee of the Head Injury Interdisciplinary Special Interest Group of the American Congress of Rehabilitation Medicine (1993). Definition of mild traumatic brain injury. *Journal of Head Trauma Rehabilitation, 8,* 86–87

Table 6–5   Stages of Recovery

1. Coma: unresponsive, eyes closed

2. Vegetative state: no cognitive responses; gross wakefulness; sleep-wake cycles

3. Minimally conscious state: purposeful wakefulness; responds to some commands

4. Confusional state: recovered speech; posttraumatic amnesic (PTA); severe attentional deficits; agitated; hypoaroused; possible labile behavior

5. Postconfusional, evolving independence: resolution of PTA; cognitive improvement; achieving independence in daily self-care; improving social interaction; developing independence at home

6. Social competence, community re-entry: recovering cognitive abilities; goal directed behaviors; social skills; personality; developing independence in the community; returning to academic or vocational pursuits

From Sohlberg, M. M., & Mateer, C. A. (2001). *Cognitive rehabilitation: An integrative neuropsychological approach.* NY: Guilford Press, with permission.

after the injury. Multiple processes may be disrupted, including attention, memory, organization, reasoning, executive functioning, communication, and social skills. Recovery following TBI progresses through a series of predictable stages (**Table 6–5**). However, it is important to emphasize that recovery is specific to individual circumstances and therefore may vary in both extent and rate. Preinjury abilities, personality of the individual, and severity of the injury all influence recovery. What follows is a brief review of common sequelae that speech–language pathologists are confronted with as they manage individuals with TBI.

Coma

Coma is the term applied to the condition in which a patient displays minimal, if any, purposeful response to the external environment (Eisenberg & Weiner, 1987). Coma is relatively common and believed to result from damage to the central portions of the brainstem. In deep coma a patient may demonstrate no discernible behavioral responses to touch, pain, sound, or movement, although autonomic physiologic responses (those not under voluntary control) such as blood pressure or heart rate sometimes change with various sensory stimulation. In lighter stages of coma the patient may respond to external stimuli but responses may be generalized, for example, whole body movements or nonspecific motor responses. An intense level of stimulation may be required to elicit such responses. Duration of coma has some prognostic implications in terms of long-term recovery. However, the predictive capability is not perfect inasmuch as some individuals who undergo lengthy comas may demonstrate good recovery, and other individuals who experience no loss of consciousness may be left with extensive physical and cognitive deficits. The term *persistent vegetative state* (PVS) is applied to those individuals who survive but never regain any degree of consciousness in the sense of higher cortical function; they neither speak nor follow commands, but do regain the alerting mechanism (Eisenberg & Weiner, 1987; Jennett, 1996; Jennett & Plum, 1972; Levin & Eisenberg, 1996). There is some disagreement as to the timeline for the appropriate application of this label. For example, the American Neurological

Association (1993) advocates the use of this term after an individual has been in that state for 1 month, whereas the Multisociety Taskforce on Persistent Vegetative State (1993) considers the use of this term appropriate once the individual who is vegetative has reached 1 month post-onset of injury.

Cognitive Disturbances

Several areas of cognition may be disrupted following TBI, including orientation, attention, memory, and executive functioning. Although each of these processes is discussed separately, it is important to emphasize that in normal cognitive functioning these processes are related and interdependent (Sohlberg & Mateer, 2001).

Orientation/Arousal

Orientation refers to a person's awareness of four spheres: person, place, time, and circumstance. Orientation to person pertains to autobiographic memory, that is, information that was acquired and stored prior to the onset of the injury. This information does not need to be relearned or acquired but simply retrieved. This aspect of orientation typically returns rapidly during recovery. Orientation to time, place, and circumstances requires the capacity to take in, store, and recall new information presented after injury. Of these three aspects of orientation, recalling circumstances returns first, followed by place and time (High, Levin, & Gary, 1990). Time (year, month, season, time of day) constantly changes, and therefore information must be continually updated, requiring an increased level of awareness and the ability to sequence and order ongoing events. The frontal lobes, which are commonly damaged in TBI, have been implicated in this process of time tagging.

Attention

Attentional problems may be mild or severe and often resolve but can also be present years after injury. Concentration problems are a common post-TBI complaint of long-term survivors. Five dimensions of attention that have been described are (1) focused attention, which is the ability to respond discretely to specific visual, auditory, or tactile stimuli, for example, visually tracking an object; (2) sustained attention or vigilance, which is the ability to maintain a consistent behavioral response during continuous repetitive activities for more than a few minutes or seconds, for example, sorting shapes correctly; (3) selective attention, which is the ability to maintain a behavioral set in the presence of distracting extraneous stimuli, for example, reading the newspaper with a television or music playing in the background; (4) alternating attention, which is the ability to shift the focus of attention and move between tasks with different behavioral requirements, for instance, a waitress serving tables and also working the cash register; and (5) divided attention, which is the ability to respond simultaneously to multiple task demands, such as driving while talking on a cell phone.

Memory

Just as there are many definitions of attention, the same is true with memory. Most definitions or models of memory involve the dimensions of attention, *encoding* (i.e., coding of information to facilitate later recall), storage, and *consolidation* (i.e., integrating new memories with old). Although memory deficits may occur in isolation, they are typically accompanied by deficits of other cognitive abilities such as orientation, attention, and language. Using this generic model of memory, various deficits can be classified by stage of memory implicated, for example, memory problems secondary to attention deficits. Difficulty with any level of attention prohibits complete processing of information for subsequent recall. Memory problems that are secondary to encoding deficits may result from impaired language or perceptual ability; in other words, if the individual does not understand or perceive what was presented, memory of that information is reduced. Memory problems related to storage may be the result of a decreased ability to put or keep information in memory. The distinction between long- and short-term memory is based on the duration of memory store and the capacity of the storage. Long-term memory holds information indefinitely and has unlimited capacity. By comparison, short-term memory is of short duration and limited capacity. Working memory is similar to short-term memory, with the exception that working memory is dynamic, that is, it is a system that allows information that is presently in use to be held and manipulated. Individuals demonstrating storage problems may have normal short-term and working memory, though their long-term memory may be reduced due to a progressive deterioration of retained information over time.

Executive Functioning

The frontal lobes coordinate input from all other regions of the brain and are important for coordinating and actualizing activities involved in cognitive processing, often referred to as executive functioning. Executive functioning metacognition, or self-regulation (Kennedy & Coelho, 2005), more than any other cognitive dimension, determines the extent of social and vocational recovery (Sohlberg & Mateer, 2001; Ylvisaker, Szekeres, & Feeney, 1998). Executive functioning is not a discrete process but rather an umbrella function that interacts with all realms of cognition. Executive functioning may be considered a composite of those activities related to goal directed behavior, including initiation, planning, sequencing, organization, and regulation of behavior. Individuals with deficits in the area of executive functioning may be able to perform single-step operations but may be unable to plan, sequence, and monitor multistep activities; for example, they may be able to answer the phone in an office but be unable to function as an office manager.

Awareness of Deficits

Unawareness of deficits, or anosognosia, is a common problem following brain injury—some reports are as high as 40%—and can be a significantly limiting factor to recovery (Sohlberg, 1996). The degree of cognitive impairment and site of lesion are predictive of awareness deficits in the stroke population, with anosognosia being more common after anterior lesions and cortical lesions versus subcortical lesions (Wagner & Cushman, 1994). Unawareness should be distinguished from denial, which is a subconscious process that spares patients the psychological pain of accepting the serious consequences of a brain injury and its unwanted effects on their life

(Crosson, Barco, Velozo, Bolesta, Cooper, Werts, & Brobeck, 1989). There are a variety of models of unawareness. The first model includes potential sources of unawareness such as (1) the individual may not have enough information or the ability to comprehend the information; (2) the individual may have the information, but not be able to appreciate the implications of this information; or (3) the individual has the information and is able to acknowledge the implications, but ignores the information to lessen the emotional pain (Langer & Padrone, 1992). The second model pertains to types of awareness, including (1) intellectual awareness, which refers to the individual's ability to understand that a particular function is impaired; (2) emergent awareness, which is the ability to recognize a problem while it is actually happening; this incorporates the ability to monitor the relationship between one's actions and the environment; and (3) anticipatory awareness, which is the ability to anticipate that a problem will occur as the result of some deficit, and depends on intact intellectual and emergent awareness (Crosson et al, 1989). The final model involves varieties of awareness deficits, that is unawareness due to (1) cognitive impairments, in particular problems with memory and reasoning; (2) psychological reactions; and (3) an inability to recognize deficits in functioning due to severity of brain damage (Giacino & Cicerone, 1998).

Language Disturbances

Aphasia

McKinley, Brooks, Bond, Martinage, and Marshall (1981) have noted that language is disturbed in 75% or more of individuals with TBI. The nature of this language disturbance in TBI, that is, whether it is aphasic or nonaphasic, is not clear-cut. Aphasia is defined as an acquired impairment of language processes underlying receptive and expressive modalities caused by damage to areas of the brain that are primarily responsible for language function (Davis, 1993). Aphasia is manifested in grammatical disturbances, deficits of word retrieval, auditory comprehension, reading, and writing, in the presence of relatively intact cognitive abilities (e.g., orientation, attention, memory). Although aphasia commonly occurs after stroke, aphasia may also result from TBI, but the incidence reported in the TBI literature varies greatly. Reports range from approximately 2% (Heilman, Safran, & Geschwind, 1971; Schwartz-Cowley & Stepanik, 1989) to nearly 50% (Levin, Grossman, & Kelly, 1976; Thomsen, 1975). Sarno, Buonaguro, and Levita (1986) reported on a group of 125 closed head injured patients admitted to a rehabilitation center. The population studied fell into three groups: those with classic aphasia (30%), those with dysarthria accompanied by subclinical aphasia (34%), and those with subclinical aphasia (36%). The authors classified patients as aphasic if their use of speech for expression or reception was impaired. Subclinical aphasia referred to evidence of linguistic processing deficits on formal testing in the absence of clinical manifestations of linguistic impairment.

The apparent discrepancies regarding the incidence of aphasia following TBI are difficult to resolve owing to the lack of consistency in the descriptions of the head-injured patients studied, the different measures employed to document the presence of aphasia, as well as the varied definitions of aphasia applied. An examination of specific linguistic deficits following TBI that are reported in the literature indicates that

anomia, difficulty retrieving words, (Heilman et al, 1971; Levin et al 1976; Levin, Grossman, Rose, & Teasdale, 1979; Levin, Grossman, Sarwar, & Meyers, 1981; Sarno, 1980; Sarno et al, 1986; Thomsen, 1976), and impaired auditory comprehension (Levin et al, 1976; Sarno et al, 1986) are the most commonly observed symptoms. Holland (1982) noted that there is overlap in these deficit areas between aphasic and TBI patients as well as in the associated reading and writing deficits both groups often demonstrate. However, it is the qualitative differences in the naming errors between the two groups that may be most useful in distinguishing between aphasic and nonaphasic responses. Both aphasic and TBI individuals produce circumlocutions and various paraphasias, and have reduced fluency in the generation of category-specific words; TBI individuals, however, demonstrate additional naming errors. For example, TBI individuals may also produce naming errors related to their personal situations or make errors of confabulation (bizarre responses related to the patient's disorientation). Milton, Turnstall, and Wertz (1983) have described a system for qualitatively evaluating naming behavior for TBI individuals. The system permits descriptions of correct responses, and, when responses are incorrect, descriptions of their semantic, phonemic, and other relationships to the target. For example, for the target stimulus "apple" semantically related responses might include such responses as "fruit," "Granny Smith," or "pear." Phonemically related responses might include such responses as "able" or "ubel." Other responses might include such things as "saw" or "We grew them in our backyard." Use of such a system provides the clinician with far more information useful for treatment planning than a basic plus/minus scoring system.

Confused Language

In addition to specific linguistic deficits, individuals with TBI may also demonstrate significant problems in the area of what has been termed *confused language* (Groher, 1977; Halperin, Darley, & Brown, 1973; Levin et al, 1979; Prigatano, 1986). Confused language is described as receptive/expressive language that may be phonologically, syntactically, and semantically intact, yet lacking in meaning because responses are irrelevant, confabulatory, circumlocutory, or tangential in relation to a specific topic, and lacking a logical sequential relationship between thoughts (Hagan, 1984). Such language dysfunction may be mistaken for a fluent aphasia but is more appropriately considered cognitively based as opposed to linguistically based, that is, as a symptom of cognitive rather than linguistic deficits. More recent considerations of language disruption following TBI have advocated using the term *cognitive-communicative disorders* because it is thought to be a more accurate description of such impairments. Cognitive-communicative disorders involve difficulty with any aspect of communication secondary to cognitive dysfunction (e.g., attention, memory, executive functions) (American Speech–Language-Hearing Association, 2004).

Pragmatics

Occasionally individuals with TBI exhibit language disorders most consistent with aphasia, and many, particularly in the acute stages of recovery, demonstrate language behavior consistent with confused language. However, the primary basis of language dysfunction in the majority of individuals with TBI pertains to disordered language use or pragmatics. Pragmatics refers to a system of rules that structures the use of language in social context. Holland (1982) has observed that whereas aphasic individuals may communicate better than they talk, individuals with TBI appear to talk better than they communicate.

Pragmatic deficits are most prevalent in those individuals with frontal lobe injuries. The frontal lobes are involved in coordinating and actualizing many functions involved in cognitive processing such as attention, motivation, regulation, and self-monitoring (Stuss & Benson, 1997). Alexander, Benson, and Stuss (1989) note that individuals with prefrontal injury frequently demonstrate problems with disorganized discourse, inappropriate social interactions (e.g., difficulty interpreting social cues), and abstract forms of language (e.g., irony or sarcasm).

Speech Disturbances

Dysarthria

Yorkston, Beukelman, and Bell (1988) have noted that the incidence of dysarthria following TBI is not well documented. Additionally, the characteristics of the dysarthria in individuals with TBI are poorly described owing to the limited number of studies that have been undertaken. Rusk, Block and Lowmann (1969) observed dysarthria in approximately 30% of 96 head-injured patients they studied. This is consistent with the findings of Sarno, Buonaguro, and Levita (1986), who noted that 34% of the 125 TBI patients in their study demonstrated dysarthria. Thomsen (1976) observed that in a group of head-injured individuals monitored longitudinally, those with dysarthria showed little improvement up to 15 years after onset. In a similar study of head-injured patients with dysarthria, Rusk et al reported that half had improved and half had not 5 to 15 years after injury.

Although there are no reports in the literature regarding the incidence of specific types of dysarthria following TBI, a few studies suggest a variety of dysarthric characteristics that may be present depending on the nature and location of the brain injury as well as the severity. Ataxic dysarthria has been the predominant dysarthria reported among individuals with TBI in a few studies (Simmons, 1983; Yorkston & Beukelman, 1981; Yorkston, Beukelman, Minifie, & Sapir, 1984). Ataxic dysarthria results from damage to the cerebellum. The cerebellum appears to regulate the force, speed, range, timing, and direction of movements originating in the other motor systems of the brain. Primary characteristics of ataxic dysarthria are marked breakdown in the articulation of consonants and vowels, abnormalities in the prosody of speech, dysrhythmia, slow rate, and harsh vocal quality.

Flaccid dysarthria as well as mixed dysarthrias (flaccid-spastic, spastic-ataxic) have also been described in individuals with TBI (Netsell & Daniel, 1979; Yorkston & Beukelman, 1981). Flaccid dysarthria results from damage to motor units required for speech, resulting in weakness, loss of muscle tone, reduced reflexes, and paralysis. Primary characteristics of flaccid dysarthria are hypernasality, nasal emission, and breathiness. Spastic dysarthria results from damage to the upper motor neurons and impairs movements necessary for efficient speech production. Spastic muscles are stiff, move sluggishly, and tend to be weak. The resulting speech is slow and is produced effortfully with imprecise articulation, low pitch, and harsh vocal quality.

Mutism

Levin, Madison, Bailey, Meyer, Eisenberg, and Guinto (1983) have defined a condition called mutism, secondary to severe TBI but not attributable to cranial nerve injury, in which the patient is speechless in the presence of an ability to comprehend simple commands and to communicate nonverbally. These investigators observed the incidence of mutism in a group of 350 TBI patients to be approximately 3%. Two types of mutism were identified, one associated with lesions to the left basal ganglia (subcortical structures deep within the brain) believed to have a better prognosis, and another associated with severe diffuse brain injury, considered to be a permanent condition.

Apraxia of Speech

Apraxia of speech (AOS) is not typically reported in demographic studies of TBI, but it does occur frequently enough to be a consideration in the management of communication following TBI (Yorkston and Beukelman, 1991). Clinical experience and isolated case reports (McHenry & Wilson, 1994) indicate that the AOS of individuals with TBI is comparable to the AOS resulting from left hemisphere strokes, and that it usually occurs in conjunction with a language disorder.

✦ Rehabilitation of Traumatic Brain Injury

Rehabilitation has been defined as the development of an individual to the fullest physical, psychological, social, vocational, avocational, and educational potential consistent with his or her physiologic or anatomic impairment and environmental limitations (Whyte & Rosenthal, 1988). A primary objective in the rehabilitation of individuals with TBI is the improvement of social skills. The ability to communicate effectively is the basis of socially skilled behavior. Although there is no universally accepted definition of social skills, Ylvisaker, Urbanczyk, and Feeney (1992) have suggested that social skills consist of five dimensions: (1) the individual's knowledge of self; (2) the extent to which individuals attend to their personal appearance; (3) social cognition (i.e., social perception, social knowledge, and social decision making); (4) communication; and (5) the social environment (i.e., important people in the individual's natural environment). Rehabilitation of TBI is best described from the perspective of the World Health Organization's (WHO) International Classification of Functioning and Health (ICF). The WHO classification was developed to provide a standard framework for the description of health and health-related states (WHO, 2002). The original domains of "impairment," "disability," and "handicap" have been updated and expanded to "pathophysiology," "impairment," "activity/functional limitations," and "participation" to reflect the influence of idiosyncratic contextual factors, both environmental and personal. From the perspective of brain injury, *pathophysiology* is the interruption of normal physiologic processes, body functions, or structures through injury or disease. *Impairments* are losses or disorders of cognitive, emotional, or physiologic functions. *Activity/functional limitations* result from impairments, and refer to the effects of the impairments on a person's everyday life activities. *Participation* is the nature and extent of a person's involvement in life situations in relation to impairments, activity limitations,

Table 6–6 Overview of World Health Organization's (WHO) International Classification of Functioning and Health (ICF)

	Domain	Definition	Positive Aspects	Negative Aspects
Part 1: functioning and disability	Body function and structures	*Body functions* are physiologic and psychological functions of the body. *Body structures* are anatomic parts of the body (e.g., organs, limbs).	Integrity of functioning and structure	Impairment of functioning and structure
	Activities and participation	*Activity* is the ability to execute a specific task. *Participation* is the ability to be involved in a life situation.	Ability to complete specific tasks or to participate in specific situations/activities of daily living	Restriction or limitation of ability to complete specific tasks or participate in certain situations
Part 2: contextual factors	Environmental factors	External influences on functioning; includes *individual factors* such as those in the immediate environment of the individual (e.g., home, workplace) and *societal factors* such as informal social structures or systems that impact the individual (e.g., attitudes, formal and informal social rules).	Individual or societal factors that facilitate the individual's functioning	Individual or societal factors that hinder the individual's functioning
	Personal factors	Personal influences on performance that are derived from the individual's particular background; includes such things as gender, race, age, education, social background, past life events, personal behavior style, coping style, etc.	Personal factors are not classified as positive or negative in ICF, but are included to demonstrate their contribution and illustrate the impact they may have on intervention outcome.	

From World Health Organization International. (2002). Classification of Impairment, Disabilities, and Handicaps. Geneva: WHO.

health conditions, and contextual factors. The revised ICF has moved away from the "consequences of disease" classification to the current "components of health" classification (WHO, 2002) (**Table 6–6**). Historically, rehabilitation has focused on impairment and disability issues following TBI. However, in recent years this focus has shifted, with the recognition that the ultimate determination of successful rehabilitation is the reintegration of patients into their communities in a meaningful and satisfying social role (Mills et al, 1997; Ponsford et al, 1995; Sohlberg & Mateer, 2001; Ylvisaker & Gobble, 1988).

Rehabilitation Continuum

The TBI rehabilitation process involves a continuum of care. This continuum consists of five distinct stages in which a variety of services are provided on the basis of the individual's needs. The typical rehabilitation continuum stages are acute care, subacute care, inpatient rehabilitation, outpatient rehabilitation, and community reintegration.

Acute Care

Acute care takes place while the individual is in an acute care hospital. It is that point in the treatment continuum where the primary goals are, by necessity, medically oriented. Medical management at this stage includes delineation of the nature and extent of the primary brain injury, as well as attempts at minimizing the effects of secondary brain complications that develop as a consequence of metabolic disturbances or the original neuronal damage (i.e., slowly developing hemorrhages, cerebral edema, intracranial pressure, hypoxic-ischemic damage, and seizures). The role of the speech–language pathologist in the

management of individuals with TBI varies with the stage of the rehabilitation continuum. In the acute care facility the speech–language pathologist differentially diagnoses cognitive-communicative, language, speech, and swallowing disorders, and initiates diagnostic treatment. The benefits of early intervention (including speech–language pathology services) for individuals with TBI during acute hospitalization have been documented (Cope & Hall, 1982; Mackay, Berstein, Chapman, Morgan, & Milazzo, 1992). For example, Mackay and colleagues compared outcome data for a group of individuals with TBI enrolled in an early intervention program that included assessment and therapy being provided in the intensive care unit with a second group that did not undergo this treatment. Findings indicated that the group that received the early treatment had significantly shorter rehabilitation stays. Furthermore, this group was discharged with higher levels of cognitive functioning and had a significantly higher percentage of discharges home versus discharges to extended care facilities. Therefore, for the purposes of the present discussion, acute care is considered the beginning stage of the TBI rehabilitation continuum. Once life-threatening issues have been addressed and medical stability has been achieved, the patient no longer requires the intense level of care provided in the acute medical setting and is discharged to one of three settings: a subacute care facility, an inpatient rehabilitation facility, or home.

Subacute Care

When discharged to a subacute care facility, the patient may be medically stable but too weak, or unable cognitively, to fully participate in and benefit from an aggressive inpatient rehabilitation program. Subacute facilities provide skilled nursing care as well as the full complement of therapy services, which are offered on a less intensive basis [e.g., 30 minutes of physical therapy (PT), occupational therapy (OT), speech–language three times per week]. The typical length of stay in subacute facilities is generally longer than in inpatient rehabilitation hospitals. Patients in subacute facilities may eventually be discharged to inpatient rehabilitation facilities or home. Subacute facilities are typically organized to deliver services via a multidisciplinary team of professionals.

Inpatient Rehabilitation

Inpatient rehabilitation hospitals or units are intended to provide intensive multidisciplinary rehabilitation. Although several years ago the average length of stay in such facilities was much longer, currently stays for individuals with TBI may range from 3 to 10 weeks. To be a candidate for intensive inpatient rehabilitation, an individual must actively be involved in a minimum of 3 hours of therapy per day and have ongoing goals in at least two services (PT, OT, and/or speech–language pathology). An integral part of this phase of the rehabilitation process is the weekly interdisciplinary team meeting to establish and discuss the individual's rehabilitation goals, prognosis, and discharge plan. In all instances the rehabilitation program designed for patients depends on their targeted outcome. Under ideal circumstances the individual is discharged home. However, an individual with TBI who has not progressed rapidly and is not ready to return home, yet who is still considered a candidate for ongoing inpatient rehabilitation services, may then be transferred to a subacute facility.

Outpatient

In most cases the individual who is discharged home continues rehabilitation on an outpatient basis or through a home-care agency. Outpatient rehabilitation services are generally comparable to those services the individual received as an inpatient, although outpatient services may differ in intensity. For example, an individual may continue to receive services from PT, OT, and speech–language pathology but only two or three times per week. Conversely, an individual may be enrolled in an outpatient day treatment program involving 5 hours of interdisciplinary services 5 days per week. Once again the rehabilitation services are determined by the individual's needs, but may also be dictated by the resources available in given facility or region. For outpatient rehabilitation, the individual is transported from home to the outpatient facility for rehabilitation services and then returns home each day.

Home Care

When the individual receives services through a home-care agency, rehabilitation services are provided in the home by professionals. These services are usually of short duration and end as soon as the individual is ambulatory or mobile enough to be safely transported to an outpatient rehabilitation facility. One particular advantage to providing rehabilitation in the individual's home is that the service providers can see first hand the real-world obstacles that the individual is confronted with. This provides an opportunity for the clinicians to decrease the activity limitations and to increase the degree of participation.

Community Reintegration

The end point of the rehabilitation continuum of care involves community reintegration. Although in this discussion community reintegration is presented as the end of the rehabilitation continuum, we must emphasize that successful community reintegration needs to begin early in the rehabilitation process. Throughout the rehabilitation continuum all therapy goals should be influenced by the specific long-term expectations for a given individual. Regardless of whether the ultimate goal is for patients to return home and to their previous job, or to live in supervised housing and work in a sheltered workshop, those skills necessary for the successful transfer to that environment must be identified and addressed in every treatment session (DePompei & Blosser, 1991; Kneipp, 1991; Kreutzer & Wehman, 1990; Story, 1991; Wehman, 1991). Community reintegration is different for each individual with a TBI. For example, individuals with significant cognitive deficits may require a highly structured environment including job coaches, and supervision at home to provide prompts and cues that will help them compensate for their cognitive-communicative difficulties. An individual with TBI may also present with a significant dysarthria and may require support involving augmentative and alternative communication devices. In such a case it will also be necessary to provide education and training to the individual's communication partners to facilitate successful interactions.

Cognitive Rehabilitation

In this section we discuss the management of cognitive-communicative disturbances following TBI. The assessment and treatment of aphasia, dysarthria, apraxia of speech, and dysphagia is not discussed in this chapter.

The treatment of cognitive-communicative deficits that result from TBI is referred to as *cognitive rehabilitation*. This term implies an intervention regimen aimed at increasing functional abilities in everyday life by improving an individual's capacity to process and interpret incoming information (Sohlberg & Mateer, 1989). In general terms there are two approaches to cognitive rehabilitation: restorative and compensatory (Ben-Yishay & Diller, 1993). The underlying rationales of these approaches are very different. The *restorative approach* is based on the notion that neuronal growth, resulting in improvement in function, is associated with repetitive exercise of neuronal circuits. The restorative approach is sometimes referred to as the "muscle building approach" and involves repetitive exercises and drilling. In contrast, the *compensatory approach* concedes that certain functions cannot be recovered, and the development of strategies to circumvent the impaired functions is the primary goal (Benedict, 1989). This view of cognitive rehabilitation implies that "restoration" and "compensation" are distinct phases of the rehabilitation continuum. In other words, compensatory strategies should not be implemented until restorative exercises have failed. However, it has been observed that helping TBI individuals to become increasingly aware of their cognitive needs and to be strategic in approaching cognitively demanding tasks, which is typically associated with a "compensatory" approach to cognitive rehabilitation, is actually restorative. In other words, the compensatory strategy actually focuses on restoring the strategic, deliberate aspect of cognitive processing, which may be more important after the injury than before. Therefore, it is misleading to contrast "restorative" and "compensatory" as though they were not overlapping approaches. Rather, these approaches should occur simultaneously in rehabilitation (Coelho, DeRuyter, & Stein, 1996; Ylvisaker & Feeney, 1998).

Currently there is disagreement regarding the most effective approach to cognitive rehabilitation. The traditional approach, termed "process-specific," consists of hierarchically organized treatment tasks targeting distinct, theoretically motivated components of cognitive processes (Sohlberg & Mateer, 1989, 2001) and has been the most widely applied technique. In recent years context-sensitive approaches have been advocated in which treatment is provided by collaborating with people in the daily environments of the person with TBI to create positive, supported everyday routines of action and interaction in the context of daily activities (Ylvisaker & Feeney, 1998). The application of specific instructional techniques in cognitive rehabilitation is also currently being investigated (Sohlberg, Ehlhardt, & Kennedy, 2005). A great deal of research remains to be done to validate cognitive and communicative rehabilitation interventions for individuals with TBI. Concrete patient-specific decision-making is critical to the development of a body of evidence supporting interventions for this population (Ylvisaker, Coelho, Kennedy, et al., 2002).

Recently, a national trend of referencing research evidence to support clinical decision making for the management of medical conditions has surfaced. Consistent with this movement, the Academy of Neurologic Communication Disorders and Sciences (ANCDS), in conjunction with the American Speech–Language-Hearing Association (ASHA's) Special Interest Division 2 (Neurophysiology and Neurogenic Speech and Language Disorders), established committees of experts to develop evidence-based practice guidelines (EBPG) for the management of dysarthria, aphasia, dementia, apraxia of speech, and cognitive-communication disorders following TBI. The committee developing the EBPGs for TBI identified several assumptions about the nature and management of cognitive-communication disorders following TBI (Kennedy, 2002) (**Table 6–7**).

Planning for Cognitive Rehabilitation

In planning for cognitive rehabilitation it is necessary to consider the long-term needs of the individual with TBI. This process is facilitated by answering the following questions: Are the treatment goals realistic? What is the individual's capacity to benefit from treatment? According to Lezak (1987), the identification of realistic treatment goals requires the evaluation of two aspects of the TBI individual's cognitive behaviors: the capacity for taking an abstract attitude, and the status of executive functioning. Abstract attitude refers to such capacities as appreciating the point of view of others, being aware that there is a world beyond one's own personal perspective, and being free of concrete or literal interpretations of daily experience. As discussed previously, executive functioning involves those capacities necessary to have an intention and thus formulate goals, to plan and organize goal-directed behavior, to carry out an effective plan, and to monitor and self-correct one's behavior as needed (Lezak, 1982, 1983). Unfortunately, unlike some cognitive deficits that improve with rehabilitation, an impaired capacity to take an abstract attitude and impairments of executive functioning may often become chronic problems that are

Table 6–7 Assumptions About Managing Cognitive-Communication Disorders Following TBI

1. Management of cognitive-communication disorders is an integral part of speech–language pathologists' (SLPs) scope of practice. SLPs are uniquely trained to manage these disorders with clinical knowledge in the interaction between cognition and communication.

2. Managing cognitive-communication disorders is an interdisciplinary endeavor.

3. Cognitive-communication intervention does not include communication intervention for aphasia or motor-speech disorders following TBI.

4. There are numerous approaches to cognitive-communication intervention, e.g., behavioral approaches, skill training, process-specific approaches, multimodal approaches, etc.

5. Numerous service delivery models exist, e.g., inpatient medical rehabilitation, long-term care, outpatient care, job coaching, school-based services, day-treatment, transitional living programs, or individual and group therapy.

6. Improvements in impairments may or may not facilitate a change in an individual's activity or participation level and vice versa.

7. The ultimate goal of cognitive-communication intervention is to achieve the highest level of communicative participation in everyday living.

From Kennedy, M. (2002). Evidence-Based Practice Guidelines for Cognitive-Communication Disorders After Traumatic Brain Injury: Initial Committee Report. *Journal of Medical Speech–Language Pathology, 10,* ix–xiii.

resistant to treatment. Retraining these capacities requires the individual to have in mind what no longer comes to mind, or what that individual no longer appreciates as missing. Generally speaking, the major limitations to an individual's ability to profit from rehabilitation are (1) impaired executive functioning, (2) loss of abstract attitude, (3) chronic attentional and/or memory disorders, and (4) learning deficits (Lezak, 1987). In addition, disorders of behavioral self-regulation and social-interactive competence are common after TBI and may further limit an individual's capacity to benefit from cognitive rehabilitation (see Ylvisaker, Turkstra, & Coelho, 2005).

Rehabilitation following TBI should be driven by the individual's real-world problems and not deficits identified by a test, as such deficits are "often far removed from the everyday manifestations of a deficit" (Wilson, 2003, p. 25). Goal planning is a preferred alternative that has been used in rehabilitation settings for several years. This approach is based on several principles: (1) the individual with TBI should always participate in goal setting, (2) goals selected should be reasonable and client-centered, (3) the goal should contain a description of the individual's behavior when the goal is attained, (4) the method for achieving the goal should be clearly delineated, and (5) all goals should be specific and measurable with definite timelines. The list of goals will consist of both long- and short-term objectives (Houts & Scott, 1975, as cited in Wilson, 2003; McMillan & Sparkes, 1999).

✦ Stages of Recovery Following Traumatic Brain Injury

The usual course of recovery following a TBI typically involves a period of unconsciousness, followed by confusion, and a progressive return of cognitive functions. The timeline of these

Table 6–8 Ranchos Los Amigos Levels of Cognitive Functioning (RLA)

RLA Level	Assistance Required	Possible Behavioral Characteristics
Level 1: no response	Total assistance: patient expends ≤25% of the effort and requires ≥75% assistance	Complete absence of observable change in behavior when presented with visual, auditory, tactile, proprioceptive, vestibular, or painful stimuli
Level 2: generalized response	Total assistance: patient expends ≤25% of the effort and requires ≥75% assistance.	Demonstrates a generalized reflex response to painful stimuli; responds to repeated auditory stimuli; responds to external stimuli with generalized physiologic changes, gross body movements, and/or purposeful vocalization; responses may be significantly delayed
Level 3: localized response	Total assistance: patient expends ≤25% of the effort and requires ≥75% assistance	Demonstrates withdrawal or vocalization to painful stimuli; turns toward or away from auditory stimuli; blinks with strong light or follows moving object in visual field; responds to discomfort by pulling tubes or restraints; responds inconsistently to simple commands; responses are directly related to type of stimulus; may respond to some people but not to others
Level 4: confused-agitated	Maximal assistance: patient expends at least 25%, but ≤50% of the effort and requires ≥50% assistance	Alert with heightened state of activity; purposeful attempts to remove restraints or tubes, or to get out of bed; may perform motor activities such as sitting, reaching, and walking but without apparent purpose, or on another's request; may demonstrate aggressive behavior or mood swings; absent short-term memory, goal-directed behavior, problem solving, and self-monitoring; poor cooperation with treatment efforts
Level 5: confused-inappropriate-nonagitated	Maximal assistance: patient expends at least 25%, but ≤50% of the effort and requires ≥50% assistance	Alert but not agitated generally; may demonstrate agitation in response to external stimuli and/or lack of environmental structure; not oriented to person, place, or time; brief periods of nonpurposeful sustained attention; severely impaired recent memory; may confuse past and present in reaction to ongoing activity; poor goal-directed behavior, problem solving, and self-monitoring; inappropriate use of objects without external direction; unable to learn new information, but may be able to perform previously learned tasks with structure and cues; responses to simple commands without external structure are random and nonpurposeful; able to converse socially with external cues, but verbalizations may be inappropriate and confabulatory without such structure
Level 6: confused-appropriate	Moderate assistance: patient expends at least 50%, but <75% of the effort and requires ≥25% assistance.	Inconsistently oriented; able to attend to highly familiar tasks in a nondistracting environment for 30 minutes with moderate redirection; remote memory has more depth and detail than recent memory; vague recognition of some staff; able to use memory aide with maximal assistance; emerging awareness of appropriate response to self, family, and basic needs; emerging goal-directed behavior related to meeting basic personal needs; moderate assistance needed to problem solve barriers to task completion; maximal assistance for new learning with little or no carryover; unaware of impairments, disabilities, and safety risks; consistently follows simple directions; verbal expressions are appropriate in highly familiar and structured situations
Level 7: automatic-appropriate	Minimal assistance for routine activities of daily living patient: expends at least 75%, and requires 25% assistance	Consistently oriented to person and place within familiar environments; needs moderate assistance for orientation to time; able to attend to highly familiar tasks in a nondistracting environment for 30 minutes with minimal assistance to complete tasks; able to use an assistive memory device with minimal assistance; minimal assistance needed for new learning; demonstrates carryover of new learning; initiates and carries out steps to complete familiar personal routines but has shallow recall of what she/he has been doing; able to monitor accuracy and completeness of each step in routine personal and household activities of daily living (ADLs) and can modify plan with minimal assistance; superficial awareness of his/her condition but unaware of specific impairments and how they limit his/her abilities; minimal supervision for safety in home or community ADLs; unrealistic planning for the future; unable to think about consequences of decisions made; overestimates abilities; unaware of others' needs and feelings; uncooperative; unable to recognize inappropriate social interactional behavior
Level 8: purposeful and appropriate	Stand-by assistance: patient requires no more than verbal cues without physical contact, or requires help with set-up of items or assistive devices	Consistently oriented to person, place, and time; independently attends to and completes familiar tasks for 1 hour in a distracting environment; able to recall and integrate past and recent events; uses assistive memory device such as daily schedule and to-do list with stand-by-assistance; initiates and carries out steps to complete familiar personal routines with stand-by assistance and can modify plan with minimal assistance; requires no assistance once new tasks are learned; aware of and acknowledges disabilities when they interfere with task completion; thinks about consequences of a decision with minimal assistance; over- or underestimates abilities; acknowledges others' needs and feelings appropriately with minimal assistance; depressed, easily frustrated, irritable, argumentative, and self-centered; uncharacteristically dependent or independent; able to recognize inappropriate social interactional behavior with minimal assistance

From Hagan, C., Malkmus, D., & Burditt, G. (1979) Levels of Cognitive Functioning. In: *Rehabilitation of the Head Injured Adult: Comprehensive Physical Management*. Downey, CA: Professional Staff Association of Rancho Los Amigos Hospital.

stages is variable among individuals with TBI and consequently it is impossible to specify a regular course of recovery among the TBI population (Sohlberg & Mateer, 1989). A more practical approach is to discuss stages of recovery. In the subsections that follow, a variety of issues pertaining to the management of individuals with TBI, and specifically the role of the speech–language pathologist, are discussed with regard to the early, intermediate, and later stages of recovery. These stages are based loosely on ratings from the Rancho Los Amigos Levels of Cognitive Function (RLA) (Hagan, Malkmus, & Burditt, 1979) (**Table 6–8**). This scale is useful for identifying a patient's most intact level of cognitive functioning over the entire course of rehabilitation. The RLA is used to identify the patient's highest level of functioning and therefore is indicative of the best way to approach the patient throughout the continuum of intervention. The RLA represents a progression of recovery of cognitive abilities in the TBI population as manifested through behavioral change. Advantages of using the RLA include (1) that it is an assessment that does not require the patient's cooperation; (2) it provides behavioral descriptions of cognitive recovery along a severity continuum; (3) it enables professionals, from a variety of disciplines, to discuss TBI patients using common and descriptive terminology; and (4) it provides baseline information for the development of team treatment goals. For each level, assessment and treatment procedures are discussed as well as the rationale for the approaches selected. The discussion of each level is followed by a brief case study of an individual at that level of functioning.

Early Stage of Recovery (RLA II, Generalized Response; RLA III, Localized Response)

Assessment/Treatment

During this phase of recovery communicative functioning is dependent on arousal mechanisms; consequently, management procedures are often diagnostic in nature and assessment and treatment become simultaneous endeavors (Kennedy & DeRuyter, 1991). There are two types of variables that need to be considered in the assessment of minimally responsive brain-injured patients: task and performance. Task variables are within the clinician's control and include such things as (1) stimulus intensity, (2) rate of presentation, (3) type of stimulus presented and type response required (receptive versus expressive), (4) duration of task and length of testing sessions, (5) familiarity of task to patient, (6) level of task complexity, and (7) context in which stimulus is presented. Performance variables are aspects of the response the clinician observes while task variables remain constant or change. These include such factors as (1) response duration; (2) response delay; (3) ability of the patient to shift response sets from one task to the next; (4) number of times a response needs to be repeated for the response to be elicited; (5) type of response; and (6) pattern of responses, or response consistency. With regard to assessment of cognitive/communicative skills in the early stages of recovery, the speech–language pathologist must rely primarily on observational skills as TBI patients at RLA II and III are typically unable to participate in standardized testing. Attempts should be made to "standardize" the observations by presenting comparable stimulation across input modalities (e.g., auditory, visual, tactile) and consistent stimulation activities (i.e., with regard to rate, complexity, duration, intensity, etc.) across sessions. By

Table 6–9 Assessment of Individuals at Rancho Los Amigos Levels of Cognitive Function (RLA) II and III

Abilities	Methods
Alertness: amount, frequency timing, activities, body positions	Team evaluation
Arousability: types of stimulation and responses	Systematic presentation of hierarchical tasks
Sensory modalities: tactile, kinesthetic, olfactory, gustatory, auditory, visual	Observe at various times and during various tasks
Communication: following commands, type of response, communication system, basic reading	Interview family members
Presence of reflexes: oral chewing, defensiveness, whole-body reflexes	Observe individual with family, note responses
Balance: posture, head control, limb alignment, sitting, standing	Use familiar items: music, pictures
Arm and hand function: reaching, grasping, gestures	Record frequency, rate, duration, variety, and quality of responses
Tone: overall, at rest, in motion, various positions	Observe responses with cuing (manual, verbal, gestural, nonverbal)

From Kennedy, M.R.T., & DeRuyter, F. (1991). Cognitive and Language Bases for Communication Disorders. In: D.R. Beukelman and K.M. Yorkston (Eds.), Communication Disorders Following Traumatic Brain Injury: Management of Cognitive, Language, and Motor Impairments (pp. 123–190). Austin, TX: Pro-Ed.

using replicable stimulation, responses observed in one session under a specific pattern of stimulation can be attempted to be re-elicited under the same conditions during another session as a measure of the consistency of the response. The Western Neuro Sensory Stimulation Profile (Ansell & Keenan, 1989) and the JFK Johnson Rehabilitation Institute's Coma Recovery Scale (Giacino, Kezmarsky, Deluca, McKenna, & Cicerone, 1991), which were designed to assess TBI patients' arousal/attention, expressive communication, and response to auditory, visual, tactile, and olfactory stimulation, are examples of attempts at standardizing observations of lower functioning patients (**Tables 6–9** and **6–10**). It should be noted that sensory or coma stimulation has generated a great deal of controversy in the field of brain injury rehabilitation (see Zasler, Kreutzer, & Taylor, 1991 for a review and recommendations for its use).

For the purposes of establishing a system for communicative interactions, once patients with TBI are responding in a more consistent fashion, their best input modality and best response mode need to be identified. Such information should be immediately communicated to the other treating team members and the patient's family members to facilitate their interactions with the patient. DeRuyter and Becker (1988) observed that for nonspeaking individuals functioning at RLA III (localized response), the success of yes-no response systems depended on the most natural and automatic body movement. The most successful yes-no systems were head nods, with decreasing success noted for systems requiring less automatic movement and the use of other cognitive and/or motor processes (e.g., visual tracking and reading for using yes-no cards). The ability to follow verbal commands in individuals who have been unresponsive has been noted to be a significant turning point in patients progressing out of coma

Table 6–10   Commonly Used Stimuli for Evaluating Individuals at RLA II and III

Tactile	Olfactory
Shapes (cubes, balls)	Extracts
Surfaces (cloth, Velcro, cotton ball)	Perfumes and colognes
Fur	Spices
Brushes and combs	Soap
Firm touch	Vinegar
Kinesthesia	Visual
Range of motion	Objects from home
Positioning (extremities and body)	Pictures of family and individual
Auditory	Mirror
Bells	Colorful items
Chimes	ADL items
Clapping	Gustatory
Music	Extracts
Voice (familiar and unfamiliar)	Lemon
Snapping fingers	Vinegar

From Kennedy, M.R.T., & DeRuyter, F. (1991). Cognitive and Language Bases for Communication Disorders. In: D.R. Beukelman and K.M. Yorkston (Eds.), Communication Disorders Following Traumatic Brain Injury: Management of Cognitive, Language, and Motor Impairments (pp. 123–190). Austin, TX: Pro-Ed.

(Bricolo, Turazzi, and Feriotti, 1980). Ansell and Keenan (1989) have reported on patterns of communication recovery in "slow to recover patients" (at RLA II and III for extended periods of time). They observed that if responses to auditory information (following commands) began to improve, the patient had a 50% chance of progressing to RLA V. If responses to auditory and visual information returned simultaneously, the probability of improving to RLA V were considerably better. If, however, responses to visual or tactile stimulation were the only responses to emerge, the likelihood for cognitive improvement was minimal. These results are consistent with previous research that has indicated retardation of development and diminished recovery of central nervous system function in the presence of environmental and sensory deprivation (Stein, Finger, & Hart, 1983). It also emphasizes the importance of the cognitive-language system to recovery after TBI.

Case Study 1

Background   L.D. is a recent college graduate who works in the sales department of a daily newspaper. She was involved in a motor vehicle accident in which her vehicle struck a utility pole at a high speed. At the time the paramedics arrived her GCS was 6; by the time she arrived in the emergency room her GCS was 3. Examination revealed multiple trauma including facial and chest contusions that required her being intubated for assisted ventilation. Computed tomography (CT) scan revealed a basilar skull fracture and multiple contusions in both hemispheres. She was admitted to the neuro–intensive care unit (ICU) and over the next 24 hours considerable cerebral edema occurred requiring the insertion of an intracranial pressure (ICP) monitor. After approximately 5 days the brain swelling subsided and the ICP was removed. It was at this point that the initial referral for a speech–language pathology consult was made.

Assessment/Treatment   When L.D. was first seen she was still in the ICU. She was no longer intubated, but was minimally responsive (RLA II, generalized response), and had an nasogastric feeding tube in place. No consistent responses could be elicited, and consequently no formalized testing was completed. Following the initial assessment session, L.D. was scheduled for three 10- to 15-minute diagnostic treatment sessions per day. She was routinely more responsive in the early morning and was most easily aroused by auditory stimuli, particularly recordings of family members saying her name. L.D.'s eyes remaining open typically signaled changes in her level of alertness. Once a consistent response to the audio-recordings was noted, attempts were made to attain and maintain her arousal with different types of auditory stimuli.

After approximately 10 days in the ICU, L.D. was transferred to a regular room on a neurosurgical unit. Nursing, PT, and OT staff members also incorporated sensory stimulation activities into their treatment regimens. Family members were also able to provide carryover with the stimulation activities on the weekends. An important aspect of these activities was a daily journal, which was kept in L.D.'s room to record the characteristics of the stimulation applied, and the consistency of her responses. This facilitated communication between treatment team and family members. At approximately 5 weeks posttrauma, L.D.'s responsiveness had increased to the point where she was inconsistently responding via head nodding to yes-no questions and was attending to visual stimuli as well. No consistent vocalizations were noted, nor had anyone observed any verbalization. Her RLA level was rated at II to III.

After nearly 7 weeks of acute care, L.D.'s medical condition stabilized and she was transferred to a rehabilitation hospital for more aggressive rehabilitation services. She continued to be tube fed via a percutaneous endoscopic gastrostomy (PEG) that had been implanted after 12 days because L.D. had developed a severe nasal irritation from the nasogastric (NG) feeding tube. Prior to leaving the acute hospital, L.D. was seen for a swallowing evaluation [via fiberoptic endoscopic evaluation of swallowing (FEES)] that revealed aspiration of thin liquid and puree consistencies. A follow-up swallowing evaluation was recommended in approximately 2 weeks, or sooner if her cognitive status improved.

Intermediate Stage of Recovery (RLA IV, Confused-Agitated; and RLA V, Confused-Inappropriate-Nonagitated)

Assessment

As the alertness of individuals with TBI, at RLA IV (confused-agitated) and V (confused-inappropriate-nonagitated) improves, they are bombarded with a multitude of stimuli from their environment. Because they are unable to focus and sustain attention for more than a few seconds, the stimuli may be meaningless or at best confusing. Consequently, these patients may demonstrate marked agitation. Their arms, legs, trunk, and head may be in constant motion and speech is often completely irrelevant beyond a few automatic social responses. The term *confusion* is usually applied to such pervasive attentional deficits. This period is almost always reversible in TBI patients; however, in some severely injured patients confusional states may become chronic (Sohlberg &

Table 6–11 Assessment of Individuals at RLA IV and V

Abilities	Methods
Hyperattentiveness and hypoattentiveness	Team evaluation
Selectivity, attention span	Systematic presentation of hierarchical tasks
Orientation or confusion: time, place, persons, objects	Use standardized tests if able
Sequencing: in expression, thought activity activities	Present simple, motor, functional
Inhibition or disinhibition	Evaluation sessions 15 to 30 minutes long
Organization: associating, categorizing	Vary tasks to allow for attention and disinhibition
Agitation: causes, frequency, duration, what reduces it	Include behavioral reinforcements for reducing agitation
Communication: modalities, content, generalized versus focal, comprehension, use of social skills	Include familiar persons to elicit best response

From Kennedy, M.R.T., & DeRuyter, F. (1991). Cognitive and Language Bases for Communication Disorders. In: D.R. Beukelman and K.M. Yorkston (Eds.), Communication Disorders Following Traumatic Brain Injury: Management of Cognitive, Language, and Motor Impairments (pp. 123–190). Austin, TX: Pro-Ed.

Mateer, 1989). With time, less agitation is noted, but TBI patients may still be unable to maintain a coherent line of thought or maintain concentration. Severe disruption of language function at this stage is common, even in the absence of aphasia. Confused language, described previously, is the best characterization of the cognitive/communicative impairments. Impaired attentional processes, including initiation, maintenance, shifting, and inhibiting (i.e., the ability ignore

distractions), affect both language comprehension and expression. Poor topic maintenance and topic shifting in conversation and stimulus bound responses result from ideational perseveration (i.e., becoming fixated on certain ideas or thoughts), verbal disinhibition (i.e., saying whatever comes to mind), and impaired impulse control (Adamovich, Henderson, & Auerbach, 1985; Hagan, 1984). In the presence of damage to the frontal lobes, which is a relatively common consequence of TBI, it has been observed that although the structural components of language remain intact, the intent and use of language may be significantly impaired (Alexander et al, 1989; Lezak, 1976; Stuss & Benson, 1997). Language behaviors associated with frontal lobe injuries include confabulation, impaired word fluency, perseveration of thought, inappropriate turn taking, inattentiveness to listener's needs, repetitive and/or disorganized messages, and social inappropriateness due to poor self-monitoring.

Kennedy and DeRuyter (1991) noted that because individuals functioning at RLA IV and V are frequently unable to focus and sustain their attention to specific tasks, to discriminate, and to sequence and organize their responses, nonstandardized procedures must be employed during the assessment. Adamovich et al (1985) presented several activities arranged in a hierarchy from low-level (arousal and alertness) to high-level (reasoning and abstraction) cognitive tasks. **Table 6–11** summarizes important considerations for the assessment of TBI patients at this level of recovery. Although use of standardized materials is not always practical, baseline data gathered as early as possible can document the pattern of recovery and provide prognostic information. Standardized procedures should be incorporated into the evaluation process as soon as possible. The ANCDS committee developing the EBPGs for TBI has offered several guidelines for the use of standardized batteries for the assessment of cognitive-communication disorders (**Table 6–12**).

Table 6–12 Synopsis of the Evidence-Based Practice Guidelines for the Assessment of Cognitive-Communication Disorders after traumatic brain injury (TBI)

1. Clinicians should use caution in applying most published standardized tests in the assessment of persons with TBI. Most of the tests recommended by publishers, distributors, and clinicians were not developed for persons with TBI.

2. For appropriately selected assessment purposes and age groups, the committee recommends the use of six standardized tests that met the majority of the stated criteria for reliability, validity, and inclusion of individuals with TBI in the test design and standardization sample. The tests are the following:

   a. American Speech–Language-Hearing Association Functional Assessment of Communication Skills in Adults (ASHA-FACS; Frattali et al, 1995)

   b. Behavior Rating Inventory of Executive Function (BRIEF; Gioia, Isquith, Guy, & Kenworthy, 1996)

   c. Communication Activities of Daily Living, Second Edition (CADL-2; Holland et al, 1999)

   d. Repeatable Battery for the Assessment of Neuropsychological status (RBANS; Randolph, 2001)

   e. Test of Language Competence- Extended (TLC-E; WIIG & Secord, 1989)

   f. Western Aphasia Battery (WAB; Kertesz, 1982)

3. On the basis of expert opinion the committee recommends that standardized testing be considered within a broader framework that includes evaluation of the person's preinjury characteristics, stage of development and recovery, and life and communication context. Standardized tests may have limited ecologic and predictive validity beyond test settings. Standardized tests may assist clinicians in identifying underlying cognitive impairments associated with relevant everyday activities that can only be assessed through dynamic, nonstandardized evaluation procedures as well as evaluation of communication context.

4. The committee recommends that speech–language pathologists integrate their cognitive-communication assessments with those of other professionals whose scope of practice includes cognitive assessment, most notably neuropsychology. Many clinicians appear to be using parts of neuropsychological tests in their evaluations and may not recognize the significant limitations in interpreting these tests.

From Turkstra, L., Ylvisaker, M., Coelho, C., Kennedy, M., Sohlberg, M., & Avery, J. (2005). Practice Guidelines for Standardized Assessment for Persons with Traumatic Brain Injury. *Journal of Medical Speech–language Pathology*, 13: ix–xxviii.

Table 6–13   Recommendations Based on Review of the Literature for the Use of Direct Attention Training

Question	Practice Recommendation	What Clinicians Should Do
Who is a good candidate for direct attention training?	Guideline for postacute or individuals with mild injuries, with intact vigilance	Scrutinize candidacy and monitor responses to training
	Insufficient evidence to make recommendation for individuals in acute stage of recovery	Scrutinize candidacy Monitor responses to training, observed improvements may be a result of spontaneous recovery
	Unknown for use with individuals with severely impaired vigilance	Be cautious and aware of uncertainties of outcome Proceed on case-by-case basis
What are the critical features of direct attention training?	Guideline for using direct attention training in conjunction with metacognitive training (feedback, self-monitoring, and strategy training)	Use attention training in combination with self-reflective logs, anticipation/prediction activities, feedback, and strategy training
	Guideline for program individualization	Identify client strengths and needs prior to treatment; select exercises to address specific areas of weakness
	Guideline for treatment frequency	
	Guideline for complex attention tasks	Treatment should be administered a minimum of once per week
	Unknown for improving vigilance or reaction time	Use a hierarchy of tasks that emphasize working memory, mental control, and selective, alternating, and/or divided attention
		Be cautious when using remediation programs that focus on simple vigilance or reaction time
What outcomes can be expected from direct attention training?	Guideline for obtaining task specific, impairment level outcomes	Identify desired outcomes Measure performance
	Unknown for obtaining generalization to untrained, impairment level tasks	Use methods that can reliably measure clinically meaningful progress
	Uncertain for obtaining generalization to participant level tasks	

From Sohlberg, M.M., Avery, J., Kennedy, M., Ylvisaker, M., Coelho, C., Turkstra, L., & Yorkston, K. (2003). Practice Guidelines for Direct Attention Training. *Journal of Medical Speech–Language Pathology, 11*, xix–xxxix.

Treatment

In the intermediate stage of recovery, RLA IV (confused-agitated) and V (confused-inappropriate-nonagitated) traditional cognitive rehabilitation and speech–language management, as needed, may be initiated. Process-specific cognitive retraining (Sohlberg & Mateer, 1989) is frequently initiated at this stage; This treatment approach is characterized by "repeated administration of hierarchically organized treatment tasks that target distinct, theoretically motivated components of cognitive processes" (p.2). The ANCDS committee on EBPGs for TBI recently reviewed the available evidence on the effectiveness of one such technique, direct attention training (Sohlberg, Avery, Kennedy, Ylvisaker, Coelho, Turkstra, & Yorkston, 2003). **Table 6–13** summarizes the clinical recommendations based on this review. Other EBPGs will be forthcoming.

In the beginning, individuals at this stage of recovery may only be able to participate meaningfully in individual sessions, as group sessions may be too distracting or overstimulating. As the client becomes more oriented and less confused, the one-on-one sessions may be supplemented by group therapy. Group intervention is useful for assessing generalization of targeted behaviors in a more natural setting (i.e., a setting full of competing stimuli, which is less structured and controlled). Group intervention is also very useful for social skills training. Social skills include a variety of abilities (e.g., conversing, sharing, cooperating, greeting others) that enable an individual to interact effectively with peers and others at home, in school, on the job, and in other environments (Ylvisaker, Urbanczyk, & Feeney, 1992).

Individual and/or group treatment may also be supplemented by computer-assisted treatment. Computers are useful for the presentation of repetitive drills and can be programmed to provide varying levels of reinforcement. Computers can also record precise facets of the patient's response such as accuracy and delays. Computers may also provide a means of facilitating functional interactive activities such as sending and receiving email. Family or significant other training/counseling, as well as interdisciplinary consultation and dismissal/discharge planning, is also ongoing during this stage.

Case Study 2

Background   M.D. is a young man who is employed as a cabinet maker. The motorcycle he was driving was struck by a car. He was not wearing a helmet and suffered a severe closed head injury. Upon admission to an acute care hospital, M.D. was unconscious, and CT scans revealed multiple bilateral cerebral contusions to the frontal, temporal, and occipital lobes. In addition he sustained numerous orthopedic and facial injuries, along with a collapsed lung. He remained comatose for approximately 5 weeks, and once he emerged from coma remained in a confused and agitated state (RLA IV) for nearly 3 months. Once M.D. eventually progressed to RLA V (confused-nonagitated) he remained at that level for nearly 6 months and never progressed beyond RLA VI (confused-appropriate).

Assessment   At approximately 2 months post-onset, M.D. was transferred to a rehabilitation hospital. Upon admission cognitive-communicative assessment was difficult because of his agitation. With time it became apparent that he did not have dysphagia, dysarthria, or aphasia, but he did demonstrate cognitive-communicative deficits characterized by very severe impairments in attention, memory, and executive functions. M.D. also demonstrated significant problems with balance and gait, as well as visual perception.

Treatment Interdisciplinary treatment was initially focused on management of his agitation, whereas diagnostic therapy probed for cognitive abilities that could be used to develop compensatory strategies to circumvent M.D.'s significant cognitive-communicative impairments. Over the course of a few weeks it was discovered that M.D. had premorbidly enjoyed rock music, and this was incorporated into treatment as a positive reinforcement. Once M.D. had passed through the agitated stage of his recovery, it was apparent that his communicative abilities were moderately limited. Conversational speech was characterized by frequent confabulations, poor topic management, and frequent disruptive topic shifts. Functional auditory comprehension was limited to short simple messages, and reading and written expression were severely limited.

At approximately 6 months post-onset, M.D. was discharged to the home of his mother, from whom he had been estranged since he dropped out of high school at the age of 16. M.D.'s mother was obviously concerned about his well-being and took on his care and supervision. M.D. continued as an outpatient at the hospital in an interdisciplinary traumatic brain injury day treatment program that met 5 days per week. Over the next 6 months M.D. demonstrated very little progress in the cognitive-communicative domains but grew steadily stronger and began a series of job trials within the rehab facility. His performance in these trials was poor, but with moderate supervision he was able to complete certain tasks. Eventually, his former employer, a furniture maker, asked if M.D. could return to work for him. Although the rehabilitation staff was not optimistic, a job trial was arranged for M.D. at his former job site. It soon became apparent that M.D. had no safety awareness in handling tools and was unable to complete even the most basic tasks, such as sweeping the workshop, because of distractability. Although his employer wanted to keep M.D. on, it was M.D.'s inappropriate social skills and disinhibition around customers that finally led to the employer's decision that the arrangement was not feasible.

At 2 years post-onset M.D.'s mother passed away. M.D., who had continued on with a modified day treatment program focusing on vocational and social skills training, was placed in a supervised apartment and began work in a sheltered workshop. At 3 years post-onset his status was essentially unchanged, though he was being evaluated for more independent jobs in the workshop.

Later Stage of Recovery (RLA VI, Confused-Appropriate; RLA VII, Automatic-Appropriate; and RLA VIII, Purposeful-Appropriate)

Assessment

In the later stages of recovery, RLA VI (confused-appropriate), VII (automatic-appropriate), and VIII (purposeful-appropriate), an interdisciplinary collaborative approach to cognitive-communicative-behavioral evaluation is critical. For example, subtle deficits of attention and speed of performance may be delineated by neuropsychological assessment while the occupational therapist analyzes the individual's behavior during activities of daily living. The speech–language pathologist

often analyzes the effects that impaired processes have on performance in daily activities and communication (Kennedy & DeRuyter, 1991).

Evaluation of individuals at RLA VI to VIII must be tailored to the person's specific injury, severity level, and overall communicative needs. With individuals who are confused, disoriented, and have difficulty with learning (RLA V), assessment should focus on impaired processes (e.g., attention and memory) as well as attention to the impact of the deficits on everyday tasks. With regard to the direct measurement of such deficits, Levin, O'Donnell, and Grossman (1979) developed the GOAT, a brief schedule of questions to measure posttraumatic amnesia and disorientation following TBI (**Table 6–2**). Assessment of individuals at RLA VII and VIII displaying milder cognitive deficits but impairment in higher thought processes (e.g., organization, integration, executive functions) will require a more detailed task-specific evaluation in addition to determining the extent of impairment within underlying processes. The use of standardized tests is most appropriate for TBI patients in the later stages of recovery. Although there are numerous standardized batteries available that can be used for assessing individuals with TBI, few were designed specifically or normed for this population. Consequently selection of standardized assessment batteries and interpretation of test data must be done with caution (**Table 6–12**). The information collected from such tests can (1) provide baseline information to measure improvement; (2) help to differentiate deficits attributable to diffuse cognitive-communicative disorganization versus focal-specific symptoms; (3) facilitate the identification of primary and secondary processes responsible for communicative breakdown; and (4) identify that point at which remediation should begin (Kennedy & DeRuyter, 1991). Assessment tasks will logically involve many cognitive processes, making it difficult to isolate the role of a single process. However, formal assessment should attempt to estimate the degree of impairment in single critical processes such as attention (alertness, arousal, processing speed, attention span, selective attention), discrimination, sequencing, organization (association and categorization), memory processes (e.g., retention span, retrieval mechanisms, recent versus remote, episodic, procedural, semantic), organization, integration, and ability to sustain goal directed activities over time (Adamovich et al, 1985; Hagan, 1984; Kennedy & DeRuyter, 1991).

As was previously mentioned, an important aspect of the assessment process for individuals with TBI at both the intermediate and later stages of recovery is not only to assess performance in traditional testing environments but also to observe their performance during functional activities and in more natural environments. This aspect of the assessment is important because there are often significant differences between an individual's performances across the two settings. Deficits that are not evident during formal testing are often apparent in unstructured everyday environments (Starch & Falltrick, 1990). For example, an individual with TBI may demonstrate concentration abilities that are adequate for functional reading comprehension when distractions are at a minimum. However, when this same individual attempts to read in a noisy/busy environment, concentration abilities may be significantly limited, thus leaving reading comprehension nonfunctional. Such a finding would be important for the planning of treatment programs. Because such observations are common among individuals with TBI, Ylvisaker and

Feeney (1998) have described an approach to assessment and treatment planning they have termed "ongoing, collaborative, contextualized, hypothesis-testing assessment." This approach is based on the notion that vocational/academic performance and social behavior of individuals with TBI is influenced by the contexts they are in; therefore, assessments and interventions must be contextually based. Collaboration among staff members, the individual, and family members adds information and facilitates compliance for the implementation of interventions. Individuals with TBI frequently present with complex profiles (i.e., premorbid disabilities, combinations of diffuse and focal damage, cognitive and behavioral impairments), and when these individuals demonstrate difficulties in the vocational, academic, or behavioral realms, there are a variety of possible explanations and corresponding interventions that may help for their problems. Without hypothesis testing it is very difficult to interpret task failure and to recommend the most effective intervention. This assessment approach is summarized in **Table 6–14**.

Sohlberg and Mateer (1989) have noted that pragmatic deficits may be the most pervasive communication problem in adults with TBI. Traditionally, assessment of communication skills in TBI patients has involved the administration of a language battery, most of which were designed to diagnose aphasia, focusing on the assessment of vocabulary and grammatical abilities at the single word and sentence levels. Hagan (1984) has observed that individuals with TBI often appear to have minimal language impairments based on the results of such assessment batteries, yet demonstrate significant functional communication difficulties in natural environments. Several investigators have advocated the use of nonstandardized assessment procedures, specifically discourse analyses (see Coelho, 1995 and Coelho, Ylvisaker, & Turkstra, 2005 for reviews). Discourse is a series of related linguistic units that convey a message. There are various types of discourse and each type has different cognitive and linguistic demands. Types of discourse include descriptions (listing static attributes or relations), narratives (conveying actions and events that unfold in time), procedures (providing instructions or directions in a specific order), persuasion (giving reasons or facts to support an opinion), or conversation (interacting with others). It has been suggested that discourse is the most natural and basic unit of normal verbal communication (Haliday & Hasan, 1976). Furthermore, accurate production or comprehension of a narrative requires a complex interaction of linguistic, cognitive, and social abilities that are sensitive to disruption following TBI.

Discourse analyses typically begin with the elicitation of a spoken narrative, ideally at least five sentences in length. The discourse narratives are audiotaped and transcribed verbatim. Once transcribed, the narratives are divided into basic units for analysis, such as T-units (i.e., independent clause plus any dependent clauses associated with it). Depending on the type of discourse and the focus of the analysis, a variety of levels of

Table 6–14   Overview of Ongoing, Contextualized, Collaborative Hypothesis-Testing Assessment (OCCHTA)

Rationale

1. Diversity:	Individuals with TBI represent a very diverse disability group. There is no such thing as a general TBI educational/vocational/behavioral/ communication assessment.
2. Complex profiles:	Individuals with TBI have complex profiles of ability and disability (i.e., premorbid disabilities, combinations of diffuse and focal damage, cognitive and behavioral impairments) that make planning difficult.
3. Context-sensitivity:	Vocational/academic performance and social behavior of individuals with TBI, particularly those with frontal lobe injury, is strongly influenced by the contexts they are in. Clinic-based assessments should be supplemented by situational observation and contextualized hypothesis testing.
4. Collaboration:	Among staff members, the individual and family members add information to the assessment process and facilitate compliance for the implementation of interventions.
5. Change:	Change and inconsistency in the individual's performance are predictable following TBI because of neurologic improvement and sometimes delayed negative consequences of the injury and evolving psychosocial adjustments.
6. Flexibility:	Staff must approach their work with individuals with TBI in a flexible fashion when delivering support, instruction, clinical interventions, and behavior management.

Value of hypothesis testing

Individuals with TBI frequently present with complex profiles, and when these individuals demonstrate difficulties in the vocational, academic, or behavioral realms, there are a variety of possible explanations and corresponding interventions that may provide help for their problems. Without hypothesis testing it is very difficult to interpret task failure and to recommend the most effective intervention. Ylvisaker and Feeney (1998) provide the following example to illustrate the clinical utility of hypothesis testing: A student with a TBI has trouble reading a paragraph and correctly answering comprehension questions. This difficulty could be attributed to any combination of the following problems:

Physical:	fatigue, hunger, over- or undermedicated, in pain, sick, etc.
Sensory/perceptual:	unable to see print, maintain clear image, difficulty scanning left to right, etc.
Attention:	unable to sustain attention, filter out distractions, shift attention from previous to current task, etc.
Memory:	difficulty encoding information for storage, or holding information long enough to answer questions, or retrieving information from storage to answer questions, etc.
Organization:	difficulty organizing information necessary for comprehension, to understand how details relate to one another, to understand how questions relate to material read, etc.
Language:	unable to comprehend vocabulary or syntax of text or questions, etc.

From OCCHTA; and Ylvisaker, M., & Feeney, T. (1998). *Collaborative Brain Injury Intervention: Positive Everyday Routines*. San Diego: Singular.

Table 6–15   Examples of Narrative Story Analyses

Discourse Measures	Description	Example
Sentence production		
Words per T-unit	Total words in story divided by number of T-units	118 words/6 T-units = 19.7
Subordinate clauses per T-unit	Number subordinate clauses in story divided by number of T-units	3 subordinate clauses/6 T-units = 0.5
Cohesion		
Cohesive adequacy	Each occurrence of a cohesive tie judged as to its adequacy	Complete tie: "The girl was hungry. *She* ate her lunch."
Percent complete ties of total ties	Number of complete ties in story divided by total number of cohesive ties	Incomplete tie: "The boys walked home from the mall. *They* stopped at his house for a snack."
		Erroneous tie: "Dave and Joe drove to the game. *He* forgot the tickets."
Story grammar		
Number of total episodes	Total number of complete and incomplete episodes in a story	Complete episode:
		"*[Initiating event]* and this fly comes in,
		and the father's bothered by this."
		"*[Attempt]* so he decides to swat or hit the fly.
		and he hits his wife."
		"*[Direct consequence]* and she goes down."
		Incomplete episode:
		"*[Attempt]* and he hits his daughter
		[Direct consequence] and the daughter goes down to the floor."
Proportion of T-units within episode structure	Number of T-units in episode structure divided by total number of T-units in story	10 T-units in episodes/ 16 total T-units = 0.625

From Coelho, C.A., Youse, K.M., & Le, K.N. (2002). Conversational Discourse in Closed-Head-Injured and Non-Brain-Injured Adults. *Aphasiology*, *16*, 659–672.

analysis are possible. For example, in a narrative story, at the sentence level the number of T-units may be tallied as a measure of narrative length, or the number of subordinate clauses may be counted as an index of grammatical complexity. Across-sentence analyses may involve examining how speakers link meaning units across several sentences (e.g., complete or incomplete ties), referred to as intersentential cohesion. In story narrative analysis, episodes are examined as a measure of story grammar ability or discourse organization. Episode components are defined as information units pertaining to stated goals, attempts at solutions, and consequences of these attempts (**Table 6–15** lists examples of story narrative analyses). Additional analyses include productivity measures such as total words produced or total speaking time, content measures such as accurate content units, and measures of conversational speech, such as appropriateness of an utterance, or topic maintenance (**Table 6–16** lists examples of conversational analyses). A variety of pragmatic rating scales are also available, many of which may be used during observations of the individual with TBI or may be completed by family members, employers, teachers, etc. (see **Appendix 6–1** for examples of pragmatic rating scales). Regardless of the discourse genre selected or the analysis procedure applied, McDonald (2000) has stressed that communication disorders following TBI must be viewed in context, including the context of the person's sociocultural background and experiences, and specific communicative contexts the individual is likely to encounter in everyday life.

Table 6–16   Examples of Analyses for Conversation that Have Been Applied to Individuals with TBI

Response appropriateness: appropriateness of participants' utterances with conversations (Blank & Franklin, 1980; Coelho, Liles, & Duffy, 1991; Coelho, Youse, & Le, 2002)

Analysis of topic: proficiency by which participants manage conversational topics (Coelho et al, 1991; Coelho et al, 2002; Mentis & Prutting, 1991; Wozniak, Coelho, Duffy, & Liles, 1999)

Exchange structure analysis: examination of who has the knowledge in an interaction and how that information is transferred (Togher, Hand, & Code, 1997a,b, 1999)

Generic structure potential analysis: which aspects of language use are influenced by particular dimensions of the context (Togher et al, 1997b)

Mood and modality analysis: examines lexical and grammatical choices made at the clause level to establish degree of directness being expressed (Togher & Hand, 1998)

Conversation analysis (CA):   delineates the structural organization and sequential ordering of talk (Friedland & Miller, 1998)

Pragmatic rating scales: unstructured rating scales of pragmatic abilities (Ehrlich & Barry, 1989; Snow, Douglas, & Ponsford, 1998)

Social information processing: analyses that view communication, and conversation in particular, as an integral aspect of social skills (McDonald, 1993; McDonald & Pearce, 1995; Turkstra, McDonald, & DePompei, 2001; Turkstra, McDonald, & Kaufman, 1996)

Treatment

Whether treatment is based on hypothesis testing (Ylvisaker & Feeney, 1998) or a process-specific intervention (Sohlberg & Mateer, 2001), for individuals in the later stages of recovery (i.e., RLA VI, VII, and VIII) the final phase of remediation should be directed toward carryover of treatment objectives to home and community environments. Consultations with teachers, employers, and fellow workers take place in this stage of recovery. This is not to imply that programming for carryover begins during the final stages of treatment. Rather, to facilitate carryover of treatment objectives to nonclinical environments, contextualization of treatment (i.e., working on skills the individual with TBI needs, in the environment where they are needed) should take place as soon as it is feasible.

Sustained community reentry at the highest level of productivity, independence, and social adaptation that an individual is capable of is the ultimate goal of TBI rehabilitation (Malkmus, 1989). Concerns have been expressed about the generalization of treatment gains demonstrated in clinical settings. Such concerns have risen from research indicating that individuals with TBI often demonstrate chronic memory problems and/or frontal lobe injuries. It has been suggested that functional gains are most easily achieved when cognitive remediation is performed in the client's home and community involving activities of high interest to the individual (Kneipp, 1991). Numerous case reports of treatment intended to enhance daily living, educational, and vocational activities provided by professionals who travel to the TBI individual's home, school, or job have cited positive results with regard to return to school (Blosser & DePompei, 1989; DePompei & Blosser, 1987; Ylvisaker & Feeney, 1998) or gainful employment (Kneipp, 1991; Story, 1991; Wehman, 1991; Ylvisaker & Feeney, 1998).

Case Study 3

Background   S.N. is a 28-year-old woman who was involved in a motor vehicle accident. She was employed as a head nurse on a surgical unit in a large urban medical center. She was also working on a master's degree in counseling, worked part-time as a realtor, was the business manager for her brother's farm, and, working with her brother, had built her own house. Immediately following her accident, S.N. was brought to the emergency room with multiple trauma including fractures of her pelvis, both legs, clavicle, two ribs, and an arm. She was noted to be conscious at the scene of the accident and when she arrived in the emergency room. A CT scan revealed no evidence of focal lesion or obvious cerebral trauma. From that point forward all medical interventions were directed toward S.N.'s orthopedic injuries. She was hospitalized for 6 weeks and eventually returned home where she had PT through home care and eventually on an outpatient basis. At approximately 6 months postinjury, S.N. attempted to return to work on a part-time basis unsuccessfully. She noted problems with fatigue and concentration, her fellow workers noted occasional errors preparing medications for distribution, and vague chart notes. At home S.N. noted being easily distracted; for example, she was no longer able to read if the TV or radio was on. She was also having difficulty keeping up with her graduate coursework, her realty work, and could no longer keep the books for her brother's farm. Eventually she took a leave of absence from her nursing job and gave up the other endeavors. When S.N. reported these difficulties to

her neurologist, she was referred to a psychiatrist who felt her difficulties were attributable to posttraumatic stress. She was treated with antidepressants and psychotherapy for approximately 3 months. At 18 months postinjury she was referred to a rehabilitation facility for evaluation of a "suspected TBI."

Assessment   On her initial visit, S.N. was seen by a neuropsychologist and a speech–language pathologist, each of whom spent approximately 1 hour with her and noted problems with attention, memory, and organizational abilities. Problems with pragmatic skills were also noted. S.N.'s RLA level was VIII (purposeful and appropriate). When these findings were reported to her, she replied, "I'm so relieved, I knew I wasn't crazy." Subsequent diagnostic sessions focused on delineation of the functional consequences of these cognitive impairments. Upon completion of the neuropsychological and speech–language pathology assessments, both evaluators met to formulate a treatment plan for S.N. A meeting was then scheduled with S.N. to review the suggested treatment plan and to solicit her input for identification of realistic treatment goals. It was at this point in the assessment process that a significant hurdle presented itself: S.N. was adamantly opposed to recruiting employers, fellow workers, or family members into the rehabilitation process. She said, "Everything I have, I've gotten on my own, through my own hard work. I can do this on my own." After much discussion it became apparent that S.N. was very concerned about not being able to return to nursing if her employer knew she had a brain injury. Consequently, she would not agree to any observations at work or job coaching.

Treatment   Treatment objectives included targeting complex attention and concentration, memory, and social/pragmatic skills. A contract was written for a trial period of treatment. The treatment program involved individual therapy in speech–language pathology for cognitive remediation, and in psychology to address psychosocial issues. Individual therapy was supplemented by a pragmatics group, and job trials within the rehabilitation center, during which S.N. took on several volunteer assignments under the supervision of a vocational rehab counselor. All participants in the treatment program signed the contract. Team meetings, which always included S.N., were held every 2 weeks. Steady gains were made in S.N.'s cognitive functioning and in her acceptance of her cognitive limitations. After approximately 6 weeks she became an outspoken member of the pragmatics group, regularly challenging her male counterparts' notions of a woman's role in today's world. At the same time she had a very successful and meaningful experience volunteering in the recreational therapy department accompanying individuals from the transitional living unit on community outings. She was noted to have a calm and patient demeanor and many of the residents gravitated to her.

S.N.'s treatment program continued for approximately 6 months. During that time she became a strong self-advocate testifying in court in a case that was brought against her insurance company for denial of therapy coverage and failure to pay her disability that nearly led to her losing her home. During this same time S.N. reevaluated her career goals. She acknowledged that her chronic concentration and memory problems would not allow her to return to nursing in the same capacity she had prior to her injury. So she began to explore options with her treatment team and finally agreed to some community-based job trials through the Bureau of Rehabilitation Services. One of these trials, in a skilled nursing facility, led to a job offer for a part-time nursing position that S.N. eventually accepted. In that position she met a practicum coordinator for nursing assistants from a local community college who offered her a part-time teaching position. Because the physical demands of regular nursing were becoming too hard for her, S.N. accepted this position. At nearly 4 years post-onset of her TBI, S.N. was still employed at the community college supervising nursing assistants in on- and off-campus training sites.

✦ Conclusion

The success or failure of cognitive rehabilitation needs to be considered on a case-by-case basis. There are numerous factors that may affect this highly complex process (Kreutzer, Gordon, Wehman, 1998). For example, it is important to prioritize the individual's problems on the basis of relationships to functional real-world outcomes, the likelihood of success, and interrelationships between deficits. A second issue pertains to how well the problems, to be addressed in treatment, are defined. It is important to define the problem in functional terms including

the frequency, duration, and environments in which the problem occurs, as well as the relationship between the problem behavior and other problems. Description of treatment is a significant factor as well. The intervention should be defined and operationalized, including frequency and duration, to provide a record of what was done and so that it can be replicated. Providing treatment in the environment or context that the problem occurs facilitates generalization. Patient selection is another key issue in determining the effectiveness of cognitive rehabilitation. The TBI population is extremely heterogeneous; therefore, those patients who benefit and those who won't need to be described. Such descriptions should include time post-onset, severity of injury, age, and level of education. All prognostic statements need to be grounded in practice theory, and dynamics of learning and interface of individual differences require specificity (i.e., what works for one individual may not work for another). A final critical feature of cognitive rehabilitation is who is doing the treating. The disciplines providing cognitive remediation are diverse and include varying levels of expertise and training. There is need to consider credentialing, specialty recognition, and, at the very least, continuing education requirements.

Study Questions

1. Describe two types of brain damage that may result from traumatic brain injury (TBI).
2. What factors determine the severity of TBI?
3. What are the main cognitive disturbances seen after TBI?
4. Discuss the distinction between aphasia and confused language following TBI.
5. What is the purpose of the World Health Organization's (WHO) International Classification of Functioning and Health (ICF)? Define each ICF domain.
6. Describe the five stages of the TBI rehabilitation continuum.
7. Describe the *restorative* and *compensatory* approaches to cognitive rehabilitation and the underlying rationale for each.
8. Describe the notion of *goal planning* as it pertains to TBI rehabilitation.
9. What are some of the factors to consider when selecting a standardized battery for assessing an individual with TBI? Name two batteries that are appropriate for use with individuals with TBI.
10. Describe the *ongoing, collaborative, contextualized, hypothesis-testing assessment* approach. How does this approach differ from more traditional evaluation procedures?

References

Adamovich, B.L.B., Henderson, J.A., & Auerbach, S. (1985). *Cognitive Rehabilitation of Closed Head Injured Patients.* San Diego: College Hill Press

Alexander, M.P., Benson, D.F., & Stuss, D.T. (1989). Frontal Lobes and Language. *Brain and Language, 37,* 656–691

American Neurological Association Committee on Ethical Affairs. (1993). Persistent Vegetative State. *Annals of Neurology, 33,* 386–390

American Speech–Language–Hearing Association. (2004). Roles of Speech–Language Pathologists in the Identification, Diagnosis, and Treatment of Individuals with Cognitive-Communication Disorders. Position Statement. ASHA Supplement 24. Rockville, MD

Ansell, B.J., & Keenan, J.E. (1989). The Western Neuro Sensory Stimulation Profile: A Tool for Assessing Slow-To-Recover Head-Injured Patients. *Archives of Physical Medicine and Rehabilitation, 70,* 104–108

Benedict, R.H.B. (1989). The Effectiveness of Cognitive Remediation Strategies for Victims of Traumatic Brain Injury: A Review of the Literature. *Clinical Psychology Review, 9,* 605–626

Ben-Yishay, Y. & Diller, L. (1993). Cognitive Remediation in Traumatic Brain Injury: Update and Issues. *Archives of Physical Medicine and Rehabilitation, 74,* 204–213

Blank, M., & Franklin, E. (1980). Dialogue with Pre-Schoolers: A Cognitively-Based System of Assessment. *Applied Psycholinguistics, 1,* 127–150

Blosser, J.L. & DePompei, R. (1989). The Head Injured Student Returns to School: Recognizing and Treating Deficits. *Topics in Language Disorders, 9,* 67–77

Bricolo, A., Turazzi, S., and Feriotti, G. (1980). Prolonged Posttraumatic Unconsciousness. *Journal of Neurosurgery, 52,* 625–634

Coelho, C.A. (1995). Discourse Production Deficits Following Traumatic Brain Injury: A Critical Review of the Recent Literature. *Aphasiology, 9,* 409–429

Coelho, C.A., DeRuyter, F., & Stein, M. (1996). Treatment Efficacy: Cognitive-Communicative Disorders Resulting from Traumatic Brain Injury in Adults. *Journal of Speech and Hearing Research, 39,* S5–S17

Coelho, C.A., Liles, B.Z., & Duffy, R.J. (1991). Analysis of Conversational Discourse in Head Injured Adults. *Journal of Head Trauma Rehabilitation, 6,* 92–99

Coelho, C., Ylvisaker, M., & Turkstra, L.S. (2005). Nonstandardized assessment approaches for individuals with traumatic brain injuries. *Seminars in Speech and Language, 26,* 223–241

Coelho, C.A., Youse, K.M., & Le, K.N. (2002). Conversational Discourse in Closed-Head-Injured and Non-Brain-Injured Adults. *Aphasiology, 16,* 659–672

Cope, D.N., & Hall, K.H. (1982). Head Injury Rehabilitation: Benefit of Early Intervention. *Archives of Physical Medicine & Rehabilitation, 63,* 433–437

Crosson, B., Barco, P.P., Velozo, C.A., Bolesta, M., Cooper, P.V., Werts, D., & Brobeck, T.C. (1989). Awareness and Compensation in Postacute Head Injury Rehabilitation. *Journal of Head Trauma Rehabilitation, 4,* 46–54

Damico, J. (1985). Clinical Discourse Analysis: A Functional Language Assessment Technique. In: C.S. Simon (Ed.), *Communication Skills and Classroom Success: Assessment of Language-Learning Disabled Students* (pp. 165–206). San Diego: College-Hill

Davis, A. (1993). *A survey of Adult Aphasia and Related Language Disorders* (pp. 1–20). Englewood Cliffs, NJ: Prentice Hall

DePompei, R. & Blosser, J. (1987). Strategies for Helping Head-Injured Children Successfully Return to School. *Language, Speech, and Hearing Services in Schools, 18,* 292–300

DePompei, R., & Blosser, J.L. (1991). Functional Cognitive-Communicative Impairments in Children and Adolescents: Assessment and Intervention. In: J. Kreutzer & P. Wehman (Eds.), *Cognitive Rehabilitation for Persons with*

Traumatic Brain Injury: A Functional Approach (pp. 215–236). Baltimore: Paul H. Brookes

DeRuyter, F., and Becker, M.R. (1988). Augmentative Communication: Assessment, System Selection, and Usage. *Journal of Head Trauma Rehabilitation, 3*, 35–44

Ehrlich, J., & Barry, P. (1989). Rating Communication Behaviors in the Head-Injured Adult. *Brain Injury, 3*, 193–198

Eisenberg, H.M., & Weiner, R.L. (1987). Input Variables: How Information from the Acute Injury Can Be Used to Characterize Groups of Patients for Studies of Outcome. In: H.S. Levin, J. Grafman, & H.M. Eisenberg (Eds.), *Neurobehavioral Recovery from Head Injury* (pp.13–29). New York: Oxford University Press

Frattali, C., Thompson, C., Holland, A., Wohl, C., & Ferketic, M. (1995). American Speech Language Hearing Association Functional Assessment of Communication Skills for Adults. Rockville, MD: American Speech Language Hearing Association

Friedland, D., & Miller, N. (1998). Conversation Analysis of Communication Breakdown After Closed Head Injury. *Brain Injury, 12*, 1–14

Giacino, J.T., & Cicerone, K.D. (1998). Varieties of Deficit Unawareness After Brain Injury. *Journal of Head Trauma Rehabilitation, 13*, 1–15

Giacino, J.T., Kezmarsky, M.A., Deluca, J., McKenna, K., & Cicerone, K.D. (1991). *JFK Johnson Rehabilitation Institute's Center for Head Injuries Coma Recovery Scale.* Edison, NJ: JFK Johnson Rehabilitation Institute

Gioia, G.A., Isquith, P.K., Guy, S.C., & Kenworthy, L. (2000). Behavior Rating Inventory of Executive Function, Odessa, FL: Psychological Assessment Resources

Groher, M. (1977). Language and Memory Disorders Following Closed Head Trauma. *Journal of Speech and Hearing Research, 20*, 212–223

Hagan, C. (1984). Language Disorders in Head Trauma. In: A. Holland (Ed.), *Language Disorders in Adults: Recent Advances* (pp. 245–282). San Diego: College-Hill Press

Hagan, C., Malkmus, D., & Burditt, G. (1979) Levels of Cognitive Functioning. In: *Rehabilitation of the Head Injured Adult: Comprehensive Physical Management.* Downey, CA: Professional Staff Association of Rancho Los Amigos Hospital

Haliday, M.A.K., and Hasan, R. (1976). *Cohesion in English.* London: Longman Group Limited

Halpern, H., Darley, F., & Brown, J.R. (1973). Differential Language and Neurologic Characteristics in Cerebral Involvement. *Journal of Speech and Hearing Disorders, 38*, 162–173

Heilman, K.M., Safran, A., & Geschwind, N. (1971). Closed Head Trauma and Aphasia. *Journal of Neurology, Neurosurgery, and Psychiatry, 34*, 265–269

High, W.M. Jr., Levin, H.S., & Gary, H.E. (1990). Recovery of Orientation Following Closed-Head Injury. *Journal of Clinical and Experimental Neuropsychology, 12*, 703–714

Holland, A.L. (1982). When is Aphasia Aphasia? The Problem of Closed Head Injury. In: R.H. Brookshire (Ed.), *Clinical Aphasiology Conference Proceedings, 12*, 345–350. Minneapolis: BRK Publishers

Holland, A., Frattali, C., & Fromm, D. (1999). Communication Activities of Daily Living, 2nd Ed. Austin, TX: Pro-Ed

Jennett, B. (1996). Clinical and Pathological Features of Vegetative Survival. In: H.S. Levin, A.L. Benton, J.P. Muizelaar, & H.M. Eisenberg (Eds.), *Catastrophic Brain Injury* (pp. 3–14). New York: Oxford University Press

Jennett, B., & Bond, M. (1975). Assessment of Outcome After Severe Brain Damage. *Lancet, 1*, 480–487

Jennett, B., & Plum, F. (1972). Persistent Vegetative State After Brain Damage. *Lancet, 1*, 734–737

Kennedy, M. (2002). Evidence-Based Practice Guidelines for Cognitive-Communication Disorders After Traumatic Brain Injury: Initial Committee Report. *Journal of Medical Speech–Language Pathology, 10*, ix–xiii

Kennedy, M., & Coelho, C. (2005). Self-regulation after traumatic brain injury: A framework for intervention of memory and problem solving. *Seminars in Speech and Language, 26*, 242–255

Kennedy, M.R.T., & DeRuyter, F. (1991). Cognitive and Language Bases for Communication Disorders. In: D.R. Beukelman and K.M. Yorkston (Eds.), Communication Disorders Following Traumatic Brain Injury: Management of Cognitive, Language, and Motor Impairments (pp. 123–190). Austin, TX: Pro-Ed

Ketesz, A. (1982). Western Aphasia Battery. San Antonio, TX: Psychological Corporation

Kneipp, S. (1991). Cognitive Remediation Within the Context of a Community Re-Entry Program. In: J. Kreutzer & P. Wehman (Eds.), *Cognitive Rehabilitation for Persons with Traumatic Brain Injury: A Functional Approach* (pp. 239–250) Baltimore: Paul H. Brookes

Kreutzer, J., Gordon, W., & Wehman, P. (1989). Cognitive Remediation Following Traumatic Brain Injury. *Rehabilitation Psychology, 34*, 117–130

Kreutzer, J.S., & Wehman, P. (1990). *Community Reintegration Following Traumatic Brain Injury.* Toronto: Paul Brookes

Langer, K.G., & Padrone, F.J. (1992). Psychotherapeutic Treatment of Awareness in Acute Rehabilitation of Traumatic Brain Injury. *Neuropsychological Rehabilitation, 2*, 59–70

Levin, H.S., & Eisenberg, H.M. (1996). Vegetative State After Head Injury: Findings from the Traumatic Coma Data Bank. In: H.S. Levin, A.L. Benton, J.P.

Muizelaar, & H.M. Eisenberg (Eds.), *Catastrophic Brain Injury* (pp. 35–50). New York: Oxford University Press

Levin, H.S., Grossman, R.G., & Kelly, P.J. (1976) Aphasic Disorders in Patients with Closed Head Injury. *Journal of Neurology, Neurosurgery, and Psychiatry, 39*, 119–130

Levin, H.S., Grossman, R.G., Rose, J.E., & Teasdale, G. (1979). Long-Term Neuropsychological Outcome of Closed Head Injury. *Journal of Neurosurgery, 50*, 412–422

Levin, H.S., Grossman, R.G., Sarwar, M., & Meyers, C.A. (1981). Linguistic Recovery After Closed Head Injury. *Brain and Language, 12*, 360–374

Levin, H.S., Madison, C.F., Bailey, C.B., Meyer, C.A., Eisenberg, H.M., & Guinto, F.C. (1983). Mutism After Closed Head Injury. *Archives of Neurology, 40*, 601–606

Levin, H.S., O'Donnell, V.M., and Grossman, R.G. (1979). The Galveston Orientation and Amnesia Test: A Practical Scale to Assess Cognition After Head Injury. *Journal of Nervous and Mental Disease, 167*, 675–684

Lezak, M.D. (1976). *Mechanisms of Neurological Disease.* Boston: Little, Brown

Lezak, M.D. (1982). The Problem of Assessing Executive Functions. *International Journal of Psychology, 17*, 281–297

Lezak, M.D. (1983). *Neuropsychological Assessment,* 2nd ed. New York: Oxford University Press

Lezak, M.D. (1987). Assessment for Rehabilitation Planning. In: M. Meier, A. Benton, and L. Diller (Eds.), *Neuropsychological Rehabilitation.* New York: Guilford Press

Mackay, L.E., Berstein, B.A., Chapman, P.E., Morgan, A.S., & Milazzo, L.S. (1992). Early Intervention in Severe Head Injury: Long-Term Benefits of a Formalized Program. *Archives of Physical Medicine and Rehabilitation, 73*, 635–641

Malkmus, D.D. (1989). Community Reentry: Cognitive-Communicative Intervention Within a Social Skill Context. *Topics in Language Disorders, 9*, 50–66

McDonald, S. (1993). Pragmatic Language Skills After Closed Head Injury: Ability to Meet the Informational Needs of the Listener. *Brain and Language, 44*, 28–46

McDonald, S., & Pearce, S. (1995). The 'Dice' Game: A New Test of Pragmatic Language Skills After Close-Head Injury. *Brain Injury, 9*, 255–271

McHenry, M., & Wilson, R. (1994). The Challenge of Unintelligible Speech Following Traumatic Brain Injury. *Brain Injury, 8*, 363–375

McKinlay, W.W., Brooks, D.N., Bond, M.R., Martinage, D.P., & Marshall, M.M. (1981). The Short-Term Outcome of Severe Blunt Head Injury as Reported by the Relatives of the Injured Person. *Journal of Neurology, Neurosurgery, and Psychiatry, 44*, 527–533

McMillan, T., & Sparkes, C. (1999). Goal Planning and Neurorehabilitation: The Wolfson Neurorehabilitation Centre approach. *Neuropsychological Rehabilitation, 9*, 241–251

Mentis, M., & Prutting, C.A. (1991). Analysis of Topic as Illustrated in a Head-Injured and Normal Adult. *Journal of Speech and Hearing Research, 34*, 583–595

Mills, V.M., Cassidy, J.W., & Katz, D.I. (1997). *Neurologic Rehabilitation: A Guide to Diagnosis, Prognosis, and Treatment Planning.* Malden, MA: Blackwell Scientific

Milton, S.B. (1988). Management of Subtle Cognitive Communication Deficits. *Journal of Head Trauma Rehabilitation, 3*, 1–12

Milton, S.B., Turnstall, C., & Wertz, R.T. (1983). Dysnomia: A Rose by Any Other Name May Require Elaborate Description. In: R.H. Brookshire (Ed.), *Clinical Aphasiology Conference Proceedings, 14*, 137–147

Multisociety Task Force on the Persistent Vegetative State. (1993). Medical Aspects of the Persistent Vegetative State (1). Statement of a Multisociety Task Force. *New England Journal of Medicine 330*, 1499–1508

Netsell, R., & Daniel, B. (1979). Dysarthria in Adults: Physiologic Approach to Rehabilitation. *Archives of Physical Medicine and Rehabilitation, 60*, 502–508

Oder, W., Podreka, I., Spatt, J., & Goldenberg, G. (1996). Cerebral Function Following Catastrophic Brain Injury: Relevance of Single Photon Emission Computed Tomography and Positron Emission Tomography. In: H.S. Levin, A.L. Benton, J.P. Muizelaar, & H.M. Eisenberg (Eds.), *Catastrophic Brain Injury* (pp. 51–76). New York: Oxford University Press

Ponsford, J., Sloan, W., & Snow, P. (1995). *Traumatic Brain Injury: Rehabilitation for Everyday Adaptive Living.* Hove, England: Lawrence Erlbaum

Prigatano, G. (1986). *Neuropsychological Rehabilitation After Brain Injury.* Baltimore: Johns Hopkins Press

Prutting, C., & Kirchner, D. (1983). Applied Pragmatics. In T.M. Gallagher & C.A. Prutting (Eds.), *Pragmatic Assessment and Intervention Issues in Language* (pp. 29–64). San Diego: College-Hill

Randolph, C. (2001). Repeatable Battery for the Assessment of Neuropsychological Status. San Antonio, TX: Psychological Corporation

Rosenthal, M., Griffith, E.R., Kreutzer, J.S., & Pentland, B. (1999). *Rehabilitation of the Adult and Child with Traumatic Brain Injury* (3rd ed.). Philadelphia: F.A. Davis

Rusk, H., Block, J., and Lowmann, E. (1969). Rehabilitation of the Brain Injured Patient: A Report of 157 Cases with Longterm Follow-Up of 118. In: E. Walker, W. Caveness, and M. Critchley (Eds.), *The Late Effects of Head Injury.* Springfield, IL: Charles C Thomas

Sarno, M.T. (1980). The Nature of Verbal Impairment After Closed Head Injury. *Journal of Nervous and Mental Disease, 168*, 685–692

Sarno, M.T., Buonaguro, A., & Levita, E. (1986). Characteristics of Verbal Impairment in Closed Head Injury. *Archives of Physical Medicine and Rehabilitation, 67*, 400–405

Schwartz-Cowley, R., & Stepanik, M.J. (1989). Communication Disorders and Treatment in the Acute Trauma Center Setting. *Topics in Language Disorders, 9*:1, 1–11

Simmons, N. (1983). Acoustic Analysis of Ataxic Dysarthria: An Approach to Monitoring Treatment. In: W.R. Berry (Ed.), *Clinical Dysarthria.* San Diego: College-Hill Press

Snow, P., Douglas, J., & Ponsford, J. (1998). Conversational Discourse Abilities Following Severe Traumatic Brain Injury: A Follow-Up Study. *Brain Injury, 12,* 911–935

Sohlberg, M.M. (1996). Making Management of Awareness Deficits a Core Part of Cognitive Rehabilitation. In M.M. Sohlberg (Ed.), *Updates in Cognitive Rehabilitation. ASHA Special Interest Division 2 Newsletter, 6,* 6–11

Sohlberg, M.M., Avery, J., Kennedy, M., Ylvisaker, M., Coelho, C., Turkstra, L., & Yorkston, K. (2003). Practice Guidelines for Direct Attention Training. *Journal of Medical Speech–language Pathology, 11,* xix–xxxix

Sohlberg, M.M., Ehlhardt, L., & Kennedy, M. (2005). Instructional techniques in cognitive rehabilitation: A preliminary report. *Seminars in Speech and Language, 26,* 268–279

Sohlberg, M.M. & Mateer, C.A. (1989). *Introduction to Cognitive Rehabilitation Theory and Practice.* New York: Guilford Press

Sohlberg, M.M. & Mateer, C.A. (2001). *Cognitive Rehabilitation: An Integrative Neuropsychological Approach.* New York: Guilford

Starch, S. & Falltrick, E. (1990). The Importance of Home Evaluation for Brain Injured Clients: A Team Approach. *Cognitive Rehabilitation, 8,* 28–32

Stein, D.G., Finger, S., & Hart, T. (1983). Brain Damage and Recovery: Problems and Perspectives. *Behavioral and Neural Biology, 37,* 185–222

Story, T.B. (1991). Cognitive Rehabilitation in Home and Community Settings. In: J. Kreutzer & P. Wehman (Eds.), *Cognitive Rehabilitation for Persons with Traumatic Brain Injury: A Functional Approach* (pp. 251–268). Baltimore: Paul H. Brookes

Stuss, D.T., & Benson, D.F. (1997). Frontal Lobe Functions. In: M.R. Trimble, J.L. Cummings (Eds.), *Contemporary Behavioral Neurology* (pp. 169–187). *Blue books of practical neurology, vol. 16.* Boston: Butterworth-Heinemann

Stuss, D.T., Winocur, G., & Robertson, I.H. (1999). *Cognitive Neurorehabilitation.* Cambridge, England: Cambridge University Press

Thomsen, I.V. (1975). Evaluation and Outcome of Aphasia in Patients with Severe Closed Head Trauma. *Journal of Neurology, Neurosurgery, and Psychiatry, 38,* 713–718

Thomsen, I.V. (1976). Evaluation and Outcome of Traumatic Aphasia in Patients with Severe Verified Lesions. *Folia Phoniatrica, 28,* 362–377

Togher, L., & Hand, L. (1998). Use of Politeness Markers with Different Communication Partners: An Investigation of Five Subjects with Traumatic Brain Injury. *Aphasiology, 12,* 755–770

Togher, L., Hand, L., & Code, C. (1997a). Measuring Service Encounters in the Traumatic Brain Injury Population. *Aphasiology, 11,* 491–505

Togher, L., Hand, L., & Code, C. (1997b). Analyzing Discourse in the Traumatic Brain Injury Population: Telephone Interactions with Different Communication Partners. *Brain Injury, 11,* 169–189

Togher, L., Hand, L., & Code, C. (1999). Exchanges of Information in the Talk of People with Traumatic Brain Injury. In: S. McDonald, L. Togher, & C. Code (Eds.), *Communication Skills Following Traumatic Brain Injury* (pp. 113–145). Hove, UK: Psychology Press

Turkstra, L.S., McDonald, S., & DePompei, R. (2001). Social Information Processing in Adolescents: Data from Normally-Developing Adolescents and Preliminary Data from Their Peers with Traumatic Brain Injury. *Journal of Head Trauma Rehabilitation, 16,* 469–483

Turkstra, L.S., McDonald, S., & Kaufman, P. (1996). Assessment of Pragmatic Communication Skills in Adolescents After Traumatic Brain Injury. *Brain Injury, 10,* 329–345

Turkstra, L., Ylvisaker, M., Coelho, C., Kennedy, M., Sohlberg, M., & Avery, J. (2005). Practice Guidelines for Standardized Assessment for Persons with Traumatic Brain Injury. *Journal of Medical Speech–language Pathology, 13,* ix–xxvii

Wagner, M.T., & Cushman, L.A. (1994). Neuroanatomic and Neuropsychological Predictors of Unawareness of Cognitive Deficit in the Vascular Population. *Archives of Clinical Neuropsychology, 9,* 57–69

Wehman, P.H. (1991). Cognitive Rehabilitation in the Workplace. In: J. Kreutzer & P. Wehman (Eds.), *Cognitive Rehabilitation for Persons with Traumatic Brain Injury: A Functional Approach* (pp. 269–288). Baltimore: Paul H. Brookes

Whyte, J. & Rosenthal, M. (1988). Rehabilitation of the Patient with Head Injury. In: J.A. DeLisa (Ed.), *Rehabilitation: Principles and Practice* (pp. 246–259). Philadelphia: Lippincott

Wiig, E., & Secord, W. (1989). Test of Language Competence-Expanded Edition. San Antonio, TX: Psychological Corporation

Wilson, B.A. (2003). Goal Planning Rather than Neuropsychological Tests Should Be Used to Structure and Evaluate Cognitive Rehabilitation. *Brain Impairment, 4,* 25–30

World Health Organization International. (2002). Classification of Impairment, Disabilities, and Handicaps. Geneva: WHO

Wozniak, R.J., Coelho, C.A., Duffy, R.J., & Liles, B.Z. (1999). Intonation Unit Analysis of Conversational Discourse in Closed Head Injury. *Brain Injury, 13,* 191–203

Ylvisaker, M., Coelho, C., Kennedy, M., Sohlberg, M.M., Turkstra, L., Avery, J., & Yorkston, K. (2002). Reflections on Evidence-Based Practice and Rational Clinical Decision Making. *Journal of Medical Speech–language Pathology, 10,* xxv–xxxiii

Ylvisaker, M., & Feeney, T. (1998). *Collaborative Brain Injury Intervention: Positive Everyday Routines.* San Diego: Singular

Ylvisaker, M., & Gobble, E.M. (1988). *Community Re-Entry for Head Injured Adults.* Boston: Little, Brown

Ylvisaker, M., Szekeres, S., & Feeney, T. (1998). Cognitive rehabilitation: Executive functions. In M. Ylvisaker (Ed.), *Traumatic brain injury rehabilitation: Children and adolescents* (pp. 221–269). Newton, MA: Butterworth-Heinemann

Ylvisaker, M., Turkstra, L.S., & Coelho, C. (2005). Behavioral and social interventions for individuals with traumatic brain injury: A summary of the research with clinical implications. *Seminars in Speech and Language, 26,* 256–267

Ylvisaker, M., Urbanczyk, B., & Feeney, T. (1992). Social Skills Following Traumatic Brain Injury. *Seminars in Speech and Language, 13,* 308–322

Yorkston, K.M., & Beukelman, D.R. (1981). Ataxic Dysarthria: Treatment Sequences Based on Intelligibility and Prosodic Considerations. *Journal of Speech and Hearing Disorders, 46,* 398–404

Yorkston, K.M., & Beukelman, D.R. (1991). Motor Speech Disorders. In: D.R. Beukelman & K.M. Yorkston (Eds.), *Communication Disorders Following Traumatic Brain Injury: Management of Cognitive, Language, and Motor Impairments* (pp. 251–316). Austin, TX: Pro-Ed

Yorkston, K.M., Beukelman, D.R., & Bell, K.R. (1988). *Clinical Management of Dysarthric Speakers.* San Diego: College-Hill Press

Yorkston, K.M., Beukelman, D.R., Minifie, F., & Sapir, S. (1984). Assessment of Stress Patterning in Dysarthric Speakers. In: M. McNeil, A. Aronson, & J. Rosenbek, (Eds.), *The Dysarthrias: Physiology, Acoustics, Perception, Management.* Boston: College-Hill Press

Youse, K.M., Le, K.N., Cannizzaro, M.S., & Coelho, C.A. (2002). Traumatic Brain Injury: A Primer for Professionals. *ASHA Leader, 7 (12),* 4–7

Zasler, N.D., Kreutzer, J.S., & Taylor, D. (1991). Coma Stimulation and Coma Recovery: A Critical Review. *NeuroRehabilitation, 1,* 33–40

Appendix 6–1   Examples of Pragmatic Rating Scales

Pragmatically oriented discourse analysis as suggested by Damico (1985)

Does client:

Give sufficient information when giving instructions or directions?

Use specific vocabulary (thing, stuff, "whatchamacallit")?

Perseverate or provide too much redundancy when talking?

Need a lot of repetition before even simple instructions are understood?

Give inaccurate messages; seem to talk when he or she "doesn't know what he or she is talking about"?

Make rapid and inappropriate changes in conversational topic without clues to the listener?

Seem to have an independent conversational agenda or give inappropriate and unpredictable responses?

Fail to ask relevant questions to clarify unclear messages, so that communication frequently breaks down?

Use language that is inappropriate for the social situation?

Produce speech that is frequently disrupted by repetitions, unusual pauses, and hesitations?

(Continued)

Appendix 6–1 *(Continued)*

Use many false starts, self-repetitions, and revisions in talking?

Produce long pauses or delays before responding?

Lack forethought and planning in telling stories and giving instructions?

Fail to attend to cues for conventional turns, interrupting frequently or failing to hold up his or her end of the conversation?

Use inconsistent or inappropriate eye contact in conversation?

Use inappropriate intonation?

Prutting and Kirchner's (1983) Pragmatic Protocol

Communicative Act	Appropriate	Inappropriate	NA

Utterance act

A. Verbal or paralinguistic

   1. Intelligibility

   2. Vocal intensity

   3. Voice quality

   4. Prosody

   5. Fluency

B. Nonverbal

   1. Physical proximity

   2. Physical contacts

   3. Body posture

   4. Foot or leg movements

   5. Hand or arm movements

   6. Gestures

   7. Facial expression

   8. Eye gaze

Propositional act

A. Lexical selection and use

   1. Specificity and accuracy

B. Specifying relationships between words

   1. Word order

   2. Given and new information

C. Stylistic variations

   1. Varying the communicative style

Illocutionary and perlocutionary acts

A. Speech acts

   1. Speech act pair analysis

   2. Variety of speech acts

B. Topic

   1. Selection

   2. Introduction

   3. Maintenance

   4. Change

C. Turn-taking

   1. Initiation

   2. Response

   3. Repair and revision

   4. Pause time

   5. Interruption and overlap

   6. Feedback to speakers

   7. Adjacency

   8. Contingency

   9. Quantity and conciseness

Appendix 6–1   *(Continued)*

Rating of Communication Behaviors from Ehrlich and Barry (1989)

Intelligibility: scale 1–9

1. Speech is severely distorted and consistently requires repetition
3. Speech is moderately distorted; can be understood about 30 to 40% of the time
5. Speech is mildly distorted; requires repetition about10% of the time
7. Speech is minimally impaired but is generally intelligible
9. No discernible speech impairment; always understood

Eye gaze: scale 1–9

1. Consistently no appropriate eye gaze with another person
3. Severely restricted eye gaze.
5. Appropriate eye gaze 50% of the time
7. Appropriate eye gaze 75% of the time
9. Consistent use of appropriate eye gaze

Sentence formation: scale 1–9

1. Consistently uses ungrammatical sentences; only short phrases and "telegraphic"
3. Omits grammatical function words often; average sentence length is reduced most of the time
5. Uses mainly simple sentences; infrequent embedding and clauses
7. Uses varied sentence patterns 75% of the time
9. Mature and varied sentence patterns consistently used

Coherence of narrative: scale 1–9

1. Consistently random and diffuse expression; incomplete thoughts
3. Disjointed verbal style; limited connection between ideas
5. Thoughts are expressed with a moderate amount of irrelevant and extraneous remarks, and are considered incomplete 50% of the time
7. Ideas are expressed in some order about 75% of the time; notice occasional incomplete thoughts
9. Shows a well-executed expression of ideas most of the time; well-formed narrative

Topic: scale 1–9

1. Rapid and abrupt shifting from topic to topic within a short time
3. Able to maintain topic for at least 30 seconds
5. Can maintain the topic for several minutes, but demonstrates difficulty in changing topics
7. Can appropriately maintain the topic most of the time; infrequently (25% of the time) shows slowness and difficulty in change of topic
9. Demonstrates no problem in maintenance and change of topic

Initiation of communication: scale 1–9

1. Infrequently initiates talk; only responds to others' questions
3. Seldom initiates talk (about 25% of the time)
5. Limited initiation of talk (about 50% of the time)
7. Minimal problem in initiating conversational talk
9. Freely initiates talk; good balance of communication most of the time

7

Dementia: Diagnostic Approaches and Current Taxonomies

Jennifer Horner, Michele L. Norman, and Danielle N. Ripich

✦ **Overview of Dementia Taxonomies**
✦ **Diagnostic Approaches**
✦ **Neurodegenerative Dementias**
✦ **Subcortical Dementia and Associated Disorders**

Speech–language pathologists who work with elderly patients must have an understanding of diagnostic approaches and current taxonomies pertaining to the dementias to understand advances in research, to interpret studies of cognition and sub-typing of these disorders, and to treat those patients who have a reasonable chance of benefiting. Speech–language pathologists are called upon rarely, if ever, to render a diagnosis of "demen-tia." Nevertheless, they are responsible for diagnosing aphasia, cognitive impairments, dysarthria, and related disorders, as well as for counseling patients and families, and tracking the course of the dementing illness. Diagnosis of dementia is a challenging and evolving endeavor, one that requires a team approach, usu-ally with a specialized neurologist at the helm.

As defined by the *Diagnostic and Statistical Manual of Men-tal Disorders,* fourth edition text revision (DSM-IV-TR), the term *dementia* refers to "multiple cognitive deficits mani-fested by both (1) memory impairment [and] . . . (2) one (or more) of the following cognitive disturbances: (a) aphasia . . . , (b) apraxia . . . , (c) agnosia . . . , (d) disturbance in executive functioning (i.e., planning, organizing, sequencing, abstract-ing)" (American Psychiatric Association, 1994, 2000). In addition, the patient's cognitive impairment must cause a sig-nificant decrement in functional ability in everyday activities. A gradual and continuing course of dementia is required, and the dementia is not attributable to other central nervous system or systemic conditions, delirium, depression, or other major psychiatric illness (American Psychiatric Association, 1994, 2000). Dementia affects 1.5% of the population older than 65 worldwide. Incidence and prevalence increase with advancing age, ultimately affecting approximately 30% of persons over age 85 (Ritchie & Lovestone, 2002). Alzheimer's disease accounts for 55 to 77% of all cases (Daffner, 1996). Various sources cite vascular disease (Ritchie & Lovestone, 2002), Lewy body disease (McKeith, Galasko, Kosaka, Perry,

Dickson, Hansen, et al., 1996), and dementia caused by fron-totemporal lobar degeneration (Tolnay & Probst, 2001) as the second most prevalent cause of dementia.

This chapter discusses contemporary approaches to dementia. The first section discusses how the dementias are classified, explaining how and why the taxonomy has changed over time. The second section discusses dementia diagnosis, emphasizing the contributions of four complementary scientific approaches: clinical studies of behavior and cognition, neuroradiologic studies of brain structure and function, postmortem studies of brain pathology, and genetic studies of disease origin. The third section describes subtypes of the neurodegenerative demen-tias: Alzheimer's, vascular, Lewy body, and frontotemporal lobar. Two additional entities of particular importance to speech–language pathologists are described: primary progres-sive aphasia and mild cognitive impairment. The fourth section describes several major diseases commonly associated with subcortical dementia—Parkinson's disease, Huntington's dis-ease, progressive supranuclear palsy, and Creutzfeldt-Jakob disease—and selectively illustrates a few additional conditions associated with dementing illness. Wilson's disease results from a metabolic abnormality; human immunodeficiency virus (HIV) encephalopathy, from a viral condition; parkinsonism, from repeated head trauma; and Wernicke's encephalopathy, from nutritional deficiency associated with chronic and excessive alcohol use.

✦ Overview of Dementia Taxonomies

In the late 1800s, when the average life span was much shorter than it is today, dementia was a unitary concept (Turner, Moran, & Kopelman, 2002). With advances in public health and medicine in the 1900s, the average life span increased dramatically, and the characterization of dementing illnesses changed. As recently as the 1960s, the dementias were classified as either presenile (onset before age 65) or senile (onset after age 65). This taxonomy fell to the wayside when neurologists realized that the underlying disease, not age, was the relevant issue. In the more recent past, the dementias were classified as either cortical or subcortical. This taxonomy is somewhat controversial, because, during the Decade of the Brain (1990–1999), advances in the cognitive neurosciences led to an appreciation that neither the *causes* nor the *effects* of certain diseases (such as Alzheimer's disease or vascular disease) are confined to one particular brain region.

Today, neurologists, neuropsychologists, speech–language pathologists, neuropathologists, neurogeneticists, and others are in the process of refining the categories they use to describe this complex array of disorders. The taxonomy is imperfect because some dementias are classified by a specific disease name (e.g., Huntington's disease), others by the appearance of brain tissue at autopsy (e.g., proliferation of neurofibrillary tangles), and still others by the underlying causal mechanism. Price (1996) classified the dementias according to their *causes* and identified 11 categories: degenerative disorders (e.g., Alzheimer's), vascular disease (e.g., lacunar state), myelinoclastic disorders (e.g., multiple sclerosis), trauma (e.g., subdural hematoma), neoplasms (e.g., glioma), hydrocephalus (e.g., normal pressure hydrocephalus), inflammatory conditions (e.g., systemic lupus erythematosus), infections (e.g., syphilis), metabolic disorders (e.g., vitamin deficiency states), toxic states (e.g., alcohol-related syndromes), and psychiatric disorders (e.g., depression) (Price, 1996; Ronthal, 1996). For specialists who are oriented to behavior and cognition, this state of affairs can be confusing, because the actual *clinical* presentation of patients from *different* neurologic categories often appear more *similar* than dissimilar. With this caveat in mind, this section describes a current taxonomy of the dementias, emphasizing the different lines of research.

There are both reversible and irreversible dementias. The irreversible dementias are broadly classified as Alzheimer's dementia (AD), vascular dementia (VaD), frontotemporal lobar dementia (FTD), and Lewy-body dementia (LBD) (Knopman, DeKosky, Cummings, Chui, Corey-Bloom, Relkin et al., 2001). Reversible, or treatable, dementias include those resulting from conditions such as drug toxicity, metabolic imbalances, infections, tumors, normal-pressure hydrocephalus, and alcohol intoxication. Daffner (1966) estimated that as many as 10 to 15% of dementias have a reversible etiology, thus stressing the importance of early and accurate diagnosis. For example, cognitive decline associated with depression, or "pseudodementia," is classified as a reversible dementia (Burke, Sengoz, & Schwartz, 2000; Caine, 1981; Mayeux, Stern, Rosen, & Leventhal, 1981; Ritchie, Gilham, Ledésert, Touchon, & Kotzi, 1999; Wells, 1979). Importantly, depression is present in about half of all dementias (Fitz & Teri, 1994) and differential diagnosis between dementia and pseudodementia may be difficult (Lopez, Becker, Klunk, Saxton, Hamilton, Kaufer et al., 2000; Lopez, Gonzalez, Becker, et al., 1995; Ritchie & Lovestone, 2002; Swainson, Hodges, Galton, Semple, Michael, Dunn et al., 2001).

A separate set of dementias is the so-called subcortical dementias. Some subcortical dementias are irreversible, for example, dementia in Parkinson's disease (PD) (Bamford, Caine, Kido, Cox, & Shoulson, 1995; Friedman, 1996; Mayeux, 1984; Seltzer, Vasterling, Mathias, & Brennan, 2001), Huntington's disease (HD) (Bamford et al., 1995; Kirkwood, Su, Conneally, Foroud, 2001; Koroshetz, 1996), progressive supranuclear palsy (PSP) (Litvan, 2001), and Creutzfeldt-Jakob disease (CJD) (Knopman et al., 2001; Spencer, Knight, & Will, 2002). Palliative treatments, however, may be available. A less favorable prognosis is also associated with dementia due to metastatic tumors (Fischbein, Dillon, & Barkovich, 2000), posttraumatic parkinsonism (e.g., "pugilistic encephalopathy") (Macklis, 1996), multisystem atrophy (due to idiopathic olivopontocerebellar atrophy, striatonigral degeneration, and Shy-Drager syndrome) (Dawson, 1996; Macklis, 1996; Ravin, 1996), encephalopathy due to HIV (Evans, 1996; Fischbein et al., 2000), encephalopathy associated with dialysis (Rob, Niederstadt, & Reusche, 2001), and encephalopathy associated with vitamin deficiency due to chronic alcoholism (Charness, 1996; Dawson, 1996; Fischbein et al., 2000). Other subcortical dementias are reversible, at least in part. For example, if diagnosis is accurate and timely, Wilson's disease (associated with excess copper deposits in the brain), and neurosyphilis are treatable (Fischbein et al., 2000).

In summary, the taxonomies associated with dementing illnesses have changed as scientific advances have been realized. Age (before or after age 65) is no longer a definitional criterion. The location of the neuropathology (cortex or subcortex) is no longer used as a major categorical distinction (although the early manifestation of motor-sensory signs remains helpful for diagnosing subcortical disease states, as will be explained further below). The (ir)reversibility of the underlying condition is important to clinical neurologists and speech–language pathologists in light of our overriding concern: whether or not we can do anything to help remediate or ameliorate the signs and symptoms of dementia, on behalf of our patients. With this background in mind, this chapter now embarks on a discussion of diagnostic approaches, and later, an exploration of the differentiating features of the most prevalent types of dementia.

✦ Diagnostic Approaches

The various dementias are *clinical syndromes* defined by age of onset, prominent clinical signs, and pattern of progression. Clinical neurobehavioral examinations by neurologists, speech–language pathologists, and neuropsychologists provide the primary data on which the clinical diagnosis of dementia rests. Neuroradiologic studies, in contrast, examine the brain in vivo for structural and functional changes. Computed tomography (CT) and magnetic resonance imaging (MRI) provide static images of brain structure that are important to differential diagnosis. Magnetic resonance angiography (MRA), positron emission tomography (PET), and single photon emission computed tomography (SPECT) provide dynamic images of blood flow and oxygen metabolism (Zamani, 1996). For example, when examining patients with suspected dementia, CT is used to detect hydrocephalus, infarctions, hemorrhages, and brain tumors (Zamani, 1996). MRI views the brain in several different planes, and is superior to CT in detecting diffuse axonal injury after trauma, intracranial infections, encephalitis, and deep brain lesions (e.g., basal ganglia, thalamus) (Zamani, 1996). Both CT and MRI provide images of atrophy due to neuronal loss, which is manifest as enlargement of the ventricles and widening of the convolutions on the brain surface. PET and SPECT, in contrast, provide estimates of overall brain metabolism as well as depletion of neuronal activation in specific brain regions (Starkstein, Vasquex, Petracca, et al., 1997; Zamani, 1996). Many studies report the usefulness of both static and dynamic imaging approaches for early detection of dementing illnesses, for differential diagnosis of the dementias, for selection of patients for clinical trials, and for following disease progression (Burton, Karas, Paling, Barber, Williams, Ballard, McKeith, Scheltens, Barkhoff, O'Brien, 2002; Devous, 2002; Duara, Barker, & Luis, 1999; Fischbein et al., 2000; Geldmacher & Whitehouse, 1997; Hsu, Du, Schuff, & Weiner, 2001; Starkstein et al., 1997).

Despite the importance of clinical and radiologic techniques for differential diagnosis, a *definitive* diagnosis of the underlying disease is often not certain until autopsy, when brain cells are examined by histopathologic techniques. In AD, the diagnostic hallmark is an overabundance of amyloid plaques (deposited between brain cells) and neurofibrillary tangles (found within the cells) (Duara et al., 1999). In LBD, the hallmark is the presence of intraneuronal inclusion bodies made up of the synuclein protein. In FTD, the hallmark is neuronal loss and focal atrophy in specific cortical regions, in some cases due to changes typical of AD and in others due to CJD or other pathologic conditions. In VaD, the lesion characteristics vary depending on whether the vascular disease is hemorrhagic or ischemic; diffuse (as in leukoencephalopathy) or focal (as in aneurysm rupture); isolated (as in a single, large vessel stroke confined to one hemisphere) or numerous (as in multiple deep white matter lacunar strokes) (Daffner, 1996).

Thus, clinicians differentiate the dementias on the basis of clinical signs and symptoms; neuroradiologists, on the basis of static images of brain structure as well as dynamic images of brain metabolism; and, neuropathologists, on the basis of postmortem analysis of brain tissue. In contrast, geneticists and microbiologists seek to understand the origins of dementia. Human geneticists study families where the disease or disease cluster has appeared. For example, in the 1980s, this type of study revealed a relationship between Down syndrome (trisomy 21) and AD in some families. Microbiologists examine chromosomes to find abnormalities (mutations) in specific genes, and, in turn, they examine neural cells to find abnormalities in their protein makeup. Genes—genetic codes—are "recipes" for proteins. The genetic code is recorded on chromosomal material and is present in the nucleus of every cell in the body. Of special interest to neurobiologists and neurogeneticists are the genes that code for the production, or breakdown, of *neural cells* (Honig, 1997; National Institute on Aging, 2000; Ritchie & Lovestone, 2002; Wisniewski, Weigiel, Morys, et al., 1994).

Finding abnormal genes, however, is just the first step in a complex biologic puzzle. Mutations in *more than one* gene may be required for the expression of a *single* clinical syndrome (so-called polygenic diseases). Conversely, mutations in a *single gene* can account for a wide *variety* of clinical syndromes. For example, mutations in the gene coding for the *tau* protein have been associated not only with FTD and AD, but also with PSP and Parkinson's disease (National Institute on Aging, 2000; Ritchie & Lovestone, 2002). Mutations in the gene coding for *amyloid* is also present in AD. Mutations in the gene coding for the *synuclein* protein have been associated with LBD, Parkinson's disease, and multisystem atrophy; mutations in the gene coding for the *prion* protein, with prion

diseases such as CJD; and, mutations in the gene coding for the *huntingtin* protein, with HD (National Institute on Aging, 2000; Ritchie & Lovestone, 2002).

To complicate matters further, epidemiologic studies suggest that one's susceptibility to disease is multifactorial, that is, it reflects genetic, environmental, experiential, nutritional, and other factors. Thus, human genetic studies are in a nascent stage. In decades to come, our understanding of the role of genetic mutations will undoubtedly play a larger role not only in the diagnosis of the dementias but also in their treatment. For now, it is merely important for the reader to be aware that these types of studies are being undertaken in tandem with other areas of science. The main areas of emphasis are as follows: clinical studies are concerned with patterns of *behavior and cognition* associated with dementing illnesses; neuroradiologic studies, with *structural and functional abnormalities* of brain tissue, both at cortical and subcortical sites; postmortem studies, with actual *pathologic changes* in the brain; and, genetic studies, with the *pathogenesis* (the origins) of the underlying disease (Ritchie & Lovestone, 2002).

As a result of these types of scientific advances, familiar distinctions such as "cortical dementia," "multiinfarct dementia," and "mixed" dementia are disappearing from the contemporary literature. As implied in the paragraphs above, recent research on AD and other progressive neurodegenerative disorders "all involve deposits of abnormal proteins in the brain" (National Institute on Aging, 2000, p. 11) and many have *both* cortical and subcortical effects (Ritchie & Lovestone, 2002). According to Ritchie and Lovestone, "as the complex interactive effects of genetic predisposition, neurochemical changes, and disease co-morbidity in the genesis of dementia syndromes are elucidated" (p. 1759), even distinctions among major clinical categories, such as AD and VaD, may be overly simplistic. Thus, even though the dementias are heterogeneous in their *clinical* presentation, recent studies have revealed commonalities in the *pathophysiology* of these neurodegenerative conditions. Therefore, the taxonomy of the dementias has changed, and this chapter has been written to reflect the taxonomy that is recognized by the neurology community.

In summary, "dementia" is a clinical diagnosis based on the signs and symptoms that manifest themselves to the examining clinician. To support the clinical diagnosis, a host of other diagnostic approaches are available. This section has described neuroradiologic, histopathologic (neuropathologic), and genetic (neuropathogenetic) approaches. Speech–language pathologists and their patients will ultimately benefit from scientific breakthroughs as they occur. Because the landscape of the dementias is changing rapidly, speech–language pathologists should strive to read the neurology and basic science literature as it unfolds.

✦ Neurodegenerative Dementias

This section describes the major neurodegenerative dementias cited above: AD, VaD, LBD, and FTD. To clarify the distinctions among "probable," "possible," and "definite" diagnoses, **Table 7–1** summarizes the major findings of various consortia. **Table 7–2** draws from the literature to summarize the major features of each category relative to onset and course, subtypes, cognitive profile, communication, associated behavior, physical signs, genetics, imaging, and definitive diagnosis.

Table 7–1 Diagnostic Criteria for Select Neurodegenerative Dementias

	Alzheimer's Dementia (AD) (NINCDS-ADRDA)	Alzheimer's Dementia (U. Pittsburgh ADRC)	Vascular Dementia (VaD) (NINCDS-AIREN)	Lewy Body Disease (LBD) (McKeith et al, 1996)
Probable	Loss of memory and deficits in two or more areas of cognition, including executive functioning; impact on daily function; progressive worsening; no disturbance of consciousness; insidious onset with slow progression	Same as NINCDS-ADRDA but the cognitive profile may show a prominent deficit in one domain (e.g., disproportionate language disturbance); may have concomitant cerebrovascular disease; or, may progress rapidly	Loss of memory and at least two other areas of cognition; decline from previous functioning; focal neurologic signs; confirmatory brain imaging; dementia must present within 3 months after the vascular event; may be stable, improving, or worsening	Progressive cognitive decline; impact on function; but memory impairment not mandatory; at least two core features must be present: fluctuating attention; recurrent hallucinations; and/or motor features of parkinsonism
Possible	Same as above, except that the presentation or course may be different from the criteria for probable AD, but the diagnosis is still one of exclusion	Same as above, except recognizes that some other disease process may contribute to the cognitive impairment, e.g., cerebrovascular disease, head injury; and there may be different cognitive subtypes depending on the relative impairment of different cortical areas	Same as above except confirmatory brain imaging may be absent; or, the onset and course may be atypical	At least one core feature must be present
Definite	Histopathologic confirmation of abundant amyloid plaques and neurofibrillary tangles; density exceeds age-matched normal brains	Histopathologic confirmation of abundant amyloid plaques and neurofibrillary tangles; density exceeds age-matched normal brains	Criteria for probable VaD satisfied and no pathologic features other than CVD are present; etiologies include multiinfarct, strategic single-infarct, small-vessel, multiple lacunes, hypoperfusion, hemorrhage	Rule out stroke or other causes; proliferation of Lewy bodies at autopsy

NINCDS-ADRDA, National Institute of Neurological and Communicative Disorders and Stroke–Alzheimer Disease and Related Disorders Association; ADRC, Alzheimer's Disease Research Center; AIREN, Association Internationale pour la Recherche et l'Enseignement en Neurosciences.

Alzheimer's Dementia (AD)

Once considered a homogeneous disorder known for its "senile" (over age 65) onset, AD is now recognized to vary in presenting symptoms, age of onset, and course of disease (Lopez et al., 2000). The contribution of the National Institute of Neurological Communicative Disorders and Stroke–Alzheimer Disease and Related Disorders Association (NINCDS-ADRDA) Work Group (McKhann, Drachman, Folstein, Katzman, Price, & Stadlan, 1984) was essential to understanding this heterogeneity. To avoid misdiagnosis, NINCDS-ADRDA differentiated possible, probable, and definite Alzheimer's disease. "Probable AD" includes "dementia established by clinical examination . . . deficits in two or more areas of cognition; progressive worsening of memory and other cognitive functions; no disturbance of consciousness; onset between ages 40 and 90, most often after age 65; and absence of systematic disorders or other brain diseases that in and of themselves could account for the progressive deficits in memory and cognition" (McKhann et al., 1984, p. 940). The NINCDS-ADRDA acknowledged that progressive deterioration could be general or specific to a cognitive domain (such as aphasia), expected to see a deterioration of activities of daily living, and recognized that plateaus could occur in the course of progression. In the NINCDS-ADRDA taxonomy, the key difference between probable and possible AD is that the former manifests "a typical insidious onset of dementia with progression" (McKhann et al., 1984, p. 942) in the absence of other diseases, whereas the term *possible AD* may be used "if the presentation or course is

somewhat aberrant" (p. 941). The term *definite AD* is reserved for cases in which a histopathologic confirmation is made (**Tables 7–1** and **7–2**).

While acknowledging that the NINCDS-ARDRA established the "gold standard" for clinical diagnosis of AD (Loewenstein, Ownby, Schram, Acevedo, Rubert, & Arguelles, 2001), the University of Pittsburgh Alzheimer's Disease Research Center (ADRC) further refined the diagnostic entity known as "probable AD." They recognized probable AD with atypical onset or presentation (e.g., disproportionate language disturbance), with atypical course (e.g., rapid progression), or with cerebrovascular disease (i.e., clinical or MRI evidence of a single ischemic event) (Lopez et al., 2000). The speed of progression of AD is of particular interest, because rapid progression is often associated with early onset and language deficits (Boller, Becker, Holland, et al., 1991; Kaszniak, Fox, Gandell, et al., 1978).

The University of Pittsburgh ADRC also revised the category of "possible AD." "Possible AD" may include "clinical evidence of some other disease process that might have *contributed to* the patient's cognitive symptomatology. This group included patients with cerebrovascular disease [CVD], head injury, depression, alcoholism, hypothyroidism, vitamin B12 deficiency, and a history of encephalitis" (Lopez et al., 2000, p. 1856, emphasis added). Furthermore, after comparing almost 1500 AD patients with normal controls, the University of Pittsburgh ADRC emphasized that distinctive cognitive profiles in AD were associated with pathology in particular cortical sites. Frontal cortical changes were correlated with behavioral

Table 7–2   Differential Diagnosis of Major Types of Neurodegenerative Dementia

	Alzheimer's Disease (AD)	Vascular Disease (VaD)	Lewy Body Disease (LBD)	Frontotemporal Lobar Dementia (FTD)
Onset and course	Insidious onset; more likely after age 65; progressive course; slow course with plateaus not unusual	Abrupt deterioration within 3 months after stroke; course may be stable, improving or worsening (stepwise or fluctuating)	Periods of normal cognition alternate with abnormal cognition in early stages; course is progressive, often rapid (1–5 years)	Insidious onset; more likely before age 65; progressive course, often slow
Subtypes	Nonfamilial or familial occurrence; onset before or after age 65; or coexistence of other conditions such as Parkinson's disease	Depends on location, type, and extent of cerebrovascular disease	Not described	Focal atrophy syndromes include FTD frontal variant, FTD temporal variant, and FTD nonfluent aphasia variant
Cognitive profile	Deficits in memory and cognition; no disturbance of consciousness; impaired function in daily life	Deficits in memory and cognition; no disturbance of consciousness; impaired function in daily life	Core features include fluctuating attention, visual hallucinations, and parkinsonism	Executive dysfunction common in the frontal lobe variant; semantic deficits in the temporal lobe variant; and, nonfluent progressive aphasia in the last variant
Communication	Aphasia is common, starting as either fluent or nonfluent; semantic system most affected; syntax and phonology later; gradual progression to mutism	Motor speech disorder; simplification of grammar and impaired writing; slowness and reduced initiation; abulic at later stages	Parkinsonian dysarthric features, e.g., hypophonia	Primary progressive aphasia (PPA) not uncommon; dysarthria unlikely; progression may be very slow
Associated behavior	Depression, insomnia, incontinence, delusions, agitation	Depression and mood changes	Periods of delirium (confusion) not uncommon as well as episodes of "going blank," daytime drowsiness, and transient confusion upon waking	Wide range of associated behaviors, most notable in the frontal lobe variant
Physical signs	In advanced disease, increased tone, myoclonus or gait disorder	Gait disorder or frequent falls; hemiparesis; motor and sensory changes in cranial nerve distributions; visual deficits; pseudobulbar signs; dysarthria	Parkinsonian features common	Not a major feature of the FTD
Genetic	Familial AD (FAD) linked to chromosomes 1, 14, and 21 (5–10% of all cases); sporadic AD linked to ApoE E4 allele on chromosome 19 in 30% of probable AD; *tau* and *amyloid* proteins affected; routine genotyping not recommended at this time	Genetic abnormalities linked to stroke risk factors, e.g., hypertension, arteriovenous malformation; routine genotyping not recommended at this time	*Synuclein* protein abnormalities linked to LBD, Parkinson's disease, and multisystem atrophy; routine genotyping not recommended at this time	Mutations on chromosome 17 and 3; abnormal *tau* protein; routine genotyping not recommended at this time
Imaging	Bilateral atrophy, medial temporal lobe, hippocampus and thalamus affected; temporoparietal hypoperfusion	Single or multiple lesions in distribution of either large or small vessels, including periventricular white matter	Bilateral frontal and temporal atrophy and insular cortex; relatively preserved medial temporal lobe, hippocampus and amygdala	Focal atrophy; frontal hypoperfusion
Definitive diagnosis	Clinical diagnosis by exclusion; dementia not attributable to other systemic disorder or brain disease; definitive examination only by postmortem examination (proliferation of amyloid plaques and neurofibrillary tangles)	Clinical diagnosis by inclusion of positive history for CVD, definitive diagnosis must rule out all other causes by postmortem examination, clinical presentation, neurologic examination and neuroimaging	Definitive diagnosis depends on presence of Lewy bodies typically in cortex, subcortex and brainstem; Alzheimer changes may co-occur, but presence of plaques and neuron loss not essential	Clinical diagnosis depends on isolated cognitive impairment (not global dementia); definitive diagnosis depends on postmortem analysis of brain tissue (e.g., Pick's bodies, neuronal loss)

CVD, cerebrovascular disease.

disinhibition and agitation; occipital lobe involvement, with visuospatial/constructional deficits; and, temporal lobe deficits, with language impairment (Lopez et al., 2000). Different patterns of performance also depended on the different levels of disease severity (Piccini, Pecori, Campani, Falcini, Piccininni, Manfred, 1998) (For a discussion about heterogeneity in AD see a review by Cummings, 2000).

Advances in our understanding of AD coincide with improving clinical diagnosis and behavioral characterization, as well as with astounding advances in the basic sciences. First, it has been known for some time that the two major abnormalities in the brains of individuals with AD are amyloid plaques and neurofibrillary tangles (National Institute on Aging, 2000; Wisniewski et al., 1994). The plaques are made up of deposits of a protein called β-amyloid; these plaques are insoluble (do not dissolve) and as a result fill up the spaces between brain neurons (National Institute on Aging, 2000). Neurofibrillary tangles are made up of a protein called *tau* that twists into paired filaments, thus interfering with the transport of nutrients and molecules within brain cells (National Institute on Aging, 2000).

Second, most cases of AD result from genetic, environmental and other factors, but the exact interplay of these factors is not fully understood (National Institute on Aging, 2000). For example, in the past, the diagnosis of AD was avoided in the presence of vascular disease. Now, it is recognized that AD and stroke can co-occur (Lopez et al., 2000; see also Heyman, Fillenbaum, Welsh-Bohmer, Gearing, Mirra, Mohs, Peterson, & Pieper, 1998). In fact, the important "Nun Study" published in JAMA, in 1997 showed that a history of vascular disease may predispose individuals to an increased risk of developing AD later in life (Snowdon, Greiner, Mortimer, Riley, Greiner, & Markesbery, 1997; Tatemichi, Desmond, Mayeux, Paik, Stern, Sano, 1992).

Third, two basic categories of Alzheimer's disease are now recognized: nonfamilial or sporadic AD, and familial AD (FAD). FAD is an early-onset variety (presenting between ages 30 to 60), and is associated with abnormalities on chromosomes 1, 14, and 21 (National Institute on Aging, 2000). For example, mutations in genetic structure on chromosome 21 are associated with abnormalities of *amyloid precursor protein* (APP), which causes plaque formation (Honig, 1997). Notably, only 5 to 10% of all cases of AD worldwide are this familial type, and only 2 to 3% of FAD cases are due to APP mutations (Honig, 1997). According to the National Institute on Aging's (2000) progress report, "the total known number of these [APP-FAD] cases is small (between 100 and 200 worldwide), and there is as yet no evidence that any of these mutations play a major role in the more common, sporadic or non-familial form of late-onset AD" (p. 9). Due to the rarity of APP-FAD cases, little is known about their neuropsychological profiles (Warrington, Agnew, Kennedy, Rossor, 2001).

Nonfamilial or sporadic AD presents after age 60 and also is linked to genetic mutations. An important study at Duke University Medical Center identified that an increased risk experiencing AD later in life was associated with the apolipoprotein E *(ApoE)* gene on chromosome 19 (Honig, 1997; National Institute on Aging, 2000; Strittmatter, Saunders, Schmechel, Pericak-Vance, Enghild, Salvesen, Roses, 1993). There are three common variants, or "alleles," of the *ApoE* gene, numbered 2, 3, and 4. Strittmatter and colleagues recognized that inheritance of *ApoE* E4 was associated with the level of risk for acquiring AD, depending on the *number of copies* of E4 that were present.

Two important findings have emerged from this line of research. First, "the inheritance of one or two ApoE E4 alleles does not predict AD with certainty." In other words, "ApoE E4 increases the *risk* of developing AD; it does not *cause* the disease" (National Institute on Aging, 2000, p. 10; see Roses, 1995). According to the American College of Medical Genetics/American Society of Human Genetics Working Group (ACMG/ASHG) on ApoE and Alzheimer Disease (1995), the *ApoE-E4* gene occurs in 34 to 65% of individuals clinically diagnosed as having AD. Second, "the more [copies of the] ApoE E4 alleles inherited, the lower the age of onset" National Institute on Aging, 2000, p. 9). Third, the presence of *ApoE* E2 may actually *protect* against AD, that is, not only lower the risk of developing AD but also encourage a later age of onset of the disease (National Institute on Aging, 2000). According to the ACMG/ASHG, testing for the abnormal protein *E2* is ill-advised, however, because many unaffected adults also have the *ApoE* gene. Finally, researchers at Harvard University and the Massachusetts General Hospital reported that a previously unidentified region of genetic material on chromosome 12 may be associated with late-onset AD, as well as with LBD (Tanzi, 1999).

In summary, Alzheimer's dementia is defined clinically by its insidious, progressive course of cognitive disability; neuropathologically, by plaques and tangles; neuroradiologically, by progressive, global atrophy (implying neuronal loss, particularly toward the end stage); and biologically, by genetic abnormalities is some patients. The dementia is heterogeneous, its underlying cause is illusive, and its cure is as yet undiscovered. The fact that CVD co-occurs with or predisposes individuals to AD is a scientific puzzle that has captured the attention of many research scientists. Speech–language pathologists who work with both stroke and Alzheimer's patients are advised to follow these new advances closely. Advances in both the clinical and basic sciences can inform our practice as more is learned about the coincidence of AD and CVD.

Vascular Dementia (VaD)

A rigorous effort to identify and categorize the dementias accurately is all-important to management of these debilitating disorders. Of particular interest to many clinical researchers is the ability to distinguish between VaD and AD (Bennett, Corbett, Gaden, Grayson, Kril, & Broe, 2002; Fahlender, Wahlin, Almkvist, & Backman, 2002; Powell, Cummings, Hill, Benson, 1988;). CVD may occur alone or in combination with other dementing illnesses. In some cases, vascular disease may increase the risk for later acquisition of AD (Heyman et al., 1998; Snowdon et al., 1997). Kalaria's (2000) analysis of the autopsy literature revealed that 60 to 90% of individuals definitively diagnosed as having AD had some evidence of cerebrovascular pathology. To improve differential diagnosis, Hachinski and colleagues developed an ischemic scoring system of 13 items designed to differentiate ischemic disease and AD. In some series, the discriminative accuracy was as high as 70% (Molsa, Paljarvi, Rinne, Rinne, & Sako, 1985; Wagner & Bachman, 1996). The compelling reason for accurately differentiating VaD and AD is, simply, that CVD is preventable and treatable, whereas the degenerative dementias are not (Roman, Tatemichi, Erkinjuntti, Cummings, Masdeu, Garcia, et al., 1993).

Because CVD may predispose some elderly persons to developing AD, the need to prevent CVD and the need to identify which individuals with CVD are at particular risk for AD become very important enterprises within dementia research. Genetic studies of stroke risk factors are part of this enterprise. These studies have revealed a relationship between genes and "the expression of stroke risk factors" such as hypertension, heart disease, diabetes, and vascular malformations (National Institute of Neurological Disorders and Stroke, 2003b). Genes are also implicated in CADASIL (cerebral autosomal dominant arteriopathy with subcortical infarcts and leukoencephalopathy). "CADASIL is a rare, genetically inherited, congenital vascular disease of the brain that causes strokes, subcortical dementia, migraine-like headaches, and psychiatric disturbances" (National Institute of Neurological Disorders and Stroke, 2003b).

The differential diagnosis between AD and VaD is complicated because there is "the uncertainty of determining whether the presence of stroke in a demented patient is the cause of the dementia, a contributing factor to underlying degenerative dementia, or simply an unrelated event" (Roman et al., 1993, p. 251). The first step in this puzzle is to clarify the definition of vascular dementia. The Neuroepidemiology Branch of the National Institute of Neurological Disorders and Stroke in collaboration with the Association Internationale pour la Recherche et l'Enseignement en Neurosciences (NINDS-AIREN) offered its expert insight. First, the group eschewed the term *multiinfarct dementia* (MID) because white matter ischemic necrosis with neuronal loss—leukencephalopathy—and multiple brain infarcts are *both* causes of VaD (Roman et al., 1993). The group also opined that the term MID *incorrectly* implies that *only* multiple brain infarcts cause VaD, and emphasized that VaD encompasses "all instances of dementia associated with not only ischemic CVD [multiple infarcts] but also with hemorrhagic and hypoxic-ischemic cerebral lesions" (Roman et al., 1993, p. 251).

A second step toward clarification, also undertaken by NINDS-AIREN, was to subcategorize the vascular dementias. These subcategories were multiinfarct dementia, strategic single-infarct dementia, small-vessel disease with dementia, multiple lacunar strokes, hypoperfusion, hemorrhagic dementia, and "other" (Roman et al., 1993). Again, the classification of the various types of dementia does not automatically tell us the *cause* of the vascular disease, because the underlying pathophysiology can vary, including hypertension, vascular malformation, systemic lupus erythematosus, and infectious vasculitides (e.g., Lyme disease) (Geldmacher & Whitehouse, 1997).

From a neurobehavioral perspective, the diagnosis of VaD requires demonstrably impaired functioning in daily life associated with a loss of memory *and* deficits in at least two other cognitive domains. (Note that this definition is more stringent than the *DSM-IV-TR's* definition of dementia, because it requires "at least two" additional cognitive deficits rather than "one or more.") In addition, the disorder must represent a decline from previous functioning, and the vascular event must coincide with the dementia; specifically, dementia must present within 3 months after the clinically evident stroke. Unlike progressive decline typical of AD, the course of VaD may be stable, improving, or worsening (Roman et al., 1993).

Thus, in the NINDS-AIREN taxonomy, "probable VaD" may be diagnosed (1) if memory is impaired; (2) if two or more additional cognitive domains are impaired (orientation, attention, language, visuospatial functions, executive functions, motor control or praxis); (3) if no other impairments exist (such as that delusions or severe aphasia preclude neuropsychological testing); (4) if focal neurologic signs are present (including motor or sensory deficits, including visual deficits or dysarthria): and (5) if there is relatively abrupt onset of dementia (within 3 months of the cerebrovascular event). If the CVD is not stabilized, the dementia is likely to progress in a stepwise fashion (Roman et al., 1993).

So-called possible VaD is similar to the foregoing definition, except that confirmatory brain imaging studies may be absent, the temporal correspondence between dementia and CVD may be absent, or the onset and course might be atypical in light of known cerebrovascular disease. Finally, "definite VaD" occurs when the criteria for probable VaD are satisfied, there is histopathologic evidence of CVD by biopsy or autopsy, the plaques and tangles do not exceed those expected by age, and there are no pathologic features other than CVD capable of causing dementia (Roman et al., 1993).

Different profiles of cognitive impairment are associated with VaD as compared with other dementing illnesses. For example, using the Mini–Mental State Examination (MMSE), Jefferson, Cosentino, Ball, Bogdanoff, Leopold, Nathan, and Libon (2002) compared VaD and AD subjects. The VaD subjects performed more poorly than AD subjects on motor/constructional tasks and short-term verbal memory (working memory). In contrast, the AD subjects performed more poorly than VaD subjects on tasks involving orientation to time and declarative memory. Thus, even though the overall scores on the MMSE were not significantly different, the groups demonstrated different profiles of impairment (see also Lukatela, Cohen, Kessler, Jenkins, Moser, Stone, Gordon & Kaplan, 2000.)

Finally, there have been reports that VaD can occur after a single clinical stroke. Barba, Castro, del Mar Morin, Rodriguez-Romero, Rodriguez-Garcia, Canton, and Del Ser (2001) reported that 79 of 273 (29%) of poststroke patients had dementia 3 months after their first clinical stroke. The authors stressed that the clinical presentation of dementia in this population was not solely due to a single stroke, but was related to a larger volume of infarcts, the extent of white matter lesions, coexisting medial temporal lobe atrophy, and low education. They concluded that dementia results from the cumulative effect of these cerebral abnormalities, as confirmed by MRI. Others have suggested that the white matter changes seen in individuals with dementia are not completely explained by either advanced age or a history of clinical strokes. In Wallin, Sjogren, Edman, Blennow, and Regland's (2000) series, patients with white matter changes were significantly more likely to have diabetes mellitus, hypertension, and ischemic heart disease. Another study, by contrast, identified advanced age, nephropathy, and previous mental decline as significant correlates of VaD, but not stroke type, location, or vascular risk factors (Barba, Martinez-Espinosa, Rodriguez-Garcia, Pondal, Vivancos, & Del Ser, 2000). Despite some divergence in empirical studies, there is emerging evidence that antihypertensive medication may significantly reduce the risk for dementia (Richards, Emsley, Roberts, Murray, Hall, Gao, & Hendrie, 2000).

In summary, VaD is a category of dementing illness that represents a wide variety of etiologies, as well as cortical and subcortical neuronal impairments. VaD may present after several (or ongoing) cerebrovascular events, or after a single cerebrovascular incident. As research emerges, it appears that the extent of neuronal involvement, rather than the specific etiology or location of lesion, is the critical factor in determining whether the person affected will demonstrate dementia on clinical examination. To the extent that cerebrovascular disease can be identified and treated, VaD is unique among the dementias, because it is preventable.

Lewy Body Dementia (LBD)

Lewy body disease with dementia (LBD) is one of the most challenging of the neurodegenerative dementias. Three Lewy body syndromes have been described: movement disorder, autonomic failure, and dementia (McKeith, 2000). The diagnostic challenge arises not only because of the variant syndromes, but also because the presence of Lewy bodies is not exclusive to LBD, because Lewy bodies can coexist with the plaques and tangles of Alzheimer's disease, and because both cortical and subcortical sites are affected (NINDS, 2003a). First, Lewy bodies are pathologic markers considered essential to the diagnosis of idiopathic Parkinson's disease (McKeith et al., 1996). In LBD, however, the distribution of Lewy bodies is far more widespread than in idiopathic Parkinson's disease. Lewy bodies in Parkinson's disease are abundant in subcortical nuclei (e.g., substantia nigra), whereas in LBD, Lewy bodies extend to the temporal, frontal and parietal cortices, the limbic cortex, the brainstem, and the subcortical nuclei (McKeith et al., 1996).

Second, in LBD cases that have been autopsied, Lewy bodies are abundant, but coexisting Alzheimer pathology is commonly present as well. Despite the neuropathologic overlap, the clinical manifestation of LBD is quite different from AD. For example, Doubleday, Snowden, Varma, and Neary (2002) found inattention, incoherence, confabulatory responses, perseveration and intrusions were much more common in LBD than AD. In addition, neuroimaging studies have revealed less severe atrophy in medial temporal lobe, hippocampus, amygdala, and thalamus in LBD patients as compared with AD patients (Burton et al., 2002; Devous, 2002; Hsu et al., 2001). Third, as in other branches of dementia work, genetic studies of LBD are ongoing. As we have learned, abnormalities in the tau and amyloid proteins are typical of AD, whereas abnormal deposits of the α-synuclein protein is distinctive of LBD (NINDS, 2003a). The α-synuclein protein is also linked to Parkinson's disease and multiple system atrophy (NINDS, 2003a; see also Gasser, 2001).

In 1996, the Consortium of Dementia with Lewy Bodies outlined standard criteria for LBD to aid clinicians in differential diagnosis (McKeith et al., 1996). Progressive cognitive decline undermining everyday functioning is an essential feature of LBD, but memory impairment (in the early stages) is not. In one case study, orientation was well preserved until late in the course of the disease (Wagner & Bachman, 1996). Progression may be rapid (1 to 5 years), leading finally to global dementia and parkinsonism (McKeith et al., 1996).

To diagnose "probable LBD," at least two of the following clinical signs must be present. First, fluctuating attention is typical and is characterized by marked shifts in alertness (within or between sessions), daytime drowsiness in some, and transient confusion on waking. Second, probable LBD patients have recurrent, detailed, and persistent hallucinations, including animate and inanimate figures and scenes. According to McKeith and colleagues (1996), visual hallucinations appear "to be the only psychotic symptom that reliably discriminates [LBD] from AD or VaD" (p. 116) (see also Gurd, Herzberg, Joachim, Marshall, 2000). Third, LBD patients are likely to have motor features of parkinsonism, often mild, such

as rigidity, bradykinesia, hypophonic speech, masked facies, stooped posture, and shuffling gait (McKeith et al., 1996; see also Sulkava, 2003). Thus, core features of DLB are fluctuating attention, visual hallucinations, and parkinsonism (McKeith et al., 1996; Kuzuhara & Yoshimura, 1993). For "probable DLB," two core features must be present. For "possible DLB," one core feature must be present (McKeith et al., 1996).

The consortium also identified clinical features that supported the diagnosis of LBD (i.e., helped with the differential diagnosis from other diseases). These features included repeated falls, syncope, transient loss of consciousness, neuroleptic sensitivity, systematized delusions, and hallucinations in other modalities (McKeith et al., 1996). The diagnosis of LBD is *less* likely in the presence of stroke as determined clinically or by neuroimaging. Patients with LBD are known to be very sensitive to antipsychotic drugs; therefore, clinicians must carefully rule out medication toxicity or other causes before the diagnosis of LBD is made (Campbell, Stephens, & Ballard, 2001).

In summary, LBD is characterized by cortical and subcortical disease, has less medial temporal lobe involvement than AD, shares common neuropathologic and neurogenetic features with Parkinson's disease, and is distinguished from the other neurodegenerative diseases by fluctuating attention, visual hallucinations, and parkinsonism.

Frontotemporal Lobar Dementia (FTD)

Formerly thought of as a singular entity known as Pick's dementia, contemporary researchers now prefer the term *frontotemporal dementia* (FTD) (Neary, Snowden, Gustafson, Passant, Stuss, Black, et al., 1998; Perry & Hodges, 2000). Although Pick's disease, in some instances, can account for FTD, Pick's disease does not account for all cases of FTD. This section briefly describes Pick's disease, explains the new term FTD, identifies the advantages and disadvantages of the umbrella category FTD, and describes the variants of FTD.

Pick's disease is rare, and is characterized by a proliferation of distinctive neuronal inclusions known as Pick bodies (Kirshner, 1994). Pick dementia is characterized by euphoria, impaired insight and judgment, and early language deficit (Cummings & Benson, 1992; Wechsler, Verity, Rosenschein, Fried, & Scheibel, 1982). In later stages Klüver-Bucy syndrome (hyperoral behavior), hypersexuality, and visual agnosia have been reported (Cummings & Duchen, 1981). Despite the historical recognition of Pick's disease, the contemporary term FTD is now used. Recognizing a family of disorders under the umbrella FTD offers the advantage of avoiding any implication regarding the underlying histopathology or etiology, while simultaneously offering the disadvantage of "amalgamating patients with different syndromes" (Perry & Hodges, 2000, p. 2277).

The common thread among the different FTD syndromes is *focal atrophy*, implying neuronal loss in particular cortical regions. Mutations on chromosome 17 (Kreeger, 2000) and chromosome 3 (Gydesen, Brown, Brun, Chakrabart, Gade, Johannsen, et al., 2002) have been associated with FTD. According to Binetti, Locascio, Corkin, Vonsattel, and Growdon (2000), the FTD classification "emphasizes the belief that the topography of the atrophy is more responsible for the clinical manifestations than is the underlying histopathologic condition" (p. 228). In short, the umbrella diagnosis of FTD helps to simplify the terminology as well as to capture a range of clinical conditions, variously referred to in the literature as primary progressive aphasia, semantic dementia, frontal lobe dementia, frontal lobe dementia with amyotrophic sclerosis, frontotemporal dementia with Parkinson disease, and corticobasal degeneration (Binetti et al., 2000; Di Maria, Tabaton, Vigo, Abbruzzese, Bellone, Donati, et al., 2000; Grossman, 2002a).

There are several variants of FTD: frontal, temporal, and nonfluent aphasia (Grossman, 2002a). In FTD patients with primarily frontal lobe atrophy, personality and behavioral changes are prominent. In FTD patients with primarily temporal lobe atrophy, progressive fluent aphasia is prominent. This latter variant is also known as "semantic aphasia," which presents with fluent output and prominent anomia (Perry & Hodges, 2000). In FTD patients with nonfluent aphasia, the distinctive manifestation is a Broca's like aphasia that is progressive (Perry & Hodges, 2000).

In a study comparing AD, FTD-frontal variant, and FTD-temporal variant, Perry and Hodges (2000) found distinctive profiles. In AD subjects, episodic memory impairment was prominent, reflecting medial temporal (hippocampal) pathology known to be affected in AD (Duara et al., 1999). In contrast, in FTD-temporal variant subjects, the prominent deficit was in the realm of semantic memory (as measured using oral naming, rapid category naming, and matching conceptually related pictures). The authors make clear that this is a deficit that goes well beyond "naming problems"; that is, semantic dementia reflects not only an impairment in the ability to use words (in expression and comprehension), but also, in how words relate to one another, and how underlying concepts are structured (Duara et al., 1999; Hodges, Patterson, Ward, Garrard, Bak, Perry, & Gregory, 1999). Similarly, Hodges (2001), drawing from Warrington's (1975) early work, emphasized that semantic dementia implies not only anomia but also a breakdown in semantic memory, that is, problems not only with "word-finding," but also with word comprehension and object recognition.

Another contrast between FTD and AD patients is in their respective abilities to benefit from cues on a variety of short-term memory and explicit verbal memory tasks. Both types of tasks were decreased in both groups, but FTD patients benefited more from cues than did AD patients (Pasquier, Grymonprez, Lebert, & Van der Linden, 2001). In addition, Bathgate, Snowden, Varma, Blackshaw, and Neary (2001) found a host of behavioral changes that reliably distinguished FTD patients from AD patients, including emotional flattening, disinhibition, gluttony, wandering, as well as motor and verbal stereotypies. Studies have also compared the different subtypes of FTD. Executive functions and attention have been found to be remarkably spared in FTD-temporal lobe variant subjects (Perry & Hodges, 2000). In contrast, in FTD-frontal variant, attention, and executive function deficits are prominent (Perry & Hodges, 2000). In another report, FTD-frontal variant was marked by executive dysfunction, disinhibition, as well as antisocial and stereotypical behavior; memory was relatively spared (Hodges, 2001).

The entity of FTD expressing as progressive nonfluent aphasia is less well understood. Neary et al. (1998) described the core features as "insidious onset and gradual progression," with "nonfluent spontaneous speech with at least one of the following: agrammatism, phonemic paraphasias, anomia" (p. 1548). Supportive diagnostic features are "(1) stuttering and oral apraxia, (2) impaired repetition, (3) alexia, agraphia,

(4) early preservation of word naming, and (5) late mutism" (p. 1548). In Hodges's (2001) series, most patients with FTD-nonfluent aphasia presented with AD at autopsy, but the anatomic distribution was distinctly in the perisylvian language areas with sparing of medial temporal lobes.

Despite some methodologic variability among these studies, the data persuasively illustrate that AD and the FTD variants resulting from lobar atrophy demonstrate distinctive profiles of cognitive impairment, and that the FTD syndromes are distinguishable from AD, both behaviorally (Hsu et al., 2001) and neuroradiologically (Duara et al., 1999). As Perry and Hodges (2000) pointed out, the emergence of pharmacologic treatments for both memory and behavioral problems in these groups (and subgroups) mandates careful differential diagnosis of these subtypes of FTD. Finally, Hodges (2001) emphasized that motor neuron disease (amyotrophic lateral sclerosis, ALS) may coincide with any one of these three FTD variants. The link between FTD and ALS may be due to an abnormality on chromosome 9 (Hosler, Siddique, Sapp, Sailor, Huang, Hossain, et al., 2001; see also Hodges & Miller, 2001). Clearly, the presence of ALS will have different management implications, particularly from the speech–language pathology perspective.

In summary, FTD is an umbrella term referring to a host of clinical syndromes that share the common feature of focal cortical atrophy. There are three variants—frontal, temporal, and nonfluent aphasia—that reflect the location of the atrophy, not the underlying neuropathologic disease. The variants are particularly important to speech–language pathologists because they present with executive disability, semantic memory impairments, and Broca's-like aphasia, respectively. Finally, ALS may co-occur with FTD, which presents special challenges for communication disorders specialists and their patients.

Primary Progressive Aphasia

A clinical entity of particular interest to speech–language pathologists is that of primary progressive aphasia (PPA). This section briefly identifies the seminal work in PPA, describes the clinical manifestations of this intriguing clinical entity, and highlights the types of aphasia that can occur.

Wechsler (1977) and later Mesulam (1982) are credited with recognizing that aphasia could occur in the absence of the intellectual and behavioral disturbances associated with dementia. Whereas some PPA patients continued to progress without signs of dementia, many slowly inched toward dementia and ultimately showed global cognitive deterioration (Foster & Chase, 1983; Heath, Kennedy, & Kapur, 1983; Hier, Hagenlocker, & Shindler, 1985; Kirshner, Webb, Kelly, & Wells, 1984; Morris, Cole, Banker, & Wright, 1984). In 1987, Mesulam, and later Mesulam and Weintraub (1992) refined the diagnostic criteria for PPA, and subsequently over 160 cases with progressive aphasia have been reported since Wechsler's seminal case in 1977 (Black, 1996; see Rogers & Alarcon, 1999 for a comprehensive review).

The syndrome is characterized by isolated language disturbance for at least 2 years, and may remain an isolated impairment for as long as 20 years! (Kempler, Metter, Riege, et al., 1990). Thus, the aphasia in PPA is progressive, whereas activities of daily living, judgment, insight, and behavior are relatively, if not totally, spared. The focus of research on PPA is to determine the presence of neuropathologies that may precipitate PPA (Morris, 1993), to rule out subtle coexisting neuropsychological deficits (Kirshner et al., 1984), and to describe the aphasic manifestations (Horner, 1985; Rogers & Alarcon, 1999).

In a meta-analysis, Rogers and Alarcon (1999) observed that the aphasia does not fit neatly into existing aphasia classification schemes. They identified 37 cases of fluent progressive aphasia, 88 cases of nonfluent progressive aphasia, and 22 cases with an undetermined type of aphasia. The fluent or nonfluent profile did not predict whether the person eventually experienced global cognitive deterioration. Of 70 cases with no dementia, the aphasia had been progressive for about 5 years.

Because of the relative rarity of PPA, the literature is characterized by case studies and small series of patients, with few attempts to compare PPA directly with AD or focal stroke syndromes (Horner, 1985). Those with fluent PPA have been described as Wernicke's (Sinforiani, Mauri, Sances, & Martelli, 1991), transcortical sensory aphasia (Bianchetti, Frisoni, & Trabucchi, 1996), sensory aphasia (Ikeda, Akiyama, Iritani, Kase, Arai, Niizato, et al., 1996), anomic aphasia (Luzzatti & Poeck, 1991), pure word deafness (Philbrick, Rummans, Duffy, Kokmen, & Jack, 1994), and conduction aphasia (Kempler et al., 1990). Some of the other clinical signs in the fluent PPA group are depression, Klüver-Bucy syndrome, and visual agnosia (Rogers & Alarcon, 1999). Those with nonfluent PPA have been described as having transcortical motor aphasia (Ackermann, Scharf, Hertrich, & Dawn, 1997), aphemia (Caselli & Jack, 1992), and anomia (Karbe, Kertesz, & Polk, 1993; see also Grossman, 2002b). Some of the other clinical signs in the nonfluent PPA group are alexia and agraphia, dysphagia, dysarthria and dysprosody (Rogers & Alarcon, 1999).

The literature on PPA originally developed as a distinctive line of research. Astute behavioral neurologists such as Kirschner, Snowdon, and Kertesz, among others, have crosswalked between the study of neuropathology and clinical aphasiology in this disorder. From these studies, it is now clearer that, whereas PPA is a distinctive *clinical* entity (warranting special management approaches), it is probably fair to characterize most cases of PPA as FTD variants. Fluent PPA cases are akin to the FTD-temporal variant (semantic aphasia); nonfluent PPA cases are akin to the FTD-nonfluent aphasia variant. PPA cases with gradually appearing dementia, along with associated neuropsychiatric features, probably represent FTD-frontal variant or some combination (Kertesz, Hudson, Mackenzie, & Munoz, 1994; Kirshner, Tanridag, Thurman, & Whetsell, 1987; Snowden, Goulding, Neary, 1989; Snowden, Neary, Mann, Goulding, & Testa, 1992). Remember that FTD in general, and isolated PPA in particular, imply *focal atrophy*, but do not specify the underlying *histopathologic condition*. Postmortem examination of PPA cases has revealed a variety of underlying diseases: Pick's disease (Kertesz et al., 1994), spongiform degeneration (Kirshner et al., 1987), Alzheimer's disease (Kirshner et al., 1984), and Creutzfeldt-Jakob disease (Spencer et al., 2002).

In summary, PPA is a clinical syndrome distinguished by a progressive aphasia (of various types) that often progresses slowly, and may or may not lead to global deterioration of cognitive abilities. PPA may be caused by a wide variety of underlying diseases. These diseases, by chance or by some inherent genetic preprogramming, or by some other etiology, affect those cortical areas that are specialized for language. As with most neurodegenerative conditions, there is no cure for PPA. Nevertheless,

because other cognitive functions (including learning) are spared, remedial or compensatory speech–language pathology interventions may be indicated for many individuals with PPA. As with other communication disorders, a careful diagnostic evaluation and close follow-up by a neurologist are essential.

Mild Cognitive Impairment

This section briefly defines mild cognitive impairment (MCI), contrasts it with other disorders involving memory loss, and reports on studies that explain the potential risk of this impairment. To introduce the topic of MCI, Petersen, Stevens, Ganguli, Tangalas, Cummings, DeKosky (2001) explained that "the use of research criteria for the classification of dementia identifies three groups of subjects: those who are demented, those who are not demented, and individuals who cannot be classified because they have a cognitive (memory) impairment but do not meet criteria for dementia" (p. 1134). The last group—those who have a measurable cognitive deficit but do *not* have dementia—are referred to as having MCI. Other terms that have been used to describe this disorder are isolated memory impairment, incipient dementia, and dementia prodrome (Petersen et al., 2001). MCI should not to be confused with age-associated memory impairment, which is merely descriptive of older person's memory functioning as compared with younger normal control subjects (Petersen et al., 2001). MCI is *not dementia*, but may be a *risk factor* for the development of dementia (Chen, Ratcliff, Belle, Cauley, DeKosky, & Ganguli, 2001; Petersen et al., 2001; Thompson & Hodges, 2002).

The criteria for MCI are (1) a complaint of memory difficulty, usually corroborated by a family member or physician; (2) a measurable memory impairment as compared with age- and education-matched norms; (3) other cognitive functions are normal; and (4) intact functioning in daily life (Petersen et al., 2001).

One of the major goals of research on MCI is to determine the extent to which MCI converts to dementia, by comparison to the global incidence of AD in aging persons. The emergence of new treatments for AD make early detection of such persons imperative, so as to preserve their functioning and their ability to live at home for longer periods, as well as to realize substantial savings in medical and nursing home care (Petersen et al., 2001).

In a valuable meta-analysis, Petersen and colleagues (2001) reported results of studies that followed MCI subjects for 2 to 4 years. Those who initially presented with MCI converted to AD at rates varying from 6% to 25% per year. These figures contrast with the general incidence of AD in the general population, estimated to be 0.2% in individuals 65 to 69 years of age, to 3.9% for individuals 85 to 89 years of age. Thus, according to extant evidence, the presence of MCI is considered to be a *risk factor* for subsequent development of dementia (Bondi, Monsch, Galasko, Butters, Salmon, Delis, 1994; Small, Herlitz, Fratiglioni, Almkvist, & Backman, 1997).

In a prospective study using the Framingham Cohort, Elias, Beiser, Wolf, Au, White, and D'Agostino (2000) followed 1076 participants for 22 years. They analyzed cognitive performance during dementia-free years to determine whether any particular cognitive tasks predicted the later onset of the very earliest phase of dementia, referred to as prelinical AD (pAD). They concluded that lower abstract reasoning and retention scores obtained 10 or more years earlier were the strongest predictors of pAD.

In summary, MCI is not dementia, but may be a predictor for the later onset of dementia. Clinicians are advised to follow this literature closely, as it holds the keys to differential diagnosis for those older patients who present to our clinics with the vague complaint of memory difficulty. A referral to a neuropsychologist (for sensitive baseline testing) and a neurologist is indicated in such cases.

✦ Subcortical Dementia and Associated Disorders

This section highlights some distinctive features of subcortical disease states that often manifest as dementing illness, in contrast to the major neurodegenerative dementias reviewed earlier. This section does not review all of the subcortical disease states that might cause dementia, but rather selects the most prevalent disorders. **Table 7–3** summarizes the distinguishing features among them.

As indicated in the introduction to this chapter, the concept of subcortical dementia is somewhat controversial. Advances in the neurosciences have allowed us to recognize that the cortical–subcortical dichotomy is imperfect. Nevertheless, the so-called subcortical dementias are associated with several hallmarks. First, lesions are primarily in the basal ganglia, brainstem, and cerebellum (Darvesh & Freedman, 1996). Second, prominent clinical signs of subcortical dementia are bradyphrenia (slowing of cognition), memory and learning impairment disturbances, and frontal executive dysfunction. Third, other clinical signs are motor disturbances in gait and speech, and psychiatric disturbances (e.g., apathy, irritability, depression, psychosis, mania, and hallucinations are common). Fourth, progression may be more rapid than cognitive dysfunction of primary progressive dementia (AD) (Stern, Tang, Jacobs, Sano, Marder, Bell, Dooneief, Schofield, & Cote, 1998). Fifth, isolated disorders of aphasia, apraxia and agnosia are uncommon (Turner et al., 2002).

Thus, the main reasons for recognizing a clinical subcategory of subcortical dementia are the hallmarks of "cognitive slowness, concomitant motor abnormalities, and a relatively low frequency of aphasias and apraxias" (Turner et al., 2002, p. 151). Readers should be cautioned against thinking that there is *one specific clinical profile* associated with subcortical dementia (Turner et al., 2002). The clinical profiles differ, depending on the underlying disease, the severity of the disease, and the stage of the disease.

To emphasize this point, Turner et al. (2002) state, "Any classification of the dementias must be sensitive to the fact that [the cortical and subcortical dementias] seem to lie along a continuum involving a greater or lesser degree of cortical and subcortical pathology" (p. 151). Comparisons between Parkinson patients and Alzheimer patients provide the paradigm example. In the initial stages, Alzheimer patients are typically free of motor impairments, but manifest an insidious cognitive decline. In contrast, in the initial stages, Parkinson's patients have motor disorders (bradykinesia, tremor, and dysarthria), but no cognitive impairment. As the diseases progress, the clinical distinctiveness between Alzheimer's and Parkinson's becomes blurred. In later stages, Alzheimer's patients display bradykinetic gait and tremor (though they are rarely dysarthric), whereas many Parkinson's patients gradually acquire bradyphrenia and memory disorders (and are commonly dysarthric). Thus, although historically AD was classified as a cortical disease, and Parkinson's as a subcortical disease, in reality these clinical signs and symptoms may appear similar (depending on the stage of the disease). Furthermore, both AD and Parkinson's have a depletion of cholinergic neurons in the subcortical nucleus basalis of Meynert (Mesulam & Weintraub, 1992), and functional neuroimaging has shown severe hypoperfusion in frontal, temporal, and parietal areas in both groups of patients (Starkstein et al., 1997). In turn, dysfunction of the frontal lobe (and associated circuitry) are implicated in many of the subcortical diseases, for example, Huntington's (Backman, Robins-Wahlin, Lundin, Ginovart, & Farde, 1997), and motor neuron disease, which has been found to co-occur with FTD (Bak & Hodges, 1999) (**Table 7–3**).

Table 7–3   Differential Diagnosis of Major Types of Subcortical Dementia

	Parkinson's Disease (PD)	Huntington's Disease (HD)	Progressive Supranuclear Palsy (PSP)	Creutzfeldt-Jakob Disease (variant CJD)
Onset and course	Sporadic; gradual course	Gradual onset; progressive course	Gradual onset; rapid progression if untreated	Usually abrupt onset and rapid course; approximately one-third present with cognitive problems
Cognitive profile	Bradyphrenia, executive dysfunction, impaired recall, visuospatial disturbances, and depression	Psychiatric and cognitive impairments with recent and remote memory impairments early in disease	Cognitive slowing, inattentiveness, memory impairment; mild relative to prominent motor impairments	Psychiatric disturbances (dysphoria, withdrawal, impaired memory, aggression) appear within 6 months in the majority
Communication	Hypokinetic dysarthria (hypophonia, rapid rate, voice tremor)	Language organization and naming impaired; dysarthria	Dysarthria; ultimately, harsh guttural sounds	Dysarthria; ultimately mute
Physical signs	Bradykinesia, rigidity, tremor	Chorea with jerky, shuffling gait; postural instability; limb apraxia; dysphagia	Supranuclear gaze palsy, parkinsonism, dystonia and rigidity; dysphagia	Paresthesias and gait disturbances early; myoclonus and incontinence later
Diagnosis	Impaired dopaminergic system; abnormalities of *synuclein* protein	Autosomal dominant; or, may be idiopathic or drug-induced; mutation on chromosome 4	Pathology in reticular formation, thalamus, or hypothalamus	Unconventional infectious agent (prion disease); spongiform encephalopathy

With these observations in mind, there are several classically recognized diseases associated with the subcortex that are still recognized today (**Table 7–3**). Turner et al. (2002) provided a helpful review. In 1872, Huntington first described a progressive chorea and dementia, Huntington's disease. In 1884, Binswanger described subcortical pathology associated with cognitive decline that Olszewski later described as subcortical arteriosclerotic encephalopathy. In 1912, Wilson described progressive lenticular degeneration. Subsequently, in 1932, Von Stockert recognized cognitive impairment in Parkinson's, and, in 1974, Albert, Feldman, and Willis recognized cognitive impairment in progressive supranuclear palsy. More recently, progressive cognitive deterioration has been associated with HIV (Evans, 1996; Navia, Jordan, & Price, 1986; Turner et al., 2002).

Another contemporary example of a dementia involving subcortical structures is Creutzfeldt-Jakob disease (CJD) (Lai, 1996; Price, 1996; Spencer et al., 2002). CJD is associated with "the aberrant metabolism of the prion protein" (coded at chromosome 20) and accounts for 75% of all human prion diseases (Lai, 1996). Infectious (transmissible) and invariably fatal, CJD results from the abnormal accumulation of the prion protein in the brain. Onset can occur as early as age 16 and as late as age 82 (Lai, 1996). There are three types of CJD: sporadic, familial, and iatrogenic or "variant." Spencer et al. (2002) summarized the results of the first 100 reported cases of variant CJD. Variant CJD occurs in humans after exposure to same infectious agent that causes bovine spongiform encephalopathy ("mad-cow disease").

Spencer and colleagues (2002) retrospectively studied the prevalence of clinical signs in variant CJD that appeared early (less than 4 months), later (between 4 and 6 months), and late (after 6 months). They found that common early psychiatric signs were dysphoria, withdrawal, anxiety, irritability, insomnia, and loss of interest, and that neurologic (motor-sensory) signs did not commonly appear at this early stage. They also found that later psychiatric signs were poor memory, impaired concentration, aggression "in combination with gait disturbance, dysarthria and sensory symptoms" (p. 1482). Late-onset psychiatric signs were disorientation and agitation, whereas late-onset neurologic signs were hyperreflexia, impair coordination, myoclonus, incontinence, and eye features. The authors concluded, "The combination of psychiatric disorder with affective or psychotic features and persistent pain, dysarthria, gait ataxia, or sensory symptoms should at least raise the suspicion of variant Creutzfeldt-Jakob disease, particularly if this is combined with any suggestion of cognitive impairment" (p. 1482).

Table 7–3 summarizes the major distinguishing features of dementia in PD (Bamford et al., 1995; Boller, Passafiume, Keefe, Rogers, Morow, & Kim, 1984; Cummings, Darkens, Mendez, Hill, Benson, 1988; Friedman, 1996; Mayeux, 1984; Mayeux et al., 1981; NINDS, 2003b; Rogers, 1986; Seltzer et al., 2001), HD (Albert, Butters, & Brandt, 1981; Bamford et al., 1995; Friedman, 1996; Kennedy, Fisher, Shoulson, & Caine, 1981; Kirkwood, et al., 2001; Koroshetz, 1996; Moss & Albert, 1988; Zakzanis, 1998), PSP (Cole, 1996; Cummings & Benson, 1983; Litvan, 2001; Podoll, Schwarz, & Noth, 1991), and CJD (Koroshetz, 1996; Spencer et al., 2002; Lai, 1996).

Table 7–4 summarizes major distinguishing features of other conditions that typically have dementia as a core deficit. Included in this table are Wilson's disease (Fischbein et al., 2000; Ripich, 1991; Ripich & Ziol, 1998), HIV encephalopathy (Evans, 1996; Fischbein et al., 2000; Oeschner, Moller, & Zaudig, 1993), pugilistic parkinsonism (Macklis, 1996), and Wernicke's encephalopathy (Charness, 1996; Dawson, 1996;

Table 7–4   Other Conditions Associated with Dementia

	Wilson's Disease	**HIV Encephalopathy**	**Pugilistic Parkinsonism (Posttraumatic Dementia)**	**Wernicke's Encephalopathy (Alcohol-Related)**
Onset and course	Progressive, complete recovery possible with treatment, including liver transplantation	Virus may be present in brain cells before clinical symptoms; after encephalopathy diagnosed, median survival is 6 months	Depends on repetitiveness and extent of injury, e.g., mild concussion or multifocal injury; may culminate in diffuse cerebral atrophy, cortical and subcortical	Varies depending on chronicity and extent of alcohol use combined with thiamine deficiency and often-repeated head trauma
Cognitive profile	Impaired memory; bradyphrenia	Impaired memory, bradyphrenia, apathy; psychosis may be present	Cognitive changes, acute and chronic	Wernicke's encephalopathy is characterized by disorientation, indifference, delirium, and generalized intellectual impairments; Korsakoff's amnestic syndrome, by isolated anterograde and retrograde memory loss
Communication	Dysarthria, mixed ataxic and hypokinetic features	Grossly disturbed thinking	Bradyphrenia, dysarthria	Confused language with memory disorder; dysarthria infrequent
Physical signs	Cirrhosis of the liver; tremor and rigidity prominent	Eventually quadriparetic	Pyramidal and/or cerebellar signs; rest tremor is common	Ataxia of gait, but rarely arms; neuropathy; myopathy
Diagnosis	Autosomal recessive disorder of copper metabolism; subcortical white matter changes	Subcortical cells infected with HIV; virus present in brain cells and cerebrospinal fluid before clinical symptoms; eventually, global atrophy	By exclusion of other causes of parkinsonism, e.g., drugs or toxins, vascular disease, lesions, viral agents, metabolic diseases	Atrophy of mamillary bodies and anterior cerebellar vermis; periventricular changes; must be correlated with history of chronic alcohol consumption *and nutritional deprivation*

Samuel, D'Olhaberriague, Levine, & Brass, 1996). These diverse conditions illustrate that dementing conditions can result from metabolic, infectious, traumatic, and nutritional abnormalities. These conditions also illustrate that treatment is available in some cases. Understanding the multifaceted nature of dementing illnesses can lead to prevention in some cases, and amelioration of symptoms, in others.

✦ Conclusion

The past decade has seen advances in clinical diagnostic criteria for the dementias, improvements in static and dynamic brain imaging techniques, a wealth of new studies in neuropsychology and speech–language pathology, and breakthroughs in the understanding of the genetic origins of various diseases causing dementing illness. For example, we have seen concepts and terms disappear from the literature, such as "presenile" and "senile" dementia. We have come to realize that cerebrovascular disease and neurodegenerative disease often co-occur. We have learned that Alzheimer's disease has subtypes. In addition, we now appreciate the focal atrophy syndromes are both common and heterogeneous in clinical presentation. We no longer think of the dementias as strictly cortical or subcortical. Finally, we are beginning to learn that some types of dementia are "familial" and some are "sporadic." Though no cure is available for the neurodegenerative dementias, increased knowledge in genetics offers hope of preventive or curative interventions in the future. To offer the most effective services to individuals with dementia, it is imperative that speech–language pathologists in both clinical and academic settings stay abreast of the dementia literature.

To bring these exciting advances to the clinicians, this chapter summarized the contemporary research. Threaded through the chapter (and in the tables) are descriptions of the patterns of *behavior and cognition* associated with dementing illnesses; neuroradiologic studies showing *structural and functional abnormalities* of brain tissue (both at cortical and subcortical sites); postmortem studies, revealing actual *pathologic changes* in the brain; and, genetic studies, which seek to uncover the *pathogenesis* (the origins) of the underlying disease. Chapter 8 discusses the speech–language manifestations of these disorders in greater detail.

In light of scientific advances within the past few years, we depended heavily on recently published authoritative diagnostic guidelines. We explained that current taxonomies are moving away from a strict distinction between cortical and subcortical dementias. We emphasized that cerebrovascular disease co-occurs with and may even predispose some individuals to Alzheimer's disease, and furthermore that it is incorrect to think of multiple infarcts as the only cerebrovascular etiology of dementia. We drew on studies that explain why even a single clinical stroke may be responsible for dementia, a concept that was not recognized until recently. We emphasized the neuropathologic distinctiveness of AD, FTD, and LBD, while recognizing that clinical diagnosis may be difficult due to the overlapping nature of the cognitive and behavioral changes in individual patients, depending on the timeliness of diagnostic evaluation and the stage of the disease.

As an aid to readers, we organized our discussion (and tables) regarding different diseases in terms of the major neurodegenerative dementias, subcortical dementias, and other medical conditions. The neurodegenerative or irreversible dementias, by definition, show cognitive and behavioral changes during the course of the disease. We described the major features of AD, VaD, LBD, and several variants of FTD. Typically, AD patients show memory loss as an early sign with spared global attention. In contrast, LBD patients show fluctuating attention, hallucinations, and parkinsonism, whereas FTD patients demonstrate focal cognitive changes consistent with the cortical region affected by the disease. VaD patients are highly varied in presentation depending on the underlying etiology, the volume of white matter and cortical involvement, and the presence of coexisting medial temporal lobe atrophy.

The dementias associated with (but not exclusive to) subcortical disease—the so-called subcortical dementias—present motor signs in addition to cognitive impairments. The examples we used were PD, HD, PSP, and CJD. Finally, several other dementing illnesses were described to show that metabolic, posttraumatic, viral, and nutritional abnormalities can cause dementia. For illustration purposes we described Wilson's disease, pugilistic parkinsonism, HIV encephalopathy, and Wernicke's encephalopathy, respectively.

Finally, recognizing that speech–language pathologists engage in clinical practice with an increasing number of elderly individuals, we highlighted the literature on PPA and MCI. PPA is a fascinating disorder, because many patients with PPA do not show signs of global deterioration of cognitive function (at least, not until later). Furthermore, PPA patients have preserved insight and learning ability and often can learn compensatory strategies for their communication disabilities. Individuals with MCI, we emphasize, do not have dementia. Rather, they show memory dysfunction that cannot be explained on the basis of aging alone. Importantly, epidemiologic studies show that individuals with MCI may be a higher risk than the general population for developing AD.

Study Questions

1. Explain why speech-language pathologists (SLPs) should be knowledgeable about current diagnostic approaches and taxonomies.

2. Define dementia.

3. Discuss the problems with the current taxonomy of dementia.

4. Explain the difference among the different approaches to diagnosis (clinical, radiologic, neuropathologic, genetic).

5. Define and identify distinctive characteristics of Alzheimer's dementia (AD).

6. Define and identify distinctive characteristics of vascular dementia (VaD).

7. Define and identify distinctive characteristics of Lewy body dementia (LBD).

8. Define and identify distinctive characteristics of frontotemporal lobar dementia (LBD).

9. Define and identify distinctive characteristics of primary progressive aphasia (PPA).

10. Define and identify distinctive characteristics of mild cognitive impairment (MCI).

References

Ackermann, H., Scharf, G., Hertrich, I., & Dawn, I. (1997). Articulatory Disorders in Primary Progressive Aphasia: An Acoustic and Kinematic Analysis. *Aphasiology, 11,* 1017–1030

Albert, M.L., Feldman, R.G., & Willis, A.L. (1974). The 'Subcortical Dementia' of Progressive Supranuclear Palsy. *Journal of Neurology, Neurosurgery, and Psychiatry, 37.* 121–130

Albert, M.S., Butters, N., & Brandt, J. (1981). Patterns of Remote Memory in Amnesic and Demented Patients. *Archives of Neurology, 38,* 495–500

American College of Medical Genetics/ American Society of Human Genetics Working Group on ApoE and Alzheimer Disease. (1995). Statement on Use of Apolipoprotein E Testing for Alzheimer Disease. *Journal of the American Medical Association, 274,* 1627–1629

American Psychiatric Association. (1994). *Diagnostic and Statistical Manual of Mental Disorders,* 4th ed., rev. (pp. 133–155). Washington, DC: American Psychiatric Association

American Psychiatric Association. (2000). *Diagnostic and Statistical Manual of Mental Disorders, IV–Text Revision (DSM-IV-TR).* BehaveNet® Clinical Capsule™ Web site: http://www.behavenet.com/capsules/disorders/alzheimersTR.htm

Backman, L., Robins-Wahlin, T.B., Lundin, A., Ginovart, N., & Farde, L. (1997). Cognitive Deficits in Huntington's Disease Are Predicted by Dopaminergic PET Markers and Brain Volumes. *Brain 120,* 2207–2217

Bak, T.H., & Hodges, J.R. (1999). Cognition, Language and Behaviour in Motor Neurone Disease: Evidence of Frontotemporal Dysfunction. *Dementia and Geriatric Cognitive Disorders, 10(Suppl 1),* 29–32

Bamford, K.A., Caine, E.D., Kido, D.K., Cox, C., & Shoulson, I. (1995). A Prospective Evaluation of Cognitive Decline in Early Huntington's Disease: Functional and Radiographic Correlates. *Neurology, 45,* 1867–1873

Barba, R., Castro, M.D., del Mar Morin, M., Rodriguez-Romero, R., Rodriguez-Garcia, E., Canton, R., & Del Ser, T. (2001). Prestroke Dementia. *Cerebrovascular Disorders, 11,* 216–224

Barba, R., Martinez-Espinosa, S., Rodriguez-Garcia, E., Pondal, M., Vivancos, J., & Del Ser, T. (2000). Poststroke Dementia: Clinical Features and Risk Factors. *Stroke, 31,* 1494–1501

Bathgate, D., Snowden, J.S., Varma, A., Blackshaw, A., & Neary, D. (2001). Behaviour in Frontotemporal Dementia, Alzheimer's Disease and Vascular Dementia. *Acta Neurologica Scandinavica, 103,* 367–378

Bennett, H.P., Corbett, A.J., Gaden, S., Grayson, D.A., Kril, J.J., & Broe, G.A. (1977). Subcortical Vascular Disease and Functional Decline: A 6-Year Predictor Study. *Journal of the American Geriatrics Society, 50,* 1969–1977

Bianchetti, A., Frisoni, G.B., Trabucchi, M. (1996). Primary Progressive Aphasia and Frontal Lobe Involvement. *Neurology, 46,* 289–291

Binetti, G., Locascio, J.J., Corkin, S., Vonsattal, J.P., & Growdon, J.H. (2000). Differences Between Pick Disease and Alzheimer Disease in Clinical Appearance and Rate of Cognitive Decline. *Archives of Neurology, 57,* 225–232

Black, S.E. (1996). Focal Cortical Atrophy Syndromes. *Brain and Cognition, 31,* 188–229

Boller, F., Becker, J.T., Holland, A.L., et al. (1991). Predictors of Decline in Alzheimer's Disease. *Cortex, 27,* 9–17

Boller, F., Passafiume, D., Keefe, N.C., Rogers, K., Morrow, L., & Kim, Y. (1984). Visuospatial Impairment in Parkinson's Disease: Role of Perceptual and Motor Factors. *Archives of Neurology, 41,* 485–490

Bondi, M.W., Monsch, A.U., Galasko, D., Butters, N., Salmon, D.P., & Delis, D.C. (1994). Preclinical Cognitive Markers of Dementia of the Alzheimer Type. *Neuropsychology, 8,* 374–384

Burke, D., Sengoz, A., & Schwartz, R. (2000). Potentially Reversible Cognitive Impairment in Patients Presenting to A Memory Disorders Clinic. *Journal of Clinical Neuroscience, 7,* 120–123

Burton, E.J., Karas, G., Paling, S.M., Barber, R., Williams, E.D., Ballard, C.G., McKeith, I.G., Scheltens, P., Barkhof, F., & O'Brien, J.T. (2002). Patterns of Cerebral Atrophy in Dementia with Lewy Bodies Using Voxel-Based Morphometry. *Neuroimage, 17,* 618–630

Caine, E.D. (1981). Pseudodementia. *Archives of General Psychiatry, 38,* 1359–1364

Campbell, S., Stephens, S., & Ballard, C. (2001). Dementia with Lewy Bodies: Clinical Features and Treatment. *Drugs and Aging, 18,* 397–407

Caselli, R.J., & Jack, C.R. (1992). Asymmetric Cortical Degeneration Syndromes: A Proposed Clinical Classification. *Archives of Neurology, 49,* 770–780

Charness, M.E. (1996). Neurologic Complications of Alcoholism. In: M.A. Samuels, & S. Feske (Eds.), *Office Practice of Neurology* (pp. 1047–1055). New York: Churchill Livingstone

Chen, P., Ratcliff, G., Belle, S.H., Cauley, J.A., DeKosky, S.T., & Ganguli, M. (2001). Patterns of Cognitive Decline in Presymptomatic Alzheimer Disease: A Prospective Community Study. *Archives of General Psychiatry, 58,* 853–858

Cole, D.G. (1996). Progressive Supranuclear Palsy. In: M.A. Samuels, & S. Feske (Eds.), *Office Practice of Neurology* (pp. 641–644). New York: Churchill Livingstone

Cummings, J.L. (2000). Cognitive and Behavioral Heterogeneity in Alzheimer's Disease: Seeking the Neurobiological Basis. *Neurobiology of Aging, 21,* 845–861

Cummings, J.L., & Benson, D.F. (1983). *Dementia: A Clinical Approach.* Stoneham, MA: Butterworth

Cummings, J.L., & Benson, D.F. (1992). *Dementia: A Clinical Approach.* Boston: Butterworth

Cummings, J.L., Darkins, A., & Mendez, M., Hill, M.A., & Benson, D.F. (1988). Alzheimer's Disease and Parkinson's Disease: Comparison of Speech and Language Alterations. *Neurology 38,* 680–684

Cummings, J.L., & Duchen, L.W. (1981). The Kluver-Bucy Syndrome in Pick's Disease. *Neurology, 31,* 1415–1422

Daffner, K.R. (1996). Alzheimer's Disease and Related Disorders. In: M.A. Samuels, & S. Feske (Eds.), *Office Practice of Neurology* (pp. 710–715). New York: Churchill Livingstone

Darvesh, S., & Freedman, M. (1996). Subcortical Dementia: A Neurobehavioural Approach. Brain and Cognition, 31, 230–249

Dawson, D.M. (1996). Progressive Ataxia. In: M.A. Samuels, & S. Feske (Eds.) *Office Practice of Neurology* (pp. 647–651). New York: Churchill Livingstone

Devous, M.D., Sr. (2002). Functional Brain Imaging in the Dementias: Role in Early Detection, Differential Diagnosis, and Longitudinal Studies. *European Journal of Nuclear Medicine and Molecular Imaging, 29,* 1685–1696

Di Maria, E., Tabaton, M., Vigo, T., Abbruzzese, G., Bllone, E., & Donati, C., et al. (2000). Corticobasal Degeneration Shares a Common Genetic Background with Progressive Supranuclear Palsy. *Annals of Neurology, 47,* 374–377

Doubleday, E.K., Snowden, J.S., Varma, A.R., & Neary, D. (2002). Qualitative Performance Characteristics Differentiate Dementia with Lewy Bodies and Alzheimer's Disease. *Journal of Neurology, Neurosurgery, and Psychiatry, 72,* 602–607

Duara, R., Barker, W., & Luis, C.A. (1999). Frontotemporal Dementia and Alzheimer's Disease: Differential Diagnosis. Dementia and Geriatric Cognitive Disorders, 10(suppl 1), 37–42

Elias, M.F., Beiser, A., Wolf, P.A., Au, R., White, R.F., & D'Agostino, R.B. (2000). The Preclinical Phase of Alzheimer Disease: A 22-Year Prospective Study of the Framingham Cohort. *Archives of Neurology, 57,* 808–813

Evans, B.K. (1996). HIV Infection and Diseases of the Brain. In: M.A. Samuels, & S. Feske (Eds.), *Office Practice of Neurology* (pp. 428–433). New York: Churchill Livingstone

Fahlander, K., Wahlin, A., Almkvist, O., & Backman, L. (2002). Cognitive Functioning in Alzheimer's Disease and Vascular Dementia: Further Evidence for Similar Patterns of Deficits. *Journal of Clinical and Experimental Neuropsychology, 24,* 734–744

Fischbein, N.J., Dillon, W.P., & Barkovich, A.J. (2000). *Teaching Atlas of Brain Imaging.* New York: Thieme

Fitz, A.G., & Teri, L. (1994). Depression, Cognition and Functional Ability in Patients with Alzheimer's Disease. *Journal of the American Geriatrics Society, 42,* 186–191

Foster, N.L., & Chase, T.N. (1983). Diffuse Involvement in Progressive Aphasia. *Annals of Neurology, 13,* 224–225

Friedman, J.H. (1996). Mental Changes in Parkinson's Disease. In: M.A. Samuels, & S. Feske (Eds.), *Office Practice of Neurology* (pp. 633–637). New York: Churchill Livingstone

Gasser, T. (2001). Molecular Genetics of Parkinson's Disease. *Advances in Neurology, 86,* 23–32

Geldmacher, D.S., & Whitehouse, P.J. (1997). Differential Diagnosis of Alzheimer's Disease. *Neurology, 48(suppl 6),* S2–S9

Grossman, M. (2002a). Frontotemporal Dementia: A Review. *Journal of the International Neuropsychology Society, 8,* 566–583

Grossman, M. (2002b). Progressive Aphasic Syndromes: Clinical and Theoretical Advances. *Current Opinion in Neurology, 15,* 409–413

Gurd, J.M., Herzberg, L., Joachim, C., & Marshall, J.C. (2000). Dementia with Lewy Bodies: A Pure Case. *Brain and Cognition, 44,* 307–323

Gydesen, S., Brown, J.M., Brun, A., Chakrabarti, L., Gade, A., Johannsen, P. et al. (2002). Chromosome 3 Linked Frontotemporal Dementia (FTD-3). *Neurology, 59,* 1585–1594

Hachinski, V.C., Iliff, L.D., Zilhka, E., Du Boulay, G.H., McAllister, V.L., Marshall, J., Rusell, R.W., and Symon, L., (1975). Cerebral blood flow in dementia. *Archives of Neurology,* 32 (9), 632–637

Heath, P.D., Kennedy, P., & Kapur, N. (1983). Slowly Progressive Aphasia Without Generalized Dementia. *Annals of Neurology, 13,* 687–688

Heyman, A., Fillenbaum, G.G., Welsh-Bohmer, K.A., Gearing, M., Mirra, S.S., Mohs, R.C., Peterson, B.L., & Pieper, C.F. (1998). Cerebral Infracts in Patients with Autopsy-Proven Alzheimer's Disease: CERAD, Part XVIII. Consortium to Establish a Registry for Alzheimer's Disease. *Neurology, 51,* 159–162

Hier, D.B., Hagenlocker, K., & Shindler, A.G. (1985). Language Disintegration in Dementia: Effects of Etiology and Severity. *Brain and Language, 25,* 117–133

Hodges, J.R. (2001). Frontotemporal Dementia (Pick's Disease): Clinical Features and Assessment. *Neurology, 56(suppl 4)*, S6–S10

Hodges, J.R., & Miller, B. (2001). The Classification, Genetics and Neuropathology of Frontotemporal Dementia. Introduction to the Special Topic Papers: Part I. *Neurocase, 7*, 31–35

Hodges, J.R., Patterson, K., Ward, R., Garrard, P., Bak, T., Perry, R., & Gregory, C. (1999). The Differentiation of Semantic Dementia and Frontal Lobe Dementia (Temporal and Frontal Variants of Frontotemporal Dementia) from Early Alzheimer's Disease: A Comparative Neuropsychological Study. *Neuropsychology, 13*, 31–40

Honig, L.S. (1997). Genetics of Alzheimer's Disease. *Neurophysiol Neurogenic Speech Lang Disord (ASHA Special Interest Division 2) 7*, 6–10

Horner, J. (1985). Language Disorder Associated with Alzheimer's Dementia, Left Hemisphere Stroke, and Progressive Illness of Uncertain Etiology. In: R.H. Brookshire (Ed.). *Clinical Aphasiology, 15*, 149–158.

Hosler, B.A., Siddique, T., Sapp, P.C., Sailor, W., Huang, M.C., Hossain, A., et al. (2000. Linkage of Familial Amyotrophic Lateral Sclerosis with Frontotemporal Dementia to Chromosome 9q21-q22. *Journal of the American Medical Association, 284*, 1664–1669

Hsu, Y.Y., Du, A.T., Schuff, N., & Weiner, M.W. (2001). Magnetic Resonance Imaging and Magnetic Resonance Spectroscopy in Dementias. *Journal of Geriatric Psychiatry and Neurology, 14*, 145–166

Ikeda, K., Akiyama, H., Iritani, S., Kase, K., Arai, T., Niizato, K., et al. (1996). Corticobasal Degeneration with Primary Progressive Aphasia and Accentuated Cortical Lesion in Superior Temporal Gyrus: Case Report and Review. *Acta Neuropathology (Berlin), 92*, 534–539

Jefferson, A.L., Cosentino, S.A., Ball, S.K., Bogdanoff, B., Leopold, N., Kaplan, E., & Libon, D.J. (2002). Errors Produced on the Mini-Mental State Examination and Neuropsychological Test Performance in Alzheimer's Disease, Ischemic Vascular Dementia, and Parkinson's Disease. *Journal of Neuropsychiatry and Clinical Neuroscience, 14*, 311–320

Kalaria, R.N. (2000). The role of Cerebral Ischemia in Alzheimer's Disease. *Neurobiology of Aging, 21*, 321–330

Karbe, H., Kertesz, A., & Polk, M. (1993). Profiles of Language Impairment in Primary Progressive Aphasia. *Archives of Neurology, 50*, 193–200

Kaszniak, A.W., Fox, J., Gandell, D.L., et al. (1978). Predictors of Mortality in Presenile and Senile Dementia. *Annals of Neurology, 3*, 246–252

Kempler, D., Metter, E.J., Riege, W.H., et al. (1990). Slowly Progressive Aphasia: Three Cases with Language, Memory, CT and PET Data. *Journal of Neurology, Neurosurgery, and Psychiatry, 53*, 987–993

Fisher J.M., Kennedy J.L., Caine E.D., Shoulson I. (1983). Dementia in Huntington disease: A cross-section analysis of intellectual decline. *Advances in Neurology, 38*, 229–238

Kertesz, A., Hudson, L., Mackenzie, I., & Munoz, D.G. (1994). The Pathology and Nosology of Primary Progressive Aphasias. *Neurology, 44*, 2065–2072

Kirkwood, S.C., Su, J.L., Conneally, P., & Foroud, T. (2001). Progression of Symptoms in the Early and Middle Stages of Huntington Disease. *Archives of Neurology, 58*, 273–278

Kirshner, H.S. (1994). Progressive Aphasia and Other Focal Presentations of Alzheimer Disease, Pick Disease, and Other Degenerative Disorders. In: V.O. Emery, & T.E. Oxman (Eds.), *Dementia: Presentations, Differential Diagnosis, and Nosology*, pp. 108–122. Baltimore: Johns Hopkins University Press

Kirshner, H.S., Tanridag, O., Thurman, L., & Whetsell, W.O., Jr. (1987). Progressive Aphasia Without Dementia: Two Cases with Focal Spongiform Degeneration. *Annals of Neurology, 22*, 527–532

Kirshner, H.S., Webb, W.G., Kelly, M.P., & Wells, C.E. (1984). Language Disturbance: An Initial Symptom of Cortical Degenerations and Dementia. *Archives of Neurology, 41*, 491–496

Knopman, D.S., DeKosky, S.T., Cummings, J.L., Chui, H., Corey-Bloom, J., Relkin, N., et al. (2001). Practice Parameter: Diagnosis of Dementia (An Evidence-Based Review): Report of the Quality Standards Subcommittee of the American Academy of Neurology. *Neurology, 56*, 1143–1153

Koroshetz, W.J. (1996). Huntington's Disease. In: M.A. Samuels, & S. Feske (Eds.), *Office Practice of Neurology*, pp 654–661. New York: Churchill Livingstone

Kuzuhara, S., & Yoshimura, M. (1993). Clinical and Neuropathological Aspects of Diffuse Lewy Body Disease in the Elderly. *Advances in Neurology, 60*, 464–469

Lai, E.C. (1996). Prion Diseases. In: M.A. Samuels, & S. Feske (Eds.), *Office Practice of Neurology*, pp. 442–444. New York: Churchill Livingstone

Litvan, I. (2001). Diagnosis and Management of Progressive Supranuclear Palsy. *Seminars in Neurology, 21*, 41–48

Loewenstein, D.A., Ownby, R., Schram, L., Acevedo, A., Rubert, M., & Arguelles, T. (2001). An Evaluation of the NINCDS-ADRDA Neuropsychological Criteria for the Assessment of Alzheimer's Disease: A Confirmatory Factor Analysis of Single Versus Multi-Factor Models. *Journal of Clinical and Experimental Neuropsychology, 23*, 274–284

Lopez, O.L., Becker, J.T., Klunk, W., Saxton, J., Hamilton, R.L., Kaufer, D.I., et al. (2000). Research Evaluation and Diagnosis of Probable Alzheimer's Disease over the Last Two Decades: I. *Neurology, 55*, 1854–1862

Lopez, O.L., Gonzalez, M.P., Becker, J.T., et al. (1995). Symptoms of Depression Alzheimer's Disease, Frontal Lobe-Type Dementia, and Subcortical Dementia. *Annals of the New York Academy of Science, 769*, 389–392

Lukatela, K.A., Cohen, R.A., Kessler, H.A., Jenkins, M.A., Moser, D.J., Stone, W.F., Gordon, N.F., & Kaplan, R.F. (2000). Dementia Rating Scale Performance: a Comparison of Vascular and Alzheimer's Dementia. *Journal of Clinical and Experimental Neuropsychology, 22*, 445–454

Luzzatti, C., & Poeck, K. (1991). An Early Description of Slowly Progressive Aphasia. *Archives of Neurology, 48*, 228–229

Macklis, J.D. (1996). Secondary Parkinsonism. In: M.A. Samuels, & S. Feske (Eds.), *Office Practice of Neurology*, pp. 644–647. New York: Churchill Livingstone

Mayeux, R. (1984). Behavioral Manifestations of Movement Disorders: Parkinson's and Huntington's Disease. *Neurology Clinics, 2*, 527–540

Mayeux, R., Stern, Y., Rosen, J., Leventhal, J. (1981). Depression, Intellectual Impairment, and Parkinson Disease. *Neurology, 31*, 645–650

Mesulam, M.M. (1982). Slowly Progressive Aphasia Without Generalized Dementia. *Annals of Neurology, 11*, 592–598

Mesulam, M.M. (1987). Primary Progressive Aphasia—Differentiation from Alzheimer's Disease. *Annals of Neurology, 22*, 533–534

Mesulam, M.M., & Weintraub, S. (1992). Spectrum of Primary Progressive Aphasia. In: M.N. Rossor (Ed.), *Bailliere's Clinical Neurology, Vol. 1, Unusual Dementias* (pp. 583–609). London: Bailliere Tindall

McKeith, I.G. (2000). Clinical Lewy Body Syndromes. *Annals of the New York Academy of Science, 920*, 1–8

McKeith, I.G., Galasko, D., Kosaka, K., Perry, E.K., Dickson, D.W., Hansen, L.A., et al. (1996). Consensus Guidelines for the Clinical and Pathologic Diagnosis of Dementia with Lewy Bodies (DLB)—Report of the Consortium on DLB International Workshop. *Neurology, 47*, 1113–1124

McKhann, G., Drachman, D., Folstein, M., Katzman, R., Price, D., & Stadlan, E.M. (1984). Clinical Diagnosis of Alzheimer's Disease: Report of the NINDCS-ADRDA Work Group Under the Auspices of Department of Health and Human Services Task Force on Alzheimer's Disease. *Neurology, 34*, 939–944

Molsa, P.K., Paljarvi, L., Rinne, J.O., Rinne, U.K., & Sako, E. (1985). Validity of Clinical Diagnosis in Dementia: A Prospective Clinicopathological Study. *Journal of Neurology, Neurosurgery, and Psychiatry, 48*, 1085–1090

Morris, J.C. (1993). The Clinical Dementia Rating Scale (CDR): Current Version and Scoring Rules. *Neurology, 43*, 2412–2414

Morris, J.C., Cole, M., Banker, B.Q., Wright D. (1984). Hereditary Dysphasic Dementia and the Pick-Alzheimer Spectrum. *Annals of Neurology, 16*, 455–466

Moss, M.B., & Albert, M.S. (1988). Alzheimer's Disease and Other Dementing Disorders. In: M.S. Albert & M.B. Moss (Eds.), *Geriatric Neuropsychology* (pp. 145–178). New York: Guilford Press

National Institute on Aging. (2000). National Institutes of Health: *Progress Report on Alzheimer's Disease: Taking the Next Steps*. Washington, DC: National Institutes of Health

National Institute of Neurological Disorders and Stroke. (2003a). Dementia with Lewy Bodies. http://www.ninds.nih.gov/health_and_medical/disorders/dementiawithlewybodies_doc.html

National Institute of Neurological Disorders and Stroke. (2003b). Stroke: Hope Through Research. http://www.ninds.nih.gov/health_and_medical/pubs/stroke_hope_through_research.htm#Genetic. Washington, DC: National Institutes of Health

Navia, B.A., Jordan, B.D., & Price, R.W. (1986). The AIDS Dementia Complex. *Annals of Neurology, 19*, 517–535

Neary, D., Snowden, J.S., Gustafson, L., Passant, U., Stuss, D., Black, S., et al. (1998). Frontotemporal Lobar Degeneration: A Consensus on Clinical Diagnostic Criteria. *Neurology, 51*, 1546–1554

Neary D., Snowden J.S., Mann D.M. (2000). Classification and description of frontotemporal dementias. *Annals of the New York Academy of Sciences, 920*, 46–51

Oechsner, M., Moller, A.A., & Zaudig, M. (1993). Cognitive Impairment, Dementia and Psychosocial Functioning in Human Immunodeficiency Virus Infection. A Prospective Study Based on DSM-III-R and ICD-10. *Acta Psychiatric Scandinavica, 87*, 13–17

Pasquier, F., Grymonprez, L., Lebert, F., & Van der Linden, M. (2001). Memory Impairment Differs in Frontotemporal Dementia and Alzheimer's Disease. *Neurocase, 7*, 161–171

Perry, R.J., & Hodges, J.R. (2000). Differentiating Frontal and Temporal Variant Frontotemporal Dementia from Alzheimer's Disease. *Neurology, 54*, 2277–2284

Petersen, R.C., Stevens, J.C., Ganguli, M., Tangalos, E.G., Cummings, J.L., DeKosky, S.T. (2001). Practice Parameter: Early Detection of Dementia: Mild Cognitive Impairment (and Evidence-Based Review). *Neurology, 56*, 1133–1142

Philbrick, K.L., Rummans, T.A., Duffy, J.R., Kokmen, E., Jack, C.R., Sr. (1994). Primary Progressive Aphasia: An Uncommon Masquerader in Psychiatric Disorders. *Psychosomatics, 35*, 138–141

Piccini, C., Pecori, D., Campani, D., Falcini, M., Picininni, M., Manfredi, G. (1998). Alzheimer's Disease: Patterns of Cognitive Impairment at Different Levels of Disease Severity. *Journal of the Neurological Sciences, 156,* 59–64

Podoll, K., Schwarz, M., & Noth, J. (1991). Language Functions in Progressive Supranuclear Palsy. *Brain, 114,* 1457–1472

Powell, A.L., Cummings, J.L., Hill, M.A., & Benson, D.F. (1988). Speech and Language Alterations in Multi-Infarct Dementia. *Neurology, 38,* 717–719

Price, B.H. (1996). Differential Diagnosis of Dementia. In: M.A. Samuels, & S. Feske (Eds.), *Office Practice of Neurology,* pp 705–710. New York: Churchill Livingstone

Ravin, P. (1996). Multiple System Atrophy: Striatonigral Degeneration and Shy-Drager Syndrome. In: M.A. Samuels, & S. Feske (Eds.), *Office Practice of Neurology,* pp 637–640. New York: Churchill Livingstone

Richards, S.S., Emsley, C.L., Roberts, J., Murray, M.D., Hall, K., Gao, S., & Hendrie, H.C. (2000). The association Between Vascular Risk Factor-Mediating Medications and Cognition and Dementia Diagnosis in a Community-Based Sample of African-Americans. *Journal of the American Geriatrics Society, 48,* 1035–1041

Ripich, D.N. (1991). Language and Communication in Dementia. In: D. Ripich (Ed.), *Handbook of Geriatric Communication Disorders* (pp. 255–283). Austin, TX: Pro-Ed

Ripich, D.N., & Ziol, E. (1998). Dementia: A Review for the Speech–Language Pathologist. In: A.F. Johnson & B.H. Jacobson (Eds.), *Medical Speech–Language Pathology: A Practitioner's Guide* (pp. 467–494). New York: Thieme

Ritchie, K., Gilham, C., Ledésert, B., Touchon, J., Kotzi, P.O. (1999). Depressive Illness, Depressive Symptomatology and Regional Cerebral Blood Flow in Elderly People with Sub-Clinical Cognitive Impairment. *Age and Ageing, 28,* 385–391

Ritchie, K., & Lovestone, S. (2002). The Dementias. *Lancet 360,* 1759–1766

Rob, P.M., Niederstadt, C., & Reusche, E. (2001). Dementia in Patients Undergoing Long-Term Dialysis: Aetiology, Differential Diagnoses, Epidemiology and Management. *CNS Drugs 15,* 691–699

Rogers, D. (1986). Bradyphrenia in Parkinsonian Patients. *Neurology, 45,* 447–450

Rogers, M.A., & Alarcon, N.B. (1999). Characteristics and Management of Primary Progressive Aphasia. *Neurophysiol Neurogenic Speech–Language Disorders (ASHA Special Interest Division 2), 9,* 12–25.

Roman, G.C., Tatemichi, T.K., Erkinjuntti, T., Cummings, J.L., Masdeu, J.C., Garcia, J.H., et al. (1993). Vascular Dementia: Diagnostic Criteria for Research Studies—Report of the NINDS-AIREN International Workshop. *Neurology, 43,* 250–260

Ronthal, M. (1996). Confusional States and Metabolic Encephalopathy. In: M.A. Samuels, & S. Feske (Eds.), *Office Practice of Neurology,* pp. 715–718. New York: Churchill Livingstone

Roses, A.D. (1995). Apolipoprotein E Genotyping in the Differential Diagnosis, not Prediction, of Alzheimer's Disease. *Annals of Neurology, 38,* 6–14

Samuel, N., D'Olhaberriague, L., Levine, S.R., & Brass, L.M. (1996). Illicit Drugs and Stroke. In: M.A. Samuels, & S. Feske (Eds.), *Office Practice of Neurology,* pp. 305–309. New York: Churchill Livingstone

Sapin, L.R., Anderson, F.H., & Pulaski, P.D. (1989). Progressive Aphasia Without Dementia: Further Documentation. *Annals of Neurology, 25,* 411–413

Seltzer, B., Vasterling, J.J., Mathias, C.W., & Brennan, A. (2001). Clinical and Neuropsychological Correlates of Impaired Awareness of Deficits in Alzheimer Disease and Parkinson Disease: A Comparative Study. *Neuropsychiatry Neuropsychology and Behavioral Neurology, 14,* 122–129

Sinforiani, E., Mauri, M., Sances, G., & Martelli, A. (1992). Slowly Progressive Aphasia: Report of a Case. *Acta Neurology (Napoli), 14,* 51–55

Small, B.J., Herlitz, A., Fratiglioni, L., Almkvist, O., & Backman, L. (1997). Cognitive Predictors of Incident Alzheimer's Disease: A Prospective Longitudinal Study. *Neuropsychology, 11,* 412–420

Snowden, J.S., Neary, D., Mann, D., Goulding, P.J., & Testa, H.J. (1992). Progressive Language Disorder Due to Lobar Atrophy. *Annals of Neurology, 31,* 174–183

Snowdon, D.A., Greiner, L.H., Mortimer, J.A., Riley, K.P., Greiner, P.A., & Markesbery, W.R. (1997). Brain Infarction and the Clinical Expression of Alzheimer Disease: The Nun Study. *Journal of the American Medical Association, 277,* 813–817

Spencer, M.D., Knight, R.S.G., & Will, R.G. (2002). First Hundred Cases of Variant Creutzfeldt-Jakob Disease. Retrospective Case Note Review of Early Psychiatric and Neurological Features. *British Medical Journal, 324,* 1479–1482

Starkstein S.E., Sabe L., Vazquez S., Teson A., Petracca G., Chemerinski E., Di Lorenzo G., Leiguarda R. (1996). Neuropsychological, psychiatric, and cerebral blood flow findings in vascular dementia and Alzheimer's disease. *Stroke, 27(3),* 408–414

Stern, Y., Tang, M.X., Jacobs, D.M., Sano, M., Marder, K., Bell, K., Dooneief, G., Schofield, P., & Cote, L. (1998). Prospective Comparative Study of the Evolution of Probable Alzheimer's Disease and Parkinson's Disease Dementia. *Journal of the International Neuropsychology Society, 4,* 279–284

Strittmatter, W.J., Saunders, A.M., Schmechel, D., Pericak-Vance, M., Enghild, J., Salvesen, G.S., & Roses, A.D. (1993). Apolipoprotein E: High-Avidity Binding to Beta-Amyloid and Increased Frequency of Type 4 Allele in Late-Onset Familial Alzheimer's Disease. *Proceedings of the National Academy of Sciences of the United States of Amnerica, 90,* 1977–1981

Sulkava, R. (2003). Differential Diagnosis Between Early Parkinson's Disease and Dementia with Lewy Bodies. *Advances in Neurology, 91,* 411–413

Swainson, R., Hodges, J.R., Galton, C.J., Semple, J., Michael, A., Dunn, B.D., et al. (2001). Early Detection and Differential Diagnosis of Alzheimer's Disease and Depression with Neuropsychological Tasks. *Dementia and Geriatric Cognitive Disorders, 12,* 265–280

Tanzi, R.E. (1999). A genetic Dichotomy Model for the Inheritance of Alzheimer's Disease and Common Age-Related Disorders. *Journal of Clinical Investigation, 104,* 1175–1179

Tatemichi, T.K., Desmond, D.W., Mayeux, R., Paik, M., Stern, Y., Sano, M., et al. (1992). Dementia After Stroke: Baseline Frequency, Risks, and Clinical Features in a Hospitalized Cohort. *Neurology, 42,* 1185–1193

Thompson, S.A., & Hodges, J.R. (2002). Mild Cognitive Impairment: A Clinically Useful but Currently Ill-Defined Concept? *Neurocase 8,* 405–410

Tolnay, M., & Probst, A. (2001). Frontotemporal Lobar Degeneration. An Update on Clinical, Pathological and Genetic Findings. *Gerontology, 47,* 1–8

Turner, M.A., Moran, N.F., & Kopelman, M.D. (2002). Subcortical Dementia. *British Journal of Psychiatry, 180,* 148–151

Wagner, M.T., & Bachman, D.L. (1996). Neuropsychological Features of Diffuse Lewy Body Disease. *Archives of Clinical Neuropsychology, 11,* 175–184

Wallin, A., Sjogren, M., Edman, A., Blennow, K., & Regland, B. (2000). Symptoms, Vascular Risk Factors and Blood-Brain Barrier Function in Relation to CT White-Matter Changes in Dementia. *European Neurology, 44,* 229–235

Warrington, E.K. (1975). Selective Impairment of Semantic Memory. *Quarterly Journal of Experimental Psychology, 27,* 635–657

Warrington, E.K., Agnew, S.K., Kennedy, A.M., & Rossor, M.N. (2001). Neuropsychological Profiles of Familial Alzheimer's Disease Associated with Mutations in the Presenilin 1 and Amyloid Precursor Protein Genes. *Journal of Neurology, 248,* 45–50

Wechsler, A. (1977). Presenile Dementia Presenting as Aphasia. *Journal of Neurology, Neurosurgery, and Psychiatry 40,* 303–305

Wechsler, A.F., Verity, A., Rosenschein, S., Fried, I., Scheibel, A.B. (1982). Pick's Disease: A Clinical, Computed Tomographic and Histological Study with Golgi Impregnation Observations. *Archives of Neurology, 39,* 287–290

Wells, C.E. (1979). Pseudodementia. *American Journal of Psychiatry, 136,* 895–900

Whitehouse, P.J., Price, D.L., Clark, A.W., et al. (1981). Alzheimer's Disease: Evidence for Selective Loss of Cholinergic Neurones in the Nucleus Basalis. *Annals of Neurology, 10,* 122–126

Wisniewski, H.M., Weigiel, J., Morys, J., et al. (1994). Alzheimer Dementia Neuropathology. In: V.O. Emery, & T.E. Oxman (Eds.), *Dementia: Presentations, Differential Diagnosis, and Nosology,* pp. 79–94. Baltimore: Johns Hopkins University Press

Zakzanis, K.K. (1998). The Subcortical Dementia of Huntington's Disease. *Journal of Clinical and Experimental Neuropsychology, 20,* 565–578

Zamani, A.A. (1996). Neuroimaging: Radiology, Magnetic Resonance Imaging, Positron Emission Tomography, and Single-Photon Emission Computed Tomography. In: M.A. Samuels, & S. Feske (Eds.), *Office Practice of Neurology,* pp 178–183. New York: Churchill Livingstone

8

Dementia: Communication Impairments and Management

Michele L. Norman, Jennifer Horner, and Danielle N. Ripich

✦ **Communication Skills in Persons with Dementia**

✦ **Assessment and Diagnosis**

✦ **Intervention for Persons with Dementia**

✦ **Ethics of Caring for Persons with Dementia**

Dementia is a symptom of a variety of diseases that affects 1.5% of the population over age 65. As the number of persons in this age group steadily increases (Hobbs & Damon, 1996), those 85 and over have become the fastest growing portion of the population (Day, 1996). Likewise, the number of older adults with dementing illnesses increases. For example, Alzheimer's disease, which accounts for over 50% of all cases of dementia (Daffner, 1996), is the eighth leading cause of death in the United States and is the sixth leading cause of death among those 85 and older (Anderson, 2001). The rising number of persons affected by dementia makes it imperative for speech–language pathologists (SLPs), who are charged with the task of treating communication disorders, to become more familiar with the communication changes that occur in this population at various stages. Considering the prevalence of Alzheimer's disease, this chapter describes dementia and the communication impairments evidenced in the disease, reviews evaluation tools and intervention strategies appropriate for this population, and discusses ethical issues to be considered when working with this population.

✦ Communication Skills in Persons with Dementia

Cognitive-Communicative Impairments

Cognitive deterioration is a hallmark of dementia. Such changes in memory, attention, and language become more noticeable over time. As the disease progresses, the cognitive-linguistic and intellectual changes experienced by the person with dementia impede the ability to communicate and function effectively. Collectively, the deficits caused by these changes are referred to as *cognitive-communicative impairments*. Using this term informs others that there are nonlinguistic as well as linguistic cognitive deficits that impair communication (ASHA, 1987). Following is a summary of the cognitive-communicative impairments evidenced at each stage of the disease.

Early Stage

The onset of Alzheimer's disease is gradual and it is often difficult to determine when the changes began to occur. Usually, slight changes in mood and occasional memory loss are attributed to "old age." However, the changes that occur in a neurologically based disease process such as Alzheimer's disease tend to occur more frequently and are more severe. In early stages, linguistic changes may be subtle markers of possible dementia. During this stage, dementia is classified as mild, and syntactic and phonologic processes are typically spared. Memory is impaired and some personality changes, as well as cognitive-linguistic changes occur (Bayles & Kaszniak, 1987; Cummings & Benson, 1983, Kempler, 1995). Sometimes displays of hostility, irritability, or frustration occur (Cummings & Benson, 1983). Also, persons with dementia demonstrate difficulty with naming and word finding. Although they are able to maintain conversations, staying on the topic and organizing ideas coherently during discourse maybe difficult (Bayles & Kaszniak, 1987; Kempler, 1995). Generally, the cumulative effect of these atypical behaviors prompts many people to seek care.

Middle Stages

As the disease progresses disparities in performance become more apparent. Memory recall is seriously impaired and personality changes are more prominent. Language skills have become poorer, making it more difficult for the patient to communicate (Bayles & Kasizniak, 1987; Kempler, 1995). Although persons with dementia respond to questions and know when they should talk, their speech is often empty and filled with stereotypical responses like, "I'm fine, how are you?" During this stage, they usually need assistance with tasks they once performed with ease, and they become more dependent on caregivers to complete routine activities of the day.

Late Stage

In the late stage of the disease, cognitive and communicative deficits advance to severe and then to profound. Eventually patients become totally dependent on caregivers and experience a myriad of problems. Persons in this stage have fewer conversations and may often become mute (Bayles & Kasizniak, 1987; Kempler, 1995). Although grammar appears to be preserved, comprehension is poor, and verbal utterances are usually composed of jargon or meaningless speech (Bayles & Kasizniak, 1987; Kempler, 1995).

Language Impairment

Language impairment is one of the cognitive disturbances evidenced in dementia, and its inclusion as one of the diagnostic criteria for various dementias demonstrates its importance (American Psychiatric Association, 1994; McKhann, Drachman, Folstein, et al, 1984; Neary, Snowden, Gostafson, et al, 1998; Roman, Tatemichi, Erkinjuntti, et al, 1993). The degenerative nature of dementing illnesses makes it difficult to categorize the language impairments demonstrated. Some researchers (Cummings, Benson, Hill, & Read 1985; Faber-Langendoen, Morris, Knesevich, et al, 1988) described the language disturbances they have encountered in persons with dementia as *aphasia* and strongly advocate for the use of the term. Later researchers (Emery, 2000; Vuorinen, Laine, & Rinne, 2000; Ripich, Carpenter, & Ziol, 1997; Ripich, Petrill, Whitehouse, & Ziol, 1995) have described the nature of the language impairments without reference to any preexisting classifications. Regardless of the terminology, differential diagnosis can be made through the evaluation of memory, verbal and nonverbal skills, and behavior, along with a thorough case history. The clinician will find it much more beneficial to evaluate and describe the cognitive-linguistic impairments in persons with dementia than to determine if the disturbances match preexisting classifications. If the clinician focuses on a specific classification, an inappropriate intervention may be selected when the management plan is developed.

The linguistic abilities of persons with dementia allow clinicians to (1) identify dementia as a diagnosis (Bayles & Boone, 1982), (2) differentiate dementia from other neurogenic communication disorders (Bayles, 1986; Deal, Wertz, & Spring, 1981; Halpern, Darley, & Brown, 1973; Holland, McBurnery, Moossy, et al, 1985; Horner & Heyman, 1981; Watson & Records, 1978), and (3) be descriptive of the unique features of language in persons with dementia (Appell, Kertez, & Fisman, 1982; Barker & Lawson, 1968; Obler, 1983; Schwartz, Marin, & Saffran, 1979; Whitaker, 1976). Differences on various language tasks performed by persons with dementia are noted. Although deterioration in phonology, syntax, and semantics have been well documented (Bayles, 1982; Bayles, Boone, Tomoeda, et al, 1989; Murdoch, Chenery, Wilks, et al, 1987; Schwartz et al,

1979), the degree of decline in *communication abilities* seems to exceed the decline in any one specific language area (Fromm & Holland, 1987; Ripich & Terrell, 1988; Ulatowska, Haynes, Donnell, et al, 1986). Therefore, a complete description of communication competence rather than linguistic knowledge is necessary. Descriptions should include information regarding the abilities and deficits evident in each language area, especially pragmatics, which is usually the most apparent.

Pragmatics

Functional language use, or pragmatics, is perhaps the most critical area for assessment and intervention. Although this area appears to contribute most to the communicative deficit in dementia and measures of pragmatics appear to be the most sensitive to discrimination among etiologies (Deal et al, 1991), the documentation of pragmatic deficits is limited (Kempler, 1995). Some of the pragmatic deficits that can be expected are poor topic maintenance; brief, but frequent turn-taking; more directives; breakdowns in cohesion and coherence vague speech; difficulty in maintaining eye contact; and difficulty taking conversational turns (Hutchinson & Jensen, 1980; Irigaray, 1973; Ripich & Terrell, 1988; Ripich, Terrell, & Spinelli, 1983; Ripich, Vertes, Whitehouse, et al, 1988). These deficits vary in severity according to the stage of disease process. The pragmatic deficits noted in Alzheimer's disease patients may be dependent on the nature of the discourse genre and task (Kimbarow & Ripich, 1989). Discourse in this population is described as having less cohesion (Ripich & Terrell, 1988), disordered and diminished content (Bayles, 1982; Kirshner, Webb, & Kelly, 1984), and high use of indefinite reference (Irigaray, 1973; Kempler, 1988; Obler, 1983; Ripich & Terrell, 1988), as well as being confusing and lacking coherence (Appell et al, 1982). Bayles (1984) anecdotally reports that requests are often missing; however, confirmation and clarification requests have been reported to occur more frequently when compared with normal elderly (Ripich et al, 1988).

Lexical-Semantics

Lexical-semantic impairments in Alzheimer's disease are characterized by limited vocabulary (De Ajuriaguerra & Tissot, 1975; Ernest, Dalby, & Dalby, 1970) and naming difficulty (Bayles & Tomoeda, 1991; Huff, Corkin, & Growdon, 1986; Kaszniak & Wilson, 1985; Neils, Boller, & Cole, et al, 1987), which are likely caused by a breakdown in cognitive processing perhaps at the prespeech level (Allison, 1962; Appell et al, 1982; Grossman, 1978; Irigaray, 1967; Obler, 1981; Schwartz et al, 1979; Warrington, 1975). In fact, lexical difficulty is one of the earliest deficits observed in persons with dementia (Kempler, 1995). Anomia, or word-finding difficulty, has been the subject of the most research in language and dementia (Appell et al, 1982; Bayles & Boone, 1982; Bayles, Tomoeda, & Caffrey, 1983; Kirshner et al, 1984, Skelton-Robinson & Jones, 1984). Even so, the nature of the anomic disorder in Alzheimer's disease and the relative contribution of perceptual, conceptual, and linguistic factors remain controversial (Hart, 1988). The majority of researchers appear to support the view that the primary breakdown in word retrieval is cognitively based as opposed to perceptual. However, a dispute remains regarding the nature of the cognitive deficit as being either a processing limitation or failure of the underlying lexical representation (Grober, Buschke, & Kawas, 1985; Schwartz et al, 1979).

Table 8–1 Language and Communication Changes that Occur in Alzheimer's Disease

Changes	Early Stages (Mild)	Middle Stages (Moderate)	Late Stages (Severe to Profound)
Pragmatic	Has difficulty using pronominal reference; being cohesive; giving instructions; storytelling; understanding humor, sarcasm, and analogies; understanding abstract expressions and inferential meanings; initiating conversation; maintaining topic	Demonstrates poor use of pronominal reference, cohesion, topic maintenance, sensitivity to conversational partners	Lack of coherence
			Difficulty maintaining eye contact
		Expresses fewer ideas	Expresses few to no related ideas
		Frequently repeats ideas	Uses fewer words and utterances
	Uses vague language	Relies on stereotypical utterances	Perseverative
	Frequently requests for clarification/confirmation		Output may be meaningless or bizarre
			May become mute
Semantic	Has difficulty with word finding, generative naming, abstract/complex concepts	Demonstrates poor word fluency, confrontation naming	Demonstrates paraphasia, echolalia, palilalia, poor comprehension, severely impaired naming
	Uses circumlocution or gestures more frequently	Has diminished vocabulary	Uses jargon and rambling speech
		Increases use of circumlocution and unrelated word substitutions	
		Frequently uses empty speech	
Syntactic	No errors generally	Occasional grammatical errors	Grammar generally preserved
		Difficulty with comprehension of complex structures	Some uses of elliptical clauses
			May use sentence fragments
			Poor comprehension of grammatical structures
Phonologic	No errors generally	No errors generally	Errors more frequent, but no non-native language sound combinations

Adapted from Ripich, D.N., & Ziol E. (1998). Dementia: A Review for the Speech–Language Pathologist. In: A.F. Johnson, & B.H. Jacobson (Eds.), *Medical Speech–Language Pathology: A Practitioner's Guide* (pp. 467–494). New York: Thieme

Syntactic

Many investigators report relatively intact syntax in dementia (Appell et al, 1982; Bayles & Boone, 1982; Obler, 1981; Schwartz et al, 1979; Whitaker, 1976). However, syntactic errors such as missing phrases and sentences, as well as breakdown in phrase markers and grammatical agreement have been reported (Constantinidis, 1978). Also, Irigaray (1967) described poor noun choice and incorrect verb tense in Alzheimer's disease patients. In addition to these problems, it appears that comprehension of syntax is relatively more impaired than production (Emery, 1988; Linebarger, Schwartz, & Saffran, 1983). One theory for the differences in reported syntactic performance is that the automatic nature of syntactic structures does not require a great deal of attention by the speaker and are maintained. In other words, syntax may be a relatively automatic cognitive function that is preserved in the midst of a more general cognitive decline (Kempler, Curtiss, & Jackson, 1987). Supporting this view, Whitaker (1976) presented a case study of a woman with severe dementia (not Alzheimer's disease) who spontaneously corrected errors of syntax and phonology when repeating sentences even though her language was restricted to echolalia and she was unresponsive to commands.

Phonologic

Phonologic deficits in persons with dementia rarely occur. Although phoneme errors have been reported in several investigations (Constantinidis, 1978; Ernest et al, 1970), these appear to be indicative of a "higher" semantic or syntactic problem, and not a problem with the individual "speech sounds" or morpho-phonemics (individual language units

signaling a change in meaning). However, there have been no firm findings to support this possibility. **Table 8–1** provides a synopsis of the language and communicative impairments evidenced during each stage of Alzheimer's disease.

In an effort to provide clinicians with a overview of evaluation tools available for assessing persons with dementia, the following section summarizes some of the major diagnostic screening tests, rating scales, and test batteries that are used to measure and describe the wide range of behavioral, neuropsychological, and cognitive-linguistic impairments associated with dementing illnesses.

✦ Assessment and Diagnosis

Owing to the complexity of differential diagnosis among the dementias, a comprehensive evaluation for dementia should include (1) a careful and thorough case history, (2) a neurologic and medical diagnostic battery and clinical examination (including neuroimaging and laboratory tests), (3) a behavioral assessment, and (4) a language and communication assessment. Dementia is a symptom complex that includes physical, social, cognitive, and communication features. As a result, multiple perspectives are required for an adequate assessment. Ideally, an interdisciplinary team represented by neurology, neuropsychology, psychiatry, nursing, social work, speech–language pathology, audiology, physical therapy, and occupational therapy should provide these perspectives.

From the SLP's perspective, comprehensive assessment and correct diagnosis of Alzheimer's and other forms of dementia are critical for prognosis, treatment, and case management. Typically, the initial interdisciplinary diagnostic workup and assessment precedes the SLP's intervention. Because the rate of progression is variable among the various diagnostic subgroups, systematic reassessment is required. Assessment must be viewed as a dynamic and ongoing process (Sohlberg & Mateer, 1989).

This section reviews several instruments available for evaluating a person with suspected dementia. The emphasis is on tests that have been developed and validated with samples of dementia patients. Supplementary tests of particular interest to SLPs are also described. **Table 8–2** lists the commonly used

Table 8–2 List of Commonly Used Neurobehavioral and Communication Instruments for Assessing Individuals with Dementia

Screenings	Mini–Mental State Examination (MMSE)	Folstein et al, 1975
	Standardized Mini-Mental State Examination (SMMSE)	Molloy & Standish, 1997
	Alzheimer's Quick Test (AQT)	Wiig et al, 2002
	Blessed Orientation and Memory Examination	Blessed et al, 1968
	Blessed-Roth Dementia Scale	Lam et al, 1997
	Mental Status Questionnaire	Kahn et al, 1960; Goldfarb, 1975
	Kokmen Short Test of Mental Status	Kokmen et al, 1991
	7-Minute Screen	Solomon et al, 1998
	Memory Impairment Screen	Buschke et al, 1999; Petersen et al, 2001; Wilder et al, 1995
Scales	Clinical Dementia Rating Scale (CDR)	Hughes et al, 1982
	Mattis Dementia Rating Scale	Mattis, 1976
	Brief Cognitive Rating Scale (BCRS)	Sclan & Reisberg, 1992
	Functional Assessment Stages (FAST)	Reisberg et al, 1984
	Global Deterioration Scale (GDS)	Reisberg et al, 1982
	Informant Questionnaire on Cognitive Decline of the Elderly (IQCODE)	Fuh et al, 1995
Neurologic	Hachinski Scale	Hachinski et al, 1974
Neuropsychiatric	Hamilton Depression Scale	Hamilton, 1967
	Present State Examination	Wing et al, 1974
	Behavioral Problem Checklist	Teri et al, 1992
Neuropsychological	Consortium to Establish a Registry for Alzheimer's Disease (CERAD)	Morris et al, 1989
	Halstead-Reitan Neuropsychological Test Battery	Reitan & Wolfson, 1985
	Wechsler Adult Intelligence Scale III	Wechsler, 1997
	Wechsler Memory Scale–III	Wechsler, 1997
	Wisconsin Card Sorting Test, Revised (WCST–R)	Heaton, 1993
	Fuld Object-Memory Evaluation	Loewenstein et al, 1995
Cognitive-linguistic	Arizona Battery for Communication Disorders of Dementia (ABCD)	Bayles & Kaszniak, 1987; Bayles & Tomoeda, 1993
	Functional Linguistic Communication Inventory (FLCI)	Bayles & Tomoeda, 1994
	Cognistat (Neurobehavioral Cognitive Status Examination, 1983)	Kiernan et al, 1995
	Cognitive-Linguistic Quick Test	Helm-Estabrooks, 2001
	Ross Information Processing Assessment Geriatric (RIPA-G)	Ross-Swain & Fogle, 1996
Language	Boston Diagnostic Aphasia Examination (BDAE)	Goodglass et al, 2000
	Western Aphasia Battery (WAB)	Kertesz, 1982; Shewan & Kertesz, 1980
	Porch Index of Communicative Abilities (PICA)	Porch, 1967
	Boston Naming Test (BNT)	Kaplan et al, 1983
	Discourse Abilities Profile (DAP)	Terrell & Ripich, 1989
	Discourse Comprehension Test	Brookshire & Nicholas, 1993; Welland et al, 2002
	FAS Word Fluency	Borkowski et al, 1967
	Peabody Picture Vocabulary Test, 3rd ed.	Dunn & Dunn, 1997
	Auditory Comprehension Test of Sentences (ACTS)	Shewan, 1979
	Token Test (TT)	DeRenzi & Faglioni, 1978
	Revised Token Test (RTT)	McNeill & Prescott, 1982
	Reporter's Test	DeRenzi & Ferrari, 1978

neurobehavioral and communication instruments for assessing individuals with dementia.

Understanding the characteristics of one's test battery is essential to avoid mislabeling a patient's disorder. When assessing patients suspected of having dementia, clinicians are advised to use tests that are norm-referenced to the appropriate age-, gender-, and education-matched adults. Ideally, the diagnosis of dementia should only be applied when the results of a test (or a test battery) have a high sensitivity and a high specificity for dementia. Sensitivity refers to the true-positive rate, that is, the rate at which subjects who have the disorder are accurately diagnosed as having the disorder. Higher sensitivity leads, therefore, to fewer errors of exclusion (fewer false-negatives). Specificity refers to the true-negative rate, that is, the rate at which subjects who do not have the disorder are accurately diagnosed as not having the disorder—higher specificity leads, therefore, to fewer errors of inclusion (fewer false-positives). The reader is referred to the Report of the Quality Standards Subcommittee of the American Academy of Neurology (Petersen, Stevens, Ganguli, et al, 2001). This evidence-based report compares the sensitivity and specificity of various instruments for detecting mild cognitive impairment and offers practice recommendations.

Geriatric Screening Instruments

A widely used instrument designed to assess general cognitive ability is the Mini–Mental Status Examination (MMSE; Folstein, Folstein, & McHugh, 1975), for which sensitivity and specificity data are available (Ganguli, Belle, Ratcliff, et al, 1993; Kukull, Larson, Terri, et al, 1994), as well as norms (Crum, Anthony, Bassett, & Folstein, 1993). The MMSE screens orientation, attention, recent verbal memory, naming, repetition, comprehension, reading, and writing. In 1997, Molloy and Standish developed a Standardized Mini-Mental State Examination (SMMSE). More recently, Folstein, Folstein, McHugh, and Fanjiang (2000) have published their own standard version of the MMSE. Wiig and colleagues (2002) developed the Alzheimer's Quick Test (AQT), which is designed to assess temporal-parietal function using timed naming and working memory tasks, among others. The AQT is reported to be free of gender, educational or cognitive-linguistic influences.

Others instruments have proven useful to neurologists, neuropsychologists, and SLPs (Ripich, 1991; Ripich & Ziol, 1998). These include mental status tests such as the Blessed Orientation and Memory Examination (Blessed, Tomlinson, & Roth, 1968), the Mental Status Questionnaire (Goldfarb, 1975; Kahn, Goldfarb, Pollack, & Peck, 1960), the Kokmen Short Test of Mental Status (Kokmen, Smith, Petersen, et al, 1991), the 7-Minute Screen (Solomon, Hirschoff, Kelly, et al, 1998; Solomon & Pendelbury, 1998), the Memory and Behavior Problem Checklist (Teri, Truax, Logsdon, Uomoto, Zarit, & Vitaliano, 1992), and Buschke's Memory Impairment Screen (Buschke, Kulansky, Katz, et al. 1999). (See also Petersen et al, 2001; Wilder, Cross, & Chen et al, 1995)

Dementia Rating Scales

Dementia rating scales are also widely used. The Clinical Dementia Rating Scale (CDRS; Hughes, Berg, Danzinger, Coben, & Martin, 1982) is a quasi-structured interview with a five-point rating scale of everyday functioning by a caregiver informant with 0 representing normal, 0.5 questionable dementia, and ratings of 1, 2, and 3 reflecting mild, moderate, and severe dementia, respectively (Horner, Heyman, Dawson, & Rogers, 1988; Juva, Sulkava, Erkinjuntti, et al, 1995; Morris, Heyman, Mohs, et al, 1989). A more comprehensive test is the Mattis Dementia Rating Scale (Mattis, 1976; Monsch, Bondi, Salmon, et al, 1995). According to Ripich (1991), "Although it is not useful for differential diagnosis, it has the advantage of measurement through the late stages of the disease when patients often become untestable by other instruments" (p. 267). Reisberg and colleagues have developed several useful scales. The Brief Cognitive Rating Scale (BCRS; Reisberg, 1983) "is a rapid structured instrument for use in assessing cognitive decline regardless of etiology" (Ripich, 1991; p. 267). The Functional Assessment Stages Test (FAST; Reisberg, Ferris, Anand, DeLeon, Schneck, Buttinger, & Borenstein, 1984) "distinguishes 15 distinct progressive characteristics of [dementia]" (Ripich, 1991; p. 267). The Global Deterioration Scale (GDS; Reisberg, Ferris, DeLeon, & Crook, 1982) for age-related cognitive decline and Alzheimer's disease "is a scale of seven stages designed to parallel the seven levels within each of the five axis categories of the BCRS" (Ripich, 1991; p. 267).

In addition to the CDRS, cited by the Quality Standards Committee of the American Academy of Neurology (Petersen et al, 2001), informant-based instruments are the Informant Questionnaire on Cognitive Decline in the Elderly (IQCODE; Fuh, Teng, Lin, et al, 1995), the Blessed-Roth Dementia Scale (BRDS; Lam, Chiu, Li, et al. 1997), and a behavioral rating scale developed by the Consortium to Establish a Registry for Alzheimer's Disease (CERAD; Tariot, Mack, Patterson, et al, 1995).

Neurologic and Neuropsychiatric Examinations

Because depression is common in dementia, or may be an independent problem that mimics dementia, some clinicians administer the Hamilton Depression Scale (Hamilton, 1967). An instrument designed to identify anxiety, depression, delusions, and hallucinations is the Present State Examination (Wing, Cooper, & Sartorius, 1974). To identify clinical signs that may be indicative of cerebrovascular disease, the Hachinski Scale (Hachinski, Lassen, Marshall, 1974; Wagner, Oesterreich, & Hoyer, 1985) has been used.

Neuropsychological Instruments

Full neuropsychological batteries and supplementary instruments should be administered by neuropsychologists who are specially trained to interpret them. These include the CERAD battery (Morris et al, 1989), for which norms are available, (Welsh, Butters, Mohs, Beekly, Edland, Fillenbaum, & Heyman, 1994), the Halstead-Reitan Neuropsychological Test Battery (Reitan & Wolfson, 1985), the Wechsler Adult Intelligence Scale–III (WAIS-3; Wechsler, 1981, 1997), and the Wechsler Memory Scale–III (WMS-3; Russell, 1988; Wechsler, 1987). A widely used supplementary test to assess new learning is a 1993 revision of the Wisconsin Card Sorting Test (WCST; Heaton, 1993) and, to assess memory, the Fuld Object-Memory Evaluation (Loewenstein, Duara, Arguelles, et al, 1995).

Cognitive-Linguistic Tests

Tests for dementia that are appropriate for administration and interpretation by SLPs are few in number. These are important because they are validated by individuals with dementia, and provide norms on age-matched cognitively normal individuals. The Arizona Battery of the Communication in Dementia (ABCD; Bayles & Tomoeda, 1993) is a comprehensive battery designed for mildly demented patients and includes memory, language, and visuospatial abilities (Bayles & Kaszniak, 1987; Bayles & Tomoeda, 1993). Bayles and Tomoeda also designed the Functional Linguistic Communication Inventory (FLCI; Bayles & Tomoeda, 1994) with moderate and severe dementia patients in mind. The FLCI takes about 30 minutes to administer and allows for staging the severity of dementia.

Cognistat, formerly the Neurobehavioral Cognitive Status Examination (Kiernan, Mueller, & Langston, 1995; Kiernan, Mueller, Langston, & Van Dyke, 1987; Roper et al, 1996; Schwamm, Van Dyke, Kiernan, Merrin, & Mueller, 1987), includes subtests of naming, spontaneous speech, comprehension, and oral repetition, in addition to tasks involving orientation, verbal and visual recall, visual-constructive ability, and verbal reasoning. The Cognistat has screening items that allow for rapid administration (about 20 minutes).

In 1996, Ross-Swain and Fogle developed the Ross Information Processing Assessment for geriatric individuals (RIPA-G). The RIPA-G is designed to be used as part of a comprehensive battery and includes subtests of immediate memory, recent memory, temporal orientation, spatial orientation, orientation to the environment, recall of general information, problem solving (both abstract and concrete), organization, and auditory processing. Finally, Helm-Estabrooks (2001) published the Cognitive-Linguistic Quick Test (CLQT), which has a range of linguistic and nonlinguistic tasks and provides geriatric norms.

Language Tests

Several additional tests of language and communication that are widely used but were not originally validated for use with dementia include the third edition of the Boston Diagnostic Aphasia Examination (BDAE-3; Goodglass, Kaplan, & Barresi, 2000), the Porch Index of Communicative Abilities (PICA; Porch, 1967), and the Western Aphasia Battery (WAB; Horner, Dawson, Heyman, & Fish, 1992; Kertesz, 1979, 1982; Shewan & Kertesz, 1980). The Discourse Abilities Profile (DAP), designed by Terrell and Ripich (1989), samples narrative and procedural discourse, and spontaneous conversation. The DAP provides for an overall rating of performance as well as consideration of linguistic, paralinguistic, and nonlinguistic factors. Finally, Welland, Lubinski, and Higginbotham (2002) reported the usefulness of the Discourse Comprehension Test, originally developed by aphasiologists Brookshire and Nicholas (1993) for differentiating early and middle-stage AD patients from non–brain-damaged control subjects.

The Boston Naming Test (Kaplan, Goodglass, & Weintraub, 1983) has proven to be popular in language and neuropsychology research studies, even though it was not originally standardized on dementia subjects (Fisher, Tierney, Snow, & Szalai, 1999; Welch, Doineau, Johnson, & King, 1996). The FAS Word Fluency Measure involves rapid naming of words beginning with the letters F, A, and S, and is sensitive to brain damage of all types (Borkowski, Benton, & Spreen, 1967).

Other supplementary tests that SLPs find useful are the Peabody Picture Vocabulary Test (Dunn & Dunn, 1997); the Auditory Comprehension Test of Sentences (ACTS; Shewan, 1979); the Token Test, (DeRenzi & Faglioni, 1978); the Revised Token Test (RTT; McNeil & Prescott, 1982), which is standardized and normed on 20- to 80-year-olds; and the Reporter's Test (DeRenzi & Ferrari, 1978).

In the interest of providing clinicians an understanding of diagnostic approaches, we summarized a range of behavioral scales, tests, and neuropsychological batteries. This was not an exhaustive catalogue but rather was a sampling of those instruments that are reportedly frequently in the contemporary literature. We described tests of communication function that have been validated for use with dementia, as well as supplementary tests of naming, comprehension, and discourse. Likewise, the following section reviews various interventions that are appropriate for persons with dementia and their caregivers.

✦ Intervention for Persons with Dementia

As a result of the degenerative nature of Alzheimer's disease, persons with the disease are initially cared for by family and eventually need institutionalization for long-term care. Primary caregivers maintain that communication is the single most distressing problem they face, and the patients experience a gradual erosion of sociability. Therefore, the goal of quality caregiving should be to prolong and promote communication between these patients and primary caregivers for as long as possible and on as high a level as possible. Researchers report that family caregivers are sensitive to the communication problems and can identify the progression of the symptoms (Bayles & Tomoeda, 1991; Orange, 1991). However, these caregivers need adequate training to communicate effectively with this increasing patient population. Developing the communication skills of professionals such as nurses, social workers, and physicians as well as direct caregivers can enhance the quality of life for the person with dementia (Carroll, 1989; Clark, 1991; Poulshock & Deimling, 1984).

A considerable need exists for SLPs and other health care professionals to shift from a more traditional medical model based on assessing pathology and restoring function to a more holistic model based on maintaining function (Clark, 1995). The American Speech–Language-Hearing Association (ASHA, 1988a,b) stresses the need for improving the quality of life and quality of care, which are rights of every individual including those who suffer from dementing disease, in the assessment and management of persons with Alzheimer's disease and related disorders. The components of quality of life include physical, mental, and spiritual health; cognitive ability; family and social relations; work and hobby activities; economic success and subjective well-being (Whitehouse & Rabins, 1992). Because social interaction and interpersonal relations are a component of quality of life (Ishii-Kuntz, 1990; LaMendola & Pellegrini, 1979; Larson, 1978), ASHA encourages SLPs to provide programs to maintain functional communication for as long as possible. An innovative and flexible treatment program designed for persons with dementia will address these quality of life issues. These treatment programs can be implemented by direct intervention, which entails working with the patient, and/or indirect intervention, which are intended for caregivers of persons with dementia.

Table 8–3 Direct Clinical Interventions for Groups

Intervention	Authors	Goals	Measures/Data	Results	Advantages/Limitations
Reality orientation	Folsom & Folsom, 1974 Green et al., 1983	To reinforce awareness by calling attention to upcoming events or current environment	Measures verbal orientation, affect, functional behavior	Numerous studies report increase in verbal orientation, improved affect, decreased mood, no functional behavior changes noted	Easily implemented Easily adapted to events and settings Criticized as having little theoretical basis and not impacting functional behavior
Validation therapy	Feil, 1992	To help validate feelings To identify four stages of conflict To intervene appropriately at each stage	No quantitative measures or data	Anecdotal reports show improved affect, positive behaviors during group sessions	Used in over 500 institutions in the U.S. May be best used with late-stage patients
Reminiscence therapy	Harris, 1997, 1998; Nomura, 2002	To improve communication and discourse skills memory recall of personal events To maintain cognitive stimulation	Varies depending on the goal of therapy	Improved MMSE score for persons with dementia in day-care setting participating in reminiscence groups	Reminiscence therapy can be conducted in a naturalistic environment Activities can be tailored to meet the needs of individuals or groups Culturally and linguistically appropriate Recall of unpleasant events is a possible risk

Direct Intervention

With direct intervention, the communication specialist works with persons with dementia on the goals of maintaining residual functional communication (Clark, 1995). In this subsection, we briefly review direct approaches that have been used in treating persons with dementia in both group and individual sessions. Many of the group treatment strategies can be taught to caregivers to use with the person with Alzheimer's disease in other settings. Likewise, many of the individual treatments can be adapted for small group settings.

Group Treatment

Group treatment even at more advanced stages of dementia provides opportunities to interact socially in a structured and supportive environment. Consisting of simple, informative sessions that review previous life experiences, group treatment has been successful for persons in the moderate stages of Alzheimer's disease (Hughston & Merriam, 1982). Group sessions can include basic cognitive or sensory activities structured for success such as identifying textures and scents, and word, object, and melody recognition tasks.

The SLPs who are treating persons with Alzheimer's disease in groups need to assess baseline communicative abilities and determine outcomes (e.g., initiation, verbal and nonverbal responses, total words, total utterances, content, generalization, affect, interaction with other residents, interaction with staff, etc.), which can be measured through discourse (Terrell & Ripich, 1989). These outcomes should be used to establish goals that are realistic, functional, tailored to the cognitive level of the group participant, and focused on optimal functioning and maintenance of communicative skills. To be "reimbursable" by Medicare and medical or private insurance, goals must be designed to achieve measurably *functional* gains within a reasonable period of time. Additionally, facilitators,

other than SLPs, need to be familiar with the communication level of participants to engage group members in the activity, cue appropriately, and promote interaction. Clinical interventions for groups are summarized in **Table 8–3**.

Reality Orientation

Reality orientation (RO; Folsom & Folsom, 1974) consists of two approaches: (1) the one-on-one basic approach, in which awareness of barriers in the environment, correction for sensory deficits, attention to nonverbal communication, and structuring communicative exchanges by the caregiver is addressed with each encounter; and (2) formal RO classes in small groups, in which signs and information boards are recommended with activities that are structured for success (Stephens, 1969). Although sometimes criticized through the years, it has been frequently taught, and some techniques are still used.

Reality orientation can be multifaceted and adapted to many settings and individuals while respecting the individuality and dignity of the person with dementia. Respectfully calling the person's attention to upcoming holidays and events can promote activity and interest (Miller & Morris, 1993). As in any treatment method the attitudes, values, and principles of the caregivers will determine how effective the approach is in a client-centered environment.

Validation Therapy

As a response to the negative reaction to RO, Feil (1992) developed validation therapy with the goals of stimulating verbal and nonverbal communication, restoring dignity and well-being, and resolving meaning in life for the person with dementia, particularly for those in later stages (Feil, 1992). Rather than confront or correct persons with dementia, the

SLP empathically "validates" or confirms a person's emotional states and helps resolve past conflicts.

Reminiscence Therapy

Reminiscence is a naturally occurring process that entails the review of life events. As a therapeutic approach reminiscence may be particularly appealing for persons with dementia as an opportunity to communicate with others because it focuses on long-term memory (Harris, 1997, 1998; Harris & Norman, 2002; Zgola & Coulter, 1988). Reminiscence can be encouraged informally by requesting advice, looking at family photographs, looking at old magazines such as *Life*, and discussing hobbies, military experiences, and past jobs. Discussions of traditional foods and celebrations, hobbies, school experiences, songs, and pets and artifacts such as tools and household objects borrowed from a local museum have been used in a group to provide sensory stimulation and to recall competencies and achievements from the past (Zgola & Coulter, 1988). Triggers such as music, food, poems, faces, colors, objects, and smells can be useful for recall. Reminiscence activities are adaptable to meet the needs of the participants, making the intervention both culturally and linguistically appropriate.

In a group, reminiscence has many benefits, such as developing relationships; entertaining peers; enhancing status of participants; assisting with identity formation; facilitating resolution, reorganization, and reintegration of life; and establishing a sense of personal continuity (Anderson, 1983). Furthermore, reminiscence has been associated with improved self-esteem in nursing home residents (Osborn, 1989). Ziol, Dobres, and White (1996) developed a group program with a variety of communication activities that incorporate aspects of RO and reminiscence for those at mild and moderate stages with suggested variations in the activities for those at later stages.

Individual Treatment

Individual treatment allows the clinician to develop personalized activities designed to enhance communication for as long as possible. The person with dementia is taught strategies to compensate for deficits in memory, such as orientation, word finding, naming, and recall. Compensatory strategies are also provided to assist with new learning. Although caregivers are not trained in the strategies, they can be present during an individual session to observe the strategies the person with dementia is learning. Caregiver presence at some sessions may be beneficial because it provides a mutual understanding of the communication goals established and the strategies developed to achieve them. **Table 8–4** summarizes the clinical interventions for individuals.

Memory and Communication Compensations

Training in memory and communication strategies and compensations are appropriate particularly in early stages when persons with dementia are more aware of communication breakdown. During this stage the SLP can reassure and train the client to ask for repetition or review and compensate with circumlocution, gesture, and associated words for semantic deficits. A memory notebook with autobiographical information,

calendar, and sections for things to do, maps, and daily logs (Mateer & Sohlberg, 1988) can draw upon more intact procedural memory abilities to compensate for short-term memory failure. Bourgeois (1992) demonstrated the use of developing memory wallets with pictures and sentences about familiar persons, places, and events. The use of external strategies such as written Post-it notes, alarms, daily pill organizers, or audio- and videotapes can help to maintain independent function for as long as possible.

Engaging persons with dementia with collections of pictures of familiar categories (e.g., flowers, boating, fishing, golfing, home decorating, local landmarks, etc.) can decrease agitated behavior and increase interaction (Denis, personal communication, 1996). These "Look Books," strategically placed within the environment, can be used informally to distract or serve as a focus for reminiscence in a group setting.

Montessori-Based Activities

Montessori methods are structured to provide successful skills performance involving multisensory experiences of daily activities for persons with dementia and help them maintain current abilities. They provide opportunities for interaction between persons with dementia and caregivers and maintain the quality of life. Improvements in constructive engagement and decreases in passivity and disruptive behaviors have been reported (Judge, Camp, & Orsulic-Jeras, 2000).

Spaced Retrieval

In spaced retrieval, persons with dementia and MMSE scores between 9 and 25 are given strategies to assist new learning and retention by recalling information or motor tasks over increasingly longer intervals. Training sessions, which provided repetitive success, are designed around daily living tasks (Brush & Camp, 1998). If the patient fails to recall, the trainer returns to the previous success interval level and moves ahead more slowly. The approach is easily modified to fit the individual's functional living needs and can be used even in late stages to help recall the caregiver's name or one-step motor tasks.

Errorless Learning with Quizzes

In errorless learning, taped narratives with questions are structured to maximize success in answering quiz questions (Arkin, 1991). The tape always provides the correct answer after a pause to verify successful recall of information.

Indirect Intervention

With indirect intervention, caregivers of persons with dementia are trained to apply strategies to improve communication interaction. Communication breakdown is consistently listed among the top stressors in caregiver surveys of stress, strain, and burden (Kinney & Stephens, 1989; Rabins, 1982; Zarit, 1982). It would appear that caregiver training in facilitating strategies could provide useful tools to the caregiver communication partner. Care of persons with Alzheimer's disease could be improved significantly by enhancing the communication skills of caregivers. The ability of caregivers to draw on strategies and techniques for dealing with communication

Table 8–4   Direct Clinical Interventions for Individuals

Intervention	Authors	Goals	Measures/Data	Results	Advantages/Limitations
Memory compensations Notebooks, wallets, notes, and look books	Bourgeois, 1992 Bourgeois, Dijkstra, Burgio & Allen-Burge, 2001	To create wallets containing relevant pictures and written information To train patients to self-prompt To improve conversational content using familiar persons, places, and events To improve the use of factual information	Seven discourse measures scored for baseline conversations, training conversations, maintenance-phase conversation	Some showed decline in nonproductive statements, maintenance of performance levels, novel utterances were similar to baseline levels	Used to improve factual information in conversations with little systematic training Patients required minimal training Patients responded to prompts to look at or read their wallets May not be useful in later stage of dementia
Montessori-based activities	Judge, Camp, & Orsulic-Jeras, 2000	To provide successful skills performance that involve multisensory experiential activities	Constructive engagement in daily activities Passive behavior and disruptive behaviors assess change resulting from Montessori-based tasks	Improvements in constructive engagement Decreases in passivity and disruptive behaviors	Activities: Work well in the daily routine Help maintain current abilities Provide opportunities for interaction between persons with dementia and caregivers Help maintain the quality of life Can be adapted to group exercises
Spaced retrieval	Brush & Camp, 1998	Persons with dementia and MMSE scores between 9 and 25 are given strategies Goals: to assist new learning to retain information or motor tasks by recalling information or motor tasks over increasingly longer intervals	Training sessions are designed around activities of daily living and are designed to provide repetitive success If the patient fails to recall, the trainer drops back to the previous success interval level and moves ahead more slowly	Variable results reported with subjects across early, middle, and late stages	Easily modified to fit the individual's functional living needs Can be used even in late stages to help recall caregiver's name or one-step motor task May require significant time from the trainer to establish the recall information or motor task Family caregivers can be trained in this method Persons with dementia may learn a limited number of associations Previously learned information may interfere with severe episodic memory impairments
Errorless learning with quizzes	Arkin, 1991	To maximize success in answering quiz questions	Successful recall of information	Narratives and quizzes were more successful than the repetition Middle- and late-stage patients showed improvements	Shows greater success than spaced retrieval Can be used by family members

problems in these persons would reduce their own stress and frustration, and improve their competence in delivering quality care. In addition, the caregivers would be better able to promote the use of residual functional communication abilities, to provide appropriate social communication opportunities, and possibly to keep family members at home longer. Nurses and nursing assistants could also benefit from improved communication with their patients with Alzheimer's disease. Several caregiver training programs are discussed in the remainder of the chapter.

Caregiver Training Programs

Communication training for caregivers can increase knowledge, improve communication satisfaction, and decrease hassles related to communication breakdown. Education in

specific communication strategies can alter attitudes toward persons with Alzheimer's disease. Providing adequate training to caregivers is essential to quality-of-life issues. Additional benefits may be caregivers' greater satisfaction and sense of accomplishment in their critical day-to-day activities. Caregivers can benefit from training in communication strategies, and this training may improve the quality of life for persons with Alzheimer's disease. After briefly reviewing a training program developed by Clark and Witte (1989), we will discuss the FOCUSED Program.

Making Family Visits Count

Clark and Witte (1989) developed this communication training program for family members to improve quality and satisfaction in visits to relatives in nursing homes. In small practice groups, family members view prepared videotapes, taking note of facilitative communicative techniques and learning how to individualize strategies. In a communication stress management program for caregivers, Clark (1991) teaches family members to understand the nature and progression of language changes in Alzheimer's disease and increase and apply problem-solving skills to reduce caregiver stress and burden. Caregivers learn appropriate expectations and the importance of maintaining the person with dementia in communicative situations.

The Focused Program

To improve communication with persons with dementia, Ripich and Wykle (1990a,b) developed the *Alzheimer's Disease Communication Guide: The FOCUSED Program for Caregivers* (Ripich, 1996; Ripich & Wykle, 1990a,b). The acronym FOCUSED organized strategies based on the seven major elements for communication maintenance for easy recall: face-to-face, orient, continue, unstick, structure, exchange, and direct. This program consists of didactic materials to better prepare family and professional caregivers to communicate with persons with Alzheimer's disease. This program was based on an interactive discourse model of conversational exchanges (Terrell & Ripich, 1989). The key points of the program are indicated in **Table 8–5**.

The training program is divided into five 2-hour modules for family or professional caregivers with an optional module for professional caregivers on cultural differences:

Module 1. Alzheimer's disease and the associated communication and language decline: This module discusses characteristics, pathology, and incidence of Alzheimer's disease. The components and processes of language are presented. Participants learn how physicians make a diagnosis of probable Alzheimer's disease and how language in aphasia and Alzheimer's disease differ.

Module 2. The differences between memory decline in normal aging and Alzheimer's disease and the effects of depression on the person with Alzheimer's disease: In this module the caregiver is taught to understand changes in memory in the normal elderly, to recognize symptoms of depression, and to differentiate these symptoms from those of dementia. Discussion of the effects of depression on the Alzheimer patient's already decreasing ability to communicate with others is included.

Module 3. Interpersonal skills and the value of effective communication skills in the care of persons with Alzheimer's disease: The critical importance of social communication to keep the person with Alzheimer's disease engaged in communication to prevent excessive functional decline and maintain abilities is discussed. Participants learn verbal and nonverbal approaches to good communication. A discussion of empathy provides a foundation for promoting sensitive interpersonal exchanges that demonstrates respect for the person with dementia and supports the self-esteem of both the caregiver and the person with Alzheimer's disease.

Module 4. The FOCUSED strategies to promote effective communication with persons with Alzheimer's disease: This is a critical module that outlines the seven-point program. The program incorporates numerous strategies into a

Table 8–5   FOCUSED Communication Strategies

F = Face-to-face communication

    Face the person with Alzheimer's disease directly

    Call his or her name

    Touch the person

    Gain and maintain eye contact

O = Orient to topic of conversation

    Orient the person with Alzheimer's disease to the topic by repeating key words several times

    Repeat and rephrase sentences

    Use nouns and specific names

C = Continue topic of conversation

    Continue the same topic of conversation for as long as possible

    Restate the topic throughout the conversation

    Indicate to the person with Alzheimer's disease that you are introducing a new topic

U = Unstick communication blocks

    Help the person with Alzheimer's disease become "unstuck" when he or she uses a work incorrectly by suggesting the intended word

    Repeat the sentence the person said using the correct word

    Ask, "Do you mean . . . ?"

S = Structure with yes/no and choice questions

    Structure your questions so that the person with Alzheimer's disease will be able to recognize and repeat a response

    Provide two simple choices at a time

    Use yes/no questions

E = Exchange conversation

    Keep up the normal exchanges of ideas we use in everyday conversation

    Keep the conversations going with comments such as, "Oh, how nice," or "That's great"

    Do *not* ask "test" questions

    Give the person with Alzheimer's disease clues as to how to answer your questions

D = Direct, short, simple sentences

    Keep sentences short, simple, and direct

    Put the subject of the sentences first

    Use and repeat nouns (names of persons or things) rather than pronouns (he, she, it, their, etc.)

    Use hand signals, pictures, and facial expressions

framework that is easy to recall and apply. A series of role-play exercises and videotaped vignettes (for the research protocol) are used to demonstrate the seven points of this communication enhancement program.

Module 5. The stages of Alzheimer's disease and concurrent communication characteristics including how to assess and recognize persons with Alzheimer's disease at each stage and maximize their communication. Though fully aware of the heterogeneity of the progress of Alzheimer's disease and the fact that dividing the progression into stages is an arbitrary device, the literature repeatedly reports three main levels of language deterioration designated as mild, moderate, and severe. In this module these stages are described, the seven points of the FOCUSED program are reviewed, and the implementation of the strategies and communication goal at each stage are discussed.

Optional module for professional caregivers. Cultural considerations in communicating with persons with Alzheimer's disease: Cultural considerations are extremely important issues in helping the professional caregiver care for the person with Alzheimer's disease. The conflicts that arise in a caregiving situation may be further complicated by the differences in cultural and socioeconomic backgrounds of extended care residents and nursing assistant staff. The resultant disparity in values and interpersonal dynamics accentuates the communication difficulties that are characteristic of persons with Alzheimer's disease. Therefore, didactic and experiential content that enhances the caregivers' understanding of cultural considerations affecting that interpersonal communication process is presented. Several investigations have been completed that examine the efficacy of the FOCUSED program and the results indicate several positive outcomes (see below).

Considerations for Service Delivery

Direct Intervention

Reality orientation has been criticized for having little theoretical basis (Hussian, 1981), for having no value (Reisberg, 1981), for showing no generalization to other areas of behavior (Burton, 1982), and for being too rigid, boring, and unstimulating (MacDonald & Settin, 1978). Reports of validation therapy show inconsistent results of improved affect or positive effects (Alprin, 1980; Dietch, Hewett, & Jones, 1989; Fritz, 1986; Peoples, 1982) when measuring communicative interaction in a group setting (Morton & Bleathman, 1991). Baines, Saxby, and Ehlert (1987) reported attendance at reminiscence sessions to be higher when compared with RO sessions. For the individual strategies, persons with dementia improved conversational content, with some subjects demonstrating improvements for up to 30 months following intervention using memory wallets (Bourgeois, 1992). Also, errorless learning and quizzes were more successful in improving memory on training task for middle- and late-stage subjects than were the repetition task and spaced retrieval (Arkin, 1991).

Indirect Intervention

A series of studies examined the effects of the FOCUSED training on various caregivers. Postintervention analysis showed significant improvements in attitude toward Alzheimer's disease patients and increased knowledge of Alzheimer's disease and of communication strategies in comparisons of pre- and posttraining assessments (Ripich, Kercher, Wykle, Sloan, & Ziol , 1999). A comparison of caregivers of persons with Alzheimer's disease revealed that African-American caregivers showed greater positive effect and significant declines in perceived daily hassles after communication training, whereas Caucasian caregivers did not (Ripich, Ziol, & Lee, 1998). Follow-up evaluations at 6 and 12 months posttraining showed decreased communication difficulties and increased knowledge of Alzheimer's disease in caregivers and

no significant changes in the control group (Ripich et al, 1998). Overall, these studies show the feasibility of FOCUSED as an effective caregiver behavioral intervention that improves communication with persons with Alzheimer's disease.

Continual Reassessment in Intervention

Continual reassessment is an important part of the intervention process in this highly variable and heterogeneous symptom complex. Evaluation at 6-month intervals provides information regarding change or maintenance of competencies. Results of minimal or no change can be a very encouraging factor for many persons with dementia and their families. Identification of further decline in an area can focus and structure case management. Furthermore, the intervention process must ideally be multidisciplinary to address the scope of problems arising from this disorder. A collaborative perspective on the person with dementia, caregiver and family counseling, education, and communication treatment provide the optimal opportunity for comprehensive support of all aspects of direct and indirect intervention.

Another integral part of the intervention process is making sure that the patient is being cared for by clinicians who understand ethics principles and who strive to maintain high ethical as well as clinical standards of care. Ethnical considerations are important not only during intervention but also throughout the case management process (i.e., referral and evaluation). The remainder of this chapter discusses ethical issues that should be considered when caring for a person with dementia.

✦ Ethics of Caring for Persons with Dementia

This section summarizes some of the ethical dimensions of our work with dementia patients. The foundations of modern clinical ethics are described briefly, followed by definitions of contemporary ethical principles. A few examples of the types of ethical difficulties that arise are then given with regard to diagnostic testing, privacy and confidentiality, patients' adjustment to their disorder, intervention, and research participation. This section is not a comprehensive review of ethics, or a comprehensive discussion of ethics problems, but rather is intended to highlight several ethical issues that arise when working with persons with dementia, or suspected dementia.

Philosophical Bases for Modern Clinical Ethics

Contemporary principles of clinical ethics are respect for autonomy, nonmaleficence, beneficence, and justice (Beauchamp & Childress, 1994). The autonomy principle derives from Kant's observation that all persons, as rational beings, are deserving of respect (Kant, 1785, p. 36). In Kantian philosophy, respect is a duty: "Act in such a way that you treat humanity, whether in your own person or in the person of another, always at the same time as an end and never simply as a means" (Kant, 1785; p. 38). In contrast, the beneficence and nonmaleficence principles derive from Bentham's observation that the pursuit of happiness, or "good," is a moral imperative. From this idea he derived the principle of utility, which requires us to act in ways that maximize good and minimize harm overall.

Bentham recognized the uncertainties involved in predicting the good (or bad) consequences of future acts, but nevertheless required that we judiciously estimate and balance potentially positive or negative outcomes before acting. Thus, these classic moral philosophers espoused two approaches to moral behavior: Kant's duty-based philosophy requires that we respect the values and decisions of others; Bentham's utility-based philosophy requires that we look ahead to the consequences of our decisions and always seek to maximize benefits over harms.

A distinct but complementary idea—the concept of virtue—was espoused by Socrates, Plato, and Aristotle. For Aristotle, "virtues are traits that make a person good and enable him to do this work well" (Pellegrino & Thomasma, 1993, p. 5). Virtue ethics emphasizes the importance of traits of character—for example, trustworthiness, compassion, prudence, and integrity—and the idea that we can nurture our character traits through diligent practice. According to Pellegrino and Thomasma (1993), Aristotelian virtue involves choice and is "a habitual disposition to act well" (p. 5).

Finally, a contemporary theory is the ethics of care. Espoused originally by Gilligan (1982), the ethics of care emphasizes the idea that moral behavior is realized through our relationships with others. In Gilligan's view (to paraphrase), the idea that we are autonomous moral agents making calculated "cost-benefit" decisions misses the point of morality. Instead, the ethics of care places empathy, concern, and responsibility for others' well-being at center stage (Mappes & DeGrazia, 2001). The ethics of care resonates with many health care professionals for two reasons. First, patients who are ill are invariably vulnerable, and they must depend on others (Pellegrino & Thomasma, 1993). Second, health care professionals have been specially educated and trained to work with, and on behalf of, sick persons. As such the quality of the relationship between carer and the cared-for has special import.

Contemporary Moral Principles

From these overlapping and complementary moral philosophies arise major biomedical ethical principles—guiding principles for clinicians when faced with complex or uncertain situations. In 1974, Congress created the National Commission for the Protection of Human Subjects of Biomedical and Behavioral Research. In 1979, the U.S. Department of Health, Education, and Welfare, on behalf of the commission, published "The Belmont Report: Ethical Principles and Guidelines for the Protection of Human Subjects of Research." The principles articulated in the Belmont report have since been applied not only in the human research context but also among the health professions as applied to the care of patients (Beauchamp & Childress, 1994; Veatch & Flack 1997).

The first principle is respect for autonomy, which acknowledges that a person has a "right to hold views, to make choices, and to take actions based on personal values and beliefs" (Beauchamp & Childress, 1994, p. 125). The second principle is that of nonmaleficence, which means we "ought not to inflict evil or harm" (p. 192) on others. The third principle is that of beneficence, which means we should act to prevent or remove harm, as well as take positive actions to do good for others. Finally, the principle of justice refers to acting in ways that are fair and appropriate, depending on what a person deserves or needs. Ethicists readily acknowledge that the principles must

be interpreted in light of the particular circumstances, and that it is not always clear how to resolve conflicts among the principles. For example if a dementia patient refuses to take an antipsychotic medication even though his physician is reasonably sure it will help him, is the physician ethically bound to defer to the patient's wishes? (How should the principles of autonomy and beneficence be balanced?) Or, if a dementia patient's family demands to have a certain of speech–language intervention, even though the clinician is reasonably sure the patient will be unable to benefit from it, and that doing therapy with this patient will waste scarce health care resources needed by others, is it ethically permissible (or, ethically required) to refuse the request? (How can the principles of autonomy, nonmaleficence, beneficence, and justice solve these problems?)

Professional Ethics

The fact that detection and treatment of the dementias is improving is, by and large, a good thing. Ironically, knowing more may actually make our work more difficult. For example, as knowledge of dementia expands, clinicians must study ever harder to stay abreast of diagnostic criteria and treatment approaches. In addition, because laypersons are increasingly knowledgeable about the dementias, and therefore more anxious about them, clinicians may feel less, rather than more, confident about their knowledge. Finally, because no single discipline can know all there is to know about the dementias, SLPs must relinquish some of their autonomy and work collaboratively with clinicians from other disciplines.

These requirements (to be competent, to respect patients' and families' choices, to work in partnership) are simultaneously clinical imperatives and ethical imperatives. Why? First, these actions and virtues are consistent with the basic moral principles as defined above. Second, they are consistent with the first principle of the Code of Ethics of the American Speech-Language-Hearing Association, which requires clinicians to "honor their responsibility to hold paramount the welfare of persons they serve professionally" (ASHA, 2003). To live up to this principle, we must not only do our work competently (in the clinical sense), but also we must do it well (in the moral sense); we must not only care *for* our patients (in the clinical sense) but also care *about* our patients (in the moral sense).

Diagnostic Testing

The first ethical quandary arises when a patient comes to our clinic and asks us to make, or contribute to, a diagnosis of progressive cognitive decline. The fact of cognitive deterioration, or merely the suspicion that one has dementia, is a personal, moral crisis for the patient. By a twist of fate, or perhaps hereditary, or both, the patient's world is at risk of being fundamentally altered in terms of his or her personal interactions, plans for the future, and overall well-being. Indeed, the threat of dementia places the person's *integrity as a person* at stake.

Before the diagnosis, the ethical issue for the clinician is that of clinical competence, and its flip side, clinical uncertainty. The clinician faces uncertainties about the instruments to use, the proper analysis of the data, and the ultimate interpretation of those data. When reviewing the patient's history, interviewing the patient, and conducting diagnostic testing, clinicians should embark on these tasks with utmost care and sensitivity. Clinicians should have enough knowledge and experience to select tests, when possible, that have known sensitivity and specificity for the diagnosis under consideration to avoid over- or underidentification of the disorder. Clinicians should know how to conduct a reliable examination and to interpret the results and make an appropriate differential diagnoses. Supplementary tests, or descriptive instruments (such as numerous instruments used by SLPs that have not been validated on dementia subjects or age-matched controls) should be used selectively. To avoid overly pessimistic appraisals of the data, clinicians should describe not only functions that are impaired, but also functions that are spared. Finally, an SLP should rarely, if ever, render a diagnosis of dementia. This is properly the realm of a specialized neurologist, who will integrate the findings of the SLP with a host of other data derived from the family history, neurologic examination, laboratory tests, brain scans, and the neuropsychology consultation.

Genetic testing and counseling usually is not within the purview of the SLP, but a working knowledge is important to understanding the significance of these types of tests. Any discussion of family history, genetic testing, and genetic counseling should normally be deferred to individuals on the team who are especially trained in human genetics. Clinicians should be aware that if a patient has been given a positive received a positive genetic test result, such as a mutation chromosome 19, this does not mean the patient has Alzheimer's dementia, or even that he definitely will acquire the disease. In most instances, a genetic mutation merely increases the *risk* for acquiring dementia, and using genetic tests for routine diagnostic purposes is not recommended at this time.

After the diagnosis of an irreversible dementia has been rendered (with a reasonable degree of clinical certainty), the issue shifts away from uncertainty toward certainty. But what is the clinician, in partnership with the patient, actually certain of at this point? The dementias are extremely heterogeneous not only in age of onset but also in rate of progression, pattern of progression, presence or absence of comorbidities, and duration of survival after the diagnosis is made. In the face of these unknowns for a given patient, clinicians nevertheless begin structuring appropriate remedial and compensatory programs of care. As in our work with other types of neurogenic speech–language disorders, the program will be individualized. When caring for dementia patients, however, goals will normally be conservative rather than ambitious; prognostic statements will be cautious rather than confident; and, the need to adapt to the ever-changing circumstances of the patient's illness will be mandatory rather than optional. Both prudence and candor in counseling demented patients about their progress, or lack thereof, require not only competence on the clinician's part but also moral courage. Sharing bad news with patients (Buckman, 1992) is a difficult but necessary part of the SLP's work with progressive neurodegenerative disorders.

Privacy and Confidentiality

Privacy and confidentiality are related ethical issues. If the patient's medical record indicates a positive history for alcoholism, psychiatric disease, or chromosomal abnormality, the clinician should regard this information as particularly sensitive. Clinicians should avoid discussing these sensitive bits of information with the patient (who may not be aware of,

or appreciate the significance of, the information) unless the information is *directly pertinent* to the diagnosis or treatment at hand. The clinician should never discuss sensitive medical details with the patient's family members without the express advance permission of the patient. For example, genetic testing has potential implications for the patient's siblings or children; as such, it is particularly sensitive information, and should not be shared with third parties (Post & Whitehouse, 1998). Similarly, as rules about the privacy of medical records are tightened, clinicians are advised to be particularly careful about sharing information with other clinicians or agencies that are not directly pertinent to speech–language pathology, or for which an explicit release of information has not been obtained (HIPAA, 2002). Attention to privacy and confidentiality is important not only because it is the law but also because it is important to the patient's dignity (Hughes & Louw, 2002).

Adjustment to the Disorder

Upon learning they have dementia, patients are certain to react to this knowledge. Patients' reactions to their dementing illness are rarely benign and often extreme. Some react bravely; some are frightened and depressed; others are anxious and hostile. In some cases, clinicians realize that referral for neuropsychiatric care is essential. If a patient seems to be coping well, but one day shares suicidal ideation with a clinician, the clinician should know to take such a situation absolutely seriously, and walk the patient immediately to the emergency room if need be. Clinicians who choose to work with such patients develop character virtues of empathy, patience, and prudence (good judgment). In short, clinicians who work with individuals with dementia have to do more than "test" and "treat" the disorder; working with dementia patients requires more than clinical competence. Sometimes helping patients and being true to our code of ethics means stepping out of our white coats and truly stepping into a relationship with the patient.

Intervention

Engaging in therapeutic intervention with persons with dementia is fraught with challenges. Again, the problem is one of uncertainty. Not only do we lack clinical evidence of effectiveness in much that we do on behalf of dementia patients (although this situation is improving), we also lack moral uncertainty about whether our efforts, albeit well meaning, are really doing them any good in the long run. In the interest of justice (or fairness) to each patient, we are ethically bound to give him an opportunity to receive services if we think he has a reasonable chance of benefiting within a reasonable period of time. On the other hand, the same ethical principle requires us to avoid treating a patient when he cannot benefit, at the risk of depriving others who also want access to our services, or misusing scarce health care dollars.

During the period that we are involved in a therapeutic endeavor with the patient, we should strive to engage him as a shared decision maker in goal setting and in choosing particular tasks. To accomplish a true partnership, clinicians should not only explain goals but also negotiate them. Frank and continuing dialogue with patients is at the heart of our ethical work with them (Post, Ripich, & Whitehouse, 1994). Having embarked on the use of certain tasks, facilitation techniques or compensatory aids, the clinician should ask the patient whether he likes them, or finds them effective. As in therapy programs with other types of patients, the clinician should keep the patient informed of his progress, in candid and supportive terms. Respect for the patient requires that we convey information in an atmosphere that supports his truly autonomous choices, even if that choice means an informed refusal of what we have offered. Finally, clinicians must recognize that our ethical duty to "do good" sometimes requires that we stipulate modest, practical goals, with carefully defined time limits. In turn, our ethical duty to "avoid harm" requires us to advise the patient gently when our services are no longer helping, and to prepare him for the discontinuance of therapy.

Research

Another area that requires particular care and attention to the ethics of our work is that of research. The dementias are intellectually challenging disease entities, in part because there is so much more to learn about them. Research is multifaceted and necessary. At the same time, persons with dementia are vulnerable, and it is our duty to protect them from any harm that may occur in the research process (Karlawish & Casarett, 2001). For example, dementia patients may confuse the roles of the clinician and the researcher, particularly if the clinician *is* the researcher.

To conceptualize the ethical dimensions of this research scenario, imagine that you are a conducting a research study on the story-retelling abilities of individuals with mild Alzheimer's dementia. You told your patient that you are inviting him to participate in research, that there is no risk to him in choosing to participate, that he has a right to refuse participation, and that he may withdraw at any time (U.S. Department of Health and Human Services, National Institutes of Health, 2001). You tailored your consent document and conversation to his level of language ability; in short, you have properly informed him (Marson, Catterjee, Ingram, & Harrell, 1996). In addition, you verified that he recognized the word *research* and that he understood the aims of your project. Nevertheless, your protocol involves speech–language test instruments and interactions that are very much like your speech–language treatment sessions. The patient may not actually perceive any difference, and, in fact, may not really appreciate the difference. This is known as the therapeutic misconception (Lidz & Appelbaum, 2002). Even though your research protocol is not intended to help him directly in any way, and you certainly did not coerce him to participate, he may believe that you would never do anything contrary to his best interests, or, because he is dependent on you for his care, that he really did not have a choice but to agree, or, that this project is, in fact, intended to help him.

This hypothetical scenario illustrates that when a dementia clinician also wears a researcher's hat, she has a heightened duty to the patient to avoid coercion or other inadvertent harms (World Medical Association, 2000). Ideally, someone other than a researcher should conduct the informed consent procedures. In addition, the patient's legally authorized surrogate decision maker should participate in these discussions (Koppelman, 2002). Finally, the clinician has a duty to reassess the validity of the patient's consent continuously throughout the research project, as a safeguard against changes in cognitive status over time. If, at any time, the clinician-researcher perceives undue risks to the patient, for example, unforeseen harm to his psychological well-being or dignity, she has a duty to hold his interests paramount and remove him from the research study.

✦ Conclusion

Dementia is a symptom of several neurodegenerative diseases of which Alzheimer's disease is the most common. Diagnostic assessment of persons with dementia determines the stage of the disease. As the dementia advances, cognitive-communicative abilities decline. Management of the disease is dependent on the stage or severity level as well as the deficits present. Intervention is an important part of management and can be provided in group or individual sessions guided by the needs of the person with dementia. Then, the SLP decides which type of intervention would most likely benefit the patients and caregivers. Once the intervention is selected, the SLP considers which strategies are most appropriate for therapy. It is important for the SLP to monitor progress monthly and reevaluate the cognitive status of the person with dementia every 6 months. Recognizing that the nature of the neurodegenerative disease will cause a decline in performance, continual reassessment should focus on recording current functional communication levels and selecting more appropriate intervention strategies as necessary.

Ethical issues in this chapter have been premised on several themes. The first is that we have an ethical duty to hold the interests of our patients paramount, a principle that is broad enough to encompass respect for autonomy, nonmaleficence, beneficence, and justice. We have an obligation to respect each patient, and to facilitate autonomy in his decision making as much as possible, be that in the clinical or research arena (Kim, Karlawish, & Caine, 2002). Finally, in the interest of fairness to all patients, we have an ethical duty to offer services when we are reasonably certain we can help, and to discontinue our services when we are reasonably certain we cannot. Some uncertainties will inevitably surround our work with dementia patients. SLPs cannot avoid uncertainty, but can master working with dementia patients by staying current in the literature, collaborating with other disciplines, adhering to ethical principles, and truly caring for their patients.

Study Questions

1. Describe the stages of language changes through the course of Alzheimer's disease.
2. What four areas should be included in a complete diagnostic evaluation for dementia?
3. Describe four evaluation tools used to assess cognition, three used to assess language, and two used to assess cognitive-linguistic skills.
4. Discuss intervention methods appropriate for individuals with dementia. Discuss intervention methods appropriate for group settings.
5. Describe the FOCUSED Program for caregivers.
6. Discuss the four principles that guide ethical practice of care for persons with dementia.

References

Allison, R.S. (1962). *The Senile Brain*. London: Edward Arnold

Alprin, S.I. (1980). Unpublished Study of Staff Attitudes After Validation. Cleveland: Cleveland State University

American Psychiatric Association. (1994). *Diagnostic and Statistical Manual of Mental Disorders*, 4th ed., rev. (pp. 133–155). Washington, DC: American Psychiatric Association

American Speech–Language-Hearing Association (ASHA). (1987). Role of Speech–Language Pathologist in the Habilitation and Rehabilitation of Cognitively Impaired Individuals. *ASHA, 29,* 53–55

American Speech–Language-Hearing Association (ASHA). (1988a). Committee on Communication Problems in Aging: The Roles of Speech–Language Pathologists and Audiologists in Working with Older Persons. *ASHA, 30,* 80–84

American Speech–Language-Hearing Association (ASHA). (1988b). Committee on Communication Problems in Aging: Provision of Audiology and Speech–Language Pathology Services to Older Persons in the nursing home. *ASHA, 30,* 72–74

American Speech–Language-Hearing Association (ASHA). (2003). Code of Ethics. *ASHA Supplement, 23,* 13–15

Anderson, J.R. (1983). A Spreading Activation Theory of Memory. *Journal of Verbal Learning Behavior, 22,* 261–295

Anderson, R.N. (2001). Deaths: Leading Causes for 1999. *National Vital Statistics Reports, 49(11),* 1–88

Appell, J., Kertesz, A., & Fisman, M. (1982). A Study of Language Functioning in Alzheimer's Patients. *Brain and Language, 17,* 73–91

Arkin, S. (1991). Memory Training in Early Alzheimer's Disease: An Optimistic Look at the Field. *American Journal of Alzheimer's Care and Related Disorders & Research, 7,* 17–25

Baines, S., Saxby, P., & Ehlert, K. (1987). Reality Orientation and Reminiscence Therapy: A Controlled Cross-Over Study of Confused Elderly People. *British Journal of Psychiatry, 151,* 222–231

Barker, M.G., & Lawson, J.S. (1968). Nominal Aphasia in Dementia. *British Journal of Psychiatry, 114,* 1351–1356

Bayles, K.A. (1982). Language Function in Senile Dementia. *Brain and Language, 16,* 265–280

Bayles, K.A. (1984). Language and Dementia. In A. Holland (Ed.), *Language Disorders in Adults*. Austin, TX: Pro-Ed

Bayles, K.A. (1986). Management of Neurogenic Communication Disorders Associated with Dementia. In: R. Chapey (Ed.), *Language Intervention Strategies in Adult Aphasia*, 2nd ed. (pp. 462–473). Baltimore: Williams & Wilkins

Bayles, K.A., & Boone, D.R. (1982). The Potential of Language Tasks for Identifying Senile Dementia. *Journal of Speech and Hearing Disorders, 47,* 210–217

Bayles, K.A., Boone, D.R., Tomoeda, C.A., et al. (1989). Differentiating Alzheimer's Patients from the Normal Elderly and Stroke Patients with Aphasia. *Journal of Speech and Hearing Disorders, 54,* 74–87

Bayles, K.A., & Kaszniak, A.W. (1987). *Communication and Cognition in Normal Aging and Dementia*. Austin, TX: Pro-Ed

Bayles, K.A., & Tomoeda, C.K. (1991). Caregiver Report of Prevalence and Appearance Order of Linguistic Symptoms in Alzheimer's Patients. *Gerontologist, 31,* 210–216

Bayles, K.A., & Tomoeda, C.K. (1993). *Arizona Battery for Communication Disorders of Dementia*. Tucson, AZ: Canyonlands Publishing

Bayles, K.A., & Tomoeda, C.K. (1994). *Functional Linguistic Communication Inventory*. Tucson, AZ: Canyonlands Publishing

Bayles, K.A., Tomoeda, C.K., & Caffrey, J.T. (1983) Language in Dementia Producing Diseases. *Communication Disorders, 7,* 131–146

Beauchamp T.L., & Childress J.F. (1994). *Principles of Biomedical Ethics*, 4th ed. New York: Oxford University Press

Blessed, G., Tomlinson, B.E., & Roth M. (1968). The Association Between Quantitative Measures of Dementia and of Senile Change in the Cerebral Grey Matter of Elderly Subjects. *British Journal of Psychiatry, 114,* 797–811

Borkowski, J.G., Benton, A.L., & Spreen, O. (1967). Word Fluency and Brain Damage. *Neuropsychologia, 5,* 135–140

Bourgeois, M.S. (1992). Evaluating Memory Wallets in Conversations with Persons with Dementia. *Journal of Speech and Hearing Research, 35,* 1344–1357

Bourgeois, M.S., Dijkstra, K., Burgio, L., & Allen-Burge, R. (2001). Memory Aids as an Augmentative and Alternative Communication Strategy for Nursing Home Residents with Dementia. *AAC Augmentative and Alternative Communication, 17,* 196–210

Brookshire, R.H., & Nicholas L.E. (1993). *The Discourse Comprehension Test*. Tucson, AZ: Communication Skill Builders/The Psychological Corporation

Brush, J.A., & Camp, C.J. (1998). Using Spaced Retrieval as an Intervention During Speech–Language Therapy. *Clinical Gerontologist, 19,* 51–64

Buckman, R. (1992). How to Break Bad News: A Guide for Health Care Professionals. Baltimore, MD: Johns Hopkins University Press

Burton, M. (1982). Reality Orientation for the Elderly: A Critique. *Journal of Advanced Nursing, 7,* 427–433

Buschke, H., Kulansky, G., Katz, M., et al. (1999). Screening for dementia with the Memory Impairment Screen. *Neurology, 52,* 231–238

Carroll, D. (1989). *When Your Loved One has Alzheimer's Disease*. New York: Harper and Row

Clark, L.W. (1991). Caregiver Stress and Communication Management in Alzheimer's Disease. In: D. Ripich, (Ed.), *Handbook of Geriatric Communication Disorders* (pp. 127–142). Austin, TX: Pro-Ed

Clark, L.W. (1995). Interventions for Persons with Alzheimer's Disease: Strategies for Maintaining and Enhancing Communicative Success. *Language Disorders, 15,* 47–65

Clark, L.W., & Witte, K. (1989). Dealing with Dementia in Long-Term Care. Miniseminar Presentation for Annual Convention on New York State Speech, Language, and Hearing Association, Kiamesha Lake, New York

Constantinidis, J. (1978). Is Alzheimer's Disease a Major Form of Senile Dementia? Clinical, Anatomical, and Genetic Data. In R. Katzman, R.D. Terry, & K.L. Bick (Eds.), *Alzheimer's Disease: Senile Dementia and Related Disorders* (pp. 15–25). New York: Raven Press

Crum, R.M., Anthony, J.C., Bassett, S.S., & Folstein, M.F. (1993). Population-Based Norms for the Mini-Mental State Examination by Age and Educational Level. *Journal of the American Medical Association, 18,* 2386–2391

Cummings, J.L., & Benson, D.F. (1983). *Dementia: A Clinical Approach*. Boston: Butterworth

Cummings, J.L., Benson, D.F., Hill, M.A., & Read, S. (1985). Aphasia in Dementia of the Alzheimer's type. *Neurology, 35,* 394–397

Daffner, K.R. (1996). Alzheimer's Disease and Related Disorders. In: M.A. Samuels & S. Feske (Eds.), *Office Practice of Neurology* (pp. 710–715) New York: Churchill Livingstone

Day, J.C. (1996). *Population Projections of the United States by Age, Sex, Race, and Hispanic Origin: 1995 to 2050*. U.S. Bureau of the Census, Current Population Reports, P25-1130. Washington, DC: U.S. Government Printing Office

De Ajuriaguerra, J., & Tissot, R. (1975). Some Aspects of Language in Various Forms of Senile Dementia: Comparisons with Language in Childhood. In: E.H. Lenneberg, & E. Lenneberg (Eds.), *Foundations of Language Development* vol. 1, (pp. 325–339). New York: Academic Press

Deal, J., Wertz, R., & Spring, C. (1981). Differentiating Aphasia and the Language of Generalized Intellectual Impairment. In: *Clinical Aphasiology Conference Proceedings* (pp. 166–173). Minneapolis: BRK Publishers

DeRenzi, E., & Faglioni, P. (1978). Normative Data and Screening Power of a Shortened Version of the Token Test. *Cortex, 14,* 41–49

DeRenzi, E., Ferrari, C. (1978). The Reporter's Test: A Sensitive Test to Detect Expressive Disturbances in Aphasia. *Cortex, 14,* 279–293

Dietch, J.T., Hewett, L.J., & Jones, S. (1989). Adverse Effects of Reality Orientation. *Journal of the American Geriatrics Society, 37,* 974–976

Dunn, L.M., & Dunn, L.M. (1997). *Peabody Picture Vocabulary Test, Revised*. Circle Pines, MN: American Guidance Service

Emery, O.B. (1988). Language and Memory Processing in Senile Dementia of the Alzheimer's Type. In: L.L. Light, & D.M. Burke (Eds.), *Language, Memory, and Aging* (pp. 221–243). New York: Cambridge University Press

Emery, V.O.B. (2000). Language Impairment in Dementia of the Alzheimer's Type: A Hierarchical Decline? *International Journal of Psychiatry in Medicine, 30,* 145–164

Ernest, B., Dalby, M., & Dalby, A. (1970). Aphasic Disturbances in Presenile Dementia. *Acta Neurologica Scandinavica, 46,* 99–100

Faber-Langendoen. K., Morris, J.C., Knesevich, J.W., et al, (1988). Aphasia in Senile Dementia of the Alzheimer Type. *Annals of Neurology, 23,* 365–370

Feil, N. (1992). Validation Therapy. *Geriatric Nursing, 13,* 129–133

Fisher, N.J., Tierney, M.C., Snow, G.W., & Szalai, J.P. (1999). Odd/Even Short Forms of the Boston Naming Test: Preliminary Geriatric Norms. *Clinical Neuropsychologist, 13,* 359–364

Folsom, J.C., & Folsom, G.S. (1974). The Real World. *Mental Health, 58,* 29–33. National Association for Mental Health

Folstein, M.F., Folstein, S.E., & McHugh, P.R. (1975). Mini-Mental State: A Practical Method for Grading the Cognitive State of Patients for the Clinician. *Journal of Psychiatric Research, 12,* 189–198

Folstein, M.F., Folstein, S.E., McHugh, P.R., & Fanjiang, T. (2000). *Mini-Mental State Examination*. San Antonio, TX: The Psychological Corporation

Fritz, A. (1986). *The Language of Resolution Among the Old-Old: The Effect of Validation Therapy on Two Levels of Cognitive Confusion*. Unpublished paper

Fromm, D., & Holland, A. (1987). Functional Communication in Alzheimer's Disease. Paper presented at the American Speech–Language–Hearing Association Conference, New Orleans

Fuh, J.L., Teng, E.L., Lin, K.N., et al. (1995). The Informant Questionnaire on Cognitive Decline in the Elderly (IQCODE) as a Screening Tool for Predominantly Illiterate Chinese Population. *Neurology, 45,* 92–95

Ganguli, M., Belle, S., Ratcliff, G., et al. (1993). Sensitivity and Specificity for Dementia of Population-Based Criteria for Cognitive Impairment. The Movies Project. *Journal of Gerontology, 48,* M152–M161

Gilligan, C. (1982). *In a Different Voice: Psychological Theory and Women's Moral Development.* Cambridge, MA: Harvard University Press

Goldfarb, A.I. (1975). Memory and Aging. In: R. Goldman & M. Rockstein (Eds.), *The Physiology and Pathology of Human Aging.* New York: Academic Press

Goodglass, H., Kaplan, E., & Barresi, B. (2000). *Boston Diagnostic Aphasia Examination,* 3rd ed. Baltimore: Lippincott Williams & Wilkins

Greene, J.G., Timbury, G.C., Smith, R., et al. (1983). Reality Orientation with Elderly Patients in the Community: An Empirical Evaluation. *Age & Aging, 12,* 38–43

Grober, E., Buschke, H., & Kawas, C., et al. (1985). Impaired Ranking of Semantic Attributes in Dementia. *Brain and Language, 26,* 276–286

Grossman, M. (1978). The Game of the Name: An Examination of Linguistic Reference After Brain Damage. *Brain and Language, 6,* 112–119

Hachinski, V.C., Lassen, N.A., & Marshall, J. (1974). Multi-Infarct Dementia: A Case of Mental Deterioration in the Elderly. *Lancet, 2,* 207–209

Halpern, H., Darley, F., & Brown, J. (1973). Differential Language and Neurological Characteristics in Cerebral Involvement. *Journal of Speech and Hearing Disorders, 38,* 162–173

Hamilton, M. (1967). Development of a Rating Scale for Primary Depression Illness. *British Journal of Social and Clinical Psychology, 6,* 278–296

Harris, J.L. (1997). Reminiscence: A Culturally and Developmentally Appropriate Language Intervention for Older Adults. *American Journal of Speech–Language Pathology, 6,* 19–26

Harris, J.L. (1998). *The Source for Reminiscence Therapy.* East Moline, IL: Lingui Systems

Harris, J.L., & Norman, M.L. (2002). Reframing Reminiscence as a Cognitive-Linguistic Phenomenon. In: J.D. Webster & B. Haight (Eds.), *Critical Advances in Reminiscence: From Theory to Application* (pp. 95–105). New York: Springer

Hart, S. (1988). Language and Dementia: A Review. *Psychological Medicine, 18,* 99–112

Heaton, R. (1993). *Wisconsin Card Sorting Test Manual.* Odessa, FL: Psychological Assessment Resource

Helm-Estabrooks, N. (2001). *Cognitive-Linguistic Quick Test.* New York: Psychological Corporation

HIPAA (Health Information Portability and Accountability Act). (2002). Standards for Privacy of Individually Identifiable Health Information. 45 CFR Parts 160 and 164; Final Rule 67 (157) Fed. Reg. 53,181–53, 273

Hobbs, F.B., & Damon, B.L. (1996). Sixty-Five (65+) in the United States. U.S. Bureau of the Census, Current Population Reports, Special Studies, P23-190. Washington, DC: U.S. Government Printing Office

Holland, A., McBurney, D.H., Moossy, J., et al. (1985). The Dissolution of Language in Pick's Disease with Neurofibrillary Tangles: A Case Study. *Brain and Language, 24,* 36–58

Horner, J., Dawson, D.V., Heyman, A., & Fish, A.M. (1992). The Usefulness of the Western Aphasia Battery for Differential Diagnosis of Alzheimer Dementia and Focal Stroke Syndromes. *Brain and Language, 42,* 77–88

Horner, J., & Heyman, A. (1981). Language Changes Associated with Alzheimer's Dementia: A Discussion Section. In: Brookshire RH (Ed.), *Clinical Aphasiology Conference Proceedings* (pp. 330–336). Minneapolis: BRK Publishers

Horner, J., Heyman, A., Dawson, D.V., & Rogers H. (1988). The Relationship of Agraphia to the Severity of Dementia in Alzheimer's Disease. *Archives of Neurology, 45,* 760–763

Huff, F.J., Corkin, S., & Growdon, J.H. (1986). Semantic Impairment and Anomia in Alzheimer's Disease. *Brain and Language, 28,* 235–249

Hughes, C.P., Berg, L., Danziger, W.L., Coben, L.A., & Martin, R.L. (1982). A New Clinical Scale for the Staging of Dementia. *British Journal of Psychiatry, 140,* 566–572

Hughes, J.C., & Louw, S.J. (2002). Confidentiality and Cognitive Impairment: Professional and Philosophical Ethics. Age Ageing, *31,* 147–150

Hughston, G.A., & Merriam, S.B. (1982). Reminiscence: A Non-Formal Technique for Improving Cognitive Functioning in the Aged. *International Journal of Aging and Human Development, 15,* 139–149

Hussian, R.A. (1981). *Geriatric Psychology: A Behavioral Perspective.* New York: Van Nostrand Reinhold

Hutchinson, J.M., & Jensen, M.A. (1980). A Pragmatic Evaluation of Discourse Communication in Normal and Senile Elderly in a Nursing Home. In: L. Obler & M. Albert (Eds.), *Language and Communication in the Elderly* (pp. 59–64). Lexington, MA: D.C. Heath

Irigaray, L. (1967). Approche Psycholinguistique de Langage des Dements. *Neuropsychologia, 5,* 25–52

Irigaray, L. (1973). *Le Langage des Dements.* The Hague: Mouton

Ishii-Kuntz, M. (1990). Social Interaction and Social Well-Being: Comparison Across Stages of Adulthood. *International Journal of Aging and Human Development, 30,* 15–35

Judge, K.S., Camp, C.J., & Orsulic-Jeras, S. (2000). Use of Montessori-Based Activities for Clients with Dementia in Adult Day Care: Effects on Engagement. *American Journal of Alzheimer's Disease, 15,* 42–46

Juva, K., Sulkava, R., Erkinjuntti, T., et al. (1995). Usefulness of the Clinical Dementia Rating Scale in Screening for Dementia. *International Psychogeriatrics, 7,* 17–24

Kahn, R., Goldfarb, A., Pollack, M., & Peck, A. (1960). Brief Objective Measures for the Determination of Mental Status in the aged. *American Journal of Psychiatry, 117,* 236–238

Kant, I. (1785). Grounding of the Metaphysics of Morals. In: D. Bonevac (Ed.). *Today's Moral Issues: Classic and Contemporary Perspectives,* 3rd ed. (pp. 33–42). London: Mayfield Publishing, 1999

Kaplan, E., Goodglass, H., & Weintraub, S. (1983). *Boston Naming Test.* Philadelphia: Lea & Febiger

Karlawish, J.H., Casarett, D. (2001). Addressing the Ethical Challenges of Clinical Trials that Involve Patients with Dementia. *Journal of Geriatric Psychiatry and Neurology, 14,* 222–228

Kaszniak, A.W., & Wilson, R.S. (1985). Longitudinal Deterioration of Language and Cognition in Dementia of the Alzheimer's Type. In: *Communication and Cognition in Dementia: Longitudinal Perspectives.* Symposium conducted at the International Neuropsychological Association, San Diego, CA

Kempler, D. (1988). Lexical and Pantomime Abilities of Alzheimer's Disease. *Aphasiology, 2,* 147–159

Kempler, D. (1995). Language Changes in Dementia of the Alzheimer's Type. In: R. Lubinski (Ed.), *Dementia and Communication* (pp. 98–114). San Diego: Singular Publishing Group

Kempler, D., Curtiss, S., & Jackson, C. (1987) Syntactic Preservation in Alzheimer's Disease. *Journal of Speech and Hearing Research, 30,* 343–350

Kertesz, A. (1979). *Aphasia and Associated Disorders.* New York: Grune & Stratton

Kertesz, A. (1982). *Western Aphasia Battery.* San Antonio, TX: Psychological Corporation

Kiernan, R.J., Mueller, J., & Langston, J.W. (1995). *Cognistat (Neurobehavioral Cognitive Status Examination).* Lutz, FL: Psychological Assessment Resources

Kiernan, R.J., Mueller, J., Langston, J.W., & Van Dyke, C. (1987). The Neurobehavioral Cognitive Status Examination: A Brief but Differentiated Approach to Cognitive Assessment. *Annals of Internal Medicine, 107,* 481–485 (Originally published by the Northern California Neurobehavioral Group, 1983)

Kim, S.Y., Karlawish, J.H., & Caine, E.D. (2002). Current State of Research on Decision-Making Competence of Cognitively Impaired Elderly Persons. *American Journal of Geriatric Psychiatry, 10,* 151–165

Kimbarow, M.L., & Ripich, D.N. (1989). Task Influences on Discourse Production in Adults. Paper presented at the annual conference of the American Speech–Language–Hearing Association, St. Louis

Kinney, J.M., & Stephens, M.A.P. (1989). Caregiving Hassles Scale: Assessing the Daily Hassles of Caring for a Family Member with Dementia. *Gerontologist, 29,* 328–332

Kirshner, H.S., Webb, W.G., Kelly, M.P., et al. (1984). Language Disturbance: An Initial Symptom of Cortical Degenerations and Dementia. *Archives of Neurology, 41,* 491–496

Kokmen, E., Smith, G.E., Petersen, R.C., et al. (1991). The Short Test of Mental Status: Correlations with Standardized Psychometric Testing. *Archives of Neurology, 48,* 725–728

Koppelman, E.R. (2002). Dementia and Dignity: Towards a New Method of Surrogate Decision Making. *Journal of Medical Philosophy, 27,* 65–85

Kukull, W.A., Larson, E.B., Terri, L., et al. (1994) The Mini-Mental State Examination Score and the Clinical Diagnosis of Dementia. *Journal of Clinical Epidemiology, 47,* 1061–1067

Lam, L.C.W., Chiu, H.F.K., Li, S.W., et al. (1997). Screening for Dementia: A Preliminary Study on the Validity of the Chinese Version of the Blessed-Roth Dementia Scale. *International Psychogeriatrics, 9,* 39–46

LaMendola, W.F., & Pellegrini, R.V. (1979). Quality of Life and Coronary Artery Bypass Surgery Patients. *Social Sciences Medicine, 13,* 457–461

Larson, R. (1978). Thirty Years of Research on the Subjective Well-Being of Older Americans. *Journal of Gerontology, 33,* 109–125

Lidz, C.W., & Appelbaum, P.S. (2002). The Therapeutic Misconception: Problems and Solutions. *Medical Care, 40,* V55–V63

Linebarger, M., Schwartz, M., & Saffran, E. (1983). Sensitivity to Grammatical Structure in So-called Agrammatic Aphasics. *Cognition, 13,* 361–392

Loewenstein, D.A., Duara, R., Arguelles, T., et al. (1995). Use of the Fuld Object-Memory Evaluation in the Detection of Mild Dementia Among Spanish and English-Speaking Groups. *American Journal of Geriatric Psychiatry, 3,* 300–307

MacDonald, M.L., & Settin, J.M. (1978). Reality Orientation vs. Sheltered Workshops as Treatment for the Institutionalized Aging. *Journal of Gerontology, 33,* 416–421

Mappes, T.A., & DeGrazia, D. (2001). *Biomedical Ethics*, 5th ed. (pp. 31–33). Boston: McGraw-Hill

Marson, D.C., Catterjee, A., Ingram, K.K., & Harrell, L.E. (1996). Toward a Neurologic Model of Competency: Cognitive Predictors of Capacity to Consent in Alzheimer's Disease Using Three Different Legal Standards. *Neurology, 46*, 666–672

Mateer, C., & Sohlberg, M. (1988). A Paradigm Shift in Memory Rehabilitation. In: H. Whitaker (Ed.), *Neuropsychological Studies of Non-Focal Brain Injury: Dementia and Closed Head Injury* (pp. 180–210). New York: Springer-Verlag

Mattis, S. (1976). Mental Status Examination for Organic Mental Syndrome in the Elderly Patient. In: L. Bellak, T.B. Karuso (Eds.). *Geriatric Psychiatry*. New York: Grune & Stratton

McKhann, G., Drachman, D., Folstein, M., et al. (1984). Clinical Diagnosis of Alzheimer's Disease: Report of the NINCDS-ADRDA Work Group under the Auspices of Department of Health and Human Services Task Force on Alzheimer's Disease. *Neurology, 34*, 939–944

McNeil, M.R., & Prescott, T.E. (1982). *Revised Token Test*. Los Angeles: Western Psychological Services

Miller, E., & Morris, R. (1993). Management of Dementia. In: E. Miller & R. Morris (Eds.), *The Psychology of Dementia*. Chichester: John Wiley & Sons

Molloy, D.W., & Standish, T.I. (1997). A Guide to the Standardized Mini-Mental State Examination. *International Psychogeriatrics, 9(suppl 1)*, 87–94

Monsch, A.U., Bondi, M.W., Salmon, D.P., et al. (1995). Clinical Validity of the Mattis Dementia Rating Scale in Detecting Dementia of the Alzheimer Type: A Double Cross-Validation and Application to A Community-Dwelling Sample. *Archives of Neurology, 52*, 899–904

Morris, J.C., Heyman, A., Mohs, R.C., et al. (1989). The Consortium to Establish a Registry for Alzheimer's Disease (CERAD). Part 1. Clinical and Neuropsychological Assessment of Alzheimer's Disease. *Neurology, 39*, 1159–1165

Morton, I., & Bleathman, C. (1991). The Effectiveness of Validation Therapy in Dementia: A Pilot Study. *International Journal of Geriatric Psychiatry, 6*, 327–330

Murdoch, B.E., Chenery, H.J., Wilks, V., et al. (1987). Language Disorders in Dementia of the Alzheimer's Type. *Brain and Language, 31*, 122–137

Neary, D., Snowden, J.S., Gustafson, L., et al. (1998). Frontotemporal Lobar Degeneration: A Consensus on Clinical Diagnostic Criteria. *Neurology, 51*, 1546–1554

Neils, J., Boller, F., Cole, M., et al. (1987). Naming Ability in Mild Alzheimer's Disease Subjects. Paper presented at the annual convention of the American Speech–Language–Hearing Association, New Orleans, LA

Nomura, T. (2002). *Evaluative Research on Reminiscence Groups for People with Dementia*. In: J.D. Webster & B.K. Haight (Eds.), *Critical Advances in Reminiscence Work: From Theory to Application* (pp. 289–299). New York: Springer

Obler, L.K. (1981). Review of *Le Langage des dements*, by L. Irgaray, 1973. The Hague: Mouton. *Brain and Language, 12*, 375–386

Obler, L.K. (1983). Language and Brain Dysfunction in Dementia. In: S. Segalowitz (Ed.), *Language Functions and Brain Organization* (pp. 267–282). New York: Academic Press

Orange, J.B. (1991). Perspectives of Family Members Regarding Communication Changes. In: R. Lubinski (Ed.), *Dementia and Communication*. Philadelphia: Mosby–Year Book

Osborn, C. (1989). Reminiscence: When the Past Eases the Present. *Journal of Gerontology Nursing, 15*, 6–12

Pellegrino, E.D., & Thomasma, D.C. (1993). The Virtues in Medical Practice. New York: Oxford University Press

Peoples, N. (1982). Validation Therapy Versus Reality Orientation as Treatment for Disoriented Institutionalized Elderly. Unpublished master's thesis. Akron, OH: University of Akron

Petersen, R.C., Stevens, J.C., Ganguli, M., et al. (2001). Practice parameter: Early detection of dementia: Mild cognitive Impairment (and Evidence-Based Review). *Neurology, 56*, 1133–1142

Porch, B.E. (1967). *Porch Index of Communicative Abilities*. Palo Alto, CA: Consulting Psychologists Press

Post, S.G., Ripich, D.N., & Whitehouse, P.J. (1994). Discourse Ethics: Research, Dementia, and Communication. *Alzheimer's Disease and Associated Disorders, 8(suppl 4)*, 58–65

Post, S.G., & Whitehouse, P.J. (Eds.). (1998). Genetic Testing for Alzheimer Disease: Ethical and Clinical Issues. Baltimore: Johns Hopkins University Press

Poulshock, S.W., & Deimling, G.T. (1984). Families Caring for Elders in Residence: Issues in the Measurement of Burden. *Journal of Gerontology, 39*, 230–239

Rabins, P. (1982). Management of Irreversible Dementia. *Psychosometics, 22*, 591–597

Reisberg, B. (1981). *Brain Failure: An Introduction to Current Concepts of Senility*. New York: Free Press/Macmillan

Reisberg, B. (1983). *Alzheimer's Disease: The Standard Reference* (pp. 178–179). New York: Free Press

Reisberg, B., Ferris, S.H., DeLeon, M.J., & Crook, T. (1982). The Global Deterioration Scale for Assessment of Primary Degenerative Dementia. *American Journal of Psychiatry, 139*, 1136–1139

Reitan, R.M., & Wolfson, D. (1985). *The Halstead-Reitan Neuropsychological Test Battery*. Tucson, AZ: Neuropsychological Press

Ripich, D.N. (1991). Language and Communication in Dementia. In: D. Ripich (Ed.), *Handbook of Geriatric Communication Disorders* (pp. 255–283). Austin, TX: Pro-Ed

Ripich, D.N. (1996). *Alzheimer's Disease Communication Guide: The FOCUSED Program for Caregivers*. San Antonio, TX: The Psychological Corporation

Ripich, D.N., Carpenter, B., & Ziol, E. (1997). Comparison of African-American and White Persons with Alzheimer's Disease on Language Measures. *Neurology, 48*, 781–783

Ripich, D.N., Kercher, K., Wykle, M., Sloan, D., & Ziol, E. (1999). Effects of Communication Training on African-American and White Caregivers of Persons with Alzheimer's disease. *Journal of Aging and Ethnicity, 1*, 1–16

Ripich, D.N., Petrill, S., Whitehouse, P., & Ziol, E. (1995). Gender Differences in AD on Standardized Language Tests. *Neurology, 45*, 299–302

Ripich, D.N., & Terrell, B. (1988). Patterns of Discourse Cohesion and Coherence in Alzheimer's Disease. *Journal of Speech and Hearing Disorders, 53*, 8–15

Ripich, D.N., Terrell, B., & Spinelli, F. (1983). Discourse Cohesion in Senile Dementia of the Alzheimer's Type. In: Brookshire, R.H. (Ed.), *Clinical Aphasiology Conference Proceedings* (pp. 316–321). Minneapolis, IN: BRK Publishers

Ripich, D.N., & Vertes, D.R., Whitehouse, P., et al. (1988). Conversational Discourse Patterns in Senile Dementia of the Alzheimer's Type. Paper presented at the American Speech–Language–Hearing Association Annual Convention, Boston

Ripich, D.N., & Wykle, M. (1990a). A Program for Nursing Assistants, with Alzheimer's Patients. Paper Presented at the American Gerontology in Higher Education Conference, Kansas City, MO

Ripich, D.N., & Wykle, M. (1990b). Developing Healthcare Professionals' Communication Skills with Alzheimer's Disease Patients. Paper Presented at the Annual Meeting of the American Society on Aging, San Francisco, CA

Ripich, D.N., & Ziol E. (1998). Dementia: A Review for the Speech–Language Pathologist. In: A.F. Johnson, & B.H. Jacobson (Eds.), *Medical Speech–Language Pathology: A Practitioner's Guide* (pp. 467–494). New York: Thieme

Ripich, D.N., Ziol, E., & Lee, M. (1998). Longitudinal Effects of Communication Training on Caregivers of Persons with Alzheimer's Disease. *Clinical Gerontologist, 19*, 37–55

Roman, G.C., Tatemichi, T.K., Erkinjuntti, T., et al. (1993). Vascular Dementia: Diagnostic Criteria for Research Studies: Report of the NINDS-AIREN International Workshop. *Neurology, 43*, 250–260

Roper, B.L., Bieliauskas, L.A., et al. (1996). Validity of the Mini-Mental State Examination and the Neurobehavioral Cognitive Status Examination in Cognitive Screening. *Neuropsychiatric Neuropsychology and Behavioral Neurology, 9*, 54–57

Ross-Swain, D., & Fogle, P.T. (1996). *Ross Information Processing Assessment, Geriatric*. Austin: Pro-Ed

Russell, E.W. (1988). Renorming Russell's Version of the Wechsler Memory Scale. *Journal of Clinical and Experimental Neuropsychology, 10*, 235–249

Sclan, S.G., & Reisberg, B. (1992). Functional Assessment Staging (FAST) in Alzheimer's Disease: Reliability, Validity, and Ordinality. *International Psychogeriatrics, 4*, 55–69

Schwamm, L.H., Van Dyke, C., Kiernan, R.J., Merrin, E.L., & Mueller, J. (1987). The Neurobehavioral Cognitive Status Examination: comparison with the Cognitive Capacity Screening Examination and the Mini-Mental State Examination in a neurosurgical population. *Annals of Internal Medicine, 107*, 486–491

Schwartz, M., Marin, O., & Saffran, E. (1979). Dissociations of Language Function in Dementia: A Case Study. *Brain and Language, 7*, 277–306

Shewan, C.M. (1979). *Auditory Comprehension Test for Sentences (ACTS)*. Chicago: Linguistics Clinical Institutes

Shewan, C.M., & Kertesz, A. (1980). Reliability and Validity Characteristics of the Western Aphasia Battery (WAB). *Journal of Speech and Hearing Disorders, 45*, 308–324

Skelton-Robinson, M., & Jones, S. (1984). Nominal Dysphasia and the Severity of Senile Dementia. *British Journal of Psychiatry, 145*, 168–171

Sohlberg, M.M., & Mateer, C.A. (1989). *Introduction to Cognitive Rehabilitation: Theory and Practice*. New York: Guilford Press

Solomon, P.R., Hirschoff, A., Kelly, B., et al. (1998). A 7-Minute Neurocognitive Screening Battery Highly Sensitive to Alzheimer's Disease. *Archives of Neurology, 55*, 349–355

Solomon, P.R., & Pendelbury, W.W. (1998). Recognition of Alzheimer's Disease: The 7-Minute Screen. *Family Medicine, 30*, 265–271

Stephens, L. (Ed.). (1969). *Reality Orientation: A Technique to Rehabilitate Elderly and Brain-Damaged Patients with a Moderate to Severe Degree of Disorientation*. Washington, DC: American Psychiatric Association

Tariot, P.N., Mack, J.L., Patterson, M.B., et al. (1995). The Behavior Rating Scale for Dementia of the Consortium to Establish a Registry for Alzheimer's Disease. *American Journal of Psychiatry, 152*, 1349–1357

Teri, L., Truax, P., Logsdon, X., Uomoto, J., Zarit, S., & Vitaliano P.P. (1992). Assessment of Behavioral Problems in Dementia: The Revised Memory and Behavior Problem Checklist. *Psychology of Aging, 7,* 622–631

Terrell, B., & Ripich, D. (1989). Discourse Competence as a Variable in Intervention. *Seminars in Speech Language Disorders, 24,* 77–92

Ulatowska, H.K., Haynes, S.M., Donnell, A.J., et al. (1986). Discourse Abilities in Dementia. Paper presented at the American Speech–Language–Hearing Association Conference, Detroit

U.S. Department of Health, Education and Welfare, National Commission for the Protection of Human Subjects of Biomedical and Behavioral Research. (1979). The Belmont Report: Ethical Principles and Guidelines for the Protection of Human Subjects of Research (National Research Act, Pub. L. 93–348)

U.S. Department of Health and Human Services, National Institutes of Health. (2001). Protection of Human Subjects. 45C.F.R. Part 46

Veatch, R.M., & Flack, H.E. (1997). *Case Studies in Allied Health Ethics.* Upper Saddle River, NJ: Prentice Hall

Vuorinen, E., Laine, M., & Rinne, J. (2000). Common Pattern of Language Impairment in Vascular Dementia and Alzheimer's Disease. *Alzheimer's Disease and Associated Disorders, 14,* 81–86

Wagner, O., Oesterreich, K., Hoyer, S. (1985). Validity of the Ischemic Score in Degenerative and Vascular Dementia and Depression in Old Age. *Archives of Gerontological Geriatrics, 4,* 333–345

Warrington, E.K. (1975). The Selective Impairment of Semantic Memory. *Quarterly Journal of Experimental Psychology, 27,* 635–657

Watson, J., & Records, L. (1978). The Effectiveness of the Porch Index of Communicative Abilities as a Diagnostic Tool in Assessing Specific Behavior of Senile Dementia. In: *Clinical Aphasiology Conference Proceedings.* Minneapolis: BRK Publishers

Wechsler, D.A. (1981). *Wechsler Adult Intelligence Scale–Revised. Test Manual.* New York: Psychological Corporation

Wechsler, D.A. (1987) *Wechsler Memory Scale–Revised.* San Antonio, TX: Psychological Corporation

Wechsler, D.A. (1997). *Wechsler Adult Intelligence Scale–III. Test Manual.* Psychological Corporation, New York

Welch, L.W., Doineau, D., Johnson, S., & King, D. (1996). Educational and Gender Normative Data for the Boston Naming Test in a Group of Older Adults. *Brain and Language, 53,* 260–266

Welland, R.J., Lubinski, R., & Higginbotham, D.J. (2002). Discourse Comprehension Test Performance of Elders with Dementia of the Alzheimer Type. *Journal of Speech–Language-Hearing Research, 45,* 1175–1187

Welsh, K.A., Butters, N., Mohs, R.C., Beekly, D., Edland, S., Fillenbaum, G., & Heyman, A. (1994). The Consortium to Establish a Registry for Alzheimer's Disease (CERAD). Part V. A Normative Study of the Neuropsychological Battery. *Neurology, 44,* 609–614

Whitaker, H.A. (1976). A Case of the Isolation of Language Function. In: H. Whitaker & H. Whitaker (Eds.), *Studies in Neurolinguistics,* vol. 2. New York: Academic Press

Whitehouse, P.J., & Rabins, P.V. (1992). Quality of Life and Dementia. *Alzheimer's Disease and Associated Disorders, 6,* 135–137

Wiig, E.H., Wiig, Neilsen, N.P., Minthon, L., Warkentin, S. (2002). *Alzheimer's Quick Test (AQT) Assessment of Temporal-Parietal Function.* Palo Alto: Psychological Corporation

Wilder, D., Cross, P., & Chen, M.P.J. (1995). Operating Characteristics of Brief Screens for Dementia in a Multicultural Population. *American Journal of Geriatric Psychiatry, 3,* 96–107

Wing, J.K., Cooper, J.E., & Sartorius, N. (1974). *The Measurement and Classification of Psychiatric Symptoms.* Cambridge: Cambridge University Press

World Medical Association. (2000). The Helsinki Declaration: Ethical Principles for Medical Research Involving Human Subjects. 52nd WMA General Assembly, Edinburgh, Scotland. http://www.wma.net/e/policy/17-c_e.html.

Zarit, J.M. (1982). Predictors of Burden and Stress for Caregivers of Senile Dementia Patients. Unpublished doctoral dissertation. University of Southern California, San Diego

Zgola, J.M., & Coulter, L.G. (1988). I Can Tell You About That: A Therapeutic Group Program for Cognitively Impaired Persons. *American Journal of Alzheimer's Disease,* 17–22

Ziol, E., Dobres, R., & White, L. (1996). *Communicative Interaction: Group Activities for Cognitively Impaired Elderly.* Bisbee, AZ: Imaginart International

Section 3

Disorders of Swallowing and Voice

9

Dysphagia: Basic Assessment and Management

Jeri A. Logemann

✦ **Nature of the Dysphagic Population in the Acute Care Setting**

✦ **Screening the Initial Referral**

✦ **In-Depth Clinical/Bedside Examination**

✦ **Selecting an Instrumental Diagnostic Procedure**

✦ **Evaluating New Diagnostic Procedures for Dysphagia**

✦ **Swallowing Therapy**

✦ **The Shaker Exercise**

✦ **Evidence-Based Practice**

✦ **Professional Interactions in Dysphagia Management**

✦ **Charting the Patient's Progress Using Outcome and Efficacy Measures**

✦ **Communication with Physicians**

This chapter presents the current status of dysphagia management in acute care hospitals, focusing on the speech–language pathologist's (SLP's) involvement from the time of the initial consultation until the patient is discharged from the acute care hospital. The types of screening and assessment tools utilized by the SLP are described in the context of cost containment and the integration of treatment into the swallowing diagnostic procedure. The SLP's involvement with other professionals in the management of dysphagia in the acute care setting is described. The competencies needed by the SLP at each stage of involvement with the dysphagic patient are outlined. In addition, protocols are presented for the screening, assessment, and treatment of the oropharyngeal dysphagic patient. Case studies are used to illustrate several critical points.

✦ Nature of the Dysphagic Population in the Acute Care Setting

Cost containment is driving every aspect of patient care in the acute care setting, as in most other levels of health care. This translates to a relatively short stay in an acute care setting for most patients with oropharyngeal dysphagia. The population of patients with dysphagia typically seen in acute care are those

who have suffered a stroke, head injury, or spinal cord injury; those with progressive neurologic disease such as Parkinson's disease, motor neuron disease, multiple sclerosis, Alzheimer's disease, etc.; and those patients receiving treatment for head and neck cancer, systemic diseases such as rheumatoid arthritis and dermatomyositis, etc. (Bhutani, 1993; Horner, Alberts, Dawson, & Cook, 1994; Lazarus, Logemann, Pauloski, Colangelo, Kahrilas, Mittal, & Pierce, 1996; Logemann, 1994; Logemann, Pauloski, Rademaker, McConnel, Heiser, Cardinale, Shedd, 1993; Logemann, Rademaker, Pauloski, Kahrilas, Bacon, Bowman, & McCracken, 1994b; Martin, Neary, & Diamant, 1997; Rademaker, Logemann, Pauloski, Bowman, Lazarus, Sisson, Milianti, Graner, Cook, Collins, Stein, Beery, Johnson, & Baker, 1993). Speech–language pathologists in acute care also often see patients on an outpatient basis who are referred for complaints of swallowing difficulty and have no known medical diagnosis. For this type of patient, the SLP often serves as a triage officer who assesses the patient's oropharyngeal swallow function as well as speech, voice, and respiratory function and makes the appropriate referrals to a physician for a final diagnosis of the underlying cause of the dysphagia. Our data show that in most cases patients with complaints of oropharyngeal swallowing difficulties most often have had neurologic damage or have undiagnosed neurologic disease including brainstem stroke, motor neuron disease, Parkinson's disease, Guillain-Barré, multiple sclerosis, or brainstem tumor.

Numerous clinical anecdotes and experience indicate that the most cost-effective care plan for the patient with a complaint of oropharyngeal dysphagia is a referral to an SLP for a modified barium swallow or videofluorographic (VFG) study of oropharyngeal swallow. Following this study, the SLP can make a referral to a particular specialty physician, usually neurology, for further diagnostic workup. Many patients of this sort are referred for VFG studies only after they have already been seen by several physicians and have had numerous medical tests at a high cost to the health care system.

Case One

A 94-year-old woman was referred by the gastroenterology service because she had a chronic bronchial infection and no known etiology for this problem. She had been treated for bronchitis for 6 months by a pulmonologist but no antibiotics were clearing the infection. The pulmonologist, becoming frustrated, referred her to an otolaryngologist for assessment to determine whether there might be some otolaryngologic reason for the bronchitis. The otolaryngologist, after examining her, referred her to gastroenterology for possible reflux disease. The gastroenterologist, after talking with her and her family, thought that dysphagia might be the reason for her bronchitis and referred her to speech–language pathology for swallowing assessment. An informal interview with the patient and observation of her behaviors revealed some degree of thoracic rigidity, a shuffling gait and a masked facies, all typical of Parkinson's disease. Videofluoroscopic examination (the modified barium swallow), revealed swallowing problems typical of Parkinson's disease including a repeated tongue pumping action making oral transit 10 to 15 seconds per swallow, a delay in triggering the pharyngeal swallow, and residue in the valleculae after the swallow indicating poor tongue-base action. This residue was chronically aspirated after the swallow. With the patient's chin down, the aspiration was eliminated. The patient was counseled that her swallowing may be of a neurologic origin and she was referred to a neurologist familiar with swallowing disorders associated with neurologic disease. She was hospitalized for an in-depth workup and found to have Parkinson's disease. Throughout her hospitalization, she was fed using the chin-down compensatory posture to facilitate her tongue-base motion and improve the clearance of the valleculae and thus reduce or eliminate the aspiration. She was placed on antiparkinsonian medications, which resulted in improvement of the pharyngeal aspects of her swallowing problem and elimination of the aspiration as viewed by repeat videofluoroscopic study. Her bronchitis cleared up when the aspiration was eliminated.

If the patient had been initially referred to an SLP in an acute care setting, those costs for numerous unnecessary referrals would have been saved and the patient would have had an earlier medical diagnosis. The competencies needed by the SLP to serve in this capacity include knowledge of neurologic disease processes and damage and their characteristic swallowing disorders at various points in recovery or degeneration, and skills in conducting and interpreting VPG studies.

The procedures described and advocated in this chapter are designed to contain costs in the current acute care environment in which rapid decision making is a fact of life, and in which assessment and treatment must be done quickly to have any significant impact on patients' swallowing function during their brief stay in the acute care setting.

✦ Screening the Initial Referral

The SLP's initial contact with a dysphagic patient is often a 10- to 15-minute bedside screening designed to determine whether the patient is exhibiting signs of an oral or a pharyngeal dysphagia or both, because the in-depth assessment procedures for the two dysphagia foci are quite different (Logemann, 1993, 1998). The screening procedure typically assesses the following patient characteristics: (1) general level of alertness; (2) general secretion levels in the mouth, throat, and chest; (3) awareness of secretions, as exhibited by attempts to wipe away drooling, throat cleaning, or coughing and attempts to clear chest secretions; (4) vocal quality (i.e., hoarse or gurgly); (5) history of any pneumonias; (6) obvious reduction in oromotor control; (7) history of neurologic insult or other neurologic or structural damage; and (8) medical diagnosis. With this information from an initial screening, the SLP may immediately recognize that the patient is at high risk for pharyngeal dysphagia because of a disorder in the triggering of the pharyngeal swallow or in any one of the neuromotor aspects that comprise the pharyngeal swallow itself, and that the patient requires an in-depth physiologic assessment to identify the physiologic or anatomic disorder responsible for the patient's dysphagia. Usually this assessment is a modified barium swallow. If the screening identifies the patient's dysphagia focus as in the oral cavity, then a detailed bedside examination will be completed to identify the nature of the problem and enable the clinician to initiate the therapy as well as to develop a compensatory diet plan to enable the patient to return to oral intake as quickly as possible. At times, the screening cannot determine the locus of the dysphagia to the SLP's satisfaction, and a modified barium swallow is recommended to define the patient's swallow physiology.

Case Two

A 93-year-old woman with Alzheimer's dementia was referred for a videofluoroscopic study of oropharyngeal swallowing because she had begun to refuse to eat and to spit food from her mouth. The preradiographic screening revealed a patient with severe dementia, unable to follow any instructions, and only variably alert. The patient refused placement of any food in her mouth when the clinician observed nursing attempting to feed her. If any food did enter her mouth, she would immediately spit it out and turn her head away. Observing this behavior, the clinician timed the attempts at food placement and found that each attempt took 2 to 3 minutes and then was unsuccessful as the patient pushed out anything that entered her mouth. The clinician then talked with the patient's referring physician about the patient's need for nonoral nutrition and also indicated that a radiographic study would be inappropriate because the patient would not get adequate nutrition or hydration even if her swallowing physiology was normal because of the behavioral and neurologic issues involved in the dementia. After this discussion, the referral for the modified barium swallow was canceled and the patient's family was counseled regarding the need for nonoral nutrition.

Case Three

A 35-year-old man who suffered a brainstem stroke was referred to a speech–language pathology service 2 days poststroke for screening for dysphagia. The chart revealed that the stroke was a large medullary lesion, that the patient had indicated complaints of dysphagia, and that the nursing staff had observed coughing during attempts to feed the patient. The diagnosis of brainstem stroke in the presence of patient complaints and observable symptoms is adequate to refer for a modified barium swallow. Brainstem stroke, particularly medullary, almost always involves damage to the timing of pharyngeal triggering, laryngeal elevation, as well as unilateral pharyngeal wall paresis and sometimes a vocal fold adductor paresis. In this case, the medical diagnosis is enough to immediately refer for a radiographic study because of the extremely high incidence of pharyngeal problems after medullary stroke. Even if the clinician could predict the types of pharyngeal problems that are present, the severity of these problems varies tremendously from patient to patient, requiring radiographic study to define them and to examine the effects of compensatory and other rehabilitation procedures on the swallow. Some of these patients can immediately return to at least partial oral intake using compensatory procedures.

The competencies needed by the SLP to screen for dysphagia include knowledge of signs and symptoms of dysphagia and medical diagnoses frequently causing dysphagia, and skill in observation of patient behavior and oromotor control.

✦ In-Depth Clinical/Bedside Examination

Once the SLP has identified the general locus of the patient's dysphagia, i.e., oral or pharyngeal, the clinician proceeds with an in-depth bedside/clinical assessment.

Review of the Patient's Medical Chart

Prior to entering the patient's room, the clinician should carefully review the patient's medical chart, focusing particularly on the medical diagnosis, any prior or recent medical history of surgical procedures, trauma, neurologic damage, etc., as well as the patient's current medications. There is a growing body of literature on the nature of swallowing disorders that result from particular medical diagnoses. Therefore, after defining the medical diagnosis, the clinician should immediately consider what physiologic or anatomic swallowing disorders are typical of that diagnosis. Unfortunately, the swallowing function of the vast majority of the patients seen by SLPs in the acute care setting is not the result of a single diagnosis. Instead, their swallowing ability reflects their medical history including all of the neurologic and structural damage they have sustained over the years, chronic medication, and other factors influencing the patient's medical status. However, knowing the medical diagnosis and recalling the particular swallowing disorders that are characteristic of that diagnosis can alert the clinician to watch for those possible swallow problems. If a consultation was made to a neurologist or otolaryngologist, the assessment report should be reviewed. History of any respiratory problems should also be identified, including the need for mechanical ventilation or a tracheostomy tube, the conditions under which it was placed (emergency or

planned), and the length of time it was present. In general, any emergency procedure such as emergency tracheostomy or intubation will tend to cause greater scar tissue than a planned procedure. Any history of gastrointestinal (GI) dysfunction should be noted. A prior history of dysphagia from an earlier stroke or head injury, for example, should be highlighted even if the patient or family indicates that the patient returned to oral intake with no apparent difficulty after the prior dysphagia. Very few patients return to entirely normal swallowing after having had a prior dysphagia. Most dysphagic patients become functional swallowers, meaning that they exhibit no aspiration, but have a slightly slower swallow with more residue than normal subjects their age and gender. Thus, it should be anticipated that a second injury causing dysphagia will result in more significant swallowing disorders than a single first-time damage.

Medical chart review should also reveal the patient's current nutritional status and the presence of any nonoral nutritional support such as a nasogastric tube, a percutaneous endoscopic gastrostomy (PEG) (placed under local anesthetic), a surgical gastrostomy, or a jejunostomy (both surgical procedures requiring general anesthesia). Intravenous feeding, as well as any other nutritional supplements, should also be noted in the patient's chart. The clinician should also be able to identify the patient's general progress as well as prognosis from this chart review. The presence of any advanced directives should also be identified. An advanced directive may be a living will or a medical power of attorney. In either case patients are generally stating their wishes regarding their care at a time of severe illness when no recovery is deemed possible.

Bedside Clinical Assessment

The bedside clinical assessment addresses the function of the patient's lips, tongue, velopharyngeal region, pharyngeal walls, and larynx, as well as the patient's awareness of sensory stimulation (Logemann, 1998). The physiology of some of these structures can be easily assessed at the bedside, whereas others can be examined accurately only in a radiographic or other instrumental study. The clinical assessment typically begins with an examination of the anatomic structure of the oral cavity including its symmetry and the presence of any scar tissue indicating surgical or traumatic damage. The oral examination should also note the presence and status of any oral secretions, especially the pooling of secretions or excessive, dried secretions. In general, the locus of excess secretions in the oral cavity indicates areas of lesser lingual control or injury.

The clinician's oromotor assessment should then progress to examination of strength, range of motion, and coordination of the lips, tongue, and palate for speech and nonspeech tasks, as well as observation of lingual function and lip closure while the patient produces any spontaneous swallows. The clinician also notes the frequency of spontaneous swallowing. There is some initial evidence that the frequency of spontaneous swallows is significantly lower in patients who are hospitalized, have dysphagia, and aspirate than in those who do not aspirate. The clinician should count swallows in a 5-minute period by observing or feeling the laryngeal motion in the patient's neck. Normal saliva swallowing occurs at the rate of about one or two per 5-minute period in awake normal adults. **Table 9–1** lists the voluntary tasks to be elicited from the patient during

Table 9–1   Voluntary Tasks to be Elicited from the Patient During the Bedside/Oromotor Assessment

Labial	Velar function
Range of motion	Elevation on prolonged /a/
Lip spread (/i/)	Retraction on prolonged /a/
Lip rounding (/u/)	Symmetry of motion
Asymmetry: right _____ left _____	Oral sensitivity—patient awareness of:
Lip closure at rest	Light touch—tongue tip
Lip closure on rapid repetitive /pa/	Light touch—left side
Lip closure during sentence repetition "*Please put the papers by the back door.*"	Lateral margin of tongue
Lingual	Posterior tongue
Range of motion	Anterior faucial arch
Protrusion	Cheek
Elevation of tip (mouth open widely)	Light touch-right side
Elevation of back (mouth open widely)	Lateral margin of tongue
Point to right side	Posterior tongue
Point to left side	Anterior faucial arch
Retraction	Cheek
Asymmetry: right _____ left _____	Laryngeal examination
Rapid repetitive lateralization	Vocal quality on prolonged /a/(hoarse, gurgly)
Rapid repetitive elevation	Strength of voluntary cough
Tip alveolar contact on repeated /ta/	Strength of throat clearing
Tip alveolar contact during sentence repetition "*Take time to talk to Tom.*"	Clarity of /h/ and /a/ during repetitive /ha/
Fine lingual shaping during sentence repetition "*Say something nice to Susan on Sunday*"	Pitch range (slide up and down scale)
	Loudness range (say name soft, conversational, loud)
Back velar contact on rapid repetitive /ka/	Respiratory assessment
Back velar contact during sentence repetition "Can you go get the garbage cans?"	Duration of phonation (prolong /o/ as long as you can)
Chewing: ability to lateralize gauze, chew on it, return it to midline, and move it to the other side	Duration of comfortable breath hold needed to use swallow maneuvers (1 second, 3 second, 5 second, 10 second)
	Coordination of respiration and swallowing: Does the patient interrupt inhalation or exhalation to swallow? Does the patient - inhale or exhale after the swallow?

the bedside/oromotor assessment. In general, at the bedside, the clinician's goals should be to assess swallow physiology without placing the patient at increased risk of food entering the airway (aspiration). Assessment of chewing and lingual control of material in the mouth can be tested safely at the bedside utilizing cloth rather than food. To this end, the clinician can bring four taste stimuli: lemon juice (sour), bitters (bitter), saline solution (salty), sugar water (sweet). In addition, the clinician should bring 4 × 4 gauze squares as well as 4 × 4's of satin and burlap. The three types of cloth represent three food consistencies (rough, burlap; smooth, satin; intermediate texture, gauze). By wrapping each 4 × 4 square of cloth around a flexible, disposable straw, the clinician can dip one end of the 4-inch roll into one of the flavors (making it as cold as desired), squeeze out the excess liquid from the cloth, and place the dampened end of the cloth containing the desired texture, flavor, and temperature into the patient's mouth. Then the clinician can observe the patient's reaction to the various combinations of stimuli and identify those particular stimuli that result in the most normal oromotor activity such as chewing, lateralizing, lifting the tongue tip, etc. Whatever combination of textures, tastes, and temperatures elicits the most normal motor activity is the one that should be introduced in any radiographic or other instrumental study to follow.

In the same way, this cloth can be used to test the patient's chewing ability by placing the damp end of the 4-inch gauze roll onto the center of the patient's tongue, and asking the patient to lateralize to each side and chew on this roll of cloth. If the patient is unable to control the cloth in the mouth for mastication, and the cloth becomes "stuck," for example two thirds of the way toward the teeth on one side, the clinician can simple pull the dry end of the gauze from the patient's mouth, replace the damp end in the middle of the tongue, and the patient can return to the task. This eliminates the need to clean the patient's mouth of food that may have gotten stuck, were food to be used in this task, and requires that the patient use all of the oromotor control needed for chewing. The risk of potentially losing food in the mouth and having it fall into the pharynx and into the open airway is eliminated. The task can be made more difficult by using chewing gum once the clinician is sure the patient will not accidentally swallow the gum. This becomes a therapy exercise then, as well as an evaluation strategy.

Respiratory Support

Respiratory support should be assessed by counting the rate of breaths per minute and by observing any obvious stressful or rapid respiration. Patients should be asked to hold their breath for a total of 1 second, then 3, 5, and 10 seconds, and the clinician should observe whether this behavior creates any respiratory distress. The duration of breath hold should be increased as tolerated by the patient. One important reason for assessing breath-hold ability is to determine whether the patient can tolerate swallow maneuvers, or other therapy procedures that increase the duration of the apneic or airway closed period during the swallow. Generally, patients need to be able to hold their breath for at least 5 seconds to use swallow maneuvers comfortably. The patient's coordination of respiration and swallowing should be examined. Most often normal adults interrupt the exhalatory phase of the respiratory cycle to swallow and return to exhalation after the swallow (Martin, Logemann, Shaker, & Dodds, 1994a). This coordination is thought to be a safer coordination than interrupting or returning to inhalation after the swallow, which might encourage inhalation of residue after the swallow.

Prolonged Phonation

Prolonged phonation on the vowel /o/ should also be examined in terms of both vocal quality and the respiratory control used. Is the patient able to take an easy inhalation followed by a slow drop of the chest and inward motion of the abdomen to produce a prolonged vowel on sustained phonation of at least 10 seconds?

Gag Reflex

The gag reflex should be tested, not to determine its presence or absence as an indicator of ability or inability to swallow, but rather to examine the pharyngeal wall motion as part of the motor response for the gag. The pharyngeal wall motion during the gag should be symmetrical. Any asymmetry may indicate a unilateral pharyngeal wall paresis. There is no evidence of a relationship between the presence and normalcy of a gag and the presence and normalcy of a swallow (Leder, 1996, 1997). The gag reflex is triggered from surface tactile sensory receptors by a noxious stimulus that does not belong in the posterior oral cavity or pharynx such as vomit or reflux. The motor response of a gag is for the pharynx and larynx to elevate and close/contract to push out any foreign body. In contrast, the swallow is triggered from deeper proprioceptive receptors as well as surface receptors, and the motor response of a swallow is a coordinated set of muscle contractions designed to carry food from the mouth through the pharynx and into the esophagus, essentially the opposite of a gag motor response. In addition, several studies have shown that the gag reflex can be eliminated by topical anesthetic, whereas the swallow remains entirely intact. If the deeper proprioceptive receptors are anesthetized, however, then the swallow will be eliminated. Thus, there is no reason to hypothesize that the gag and swallow in any way predict each other, other than to say that if a patient sustains significant neurologic damage, it is quite likely that both the gag and the swallow will be affected because of the extent of damage. Despite the lack of relationship between gag and swallow, both neurologically and physiologically, many physicians learn in their residency that the gag reflex in some way is predictive of swallow normalcy. Case four emphasizes this point.

Case Four

A 53-year-old man was referred for a modified barium swallow because he had an asymmetrical uvula and an absent gag reflex. In discussing this test with the patient and taking a brief history prior to the x-ray study, the clinician determined that the patient had no swallowing complaints and had no nasality or any other indication of velopharyngeal insufficiency or incompetence for speech. Oral examination did reveal an asymmetrical uvula but good upward-backward motion of the soft palate and visible inward motion of the lateral and posterior pharyngeal walls. Because the patient insisted, the videofluoroscopic study was completed and showed an entirely normal oropharyngeal swallow. In this case, the patient had been referred because the physician thought that an absent gag reflex indicated a swallowing problem and in combination with an asymmetrical uvula, may indicate neurologic disease. In the report of the radiographic study to the physician, the differences in the gag reflex and swallow were emphasized as was the high incidence of absent gag in normal individuals. The physician indicated that he was extremely grateful for this information.

Laryngeal Function

Laryngeal function should also be assessed by a series of voluntary tasks listed in Table 9–1, with the clinician assessing vocal quality and respiratory support during each task. Increasing loudness and increasing phonation time requires coordination between respiratory and phonatory control.

Throughout all of the oromotor testing, the clinician also assesses patients' general behavioral level, ability to discipline their own behavior and focus on the tasks, impulsiveness, and other cognitive and language characteristics that interact with swallow physiology to facilitate the eating situation. Successful eating requires functional swallowing (no aspiration and some manageable residue) and behavioral control and language ability. Two patients may exhibit the same swallow physiology but one with behavioral problems and an inability to focus on tasks will generally exhibit longer recovery to oral intake than the patient who is capable of focusing, following directions, and monitoring one's own performance.

If the patient is taking oral nutrition, the clinician should observe the patient at bedside during a meal to identify the typical postures used, the placement of the food in the mouth, the patient's general awareness of food and reaction to food, and the presence of any behavior that might indicate food entering the airway (aspiration) such as coughing, throat clearing, periods of difficulty breathing, gurgly voice, etc. (Logemann, 1990). Also, an apraxia of swallow should be noted. Generally, apraxia of swallow is observed to be characterized by searching motions in the oral cavity as food is being placed there, or simply no motion in the oral cavity in response to placement of food there.

Once the clinician has collected data on oromotor control, the patient's behavior and language levels, and any symptoms of an oropharyngeal dysphagia, the clinician may attempt some intervention strategies at the bedside. The difficulty, of course, is that if there is a pharyngeal dysphagia, the effects of any treatment strategies, as well as the identification of the actual abnormality on anatomy or physiology causing the patient's symptoms, cannot be accurately identified at the bedside.

Therefore, the clinician may believe that a therapy procedure works because the patient doesn't cough or clear any material from the airway, but in fact, food may be collecting in the pharyngeal recesses formed by the natural attachment of structures to each other, such as the pyriform sinuses or the valleculae. The patient may appear to be "swallowing" when in fact food is simply resting in these recesses, waiting for a swallow, or may be left in these recesses after an inefficient swallow.

At this point, all of the data the clinician has collected from the patient's medical chart and history, as well as direct examination, combine to identify the patient's risk level for a pharyngeal dysphagia and the need for a VFG or modified barium swallow study of the pharyngeal stage of swallowing. As a general guideline, if the patient has any of the behaviors or diagnoses listed in **Table 9–2**, the clinician should recommend a modified barium swallow or other physiologic assessment to directly examine pharyngeal physiology during swallows of various bolus types, as described below. Treatment for oral-stage problems can be initiated in parallel with conducting the VFG study of the pharyngeal stage of swallowing.

The bedside clinical assessment of oropharyngeal dysphagia is a screening test for the pharyngeal stage of swallowing, but not a definitive diagnostic test for the oral stages of swallowing in patients with neurologic lesions in the brainstem or below, that is, the final common path, and for patients with peripheral structural damage such as surgery or radiotherapy for head and neck cancer, gun shot wounds, other trauma, etc. (Kennedy, Pring, & Fawcus, 1993). For patients with cortical or subcortical neural damage, the effects on oral control may be different for speech and swallowing because these higher neural structures, although involved in both speech and swallowing, are utilized differently for the two functions. Performance on voluntary speech tasks may not reflect performance of the same structures during swallowing (Kennedy et al 1993).

Table 9–2 Diagnoses and Patient Behaviors Indicative of Increased Risk for Pharyngeal Stage Disorders and/or Aspiration

Diagnosis at Highest Risk for Pharyngeal Dysphagia	Symptoms Indicating High Risk for Pharyngeal Disorders
Parkinson's disease	Gurgly voice
Motor neuron disease	History of pneumonia
Amyotrophic lateral sclerosis (ALS)	Difficulty managing secretions
Postpolio syndrome	Increased secretions in chest
Brainstem stroke	Coughing or throat clearing during eating
Head and neck cancer patients whether treated with surgery/radiotherapy	Patient report of food "sticking" in throat
Myasthenia gravis	
Guillain-Barré	
Multiple sclerosis (if complaining of swallow problems)	
Dermatomyositis	
Scleroderma	
Oculopharyngeal muscular dystrophy	
Myotonic dystrophy	

Other Bedside Screening Tests

The clinician may wish to introduce other screening tests at the bedside to gain further evidence of the potential of a pharyngeal-stage swallowing problem. These include the blue dye test in tracheostomized patients, cervical auscultation, and the videoendoscopic assessment of pharyngeal swallow known as the fiberoptic endoscopic examination of swallowing (FEES). Each of these procedures defines symptoms of swallow disorders.

Blue Dye Test

The blue dye test involves presenting blue dyed foods to a patient with a tracheostomy and suctioning after each swallow attempt to identify the presence of any food in the airway below the larynx (Myers, 1995; Thompson-Henry and Braddock, 1995). This test has been found to have both a negative and positive error rate, that is, it misidentifies patients as aspirating who are not and misidentifies patients who are actually aspirating as not aspirating. There is no set protocol for this procedure. Generally clinicians using it prefer to introduce thin liquids, thick liquids, pureed, and mechanical soft foods, all dyed blue, to distinguish the foods from bodily secretions. If the patient loses food out the tracheostomy during or after a swallow or for a period of time after eating, aspiration is indicated and the need for VFG or definitive diagnostic study is identified.

Cervical Auscultation

Cervical auscultation involves placing a stethoscope against the patient's neck and listening to the sounds of swallow and respiration (Hamlet, Penney & Formolo, 1994; Zenner, Losinski & Mill, 1995). The inhalatory and exhalatory phases of the respiratory cycle can generally be identified with auscultation. Also the clinician can define the phase of respiration during which the patient swallows. Unfortunately, the sounds of swallowing have not yet been completely identified so that the meaning of the sounds heard by the clinician during the swallow is undetermined. Also, we do not know if clinicians can detect normal from abnormal sounds. In any case, the outcome of auscultation is the identification of a patient's risk for pharyngeal-stage dysphagia and its major symptom, aspiration. A definitive diagnostic procedure is needed to identify the exact nature of the dysphagia, to plan treatment, and to evaluate effects of treatment procedures.

Fiberoptic Endoscopic Examination of Swallowing

Fiberoptic Endoscopic Examination of Swallowing (FEES) involves nasal placement of a fiberoptic laryngoscope (generally 3.5-mm diameter) so that the tip of the laryngoscope is positioned posterior to the uvula as seen in **Fig. 9–1**. In this position, the endoscope visualizes the pharynx from above including the valleculae, the airway entrance, and the posterior and lateral pharyngeal walls (Bastian, 1993; Kidder, Langmore, & Martin, 1994; Perlman & Van Daele, 1993). During the swallow the oral stages are not visible. The bolus becomes visible as it comes over the base of the tongue and into the pharynx. When the pharyngeal swallow triggers and the pharyngeal motor response begins, laryngeal and pharyngeal elevation is

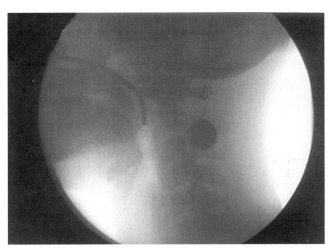

Figure 9–1 Lateral videofluorographic view of the oropharyngeal region showing the placement of the fiberoptic endoscope through the nose and over the soft palate with the tip of the endoscope at the approximate level of the inferior tip of the uvula.

partially visualized followed by a period of "white out" when nothing can be seen as the pharynx closes around the endoscopic tube. When the swallow ends and the pharynx relaxes, the pharynx can be visualized again. Any residual food left in the pharynx can be seen. Thus, the swallow itself is not visualized. Instead, FEES examines the pharynx before and after the swallow. FEES can provide information on anatomic changes in the pharynx resulting from surgery or trauma, which can be helpful to the clinician trying to understand the patient's altered anatomy. FEES can also be used to provide biofeedback for airway closure maneuvers described later, specifically the supraglottic and super-supraglottic swallow maneuvers.

A rigid endoscope placed transorally can also visualize the pharynx and larynx from above and can be used to provide biofeedback for learning the airway closure maneuvers. Other procedures (heart rate, arterial oxygen saturation, and blood pressure) have been introduced in an attempt to screen or assess swallow, but have been found to be inaccurate (Leder, 2000).

The competencies needed by the SLP in screening and clinical bedside assessment of the dysphagic patient include knowledge of the range of normal oral anatomy and range, pattern, and coordination of the lips, tongue, jaw and palate, and knowledge of the various screening procedures and their appropriateness for various patients. The SLP also should be skilled in eliciting and evaluating oromotor actions for speech and nonspeech tasks in various types of patients, and in auditory recognition of normal and abnormal articulation and voice.

✦ Selecting an Instrumental Diagnostic Procedure

In acute care, there are many diagnostic modalities available for use in evaluation of patients with dysphagia. Videofluorography is certainly the most commonly used procedure to understand the anatomy and physiology of a patient's swallow. There are times when questions about a patient's anatomy would dictate a different view of the oropharyngeal structures that could be provided through other imaging such as

videoendoscopy (Langmore, Schatz, & Olson, 1988). The superior view of the pharynx can identify changes in anatomy in postsurgical head and neck cancer patients and in trauma victims. At times, there are questions about the exact position of the epiglottis, the location of the arytenoid cartilages, and the relationship of structures in the airway that endoscopy can help us answer. If the amount of pressure generated during swallow is questionable in a patient, manometry may be needed. This GI procedure involves the patient swallowing a small 3-mm tube containing three solid-state pressure sensors that are usually positioned at the tongue base, just above the upper esophageal sphincter, and in the top of the cervical esophagus. Utilizing this technique usually involves concurrent videofluoroscopy so that the position of the sensors can be visualized in relation to structures that may be contacting the sensors and creating a pressure change during swallow (Ergun, Kahrilas, & Logemann, 1993).

There may be patients for whom there is need to visualize tongue movements in more detail. In this case, ultrasound may be helpful (Perlman & Van Daele, 1993; Shawker, Sonies, Hall, & Baum, 1984). Generally, radiology departments will allow an SLP to examine patients with ultrasound free of charge by utilizing equipment at off times. The ultrasound image allows visualization of tongue movements in the frontal or lateral plane. Ultrasound can also be used for biofeedback to better understand the patient's tongue movement and what should be done to improve it. Any of these procedures can be appropriately used in the assessment of patients with dysphagia. The key is to identify the clinical question to be answered by utilization of a particular instrument.

Modified Barium Swallow

The modified barium swallow procedure is a VFG evaluation of swallowing and is designed to identify the abnormal anatomy or physiology in the patient's oral and pharyngeal stages of swallowing that are causing the dysphagic symptoms (Logemann, 1993). In addition, the VFG study assesses the effectiveness of treatment procedures to eliminate the patient's swallowing symptoms and improve the patient's swallowing safety and efficiency. The types of swallows introduced during the VFG study should be selected based on two characteristics: (1) the bolus characteristics that create systematic changes in normal swallowing including increases in volume and viscosity, and (2) the types of stimuli the clinician believes may improve the patient's swallow physiology and thereby eliminate aspiration or significant residue. Because we know that bolus volume and viscosity can cause significant changes in normal swallow physiology, the typical modified barium swallow includes presentation of two to three swallows each of 1, 3, 5, of 10 mL, and cup drinking of thin liquids, as tolerated (Bisch, Logemann, Rademaker, Kahrilas, & Lazarus, 1994; Jacob, Kahrilas, Logemann, Shah, & Ha, 1989; Kahrilas & Logemannn, 1993; Kahrilas, Logemann, Lin, & Ergun, 1992; Kahrilas, Lin, Logemann, Ergun, & Facchini, 1993; Lazarus, Logemann, & Gibbons, 1993a; Lazarus, Logemann, Rademaker, Kahrilas, Pajak, Lazar, & Halper, 1993b; Perlman & Van Daele, 1993). The importance of beginning with small volumes (1 mL) of thin liquid is emphasized (Penington, 1993). Similarly, because bolus viscosity creates significant changes in normal swallow physiology, the patient is typically given thin liquids, pudding-type material, and something

Table 9–3 Postural Strategies and Their Known Effects on Oropharyngeal Dimension and Bolus Flow

Disorder for Which Posture Appropriate (Symptoms of Disorders)	Posture	Effects of Oropharyngeal Dimensions and Bolus Flow
Inefficient oral transit (reduced posterior lingual propulsion of bolus)	Chin up	Uses gravity to clear oral cavity from bolus
Delay in triggering the pharyngeal swallow (bolus past ramus of mandible, but pharyngeal swallow is not triggered)	Chin down	Widens valleculae to prevent bolus entering airway; narrows airway entrance, reducing risk of aspiration
Reduced posterior motion of tongue base (residue in valleculae)	Chin down	Pushes tongue base closer to the posterior pharyngeal wall
Reduced closure of laryngeal entrance and vocal folds (aspiration during the swallow)	Chin down	Puts epiglottis in more protective position; narrows laryngeal entrance.
	Head rotated to damaged side	Improves vocal fold closure by applying extrinsic pressure
Unilateral pharyngeal paresis (residue on one side of pharynx)	Head rotated to damaged side	Eliminates damaged side of pharynx from bolus path
Unilateral oral and pharyngeal weakness on the same side (residue in mouth and pharynx on same side)	Head tilt to stronger side	Directs bolus down stronger side by gravity
Reduced pharyngeal contract (residue spread throughout pharynx)	Lying down on one side	Eliminates effect of gravity on pharyngeal residue
Cricopharyngeal dysfunction (residue in pyriform sinuses)	Head rotated	Pulls cricoid cartilage away from posterior pharyngeal wall, reducing resting pressure in cricopharyngeal sphincter

requiring mastication such as a Lorna Doone cookie. The volume of the pudding is generally restricted to 1 or 3 mL and the amount of cookie presented is usually one fourth of a Lorna Doone because the volume range of thicker foods is much less than liquids, that is, 3 to 6 mL. Generally the thicker the food, the smaller the volume per swallow. The cookie is utilized to study mastication. Although patients might be able to swallow 25 mL of thin liquid, they might not be capable of swallowing 25 mL of pudding, which would require too much distention of the upper esophageal sphincter. Thus, as viscosity increases, the maximum bolus volume per swallow decreases.

Patients may need to have particular bolus tastes presented such as sour as well as other types of therapy strategies to improve their swallow. Generally, postural techniques are attempted first to eliminate aspiration or large amounts of residue because they are easy for most patients to use and do not require extra muscular work (Drake, O'Donoghue, Bartram, & Lindsay, 1997; Larnert and Ekberg, 1995; Logemann, Rademaker, Pauloski, & Kahrilas, 1994a; Rasley, Logemann, Kahrilas, Rademaker, Pauloski, & Dodds, 1993; Shanahan, Logemann, Rademaker, Pauloski, & Kahrilas, 1993; Welch, Logemann, Rademaker, & Kahrilas, 1993). Heightening sensory awareness follows postures and is designed to improve the speed of oral onset and the pharyngeal trigger of the swallow. Swallowing maneuvers and other therapy procedures may be attempted followed by presentation of swallows of thicker foods.

In many cases these strategies can be combined for best effect. For example, if a patient has difficulty in closing the entry of the larynx, the first strategy attempted would be a postural technique, that is, chin down, which narrows the airway entrance and puts the epiglottis in a more overhanging position to protect the airway. If this posture is not successful and there is any asymmetry in laryngeal function, the patient may be asked to try head rotation to the side of any laryngeal damage, thereby applying extrinsic pressure to the damaged side of the larynx to achieve improved closure. If this posture reduces but does not eliminate aspiration, the two postures may be combined with the head rotated and the chin down, thereby achieving the effects of both postures. If the patient still continues to aspirate small amounts, the super-supraglottic swallow may be attempted, which is a swallow maneuver to voluntarily close the entrance to the airway. Finally, the two postures and the super-supraglottic swallow may be combined to eliminate the patient's aspiration. Thus, therapy procedures can be assessed separately as well as in combination to identify those procedures that successfully eliminate aspiration or reduce residue and allow the patient to eat.

The goal of the radiographic study is not to eliminate oral feeding but instead to find a way in which the patient can eat successfully. **Table 9–3** presents all of the postural strategies and their known effects on the dimensions of the pharynx or the direction of bolus flow. **Table 9–4** presents sensory enhancement procedures that generally improve the oral onset of the swallow, that is, the time from the command to swallow until the oral transit is initiated, and the pharyngeal delay time (Fujiu, Toleikis, Logemann, & Larson, 1994; Logemann, 1993; Logemann, Pauloski, Colangelo, Lazarus, Fujiu, & Kahrilis, 1995; Rosenbek, Rocker, Wood, & Robbins, 1996). **Table 9–5** presents the swallow maneuvers and their known effects on swallow physiology (Kahrilas, Logemann, & Gibbons, 1992; Kahrilas, Logemann, Krugler, & Flanagan, 1991; Lazarus, 1993; Lazarus et al, 1993a; Logemann, 1993, 1995, 1997; Logemann and Kahrilas, 1990; Martin, Schleicher, & O'Connor, 1993; Ohmae, Logemann, Kaiser, Hanson, & Kahrilas, 1996; Robbins and Levine, 1993).

The outcome of the modified barium swallow should be (1) the identification of the specific anatomic or physiologic dysfunctions in the patient's oropharyngeal swallow; (2) the relationship of the physiology to the patient's symptoms, that is, the cause(s) of residue or aspiration; (3) the identification of treatment strategies to improve the pharyngeal swallow and the conditions under which the patient can eat safely, if possible; (4) the need for any nonoral supplement or nonoral nutrition if the patient aspirates and the aspiration cannot be

Table 9–4 Sensory Enhancement Procedures Designed to Improve Oral Onset of the Swallow and Reduce Pharyngeal Delay and Their Method of Presentation (All Are Helpful in Patients with Swallow Apraxia or Reduced Sensory Input)

Procedure	Method
Increase bolus volume	Present measured bolus volumes during radiographic study, beginning with 1 mL and increasing to 3, 5, 10 mL as tolerated (if no aspiration). If pharyngeal delay reduced as volume increased, provide "best" volumes during feeding and therapy.
Increase bolus viscosity	Feed patient those food viscosities that are easiest and safest to swallow.
Change bolus taste	Present liquid with a strong taste such as "sour"* lemonade or salty water.
Increase pressure of spoon on tongue	As spoon is placed in the mouth, press down firmly on the patient's tongue.
Thermal tactile stimulation	Rub a cold size 00 mirror up and down five times on each anterior face and arch.
Suck swallow	Ask patients to close their mouth and suck in their mouth as they pump their tongue and jaw up and down.
Chewing	Ask patient to "chew" liquid and paste substances.
Self-feeding	Facilitate the patient's self-feeding. The hand-to-mouth movement may constitute an alerting stimulus to ready the central nervous system to initiate a swallow.

*Do not present if patient is aspirating unless there is radiographic evidence that sour eliminates aspiration. Acidic substances are more irritating to the lungs.

stopped by any of the treatment strategies; (5) the type of swallowing therapy needed to further improve the patient's swallow; and (6) the need for and timing of reassessment of the patient's swallow. Because of the relatively short time the patient spends in acute care, the transfer of this information from the acute care clinician to the clinician in rehabilitation or home health or the skilled nursing facility is critical in order for the patient's swallowing therapy and recovery to be uninterrupted. The sequence of reevaluation is also critical so that the patient who receives nonoral nutrition in acute care in the first few days or weeks after a stroke, for example, will be evaluated 3 or 4 weeks later to determine a continued need for such nonoral nutrition. With the rapid transfer of the patient from acute care to another facility, whether it be a rehabilitation center, nursing home, or the patient's home, the transfer of information from each facility to the next and each clinician to the next is critical to ensure a smooth continuum of care and optimal recovery for the dysphagic patient (Klor and Milianti, 1995). The videofluoroscopic results including all of the recommendations and follow-up therapy notes should be transferred with the patient so that the next clinician can provide appropriate care.

Several studies indicate that patients who aspirate during radiographic study are at higher risk for developing pneumonia during the next 6 to 12 months than patients who are not found to aspirate on videofluoroscopy (Martin, Corlew, Wood, Olson, Gallipol, Wingbowl, & Kirmani, 1994b; Schmidt, Holas, Halvorson, & Redding, 1994; Taniguchi and Moyer, 1994). This is important information to pass along to the patient's physician.

Ideal Equipment for the Modified Barium Swallow

To conduct the modified barium swallow, the clinician needs a videorecorder that can be wired directly into the

Table 9–5 Swallow Maneuvers (Voluntary Changes in Selected Motor Aspects of the Oropharyngeal Swallow), Their Purpose and Instructions

Swallow Maneuvers	Purpose	Problem for which Maneuver Designed	Instructions
Supraglottic swallow	Close vocal folds before and during swallow (Martin, Schleicher, & O'Connor, 1993)	Reduced or late vocal closure	Take a breath, hold your breath, keep holding your breath while you swallow and cough or take a breath, exhale a little and hold your breath while you swallow and cough.
	Close vocal folds before and during delay	Delayed pharyngeal swallow	
Super-supraglottic swallow	Tilts arytenoid forward, and pulls false vocal folds in closing airway entrance before and during swallow	Reduced closure of airway entrance	Follow instructions as above, but bear down as you hold your breath.
Effortful swallow	Increases posterior tongue-base movement and pressure generated	Reduced posterior movement of the tongue base	Swallow hard. Squeeze hard with all your muscles as you swallow.
Mendelsohn maneuver	Laryngeal movement opens the upper esophageal sphincter; prolonging laryngeal elevation prolongs UES opening (Cook et al, 1989; Jacob et al, 1989) Normalizes coordination of pharyngeal swallow events (Lazarus, Logemann, & Gibbons, 1993a)	Reduced laryngeal movement Discoordinated swallow	

fluoroscopy equipment or can be attached by cable to the back of the fluoroscopy monitor. The latter arrangement is best because it enables the clinician to use a variety of videorecorders. If the videorecorder is wired directly into the fluoroscopy, the radiologist or technician can activate the recording at the same time as the fluoroscopy image begins. However, often the videorecorder in radiology has a different line rate per inch than standard recorders so that the videotape resulting from the study can only be played in radiology and cannot be played to educate families, physicians, nurses, and others. The videorecorder, whenever possible, should have a "jog wheel," which enables the clinician to watch the videotape of the radiographic study in slow motion, frame by frame, and forward or backward at any rate. A pause button will not enable the clinician to do the kind of slow-motion analysis needed for careful assessment of patient studies. Both ¾-inch and ½-inch (VHS) tapes are available with a "jog wheel" feature.

Additional equipment is also helpful, whenever possible. A video counter timer that records numbers on the individual frames of fields of the videotape as it is being recorded enables the clinician to make better notations and measurements of the timing of swallowing events. Another piece of equipment that adds to the ease of the test is a video character generator that enables the clinician to type the patient's name, date, condition of the study, diagnosis, or any other information onto the video screen so that it is visible and recorded at all times on the videotape. This makes finding the patient's study from a tape containing the radiographic studies of 10 or 15 other patients quite easy.

A seating device that enables the patient to be positioned easily in the radiographic equipment is also helpful. There are several chairs commercially available for this purpose. **Table 9–6** lists some of the available chairs and their manufacturers. The chair should allow the clinician (1) to change the patient's posture from true vertical to any degree including true horizontal, (2) switch from a lateral view to an anterior posterior view without moving the patient from the chair, and (3) position all types of patients whether they are conscious or not, able to follow directions or not, or have no motor control of their body. One alternative to a chair is to position the patient on a gurney or cart with a back support narrow enough to fit into the radiologic equipment. In this way, the patient can sit on the gurney with a back support in place. The back support can be shifted from true vertical to various degrees backward until the patient reaches horizontal. This type of back support on a gurney is very helpful for patients with spinal cord injuries, head injuries, or dementia who are sometimes difficult to position. One source for such back support is listed in **Table 9–6**. The challenge to the clinician is to be able to position patients for the study regardless of their physical or mental limitations.

The competencies needed to complete a modified barium swallow include knowledge of (1) normal versus abnormal radiographic anatomy of the head and neck (Logemann, 1993; Robbins, Hamilton, Lof, & Kempster, 1992; Tracy, Logemann, Kahrilas, Jacob, Kobara, & Krugler, 1989); (2) the equipment needed for the study; (3) the types and volumes of foods given; (4) the variations in normal swallow based on food characteristics and voluntary control; (5) anatomic and physiologic swallowing disorders; and (6) the range of swallow therapy options that can be introduced into the radiographic study, and their rationale and appropriateness for various

Table 9–6 Purchasing Sources for Equipment for Positioning Patients During the Radiographic Procedure

Amigo Escort Video Swallow Chair	Durable Medical Equipment Shoppe 1600 Shore Road, Unit H Naperville, IL 60540 (312) 420-7621 or (800) 225-3900
Beach chair without seat for back support on standard cart	Northern Speech Services, Inc. 117 North Elm Gaylord, MI 49735 (989) 732-3866
MAMA Systems: multiple applications and articulations (an infant/ child chair)	MAMA Systems, Inc. 4347 Silver Lake Street Oconomowoc, WI 53066 (414) 569–9188
Plywood Sacred Heart Chair (plans)	Manager, Radiation Department Sacred Heart Hospital 1545 S. Layton Boulevard Milwaukee, WI 53215 (414) 383-4490
Tumble Form Feeder Seats (Floor Sitter Wedge) small, medium, large	J.A. Preston (Distributor) P.O. Box 89 Jackson, MI 49204 (800) 631-7277
Vess Chair	Vess Chair, Inc. 2938 North 61st Street Milwaukee, WI 53210 (414) 932-2203
Video Fluoro Chair	Rehab Tech, Inc. 6469 Germantown Pike Dayton, OH 45418 (513) 866-4308
Video Fluoroscopic Imaging Chair (VIC)	Hausted, Inc. 927 Lake Road, P.O. Box 710 Medina, OH 44256-0710 (216) 723-3271; Fax: 725-0505
Video Counter Timer	Thalner Electronic Laboratory, Inc. 7235 Jackson Ann Arbor, MI 48103 (313) 761-4506
Dysphagia Cup	Jamie H. Stevens, MS, CCC, Inc. 2518 Wheaton Way, Suite 106 Bremerton, WA 98310 (206) 373-7276 /Fax: 297-8121

patients. The skills needed are in (1) positioning all types of patients in the radiographic equipment; (2) presenting food to the mouth in various ways; (3) interpreting the radiographic study accurately; (4) selecting intervention strategies for the swallow disorder and the patient's diagnosis; (5) evaluating the success of the strategies; and (6) writing a report describing the results and making recommendations.

✦ Evaluating New Diagnostic Procedures for Dysphagia

From time to time, new equipment is introduced for the evaluation of dysphagia. Sometimes this equipment does not have adequate study or data to enable prospective buyers to evaluate it in terms of its usefulness in the care of dysphagic patients. Generally, clinicians should have a clear understanding of the specific aspects of the swallow of interest, that is, the oral stage, the pharyngeal stage, the upper esophageal sphincter, etc. Any new diagnostic equipment should be evaluated in terms of the type of information it provides and the validity and reliability of that data. For example, recently the laryngeal analyzer was introduced as a way to evaluate swallowing. When the developer was asked by a large number of swallow researchers what the equipment actually displayed and what the line it produced represented in swallows, there was no clear response. One study reported that the line produced by the equipment could relate to any movement of the head or neck, whether or not it was related to swallowing (Danbolt, Hult, Grahn, & Ask, 1999). Thus, this is an example of an expensive piece of equipment that currently has no valid application to the assessment or treatment of patients with swallowing disorders. Before purchasing any piece of equipment, the clinician must clearly understand what information the equipment provides and how it can be utilized in the assessment of swallowing disorders. The phrase "buyer beware" is applicable.

✦ Swallowing Therapy

Swallowing therapy may be provided to the dysphagic patient in acute care if it is anticipated that the patient's spontaneous recovery will be slow or if there is a need to improve specified aspects of swallow physiology (Logemann, 1998; Martin et al, 1993; Ylvisaker & Logemann (1998). Swallowing therapy is designed to change the physiology of the patient's swallow and generally includes muscle exercises directed at the specific locus of the patient's physiologic abnormality.

Indirect Therapy

The swallowing therapy may be given indirectly, that is, by exercising muscle groups used in swallowing or by practicing specific neuromuscular elements of the swallow without actually using food. In this way, if the patient is aspirating, there will be no increased risk of pneumonia nor will the clinician be placed at any risk. **Table 9–7** presents a list of therapy exercises that can be done indirectly and their therapy goal. The directions for each procedure are presented as well. In general, patients are instructed to practice these procedures 10 times a day for 5 minutes each if the patient can practice independently. Otherwise, family members can be instructed to work with the patient multiple times per day. The clinician in acute care usually has difficulty reaching the patient even twice a day because of the scheduling of multiple tests and other

Table 9–7 The Goals and Instructions for Therapy Procedures Can Be Practiced Indirectly (i.e., with No Food or Liquid Given)

Procedure	Goal	Instructions
Range of motion exercises for lips, tongue, or jaw	Increase range of motion	Extend the structure in the desired direction as far as possible, hold for a second in extreme extension, relax.
Adduction exercises	Improve vocal fold movement arytenoid movement	Say "ah" with a hard attack and prolong a clear vocal quality. Repeat "ah-ah-ah" with a hard attack. Cough. Clear your throat, say "ah," and bear down say "ah" as you lift up on the arms of a chair. Turn your head to the side of the laryngeal damage and say "ah." Listen to the voice quality and maintain the quality as you say "ah" and slowly turn your head to the midline.
Effortful swallow	Improve tongue-base movement Improve pressure generation	Swallow saliva "hard" with lots of muscle effort.
Chewing on gauze	Increase tongue control for chewing	Place a 4-inch roll of gauze on the patient's tongue so that 2 inches of the gauze are in the mouth and 2 inches are hanging out. Ask the patient to move the gauze over to their teeth, chew on it, move it across their mouth and chew on it. Continue this exercise with gauze until the patient can move the gauze easily. Then move to chewing gum or food.
Bolus control exercises	Improve bolus control by the tongue	Place a lozenge in the patient's mouth. Ask the tongue patient to move the lozenge around and spit it out. When the patient can move the lozenge easily, use a glob of peanut butter, then move to pudding and further liquefy the pudding. The thicker the food, the easier the exercise. Patient can spit out the food without swallowing.
Falsetto	Increase laryngeal range of motion	Slide up the pitch scale as high as possible to the "high, squeaky" level and hold the tone for 2 seconds. Then relax.
Thermal-tactile stimulation	Improve triggering of the pharyngeal swallow	See Table 9–4 (use saliva; be sure patient's mouth is damp).
Suck swallow	Improve triggering of the pharyngeal swallow	See Table 9–4 (use saliva; be sure patient's mouth is damp).
Easy breath hold (first part of the supraglottic swallow)	Improve vocal fold closure	Take a breath in and hold your breath for 2 seconds. Relax.
Effortful breath-hold (first part of the supraglottic swallow)	Improve airway entrance closure (arytenoid and tongue base movement)	Take a breath in, hold your breath, and bear down for 2 seconds. Relax.

procedures to be completed during the acute care period. As the patient moves toward the rehabilitation phase or to a sub-acute unit, or a skilled nursing facility, there may be more time to provide multiple therapy visits per day to facilitate regular practice.

Case Five

A 70-year-old man had undergone a supraglottic laryngec-tomy a week prior to the radiographic study. This surgical pro-cedure involves removal of all or part of the hyoid bone, part of the base of the tongue surrounding the hyoid bone, the aryepiglottic folds, the false vocal folds, and the topmost por-tion of the thyroid cartilage. The base of tongue is then sutured to the top of the thyroid cartilage so that the postoperative airway entrance consists of the tongue base and the arytenoid cartilage. The patient was examined radiographically and found to have poor closure of this reconstructed airway en-trance, resulting in food reaching the top surface of the true vocal folds during the swallow. When the patient inhaled after the swallow, the material was aspirated. Attempts at a super-supraglottic swallow designed to improve tongue base and arytenoid motion were not successful in adequately protect-ing the airway though improved range of motion was seen. Therefore, the patient was given exercises to improve the air-way entrance closure. These included an effortful breath hold without swallowing. The effortful breath hold is the critical portion of a super-supraglottic swallow in which the patient holds the breath tightly and bears down, which pulls the tongue base posteriorly and the arytenoid anteriorly as well as closes the true vocal folds. After 3 weeks of practicing the pro-cedure 10 times a day for 5 minutes each time without food, the patient was returned to x-ray and the effects of the effort-ful breath hold were evaluated. Tongue-base motion had improved sufficiently as had anterior arytenoid motion to close the airway entrance prior to and during the swallow. The pa-tient was then allowed to begin oral intake using this voluntary airway protection technique. Within 3 more weeks, the patient was begun on full oral intake.

Direct Therapy

In contrast to indirect therapy, direct therapy is designed to actually change swallow physiology and the procedures are practiced utilizing food or liquid. Generally, direct therapy is not provided if a patient is aspirating. Direct therapy procedures include swallowing maneuvers that are voluntary neuromus-cular controls applied to selected aspects of the oropharyngeal swallow. There are four swallow maneuvers: (1) the supra-glottic swallow, (2) the super-supraglottic swallow, (3) the effortful swallow, and (4) the Mendlesohn maneuver. These are listed in **Table 9–5** along with the neuromuscular aspect of swallow that each maneuver is designed to improve and the instructions given to teach the maneuver. In general, swallow maneuvers require that the patient be able to follow directions and therefore are not useful with low-functioning patients or with infants and young children. Swallow maneuvers also require a level of muscle work and energy that may not be fea-sible for some patients with extreme fatigue. In general, it is best to introduce the therapy procedures and exercises that are effective and require least effort and are most easily done even by low-functioning patients.

✦ The Shaker Exercise

The Shaker exercise is a new procedure to improve elevation of the hyoid bone and larynx during swallow and thereby increase the duration and width of opening of the upper esophageal sphincter. The Shaker exercise is a simple proce-dure in which patients lie on their back and elevate their head just enough to see their feet/toes while keeping their shoulders on the bed. The head is elevated for 1 minute, followed by 1 minute of rest. The procedure is done three times with rest in between each head elevation. And finally, after the third minute of rest, patients lift their head to see their toes and then rest it back. This is repeated 30 times. The procedure is designed to strengthen the cervical muscles that in turn pull on the hyoid and larynx and thus open the upper esophageal sphincter. Available data support the effectiveness of the exercise in older normal subjects and in patients with disor-ders of the upper esophageal sphincter who have been taking nutrition nonorally for some time (Shaker, Easterling, Kern, Nitschke, Massey, Daniels, Grande, Kazandjian, & Dikeman, 2002).

How should this new procedure be assessed? The designer of the procedure, Dr. Reza Shaker, a gastroenterologist, has presented the procedure in a responsible way, first describing its physiology and theoretical effect, then examining the effec-tiveness of the therapy done for 6 weeks in normal older sub-jects, and then the same therapy for 6 weeks in dysphagic patients with upper sphincter problems. This process of study of the procedure is a good example of how new procedures should be assessed and presented. New procedures should not simply be presented in a workshop environment with no data to support them. They should be described in the literature with data to show their effectiveness, and then, if effective, educational workshops can be built around them.

Case Six

This case illustrates both the effects of a swallow maneuver and the application of that maneuver during the radiographic or other physiologic assessment. The patient is a 60-year-old woman who suffered a medullary stroke 4 days before the as-sessment. As in most medullary strokes, language and cogni-tion were not affected and she was able to follow directions. During the radiographic study, the swallow was characterized by poor laryngeal elevation and unilateral pharyngeal wall paresis as indicated by residue in one side of the pharynx. Both of these disorders resulted in reduced cricopharyngeal opening. The unilateral pharyngeal wall paresis and the reduced laryn-geal elevation resulted in 70% of the bolus remaining in the pharynx with aspiration of most of this material after the swal-low when the patient breathed. The first strategy attempted was head rotation to the damaged side of the pharynx, which resulted in improved clearance of the bolus but was not suc-cessful enough to clear all of the bolus and the patient contin-ued to aspirate. After head rotation, the Mendelsohn maneuver was taught to the patient. This maneuver is designed to increase and prolong laryngeal motion during swallow and thereby improve cricopharyngeal opening. The maneuver resulted in clearing approximately 30% more of the bolus. However, the patient still aspirated the remaining residue after the swallow. Then, head rotation and the Mendelsohn maneuver were combined. This combination resulted in clearance of the vast majority of the bolus with only approximately 20% remaining in the pharynx after the swallow. Aspiration was eliminated. The patient began small amounts of trial oral intake using both head rotation and the Mendelsohn maneuver. The SLP continued to follow the patient to assure good use of the Mendelsohn maneuver and after several days the patient was discharged to her home. She had been instructed to continue this therapy regimen and to continue nonoral intake for several more weeks. She was seen for weekly visits by the SLP and was reevaluated radiographically at the end of another 2 weeks. At that time, her swallow showed significant improvement and, using both the Mendelsohn and head rotation, she was able to take all bolus thicknesses and volumes orally and was recommended to begin oral intake. A reassessment at 3 months post-onset revealed an entirely functional swallow without using either head rotation or the Mendelsohn maneuver. She was then instructed to go ahead and begin full oral intake not using any of the therapeutic strategies.

✦ Evidence-Based Practice

Evidence-based practice involves integrating current best evidence, clinical expertise, pathophysiologic knowledge, and patient preferences in making decisions about the care of individual patients. The relevant skills include precisely defining a patient's problem (that is, careful diagnosis), proficiently searching and critically appraising relevant information from the literature, and then deciding whether, or how, to use this information in practice to design a patient's treatment plan (Jenicek, 1997; Straus, 1998). These skills are now being incorporated into the training of primary care providers and into continuing medical education (American Academy of Neurology, 1994; Tsafrir & Grinberg, 1998). Evidence-based practice is currently being advocated in all professions in health care, with the emphasis placed on peer-reviewed published evidence that a procedure is effective (Doggett, Tappe, Mitchell, Chapell, Coates, & Turkelson, 2001). The preference is that the evidence be in the form of a randomized clinical trial. There are not a large number of randomized clinical trials in our profession but there are some, and clinicians should be aware of these. There are several currently being conducted in speech–language pathology. It is also important for clinicians to know which evaluation or treatment procedures in any disorder area have no evidence to support them and to be cautious in utilizing them. Some third parties may reject a claim for payment of swallow therapy if the therapy is not evidence based. If clinicians measure the impact of a particular procedure in their daily therapy sessions, then they can share those data with the patient's third party. **Table 9–8** lists measures that can be used to ensure the effectiveness of various treatment procedures. Clinicians using non–evidence-based procedures should be ready to present data to the third party in support of the procedures (Duchan, Calculator, Sonnenmeier, Diehl, & Cumley, 2001).

In swallowing, there are currently several procedures being advocated for which there is no published evidence in peer-reviewed journals: deep pharyngeal neuromuscular stimulation (DPNS), electrical stimulation (E-Stim) to the surface of the neck, and myofascial release. There is a manuscript published on the E-stim procedure, but the data have severe limitations. The clinician must carefully evaluate the quality of the data.

Table 9–8 Measures of Swallowing Useful for Clinicians When Defining the Efficacy of Treatment During the Radiographic Study of Oropharyngeal Swallow

Efficacy Measures	Treatment Protocols
Oral transit time	Exercises to improve oral control; tongue range of motion and coordination exercises
Pharyngeal delay time (time from bolus head 1st reaching mandible till onset of laryngeal elevation assoc. w/swallow)	Therapy to improve triggering of the pharyngeal swallow; Thermal/tactile stimulation/suck swallow
Duration of velopharyngeal closure	Techniques to improve velopharyngeal closure
Duration of airway closure at entrance (between arytenoid and base of epiglottis or base of tongue)	Super-supraglottic swallow; effortful breath hold and adduction exercises
Approximate percent residue in valleculae	Effortful swallow
Approximate percent aspiration	Postures, supraglottic, super-supra-glottic and Mendelsohn maneuver
Duration of cricopharyngeal opening	Mendelsohn maneuver
Coordination of pharyngeal swallow events	Mendelsohn maneuver
Extent of laryngeal elevation*	Falsetto Mendelsohn maneuver
Extent of anterior hyoid motion*	Mendelsohn maneuver
Extent of vertical hyoid motion*	Falsetto Mendelsohn maneuver
Extent of tongue base to pharyngeal wall*	Effortful swallow, tongue-base retraction exercises
Approximate percent residue in valleculae	Effortful swallow, tongue retraction exercises
Approximate percent swallowed into esophagus divided by oropharyngeal transit time	
Oropharyngeal swallow efficiency**	
Oropharyngeal transit time: onset of posterior movement of bolus tail until it passes cricopharyngeal (CP) region	Any therapy to improve swallow function (compensatory or direct)

* To measure extent of movement, tape a dime at midline under the patient's chin or use a single vertebra as a reference distance to account for magnification.

**Rademaker et al., 1994.

If clinicians wish to use a procedure for evaluation or treatment of dysphagia that has no evidence, it becomes their responsibility to collect data on the effectiveness of the procedure in each patient with whom the procedure is used. This means measuring the outcomes and efficacy of the procedure in terms of the patient's targeted disorder and ultimate ability to return to oral feeding on various types of food. This should be documented in the patient's chart at regular intervals, even daily. Thus, utilizing an undocumented procedure adds additional responsibility to the clinician's care of a dysphagic patient.

Use of Water in Screening or Treatment of Dysphagic Patients

There are several screening procedures that involve the dysphagic patient swallowing measured amounts of water uninterrupted until the water has been completely cleared (DePippo, Holas, & Reding, 1992; Garon, Engle, & Ormiston, 1995; Nathadwarawala, McGroary, & Wiles, 1994). Generally, a negative response to this test is the patient interrupting the repeated swallows to breathe, coughing, choking while drinking, and the inability to swallow the entire measured volume in consecutive, repeated swallows. Failure results in an instrumental assessment of swallow. However, should the patient be severely dysphagic, these screening procedures can result in large volumes of water entering the airway and, rarely but possibly, respiratory arrest. In general, these procedures are not necessary to screen for swallow disorders and add an unnecessary risk. Overall, management of dysphagia should not increase the patient's risk.

Water has been recommended by one group as an important aspect of dysphagia management (Garon, Engle, & Ormiston, 1997). There are several protocols available to examine water and use it in the management of the dysphagic patient. Several procedures discuss the fact that using sterile water is safe. In fact, water, even if sterile in the cup, becomes full of anaerobic bacteria the minute it touches the mouth. Therefore, water is not sterile and runs the risk of introducing bacteria to the airway. One protocol suggests that the clinician should keep water in the room but not next to the patient's bed and that the patient should swallow the water only when a caregiver, including family members, is present. These procedures have not been evaluated with data-based approaches. In general, it is recommended that clinicians be as cautious in utilizing water in their management of dysphagic patients as they are in utilizing their food or other materials.

Throughout the process of evaluation and treatment of the dysphagic patient in acute care, or in any other health care or school setting, it is critical that the clinician be able to understand and explain the rationale for each procedure to the patient's attending physician, other health care professionals, the family, as well as the patient. Each procedure in the area of dysphagia management has or should have a strong physiologic rationale that should be communicated to other professionals to validate the procedures used.

✦ Professional Interactions in Dysphagia Management

Because of the complexity of some patients' dysphagia, a multidisciplinary team of professionals is often needed. However, in the current cost-containment environment, not every patient needs to see or should see every professional. In most cases the SLP serves as the triage person, suggesting the referrals each patient may need. A successful team depends on communication and mutual respect among all team members. It is not necessary for the team to meet every week. Communication may be effectively maintained by telephone or face-to-face discussions by various team members. Team members examine the patient from the perspective of their expertise. The patient's attending physician in concert with the patient and family is the ultimate decision maker regarding the patient's care and should be kept well informed regarding the patient's status. Other members of the team include the neurologist, otolaryngologist, gastroenterologist, pulmonologist, pharmacist, radiologist, dietitian, and occupational therapist, as well as the SLP. Patients exhibiting oropharyngeal dysphagia with no known medical diagnosis most often are found to have neurologic damage or disease, such as Parkinson's disease, motor neuron disease, brainstem stroke, brain tumor, etc. These patients should be referred to a neurologist, on the basis, often, of a modified barium swallow. In many cases the results of the modified barium swallow will point toward the underlying diagnosis because the patient's swallowing pattern is typical of a particular neurologic disease or bolus of damage. These results should be sent to the neurologist to whom the patient is referred.

The dietitian is a critical member of the dysphagia team. Once an optimal diet has been identified that can be swallowed safely and efficiently for a patient, the SLP should interact daily with the dietitian to determine whether or not the patient can sustain the intake of adequate nutrition and hydration on the targeted food types. The dietitian will normally monitor the patient's blood chemistries, calorie intake, as well as intake of nutrients to ensure that the patient is getting an adequate amount of nutrition as well as an adequate profile of nutrients. If the patient is able to manage only one consistency/viscosity such as pureed food, the dietitian should determine that the patient is able to get adequate nutrition in that one single viscosity and that the patient takes an adequate volume without fatiguing.

In many cases the patient will need nonoral supplement to get adequate calories and nutrients. Most patients with dysphagia begin oral intake on selected food types while maintaining nonoral nutrition or hydration. Patients should demonstrate adequate oral intake before discontinuing the nonoral nutrition. Generally, oral intake is given first followed by nonoral nutrition to supplement the oral intake. The particular type of nonoral nutrition is less important then the adequacy of the nutrition received. It is important for the SLP to communicate daily with the patient's attending physician to ensure that the physician understands the patient's calorie intake as well as need for any supplementation. An occupational therapist may be involved with the dysphagic patient; if self-feeding is a goal. The patient may need to improve arm and hand control for hand to mouth placement of food. The patient may also need assistive devices to improve food placement in the mouth. These are normally supplied by the occupational therapist (OT), and the patient is also trained to use them by the OT.

✦ Charting the Patient's Progress Using Outcome and Efficacy Measures

In today's health care system, each clinician is required to measure the patient's progress at each therapy session. In dysphagia this can be done in two ways: (1) by charting the measured improvement day to day in the patient's target area of dysfunction, and (2) by charting their progress toward oral intake. Efficacy measures of treatment present the measured improvement day to day in target functions. For example, the duration of a pharyngeal delay can be measured in seconds during each therapy session, and charted to reflect improvement in triggering over time. If the closure at the airway entrance is being treated, the extent of movement of the arytenoid or base or tongue or front wall of the epiglottis can be measured from one radiographic study to the next. If laryngeal elevation is the target of therapy, the extent of laryngeal elevation observed externally by motion of the thyroid cartilage can be measured in each therapy session with a millimeter ruler on the outside of the patient's neck. Efficacy measures may be temporal such as the duration of pharyngeal delay, or can be distance measures such as range of motion as in laryngeal elevation. **Table 9–7** presents a list of therapy procedures and measures of efficacy of that therapy procedure from session to session.

Outcome measures reflect the broad, ultimate goals for the patient such as safe intake of liquids or return to full oral intake. Each patient should be tracked for these outcomes to define the changes during the patient's acute hospitalization. Unfortunately, with the duration of acute care stays being reduced to a few days, in many cases these ultimate outcome measures may not be observed during the acute care hospitalization unless the patient responds immediately to the treatment procedures introduced in the radiographic study, in which case the patient can be moved quickly to at least partial oral intake. Data show that approximately 25% of patients can increase oral intake after the radiographic study, a significant reduction in cost.

✦ Communication with Physicians

Good, constant, knowledgeable communication with the dysphagic patient's attending physician and medical consultants is critical as the SLP completes the evaluation and treatment of the patient's swallowing disorders. Communication should be established at the time of the bedside or clinical assessment when the SLP makes a judgment about the need for an in-depth diagnostic study. The communication of the rationale for the diagnostic study is critical. The patient's attending physician must understand that treatment of oropharyngeal dysphagia is directed at the patient's abnormal anatomy or physiology that is creating the dysphagia. Treatment is not directed at symptoms such as aspiration or inefficient eating, but is directed at the physiology causing the symptoms.

The SLP should also keep in mind that medical training does not include information on swallowing, either normal or abnormal. The request for an in-depth diagnostic study, such as a radiographic study, should include comments such as:

After reviewing your patient's chart and completing a brief screening, it appears that the patient is at high risk for a pharyngeal dysphagia, which may include poor laryngeal elevation, poor airway closure or poor tongue-base action, none of which are visible at a screening. His diagnosis and additional medical problems would put him at risk for abnormalities in any of these areas. Because our treatment is different for each of these disorders, we need an in-depth study to define the specific physiologic abnormalities and evaluate the effects of immediate compensatory treatment which may allow him to begin oral intake right away.

Such a report by SLPs reflects their knowledge base in dysphagia and informs the physician of the goals of dysphagia evaluation and treatment, that is, the physiologic understanding of the patient's problem. A radiographic or other diagnostic study should never be requested to define the presence or absence of aspiration. Such a request will often be denied because a clinical observation at bedside may reveal the patient as aspirating or at high risk for aspiration. In the current cost-containment climate, most physicians will reject the request for a diagnostic swallowing study if it is designed to simply define the presence or absence of aspiration.

Communication with a patient's physician should not only reflect the clinician's knowledge while informing the physician about the assessments that have been completed but also be timely in relation to the patient assessments and treatments. Regular communication on the patient's progress is also critical.

Speech–language pathologists in acute care must work quickly and efficiently to be able to show improvement in efficacy and outcome measures for dysphagic patients. To be efficient and effective the clinician in the acute care setting must gain knowledge about the patient's swallow physiology quickly to target treatment to the exact disorder and move the patient as quickly as possible toward full oral intake.

Study Questions

1. Would you recommend a radiographic procedure for a patient with:
   A. Swallow apraxia
      (Why or why not?)
   B. Reduced laryngeal elevation
      (Why or why not?)
2. What types of treatment strategies might you try for the following patients and why?
   A. Alzheimer's disease with no ability to understand directions
   B. Patient with oral cancer resection
   C. Patient with a supraglottic laryngectomy
   D. Anterior left cortical stoke

3. Your patient has the following problem. Which diagnostic or screening procedures might you use?
   A. Cervical spinal cord injury with tracheostomy
   B. Delay in triggering the pharyngeal swallow
   C. Reduced range of tongue motion
4. Which postures and maneuvers would you combine for each of these patient types and why?
   A. Medullary stroke
   B. Supraglottic laryngectomy
   C. Alzheimer's disease
5. Which postures work best for these problems and why?
   A. Reduced range of vertical tongue motion
   B. Reduced airway closure
   C. Bilateral reduced pharyngeal wall function

References

American Academy of Neurology. (1994). *Assessment: Melodic Intonation Therapy*. Report of the Therapeutics and Technology Assessment Subcommittee of the American Academy of Neurology. *Neurology, 44,* 566–568

Bastian, R.W. (1993). The Videoendoscopic Swallowing Study: An Alternative and Partner to the Videofluoroscopic Swallowing Study. *Dysphagia, 8,* 359–367

Bhutani, M.S. (1993). Dysphagia in Myotonic Dystrophy. [Letter to the Editor]. *American Journal of Gastroenterology, 8,* 974–975

Bisch, E.M., Logemann, J.A., Rademaker, A.W., Kahrilas, P.J., & Lazarus, C.L. (1994). Pharyngeal Effects of Bolus Volume, Viscosity and Temperature in Patients with Dysphagia Resulting from Neurologic Impairment and in Normal Subjects. *Journal of Speech and Hearing Research, 37,* 1041–1049

Cook, I.J., Dodds, W.J., Dantas, R.O., Massey, B., Kern, M.K., Lang, I.M., Brasseur, J.G., Hogan, W.J. (1989). Opening mechanisms of the human upper esophageal sphincter. *Am J Physiol,* G748–G759

Danbolt, C., Hult, P., Grahn, L.T., & Ask, P. (1999). Validation and Characterization of the Computerized Laryngeal Analyzer (CLA) technique. *Dysphagia, 14,* 191–195

DePippo, K.L., Holas, M.A., & Reding, M.J. (1992). Validation of the 3 Oz Water Swallow Test for Aspiration Following Stroke. *Archives of Neurology, 49,* 1259–1261

Doggett, D.L., Tappe, K.A., Mitchell, M.D., Chapell, R., Coates, V., & Turkelson, C.M. (2001). Prevention of Pneumonia in Elderly Stroke Patients by Systematic Diagnosis and Treatment of Dysphagia: An Evidence-Based Comprehensive Analysis of the Literature. *Dysphagia, 16,* 279–295

Drake, W., O'Donoghue, S., Bartram, C., Lindsay, J., & Greenwood, R.(1997) . Eating in Side-Lying Facilitates Rehabilitation in Neurogenic Dysphagia. *Brain Injury, 11,* 137–142

Duchan, J. F., Calculator, S., Sonnenmeier, R., Diehl, S., & Cumley, G. D. (2001). A Framework for Managing Controversial Practices. *Language, Speech, and Hearing Sciences in the Schools, 32,* 133–141

Ergun, G.A., Kahrilas, P.J., & Logemann, J.A. (1993). Interpretation of Pharyngeal Manometric Recordings: Limitations and Variability. *Disorders of the Esophagus, 6,* 11–16

Fujiu, M., Toleikis, J.R., Logemann, J. A., & Larson, C.R. (1994). Glossopharyngeal Evoked Potentials in Normal Subjects Following Mechanical Stimulation of the Anterior Faucial Pillar. *Electroencephalography and Clinical Neurophysiology, 92,* 183–195

Garon, B.R., Engle, M., & Ormiston, C. (1995). Reliability of the 3-Oz. Water Swallow Test Utilizing Cough Reflex as Sole Indicator of Aspiration. *Journal of Neurologic Rehabilitation, 9,* 139–143

Garon, B.R., Engle, M., & Ormiston, C. (1997). A Randomized Control Study to Determine the Effects of Unlimited Oral Intake of Water in Patients with Identified Aspiration. *Journal of Neurologic Rehabilitation, 11,* 139–148

Hamlet, S., Penney, D.G., Formolo, J. (1994). Stethoscope Acoustics and Cervical Auscultation of Swallowing. *Dysphagia, 9,* 63–68

Horner, J., Alberts, M.J., Dawson, D.V., & Cook, G.M. (1994). Swallowing in Alzheimer's Disease. *Alzheimer Disease and Associated Disorders, 8,* 177–189

Jacob, P., Kahrilas, P., Logemann, J., Shah, V., & Ha, T. (1989). Upper Esophageal Sphincter Opening and Modulation During Swallowing. *Gastroenterology, 97,* 1469–1478

Jenicek, M. (1997). Epidemiology, Evidence-Based Medicine, and Evidence-Based Public Health. *Journal of Epidemiology, 7*(4), 187–197

Kahrilas, P.J., Lin, S., Logemann, J.A., Ergun, G.A., & Facchini, F. (1993). Deglutitive Tongue Action: Volume Accommodation and Bolus Propulsion. *Gastroenterology, 104,* 152–162

Kahrilas, P.J., & Logemann, J.A. (1993). Volume Accommodations During Swallowing. *Dysphagia, 8,* 259–265

Kahrilas, P.J., Logemann, J.A., & Gibbons, P. (1992). Food Intake by Maneuver: An Extreme Compensation for Impaired Swallowing. *Dysphagia, 7,* 155–159

Kahrilas, P.J., Logemann, J.A., Krugler, C., & Flanagan, E. (1991). Volitional Augmentation of Upper Esophageal Sphincter Opening During Swallowing. *American Journal of Physiology (Am J Physiol), 260*(3 pt 1), G450–456

Kahrilas, P.J., Logemann, J.A., Lin, S., & Ergun, G.A. (1992). Pharyngeal Clearance During Swallow: A Combined Manometric and Videofluoroscopic Study. *Gastroenterology, 103,* 128–136

Kennedy, G., Pring, T., & Fawcus, R. (1993). No Place for Motor-Speech Acts in the Assessment of Dysphagia? Intelligibility and Swallowing Difficulties in Stroke and Parkinson's Disease Patients. *European Journal of Disorders of Communication, 28,* 213–226

Kidder, T.M., Langmore, S.E., & Martin, B.J.W. (1994). Indications and Techniques of Endoscopy in Evaluation of Cervical Dysphagia: Comparison with Radiographic Techniques. *Dysphagia, 9,* 256–261

Klor, B., Milianti, F. (1995). Rehabilitation in Patients with G-Tubes. Presented at the 1995 ASHA convention in Orlando, FL

Langmore, S.E., Schatz, K., & Olson, M. (1988). Fiberoptic Endoscopic Examination of Swallowing Safety: A New Procedure. *Dysphagia, 2,* 216–219

Larnert, G., & Ekberg, O. (1995). Positioning Improves the Oral and Pharyngeal Swallowing Function in Children with Cerebral Palsy. *Acta Pædiatrica, 84,* 689–692

Lazarus, C.L. (1993). Effects of Radiation Therapy and Voluntary Maneuvers on Swallowing Functioning in Head and Neck Cancer Patients. *Clinics in Communication Disorders, 3,* 11–20

Lazarus, C., Logemann, J.A., & Gibbons, P. (1993a). Effects of Maneuvers on Swallowing Function in a Dysphagic Oral Cancer Patient. *Head & Neck, 15,* 419–424

Lazarus, C.L., Logemann, J.A., Pauloski, B.R., Colangelo, L.A., Kahrilas, P.J., Mittal, B.B., & Pierce, M. (1996). Swallowing Disorders in Head and Neck Cancer Patients Treated with Radiotherapy and Adjuvant Chemotherapy. *Laryngoscope, 106,* 1157–1166

Lazarus, C.L., Logemann, J.A., Rademaker, A.W., Kahrilas, P.J., Pajak, T., Lazar, R., & Halper, A. (1993b). Effects of Bolus Volume, Viscosity and Repeated Swallows in Non-Stroke Subjects and Stroke Patients. *Archives of Physical Medicine and Rehabilitation, 74,* 1066–1070

Leder, S.B. (1996) Gag Reflex and Dysphagia. *Head and Neck, 18,* 138–141

Leder, S.B. (1997). Videofluoroscopic Evaluation of Aspiration with Visual Examination of the Gag Reflex and Velar Movement. *Dysphagia, 12,* 21–23

Leder, S.B. (2000). Use of Arterial Oxygen Saturation, Heart Rate, and Blood Pressure as Indirect Objective Physiologic Markers to Predict Aspiration. *Dysphagia, 15,* 201–205

Logemann, J.A. (1990). Factors Affecting Ability to Resume Oral Nutrition in the Oropharyngeal Dysphagic Individual. *Dysphagia, 4,* 202–208

Logemann, J. (1993). *A Manual for Videofluoroscopic Evaluation of Swallowing,* 2nd ed. Austin, TX: Pro-Ed

Logemann, J.A. (1994). Management of Dysphagia Post Stroke. In: R. Chapey (Ed.), *Language Intervention Strategies in Adult Aphasia,* 3rd ed. (pp. 503–512). Baltimore: Williams & Wilkins

Logemann, J.A. (1995). Surgical Rehabilitation of Adults. In: M. Leahy (Ed.), *Disorders of Communication: The Science of Intervention,* 2nd ed. (pp. 305–326). London: Whurr

Logemann, J.A. (1997). Therapy for Oropharyngeal Swallowing Disorders. In: A. Perlman & K. Schulze-Delrieu (Eds.), *Deglutition and Its Disorders: Anatomy, Physiology, Clinical Diagnosis and Management* (pp. 449–461). San Diego, CA: Singular Publishing Group

Logemann, J.A. (1998). *Evaluation and Treatment of Swallowing Disorders,* 2nd ed. Austin, TX: Pro-Ed

Logemann, J.A., & Kahrilas, P.J. (1990). Relearning to Swallow Post CVA: Application of Maneuvers and Indirect Biofeedback: A Case Study. *Neurology, 40,* 1136–1138

Logemann, J.A., Pauloski, B.R., Colangelo, L., Lazarus, C., Fujiu, M., Kahrilis, P.J. (1995). Effects of a Sour Bolus on Oropharyngeal Swallowing Measures in Patients with Neurogenic Dysphagia. *Journal of Speech and Hearing Research, 38,* 556–563

Logemann, J.A., Pauloski, B.R., Rademaker, A.W., McConnel, F.M.S., Heiser, M.A., Cardinale, S., Shedd, D. (1993). Speech and Swallow Function After Tonsil/Base of Tongue Resection with Primary Closure. *Journal of Speech and Hearing Research, 36,* 918–926

Logemann, J.A., Rademaker, A.W., Pauloski, B.R., Kahrilas, P.J. (1994a). Effects of Postural Change on Aspiration in Head and Neck Surgical Patients. *American Academy of Otolaryngology-Head and Neck Surgery, 110,* 222–227

Logemann, J.A., Rademaker, A.W., Pauloski, B.R., Kahrilas, P.J., Bacon, M., Bowman, J., & McCracken, E. (1994b). Mechanisms of Recovery of Swallow After Supraglottic Laryngectomy. *Journal of Speech and Hearing Research, 37,* 965–974

Martin, B.J., Corlew, M.M., Wood, H., Olson, D., Gallipol, L.A., Wingbowl, M., & Kirmani, N. (1994b). The Association of Swallowing Dysfunction and Aspiration Pneumonia. *Dysphagia, 9,* 1–6

Martin, B.J.W., Logemann, J.A., Shaker, R., & Dodds, W.J. (1994a). Coordination Between Respiration and Swallowing: Respiratory Phase Relationships and Temporal Integration. *Journal of Applied Physiology, 76,* 714–723

Martin, B.J.W., Schleicher, M.A., & O'Connor, A. (1993). Management of Dysphagia Following Supraglottic Laryngectomy. *Clinics in Communication Disorders, 3,* 27–34

Martin, R.E., Neary, M.A., & Diamant, N.E. (1997). Dysphagia Following Anterior Cervical Spine Surgery. *Dysphagia, 12,* 2–8

Myers, A.D. (1995). Editorial: The Blue Dye Test. *Dysphagia, 10,* 175–176

Nathadwarawala, K.M., McGroary, A., Wiles, C.M. (1994) Swallowing and Neurological Outpatients: Use of a Timed Test. *Dysphagia, 9,* 120–129

Ohmae, Y., Logemann, J.A., Kaiser, P., Hanson, D.G., & Kahrilas, P.J. (1996). Effects of Two Breath-Holding Maneuvers on Oropharyngeal Swallow. *Annals of Otology, Otolaryngology, Rhinology, and Laryngology, 105,* 123–131

Penington, G.R. (1993). Severe Complications Following a "Barium Swallow" Investigation for Dysphagia. *Medical Journal of Australia, 159*, 764–765

Perlman, A.L., & Van Daele, D.J. (1993). Simultaneous Endoscopic and Ultrasound Measures of Swallowing. *Journal of Medical Speech Pathology, 4*, 223–232

Rademaker, A. W., Logemann, J. A., Pauloski, B. R., Bowman, J., Lazarus, C., Sisson, G., Milianti, F., Graner, D., Cook, B., Collins, S., Stein, D., Beery, Q., Johnson, J., & Baker, T. (1993). Recovery of Postoperative Swallowing in Patients Undergoing Partial Laryngectomy. *Head and Neck, 15*, 325–334

Rademaker, A.W., Pauloski, B.R., Logemann, J.A., Shanahan, T.K. (1994). Oropharyngeal Swallow Efficiency as a Representative Measure of Swallowing Function. *Journal of Speech and Hearing Research, 37*, 314–325

Rasley, A., Logemann, J.A., Kahrilas, P.J., Rademaker, A.W., Pauloski, B.R., Dodds, W.J. (1993). Prevention of Barium Aspiration During Fluoroscopic Swallowing Studies: Value of Change in Posture. *AJR, 160*, 1005–1009

Robbins, J., Hamilton, J.W., Lof, G.L., Kempster, G.B. (1992). Oropharyngeal Swallowing in Normal Adults of Different Ages. *Gastroenterology, 103*, 823–829

Robbins, J., & Levine, R. (1993). Swallowing After Lateral Medullary Syndrome Plus. *Clinics in Communication Disorders, 3*, 45–55

Rosenbek, J.C., Rocker, E.B., Wood, J.L., & Robbins, J.A. (1996). Thermal Application Reduces the Duration of Stage Transition in Dysphagia After Stroke. *Dysphagia, 11*, 225–233

Schmidt, J., Holas, M., Halvorson, C., & Redding, M. (1994). Videofluoroscopic Evidence of Aspiration Predicts Pneumonia and Death But Not Dehydration Following Stroke. *Dysphagia, 9*, 7–11

Shaker, R., Easterling, C., Kern, M., Nitschke, T., Massey, B., Daniels, S., Grande, B., Kazandjian, M., & Dikeman, K. (2002). Rehabilitation of Swallowing by Exercise in Tube-Fed Patients with Pharyngeal Dysphagia Secondary to Abnormal UES Opening. *Gastroenterology, 122*, 1314–1321

Shanahan, T.K., Logemann, J.A., Rademaker, A.W., Pauloski, B.R., & Kahrilas, P.J. (1993). Chin-Down Posture Effect on Aspiration in Dysphagic Patients. *Archives of Physical Medicine and Rehabilitation, 74*, 736–739

Shawker, T., Sonies, B., Hall, T., & Baum, G. (1984). Ultrasound Analysis of Tongue, Hyoid, and Larynx Activity During Swallowing. *Investigative Radiology, 19*, 82–86

Straus, S.E. (1998). Evidence-Based Medicine as a Tool. *Hospital Medicine, 59*, 762–765

Taniguchi, M.H., & Moyer, R.S. (1994). Assessment of Risk Factors for Pneumonia in Dysphagia Children: Significance of Videofluoroscopic Swallowing Evaluation. *Developmental Medicine and Child Neurology, 36*, 495–502

Thompson-Henry, S., & Braddock, B. (1995). The Modified Evan's Blue Dye Procedures Fails to Detect Aspiration in the Tracheostomized Patients: Five Case Reports. *Dysphagia, 10*, 172–174

Tracy, J., Logemann, J., Kahrilas, P., Jacob, P., Kobara, M., Krugler, C. (1989). Preliminary Observations on the Effects of Age on Oropharyngeal Deglutition. *Dysphagia, 4*, 90–94

Tsafrir, J., & Grinberg, M. (1998). Who Needs Evidence-Based Health Care? *Bulletin of the Medical Library Association, 86*, 40–45

Welch, M.V., Logemann, J.A., Rademaker, A.W., & Kahrilas, P.J. (1993). Changes in Pharyngeal Dimensions Effected by Chin Tuck. *Archives of Physical Medicine and Rehabilitation, 74*, 178–181

Ylvisaker, M., & Logemann, J.A. (1998). Therapy for Feeding and Swallowing Disorders After Traumatic Brain Injury. In: M. Ylvisaker (Ed.), *Traumatic Brain Injury Rehabilitation: Children and Adolescents*, 2nd ed. (pp. 85–99). Boston: Butterworth-Heinemann

Zenner, P.M., Losinski, D.S., & Mills, R.H. (1995). Using Cervical Auscultation in the Clinical Dysphagia Examination in Long-Term Care. *Dysphagia, 10*, 27–31

10

The Use of Flexible Endoscopy to Evaluate and Manage Patients with Dysphagia

Susan Langmore

- ✦ **Indications for Endoscopy**
- ✦ **Fiberoptic Endoscopic Evaluation of Swallowing Protocol**
- ✦ **Sensory Awareness**
- ✦ **Use of Endoscopy to Manage Patients with Dysphagia**
- ✦ **Case Presentation**
- ✦ **Risks Associated with Videoendoscopy**

Flexible laryngoscopy has been used by physicians and speech–language pathologists (SLPs) for many years. Although there is some overlap in our areas of interest and the procedures we use, our primary goals and objectives are very different. Physicians employ the procedure to help them arrive at medical diagnoses that may subsequently lead to medical or surgical intervention. They attempt to uncover the underlying causes of anatomic abnormality (e.g., benign or malignant tissue changes or structural abnormalities in response to trauma or congenital abnormality), abnormal movement (e.g., recurrent laryngeal nerve paralysis), or neurosensory deficit (e.g., superior laryngeal nerve dysfunction) observed endoscopically. Depending on the diagnosis, the physician may suggest medical or surgical treatment options to eliminate the cause of the swallowing problem or they may refer to an SLP for behavioral intervention.

Speech–language pathologists do not use endoscopy to make medical or surgical diagnoses. Rather, they use endoscopy to observe, explain, and document the anatomic and physiologic correlates of the underlying medical problem. Such observations may then become the basis for making decisions about whether and what type of behavioral management may be indicated in the overall treatment plan for the patient. Many swallowing disorders requiring behavioral management also may necessitate medical/surgical diagnosis and treatment. Consequently, it is standard practice in speech–language pathology to require patients who have a suspected anatomic or physiologic disorder affecting swallowing to have a medical/surgical evaluation before behavioral management is considered. Because endoscopy is performed by either professional, this may involve performing two examinations or

one joint examination, after which the endoscopic findings can be evaluated as a team. Speech–language pathologists may further employ videoendoscopy as a behavioral management tool.

This chapter briefly outlines how SLPs incorporate videoendoscopy into the evaluation and treatment of the patient with dysphagia. Complete consideration of the many theoretical, technical, and practical issues involved in dysphagia assessment and treatment is not possible here, and interested readers are encouraged to consult other works for additional detail regarding anatomy and physiology of normal and abnormal swallowing, clinical and instrumental assessment techniques, and behavioral and dietary management. We assume that readers already have a firm foundation in nonendoscopic assessment and management of swallowing disorders in adults and children. For more information regarding the role of the SLP in the assessment and management of patients with dysphagia using endoscopy, go to the American Speech–Language-Hearing Association (ASHA) Web site (www.asha.org) and review documents pertaining to endoscopy.

✦ Indications for Endoscopy

Speech–language pathologists evaluate and treat swallowing problems that primarily affect the oral and pharyngeal stages of swallowing. The first steps in the evaluation of dysphagia should include a review of the medical history, an interview with the patient, and a clinical examination of oral, laryngeal, and respiratory function. Following this, an instrumental examination is often performed.

Fluoroscopy, or the modified barium swallow (MBS), has been used as a standard examination for oropharyngeal dysphagia for many years, with endoscopy (fiberoptic endoscopic evaluation of swallowing, FEES) emerging later as a diagnostic tool. The first published study describing the endoscopic swallowing procedure was in 1988 (Langmore, Schatz, & Olson, 1988). Since that time, the merits of both examinations have been argued, and today they are both accepted as valid, sensitive, and useful examinations (Hiss & Postma, 2003; Langmore, 2003; Rao, Brady, Chaudhuri, et al., 2003).

Many abnormal findings can be gleaned from either examination, but there are also unique findings that lead the discerning clinician to choose one procedure over the other. Indications for performing an endoscopic examination versus a fluoroscopic examination are listed in **Table 10–1**. First there may be logistic or practical reasons for choosing endoscopy or fluoroscopy. For example, when the patient is critically ill,

Table 10–1 Indications for a Fiberoptic Endoscopic Evaluation Swallowing (FEES®) or Fluoroscopy Examination

Indications for a FEES examination

Need exam that day; cannot schedule fluoroscopy that day

Positioning in fluoroscopy problematic: e.g., patient bedridden, weak, has contractures, in pain, has decubitus ulcers, quadriplegic, wearing neck halo, obese, on ventilator

Transportation to fluoroscopy suite is problematic: medically fragile/unstable patient (in ICU); cardiac or other monitoring in place; on ventilator; nursing/medical care must be with patient

Transportation to hospital problematic: nursing home issues, including cost of transportation, resources needed to accompany patient, strain on patient, patient fearful of leaving familiar surroundings, etc.

Concern about excess and repeated radiation exposure

Concern about aspiration of barium, food, and/or liquid in patient with potentially profound dysphagia or very limited ability to tolerate any aspiration

Postintubation or postsurgery where vagal nerve damage is possible

Need to assess status of patient's ability to manage secretions

Want time to assess fatigue or swallow status over a meal

Want therapeutic exam: time to try out several maneuvers, several consistencies, etc.; you want to try real foods; you want caregiver to hold baby in several positions, etc.

Need repeat exam to assess change; to assess effectiveness of maneuver

Want to try biofeedback

Indications for a fluoroscopy examination

Patient will not accept/tolerate endoscopy

Oral stage problem needs to be imaged

Globus complaints: suspect esophageal stage problem or gastroesophageal reflux (GER); want to visualize esophageal motility and GE reflux (must include esophagram for complete examination)

Possible cricopharyngeal (CP) dysfunction

Need to view cervical osteophytes

Vague symptomatology from patient; need comprehensive view

Need to better identify amount of aspiration of thin liquids during the swallow

*FEES® is a copyrighted trademark of Susan E. Langmore, Ph.D. Use of the acronym FEES indicates that the endoscopic examination of pharyngeal swallowing herein performed or reported on was consistent with the procedure developed by Susan E. Langmore, Ph.D., and described in this chapter.

intubated, or requires continuous monitoring, videoendoscopy may be safer and easier for the patient to tolerate than videofluoroscopy. The portability of the endoscopic equipment allows it to be brought to the patient's bedside where the exam can be done in a safer and more comfortable environment than the fluoroscopy suite. The patient who is agitated and confused may do better with fluoroscopy, which is less invasive for the patient. There are also clinical indications for choosing one examination or the other. A common example is the patient who has a breathy or hoarse voice quality after intubation or surgery and for whom a direct look at the larynx would be beneficial. Structural and physiologic changes to the larynx that directly affect swallowing are best revealed by endoscopy. On the other hand, patients who complain of globus, or foreign-body sensation, may well have normal oral and pharyngeal swallowing, but abnormal esophageal motility or gastroesophageal reflux. Adding an esophagram to the MBS is an efficient way to detect this problem.

Children with dysphagia as well as adults benefit from endoscopy. Some advantages for infants or children are the ability to be tested in a natural seating position (even held in the parent's arms), with typical liquids or foods, and the absence of radiation exposure. Voluntary compliance and cooperation from children are not always assured, however.

The views provided by videoendoscopy and videofluoroscopy are distinctly different. Fluoroscopy provides both coronal (frontal) and sagittal (lateral) planes, imaging the shadow of oral, pharyngeal, and esophageal structures. Endoscopy offers a transverse (horizontal) view, looking directly at the nasopharynx, oropharynx, hypopharynx and larynx from above. Both views show the bolus, although the endoscopic view is obliterated for about 0.5 second during the height of each swallow, except in cases where the swallow is so weak that the air space is not obliterated. The fluoroscopic view is limited in time by radiation exposure constraints so that the fluoroscopy unit is generally turned off between every swallow and total viewing time is limited to 3 to 5 minutes. Endoscopy can provide a constant view over a prolonged period of time, including the period between swallows when important events can take place. Fluoroscopy can provide a clearer representation of subglottic aspiration, whereas endoscopy reveals the location of the bolus within the hypopharynx with more specificity.

Although there are significant differences between the two procedures, they have similar purposes and outcomes. Both fluoroscopic and endoscopic procedures can be used to detect the presence of dysphagia, both can reveal the nature of the problem, and both will allow the examiner to make the recommendations needed for adequate management of the problem.

✦ Fiberoptic Endoscopic Evaluation of Swallowing Protocol

Langmore, Schatz, and Olson (1988, 1991) published the first description of the FEES procedure for evaluating swallowing with endoscopy. This acronym was copyrighted to distinguish it from a laryngeal examination as done by an otolaryngologist and to define it as a comprehensive evaluation of oropharyngeal dysphagia. Equipment needed for a FEES examination includes a standard flexible laryngoscope attached to a video camera, a light source, a video recorder, and a monitor.

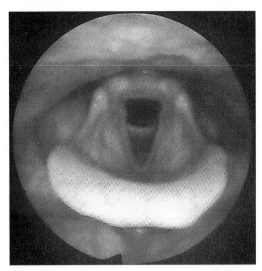

Figure 10–1 View of the hypopharynx with the tip of the endoscope positioned just superior to the epiglottis so that the entire hypopharynx and larynx can be viewed. The typical position for the endoscope just prior to the swallow, is called the "home" position.

The laryngoscope is passed transnasally to a point just above the epiglottis where the hypopharynx and larynx can be optimally viewed (**Fig. 10–1**). This is called the home position. For most of the exam this is the position of choice; however, after each swallow, the scope is briefly passed into the laryngeal vestibule so that the true vocal folds and the subglottic shelf (membranous portion of the thyroid and cricoid cartilage positioned just below the true vocal folds) can be examined more closely for evidence of penetration or aspiration (**Fig. 10–2**).

Patient comfort is paramount for this examination because the objective is to assess habitual swallowing function and to be able to keep the endoscope in place for as long as 20 to 30 minutes. Some patients request topical anesthesia to help dull the sensation inside the nose. In this case, the examiner can administer a very small amount of topical anesthetic in the nares that will be used to pass the endoscope. The use of anesthesia is discouraged for a FEES examination because

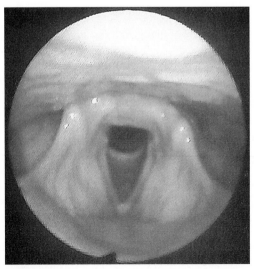

Figure 10–2 Close-up view of the larynx, including arytenoids, true vocal folds, and subglottic shelf. This view should be obtained between swallows for a brief period to inspect for signs of aspiration.

it might depress sensation in the pharynx or larynx and adversely affect swallowing function, although this has been contested by some researchers (Johnson, Belafsky, & Postma, 2003; Willging, et al., 1998).

The FEES® protocol is shown in **Table 10–2**. There are three parts to a complete FEES examination. Part I consists of a direct examination of the base of the tongue, and velopharyngeal (VP), pharyngeal, and laryngeal function. Anatomy and secretions within the hypopharynx (HP) are also noted. Part II requires the patient to eat and drink food and liquid while swallowing function is directly assessed. Part III includes the introduction of therapeutic maneuvers to try to remediate the problem.

Part I is an extension of the oral and motor clinical examination done to examine the lip, tongue, and jaw movement. This is a critical part of the examination because it helps the examiner understand the underlying anatomic or physiologic cause of the dysphagia. The endoscopic view provides a direct view of the mucosa overlying the structures of interest. The size, shape, and symmetry of the pharyngeal and laryngeal structures are observed for their effect on swallowing function. The depth of the lateral channels and resting position of the epiglottis are appreciated for their ability to contain a spilled bolus. Edema and erythema are noted. Any suspicious growths or unusual appearance of the mucosal surface would alert the SLP to a possible medical pathology and would warrant referral to otolaryngology.

The FEES protocol then directs the examiner to ask the patient to perform a variety of tasks that recruit velopharyngeal, base of tongue, pharyngeal, and laryngeal movement. Parameters of interest include strength, range, symmetry, and briskness of movement. Most of the tasks require the patient to speak, but some can be tested even in a confused or nonspeaking patient, such as breath hold or cough. Glottal closure or airway protection is tested in detail because this function is so critical for prevention of aspiration.

Over the first few minutes of the examination, the examiner observes the status of any standing secretions, the ability of the patient to swallow or clear these secretions, and the frequency of spontaneous dry swallows. The presence of pooled secretions in the larynx has been shown to be an excellent predictor of aspiration of food and liquid and is therefore an important part of the FEES examination (Donzelli, Brady, Wesling, et al., 2003; Murray, Langmore, Ginsberg, & Dostie, 1996).

At the conclusion of part I, laryngeal and pharyngeal sensation can be directly assessed with the air pulse sensory stimulator, if this equipment is available (Pentax Precision Instrument Corp., Orangeburg, NY). This equipment allows the examiner to determine the lightest force of air in millimeters of mercury that elicits a laryngeal adductor reflex when an air pulse is directed over each aryepiglottic fold. The patient's threshold response can be compared to norms to determine if it is abnormal. When added to the FEES examination, the procedure can be called a FEES sensory testing (ST) examination. If the sensory box is not available, the examiner can grossly assess sensation directly by lightly touching structures within the HP with the tip of the endoscope. However, it is advised that the examiner wait until the very end of the examination if using the "touch" method because it may not be needed. Often, by that point in the exam, the patient's response to sensory stimuli in the HP is known and direct testing is unnecessary. In addition, it is more intrusive and may generate a strong cough.

Table 10–2　The FEES® Protocol as Developed by Susan E. Langmore, Ph.D., in 2004

Patient Name:

Date:

Examiner:

I. Anatomic-Physiologic Assessment

A. Velopharyngeal Closure

Task:	Say "ee", "ss", other oral sounds; alternate oral and nasal sounds ("duh-nuh")
Task:	Dry swallow
Optional task:	Swallow liquids and look for nasal leakage

B. Appearance of Hypopharynx and Larynx at Rest

Scan around entire HP to note symmetry and abnormalities that impact swallowing and might require referral to otolaryngology or other specialty.

Optional task:	Hold your breath and blow out cheeks forcefully (pyriform sinuses)

C. Handling of Secretions and Swallow Frequency

Observe amount and location of secretions and frequency of dry swallows over a period of at least 2 minutes

Task:	If no spontaneous swallowing noted, cue the patient to swallow

Go to Ice Chip Protocol if secretions in laryngeal vestibule or if no ability to swallow saliva.

D. Base of Tongue and Pharyngeal Muscles

1. Base of Tongue

Task:	Say "earl, ball, call" or other post-vocalic "l" word several times

2. Pharyngeal Wall Medialization

Task:	Screech; hold a high pitched, strained "ee"

(Task: see laryngeal elevation task below)

E. Laryngeal Function

1. Respiration

Observe larynx during rest breathing (respiratory rate; adduction/abduction)

Tasks:	Sniff, pant, or alternate "ee" with light inhalation (abduction)

2. Phonation

Task:	Hold "ee" (glottic closure)
Task:	Repeat "hee-hee-hee" 5 to 7 times (symmetry, precision)

3. Elevation

Glide upward in pitch until strained; hold it (pharyngeal walls also recruited)

4. Airway Protection

Task:	Hold your breath lightly (true vocal folds)
Task:	Hold your breath very tightly (ventricular folds; arytenoids)
Task:	Hold your breath to the count of 7
Optional:	Cough, clear throat, Valsalva maneuver

F. Sensory Testing

Note response to presence of scope

Optional task:	Lightly touch tongue, pharyngeal walls, epiglottis, aryepiglottic (AE) folds
Optional task:	Perform formal sensory testing with air pulse stimulator

Note: Additional information about sensation will be obtained in part II and formal testing can be deferred until the end of the examination if desired.

II. Swallowing of Food and Liquid: All foods/liquids dyed green or blue with food coloring

Consistencies to try will vary depending on patient needs and problems observed; suggested consistencies to try:

✦ Ice chips:	usually 1/3 to 1/2 teaspoon, dyed green
✦ Thin liquids:	milk, juice, formula. Milk or other light-colored thin liquid is recommended for visibility. Barium liquid is excellent to detect aspiration, but retract the scope to prevent gunking during the swallow.
✦ Thick liquids:	nectar or honey consistency; milkshakes
✦ Puree	
✦ Semisolid food:	mashed potato, banana, pasta
✦ Soft solid food: (requires some chewing)	bread and cheese, soft cookie, casserole, meat loaf, vegetables
✦ Hard, chewy, crunchy food:	meat, raw fruit, green salad
✦ Mixed consistencies:	soup with food bits, cereal with milk

Amounts/Bolus Sizes

If measured bolus sizes are given, a rule of thumb that applies to many patients is to increase the bolus size with each presentation until penetration or aspiration is seen. When that occurs, repeat the same bolus size to determine if this pattern is consistent. If penetration/aspiration occurs again, do not continue with that bolus amount. The following progression of bolus volumes are suggested:

<5 cc if patient is medically fragile and/or pulmonary clearance is poor

5 cc (1 teaspoon)

10 cc

15 cc (1 tablespoon)

20 cc (heaping tablespoon, delivered)

Single swallow from cup or straw:　monitored

Single swallow from cup or straw:　self-presented

Free consecutive swallows:　　　　self-presented

Feed self food at own rate

The FEES Ice Chip Protocol

Part I:	Emphasize anatomy, secretions, laryngeal competence, sensation

Note spontaneous swallows, cued swallow

Part II:	Deliver ice chips

Note effect on swallowing, effect on secretions, cough if aspirated

When utilized, the examiner can lightly touch the lateral pharyngeal walls, base of tongue, aryepiglottic folds, and, if necessary, the tip of epiglottis. The response should be a cough or other lesser response indicating the patient felt the scope.

When all the components of part I have been tested, the FEES exam progresses to part II, in which the delivery of food and liquid is given and swallowing of these materials can be directly observed. A variety of foods and liquids in varying volumes and consistencies are given to patients and their ability to swallow them safely and adequately is noted. Every bolus is dyed green or blue so that it is more visible and distinct from surrounding mucosal surfaces. The liquid bolus to be used poses some problems. Juice or green-tinged water makes an excellent bolus for observing spillage, but if they are aspirated, they may easily be missed. When the question is whether or not the patient aspirates, the liquid to use must reflect the light and, ideally, coat the mucosal surface. Use of milk, vanilla-flavored formula, or barium liquid is recommended for this purpose. However, these liquids often coat the tip of the endoscope as well, and reduce the view. I generally use both kinds of liquids during the examination. I visualize spillage with the juice over several swallows and then, at the end of the examination, I retract the scope up to the nasopharynx as the patient swallows the barium liquid. After the swallow, I advance the scope quickly to the larynx and look for any signs of aspiration.

The FEES examination may be structured, with measured bolus sizes trialed, or the examination can be very unstructured, by simply asking the patient to eat everything on the plate in front of him and delivering no specific instructions. This is a clinical decision that the examiner must decide. Abnormal function is identified by signs such as residue, spillage, laryngeal penetration, and aspiration of material below the true vocal folds. The anatomic or physiologic cause of the swallowing problem is determined by studying the pattern of swallowing and by relating the findings back to part I of the study. This will be discussed further in the next section.

As soon as a problem is identified, part III commences. The examiner may want to intervene immediately with appropriate therapeutic alterations to observe their effect on swallowing. Interventions might include instructing the patient to assume another posture such as chin-tuck, teaching the patient a swallow maneuver such as the controlled breath hold prior to swallowing, or adjusting the bolus consistency, size, or method of delivery. Alternatively, the examiner may want to wait through several swallows before intervening in order to more accurately assess the real risk of aspiration. For example, it may be useful to see how the patient spontaneously responds to a buildup of residue before trying to reduce it. The examination ends when the examiner understands the nature of the problem, has determined which bolus amounts and consistencies can be swallowed effectively and safely, and has noted what therapeutic alterations facilitate swallowing.

Whenever possible, the patient, the family, and the nursing staff members who feed the patient are involved in the examination and participate in decision making regarding possible treatment for the swallowing problems that are observed. It has been our clinical experience that education of and collaboration with these significant persons are the most effective means of developing realistic and meaningful treatment goals and ensuring compliance with the treatment plan. Generally, we have the patient face the monitor during the entire examination so that patient education and biofeedback, using the image on the monitor, can be incorporated into the examination itself.

Scoring and Interpretation

Many of the major findings from a FEES exam can be identified during the examination by simply noting the abnormal findings as they occur. Possible observations might include spillage of pureed material to the level of the pyriforms before

the swallow, residue remaining in the right lateral channel, aspiration of liquid before the swallow, and so on. However, to interpret the examination and determine why the problems occurred, it is usually necessary to review the examination at least one time, often pausing to play back some portion in slow motion.

When scoring and reporting on a FEES exam, it is sometimes useful to describe the abnormal findings that occur over time with each consistency, for example, to describe how the patient handled pureed food, then solid food, and finally liquids. Other times, it is more useful to discuss the problems in relation to the timing of the swallow, that is, to discuss the oral preparatory phase, the transitional time or the initiation of the swallow, the effectiveness of bolus clearance, and the patient's response after the swallow. This, again, is an individual decision.

Interpretation requires the examiner to relate the individual findings to the underlying anatomy and pathophysiology that created the particular pattern observed. This not only explains the dysphagia, but also provides the rationale for the treatment plan. There are four major types of problems that occur in the oral and pharyngeal stages of swallowing that can be identified from the examination: (1) inability to prepare the food orally, (2) inability to initiate the swallow in a timely and coordinated manner, (3) inadequate airway protection or VP closure during the swallow, and (4) incomplete bolus clearance. These problems can all be revealed from a FEES examination, although problem 1 is also dependent on clinical observations of the patient.

1. *Inability to prepare the food orally.* The clinical interview, oral motor examination, and observations during eating will explain why food is not prepared well. Mastication, containment of the food in the mouth, and the ability to propel the food out of the mouth require a fairly intact tongue, some teeth that are aligned, lips that can close, a jaw that can move, and a degree of alertness and self-monitoring. If the oral stage is impaired, the pharyngeal consequences can be directly viewed endoscopically. The masticated bolus may leak over the base of tongue during mastication, may not be propelled at all, but only fall by gravity, or may not be masticated sufficiently and may stick in the valleculae.

2. *Inability to initiate the swallow in a timely and coordinated manner.* A major cause for dysphagia is mistiming of bolus propulsion and the pharyngeal response at the initiation of the swallow. This problem of mistiming, often described as a problem in delaying the pharyngeal response, is one of the most common abnormalities reported for patients with neurogenic dysphagia and is a frequent cause of aspiration (Horner, Massey, Riski, Lathrop, & Chase, 1988; Smith, Logemann, Colangelo, Rademaker, & Pauloski, 1999). This problem is visualized during the examination as material spilling into the hypopharynx prior to the initiation of the swallow (**Fig. 10–3**). If the spillage is excessive, the bolus will overflow the lateral channels or the pyriforms and enter the laryngeal vestibule. Because the swallow has not yet begun, the airway will likely be open, and thus the bolus can enter the glottis and be aspirated. All these events are directly viewed with endoscopy because the airspace has not yet closed.

   Spillage can be attributed to (1) poor oral control or sensation, allowing the bolus to fall into the pharynx too early, during the oral preparatory stage, or (2) delay initiating

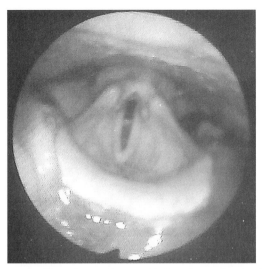

Figure 10–3 Spillage of pureed material before the swallow has begun. The material has spilled nearly to the pyriform recesses without any indication of the swallow initiation, indicating a pharyngeal delay. (See Color Plate 10–3.)

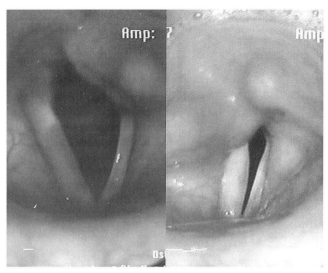

Figure 10–4 Abducted (left) and adducted (right) view of larynx with left laryngeal paralysis. Note the bowing of the affected left vocal fold visible in the abducted view. (See Color Plate 10–4.)

the swallow. The swallow reflex may not be triggered promptly because of reduced peripheral sensation, slow or incomplete transmission of sensory information, reduced processing of sensory information in the brainstem or higher brain centers, or reduced motor output from the brainstem and higher cortical centers. Pharyngeal delay time is a temporal measure of how long the bolus was in the pharynx before the swallow began. This is a well-known quantitative measure of the problem and can be readily calculated from endoscopy as well as fluoroscopy (Robbins, Levie, Maser, Rosenbek, & Kempster, 1993; Lazarus, Logemann, Rademaker, Kahrilas, Pajak Lazar, & Halper, 1993). Recent research has established that some spillage is normal, especially with solid food, and the cut-off for normal vs. pharyngeal delay has become clouded (Dua, Ren, Bardan, Xie, & Shaker, 1997; Palmer, 1998). Rather than focusing solely on a temporal measure of delay, the examiner should appreciate all the factors that allow one person to aspirate more easily than another. The length of time the bolus is in the pharynx, combined with the bolus size, along with the significant influence of anatomy on directing the path of the bolus, will cumulatively determine whether a person will run into trouble at the initiation of the swallow. For example, some persons have an epiglottis with a flattened-down tip that rests directly on the base of the tongue. Even a small amount of spillage cannot be tolerated by these individuals, because the bolus will be directed into the vestibule rather than into an open vallecular recess.

3. *Inadequate airway protection or VP closure during the swallow.* Inadequate airway protection results in aspiration of material during the swallow. The underlying pathophysiology is often thought to be weakness or incomplete movement of the laryngeal structures that participate in the swallow (i.e., epiglottic retroversion, arytenoid adduction and forward tilt, true and false vocal fold adduction). More often, however, it is really a problem of delayed airway closure and reflects a delayed or mistimed initiation of the swallow. If there is no spillage whatsoever prior to the onset of the swallow, and the bolus is still aspirated during the swallow, one can assume airway protection is compromised.

Although fluoroscopy is better for viewing aspiration of the bolus as it occurs during the swallow, endoscopy is better for judging the source of the weakness, or laryngeal incompetence. The tasks requested of the patient in the first part of the FEES examination (breath holding, etc.) assess the ability of the glottis to be closed off by vocal fold adduction. It also gives a good representation of the briskness of laryngeal movement. **Figure 10–4** is an example of a patient with incomplete vocal fold adduction who may not be able to close off the airway during the swallow. If glottic closure is normal, however, the reason for aspiration during the swallow must be tied to some other incomplete movement. Reduced arytenoid anterior tilt or incomplete epiglottal retroflexion would allow leakage into the airway during the swallow. Although closing the airway may be the primary function of these two factors, they are also part of laryngeal elevation and their movement is facilitated by good laryngeal excursion. The most direct evidence of laryngeal elevation from a FEES examination comes from the view of the epiglottis as it returns to rest when the air space reopens and white-out ends at the end of the swallow. If the examiner notes that the epiglottis did *not* retroflex, this supports the impression that reduced hyolaryngeal elevation is part of the etiology of the aspiration.

Aspiration that occurs during the swallow cannot be viewed directly with endoscopy, but it is usually apparent from residue of the bolus left in the laryngeal vestibule or on the subglottic shelf after the swallow. If there is doubt, the endoscopist can ask the patient to cough and see if any material is expelled, or the same bolus condition can be repeated. Several research studies have shown that in spite of losing the view for a brief time, endoscopy is sensitive to aspiration (Langmore et al., 1991; Leder, Sasaki, & Burrell, 1998; Madden, Fenton, Hughes, & Timon, 2000; Perie, Laccourreye, Flahault, Hazebroucq, Chaussade, & St. Guily, 1998; Schroter-Morasch, Bartolome, Troppmann, & Ziegler, 1999; Wu, et al., 1997).

4. *Incomplete bolus clearance.* This is a very common type of problem, evidenced by residue of bolus left behind after the swallow (**Fig. 10–5**). If residue is left in the HP after the

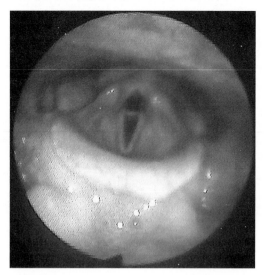

Figure 10–5 Residue of pureed material left in the valleculae and lateral channels after the swallow. (See Color Plate 10–5.)

swallow, and especially if it builds up over several swallows, it will eventually spill into the laryngeal vestibule and be aspirated when the airway reopens. The underlying pathophysiology causing the residue may be weakness of the base of the tongue or pharyngeal muscles or the presence of an obstruction in the bolus path. Although residue, the patient's reaction to the residue, and the path it eventually takes are clearly seen by endoscopy, identifying the specific source of a possible weakness is more difficult and requires some analysis. Fortunately, the location of the residue points to the source of the problem. For example, if residue is left on the base of the tongue, one can assume this region was not squeezed completely against the posterior pharyngeal wall. Research using simultaneous manometry and fluoroscopy have supported the relationship between the location of the residue and the source of the problem (Perie et al., 1998; Perlman, Grayhack, & Booth, 1992; Dejaeger, Pelemans, Ponette, & Joosten, 1997; Olsson, Castell, Johnston, Ekberg, & Castell, 1997). If residue is left in the HP because of an alteration in anatomy or an obstruction, such as a large feeding tube or a tumor, this problem is well appreciated from the endoscopic view and can be very helpful in guiding treatment strategies.

✦ Sensory Awareness

Reduced sensation is another factor that can contribute to several of the abnormal swallow patterns described above. Impaired sensation can cause loss of bolus control in the mouth, contribute to excess spillage, and reduce a patient's awareness and response to residue, penetration, or aspiration. It is not only a problem in patients with peripheral loss of sensation, however, but it is also commonly seen in patients with cortical or subcortical damage. The deficit should more properly be thought of as *reduced sensory processing* of information about the bolus, implying that the problem could originate anywhere along the neural pathway from the periphery to the higher centers that process sensory information, to the brainstem which receives this information and

incorporates it into the motor response. Further research is needed to elucidate this problem. As we understand it better, more effective treatment paradigms may emerge for dealing with this loss.

✦ Use of Endoscopy to Manage Patients with Dysphagia

Endoscopy is an extremely useful tool to guide the treatment or management of dysphagia. Because it is portable, the equipment can be brought to patients who would otherwise not have the advantage of an instrumental examination. The exam can be done in the presence of, and with the cooperation of, the patient, family, nursing staff, and anyone else involved in the patient's eating. The visual image can be discussed, the abnormal findings can be easily explained, and the entire team can be involved in making decisions as the exam progresses along. Compliance is greatly improved in such an environment.

The FEES examination is well suited to being a therapeutic examination. As soon as the patient experiences difficulty with a bolus, the examiner may alter conditions to find a safe and effective way for the patient to swallow. This may involve increasing or decreasing the bolus size, changing the consistency of the bolus, altering the method of food delivery, teaching the patient a swallow maneuver, or altering the patient's posture. All therapeutic applications can be tried without the time constraints of fluoroscopy, and their effect can be shown directly to the patient and caregivers for their understanding and input. If fatigue is a mitigating factor, there is ample time to observe the effects of fatigue on swallowing performance. Recommendations regarding diet, treatment, and management follow directly from therapeutic interventions tried during the initial assessment. Follow-up FEES examinations may be done with the sole purpose of testing the effectiveness or continued need for a therapeutic alteration.

Finally, endoscopy can be used directly as a feedback tool. If the patient is turned to face the monitor, endoscopy can provide visual biofeedback. We have employed endoscopy to teach a more protective and consistent pattern of airway closure, to help with the problem of bolus spillage, to emphasize the effects of a different posture, and to increase a patient's awareness of residue, penetration, or aspiration. Although endoscopy would not be done daily, infrequent sessions are tolerated well by most patients. The value of biofeedback cannot be underestimated, as it is an excellent tool for learning motor behaviors. Denk and Kaider (1997) found that when endoscopy was used with head and neck cancer patients to teach them swallow strategies, they progressed faster than the patients who did not have the benefit of endoscopic biofeedback.

✦ Case Presentation

A patient in the intensive care unit had coronary artery bypass graft (CABG) surgery, which was reported to be uneventful. The day following surgery, he was offered some thin liquids, and on the second day began receiving meal trays of liquids and soft foods. He coughed regularly while eating and complained of difficulty swallowing liquids. A FEES examination was done at bedside in the intensive care unit.

Findings

Before delivery of food and liquid, the larynx and hypopharynx were viewed. Reduced movement of the left vocal fold and arytenoid were noted at rest, for breath holding, and phonation. Complete closure of the airway was only achieved with great effort. In addition, left lateral pharyngeal wall contraction appeared to be reduced during a strained high-pitched "ee." Secretions were seen in the laryngeal vestibule and were aspirated, although the patient inconsistently and ineffectively attempted to clear them with throat clearing and coughing. The entire laryngeal vestibule was edematous.

Ice chips (¼ tsp.) were first delivered to the patient and were swallowed fairly successfully (no aspiration after three trials). Therefore, food and liquids were delivered to assess swallowing function. There was a consistent slight delay initiating the swallow of about 3 seconds, with pureed boluses falling midway down the lateral channels but liquid boluses falling to the pyriforms and four times spilling into the laryngeal vestibule as the swallow was initiated. On two swallows of thin liquid, aspiration occurred at the onset of the swallow. The patient coughed in response. The swallow itself was weak, with more residue on the weakened left side. Although the patient was instructed to clear this residue, seven or eight dry swallows were needed to mainly clear the bolus. On one swallow of pureed and two swallows of liquid, aspiration occurred during the swallow, evidenced by residue of material on the subglottic shelf. The patient only coughed in response to the liquid aspiration.

Use of thickened liquid did not eliminate aspiration of liquids. Head turning to the patient's affected left side reduced the residue, but moderate amount of residue still remained on the right side. More food was not given, but if it had been, the buildup of residue would have resulted in aspiration of the residue at some point.

Impressions

Severe dysphagia is characterized by the following: (1) mild delay initiating the swallow, causing excess spillage of liquid and pureed food into the hypopharynx prior to the swallow, leading to inconsistent aspiration of liquids before the swallow; (2) reduced bolus clearance due to weakened laryngeal elevation and pharyngeal constriction, especially on the left side, leading to occasional aspiration during and after the swallow; (3) reduced laryngeal closure at the level of the left vocal fold and left arytenoid, contributing to aspiration during the swallow; (4) edema of laryngeal structures likely causing sluggish laryngeal movement (elevation and closure) and reduced sensation in these structures; and (5) mildly reduced sensory awareness of residue and aspiration. The changes in anatomy and sensation may be largely related to the intubation during and postsurgery, whereas the weakness on the left side suggests possible neurologic damage to the recurrent laryngeal nerve. The delay initiating the swallow may be a temporary condition related to the recent trauma and fatigue of undergoing major surgery.

Recommendations

1. Refer the patient to otolaryngology.
2. Because of the patient's unstable medical condition at this time and his reduced response to aspiration, he is not able to take food or liquid safely by mouth. Ice chips are recommended as tolerated by the patient to help dilute and clear secretions that might otherwise accumulate in the hypopharynx and be aspirated. Delivery of oral hygiene must precede the ice chips.
3. Reevaluation (FEES) should be done in 3 days to determine if there has been a change in swallow function.
4. Direct therapy is not recommended at this time because of his weakened state and anticipated spontaneous improvement in function.
5. Consider alternative means of nutrition at this time.

Comment

Several key findings that accounted for the dysphagia were apparent from the endoscopic exam: altered anatomy, reduced movement/weakness of the left side of the larynx and pharynx (innervated by the recurrent laryngeal nerve), and mild delay initiating the swallow with spillage and aspiration of liquids before the swallow. Although the event of aspiration of pureed foods was not directly observed, it was evidenced from residue after the swallow. Further information that might be gained from a fluoroscopy study was not thought to be necessary or even useful at this time. A repeat FEES exam was indicated in a few days to determine whether the edema had subsided, whether the patient was swallowing his secretions successfully, and whether the reduced movement of the left side of the larynx and pharynx was still present. An improvement in any of these conditions would signal a possible readiness for food or liquid.

✦ Risks Associated with Videoendoscopy

The risks are negligible when performing flexible laryngoscopy, provided the clinician has received adequate training and no topical anesthetic is applied. There are no reported incidents of major problems as a consequence of performing a FEES examination after more than 15 years of use by thousands of clinicians (Aviv et al., 1998; Aviv, Kaplan, & Langmore, 2001; Willging et al., 1996). The most common problem is patient discomfort. The potential for stimulating a cough or gag response is always present but usually can be minimized with appropriate technique. If the patient's gag reflex is elevated and cannot be inhibited, the examiner may wish to use a pediatric endoscope.

If the patient is too bothered by the passage of the scope through the nares, a light administration of topical anesthesia or nasal decongestant to the nares may be needed. When topical anesthetic is applied, there is a small risk of allergic reaction to the anesthesia. Medical clearance to apply topical anesthesia or nasal decongestant should be obtained prior to using such agents for clinical purposes, and application should be limited to institutions that provide medical support should an unexpected reaction occur. Also, when applying anesthesia for FEES, only a very small amount (about 1 mL) of gel is inserted about one third of the way back in one of the nares so that only the most narrow part of the nose (usually between the median septal wall and the inferior turbinate) is numbed. By using viscous material rather than a spray, sensitivity in the pharynx and larynx for intact swallowing function is preserved, and any risks from using an anesthetic that might pass into the lungs is eliminated. Lidocaine 2% hydrochloride gel is one of the safest anesthetics available. If any reaction should occur, it will likely be a localized reaction within the nose itself (Eyre & Nally, 1971).

Three other possible risks from nasal endoscopy are nose bleed, vasovagal response, and laryngospasm. All these are largely preventable because of the nature of the examination. Well-trained clinicians carefully monitor passage of the endoscope through the nasal lumen using visual and tactile feedback to ensure there is minimal contact pressure between the endoscope insertion tube and the nasal mucosa. Resistance to insertion can be seen and felt as it occurs, and the scope position can be adjusted to avoid discomfort or nosebleed.

Risk of laryngospasm is minimal and has never been reported as long as the examiner remains above the vocal folds, as is the practice in a FEES examination. The unlikely chance of a laryngospasm is minimized by avoiding unexpected and blunt contact between the endoscope and the true vocal folds. Laryngeal structures are only intentionally touched during a FEES if sensory awareness is being tested and sensitivity is highly suspect. During the swallow, the patient may feel the endoscope, but this will not trigger a laryngospasm. Laryngospasm has been reported in the literature mainly when the stimulus is unexpected and noxious and usually when the person is in a depressed level of consciousness. A common reason for laryngospasm is when a sleeping person is wakened by a significant gastroesophageal reflux event (Bortolotti, 1989). It is most commonly reported in the literature in patients who have had general anesthesia, are beginning to awake, and are being extubated (Staffel, Weissler, Tyler, & Drake 1991). Finally, laryngospasm is commonly reported by patients who have bilateral upper motor neuron (UMN) damage, as in amyotrophic lateral sclerosis (ALS). They report that it can be a daily problem, occurring suddenly as a bit of saliva enters the airway or to spicy food that is inhaled. If laryngospasm should occur during a FEES examination, the endoscope should be withdrawn and the person instructed to relax. This will eventually cause the spasm to break. Alternatively, the Heimlich maneuver can be delivered or oxygen can be applied intraorally to break the laryngospasm.

Vasovagal response, or fainting, is usually due to patient anxiety (Kelly, 1991; Kleinknecht, Lenz, Ford, et al., 1990). This complication is preventable as long as the examiner monitors the patient carefully and conveys an air of calm reassurance. If patients faint, they should be placed in the supine position with the feet above the head. Smelling salts can be applied and medical assistance should always be sought. Vasovagal response can be dangerous in the patient who has an acute cardiac condition with predisposition to bradycardia or cardiac

dysrhythmia (Fitzpatrick, Theodrakis, Vardas, et al., 1991; Van Lieshout, Weiling, Karemaker, et al., 1991). Heart rate can be monitored during the exam in these patients and if the pulse quickens dramatically, signaling a possible vasovagal response, the exam should be terminated. I recommend that a physician or nurse be available for procedures done on patients with complex cardiac problems.

Aspiration is a potential complication that accompanies all dysphagia examinations. The FEES protocol calls for a conservative approach to this problem. If the patient has not eaten by mouth for a prolonged period or if a swallow reflex is suspected to be absent, the protocol calls for delivery of ice chips as the first external bolus to be swallowed. Only after several successful swallows of ice chips would the patient be given food or liquid that, if aspirated, would be potentially much more harmful to the lungs. It is probably worth emphasizing that the unlikely but possible risks associated with either endoscopy or fluoroscopy are far less serious than the well-known risks of aspiration, which are likely to continue if the SLP is unable to assess the problem and intervene in a meaningful way.

Transmission of infectious disease is always a concern when performing endoscopy. Endoscopes must be cleaned according to guidelines such as those developed by the Association of Professionals in Infection Control and Epidemiology and the Association for the Advancement of Medical Instrumentation (American National Standards Institute, 1996; Rutala, 1996). These guidelines change from time to time so it is important to stay current with recent developments. Use of Universal Precautions is advised to protect both the patient and the clinician (Centers for Disease Control, 1987).

✦ Conclusion

The SLP who performs endoscopy should have extensive training in normal anatomy and physiology of the upper aerodigestive tract, normal and abnormal swallow physiology, and appropriate treatments for different kinds of swallowing abnormalities. The SLP should be well aware of the variability of normal anatomic and physiologic requirements for swallowing function. Knowing the difference between normal variability and abnormal function is often the key in interpreting videoendoscopic recordings.

Videoendoscopy requires a degree of tolerance, cooperation, and stimulability on the part of the patient, given the presence of the scope. It is critical that the patient be as comfortable as possible so the foods and liquids consumed evoke natural swallowing behavior. The SLP has training in principles of behavioral modification and motor learning that are critical to using endoscopy as a biofeedback tool and to assessing the cognitive capabilities of the patient to learn swallowing maneuvers. Endoscopy is a valuable tool in the hands of the trained, competent clinician.

Study Questions

1. What are some indications for SLPs to perform a FEES rather than a modified barium swallow procedure?

2. What are the three components of a FEES protocol?

3. What are the four major types of problems seen in dysphagia?

4. What is the underlying pathophysiology behind the appearance of material spilling into the hypopharynx before the swallow is initiated?

5. How can aspiration be detected in a FEES examination if the view at the height of the swallow is obliterated by white-out?

References

American National Standards Institute. (1996). Safe Use and Handling of Glutaraldehyde-Based Products in Health Care Facilities. *ANSI/AAMI* standard 58

Aviv, J., et al. (1998). The Safety of Flexible Endoscopic Evaluation of Swallowing with Sensory Testing FEESST: An Analysis of 500 Consecutive Evaluations. *Dysphagia 13*, 130

Aviv, J.E., Kaplan, S.T., & Langmore, S.E. (2001). The Safety of Endoscopic Swallowing Evaluations. In: S.E. Langmore (Ed.), *Endoscopic Evaluation and Treatment of Swallowing Disorders*. New York: Thieme

Bortolotti, M. (1989). Laryngospasm and Reflex Central Apnoea Caused by Aspiration of Refluxed Gastric Content in Adults. *Gut 30*, 233–238

Centers for Disease Control. (1987). Recommendations for Prevention of HIV Transmission in Health Care Settings. *Morbidity and Mortality Weekly Report: CDS Surveillance Summary 36(suppl 25)*

Dejaeger, E., Pelemans, W., Ponette, E., & Joosten, E. (1997). Mechanisms Involved in Postdeglutition Retention in the Elderly. *Dysphagia 12*, 63–67

Denk, D.M., & Kaider, A. (1997). Videoendoscopic Biofeedback: A Simple Method to Improve the Efficacy of Swallowing Rehabilitation of Patients After Head and Neck Surgery. *ORL Journal of Otorhinolaryngology and Related Specialties, 59*, 100–105

Donzelli, J., Brady, S., & Wesling, M., et al. (2003). Predictive Value of Accumulated Oropharyngeal Secretions for Aspiration During Video Nasal Endoscopic Evaluation of the Swallow. *Annals of Otology, Rhinology, and Laryngology, 112*, 469–475

Dua, K.S., Ren, J., Bardan, E., Xie, P., & Shaker, R. (1997). Coordination of Deglutitive Glottal Function and Pharyngeal Bolus Transit During Normal Eating. *Gastroenterology 112*, 73–83

Eyre, J., & Nally, F.F. (1971). Nasal Test For Hypersensitivity Including a Positive Reaction to Lignocaine. *Lancet 1*, 264–265

Fitzpatrick, A., Theodrakis, G., & Vardas, P, et al. (1991). The Incidence of Malignant Vasovagal Syndrome in Patients with Recurrent Syncope. *European Heart Journal, 12*, 389–394

Hiss, S.G., & Postma, G.N. (2003). Fiberoptic Endoscopic Evaluation of Swallowing. *Laryngoscope 113*, 1386–1393

Horner, J., Massey, E.W., Riski, J.E., Lathrop, D.L., & Chase, K.N. (1988). Aspiration Following Stroke: Clinical Correlates and Outcome. *Neurology, 38*, 1359–1362

Johnson, P.E., Belafsky, P.D., & Postma, G.N. (2003). Topical Nasal Anesthesia for Transnasal Fiberoptic Laryngoscopy: A Prospective, Double-Blind, Cross-Over Study. *Annals of Otology, Rhinology, and Laryngology, 112*, 14–16

Kelly, T.J. (1991). Mechanics and Treatment of Vasovagal Syncope. *Radiology Technology, 62*, 216–218

Kleinknecht, R.A., Lenz, J., Ford, G., et al. (1990). Types and Correlates of Blood Injury-Related Vasovagal Syncope. *Behaviour Research and Therapy 28*, 289–295

Langmore, S.E. (2003). Evaluation of Oropharyngeal Dysphagia: Which Diagnostic Tool Is Superior? *Current Opinion in Otolaryngology–Head and Neck Surgery, 11*, 485–489

Langmore, S.E., Schatz, K., & Olson, N. (1988). Fiberoptic Endoscopic Examination of Swallowing Safety: A New Procedure. *Dysphagia 2*, 216–219

Langmore, S.E., Schatz, K., & Olson, N. (1991). Endoscopic and Videofluoroscopic Evaluations of Swallowing and Aspiration. *Annals of Otology, Rhinology, and Laryngology, 100*, 678–681

Lazarus, C.L., Logemann, J.A., Rademaker, A.W., Kahrilas, P.J., Pajak, T., Lazar, R., & Halper, A. (1993). Effects of Bolus Volume, Viscosity, and Repeated Swallows in Nonstroke Subjects and Stroke Patients. *Archives of Physical Medicine and Rehabilitation, 74*, 1066–1070

Leder, S.B., Sasaki, C.T., & Burrell, M.I. (1998). Fiberoptic Endoscopic Evaluation of Dysphagia to Identify Silent Aspiration. *Dysphagia 13*, 19–21

Madden, C., Fenton, J., Hughes, J., & Timon, C. (2000). Comparison Between Videofluoroscopy and Milk-Swallow Endoscopy in the Assessment of Swallowing Function. *Clinics in Otolaryngology and Allied Sciences, 25*, 504–506

Murray, J., Langmore, S.E., Ginsberg, S., & Dostie, A. (1996). The Significance of Accumulated Oropharyngeal Secretions and Swallowing Frequency in Predicting Aspiration. *Dysphagia, 11*, 99–103

Olsson, R., Castell, J., Johnston, B., Ekberg, O., & Castell, D.O. (1997). Combined Videomanometric Identification of Abnormalities Related to Pharyngeal Retention. *Academy of Radiology, 4*, 349–354

Palmer, J.B. (1998). Bolus Aggregation in the Oropharynx Does Not Depend on Gravity. *Archives of Physical Medicine and Rehabilitation, 79*, 691–696

Perie, S., Perie, S., Laccourreye, L., Flahault, A., Hazebroucq, V., Chaussade, S., & St. Guily, J.L. (1998). Role of Videoendoscopy in Assessment of Pharyngeal Function in Oropharyngeal Dysphagia: Comparison with Videofluoroscopy and Manometry. *Laryngoscope, 108*, 1712–1716

Perlman, A.L., Grayhack, J.P., & Booth, B.M. (1992). The Relationship of Vallecular Residue to Oral Involvement, Reduced Hyoid Elevation, and Epiglottic Function. *Journal of Speech and Hearing Research, 35*, 734–741

Rao, N., Brady, S.L., Chaudhuri, G, et al. (2003). Gold-Standard? Analysis of the Videofluoroscopic and Fiberoptic Endoscopic Swallow Examinations. *Journal of Applied Research, 3*, 1–8

Robbins, J., Levine, R.L., Maser, A., Rosenbek, J.C., & Kempster, G.B. (1993). Swallowing After Unilateral Stroke of the Cerebral Cortex. *Archives of Physical Medicine and Rehabilitation, 74*, 1295–1300

Rutala, W.A. (1996). APIC guideline for selection and use of disinfectants. 1994, 1995, and 1996 APIC Guidelines Committee. Association for Professionals in Infection Control and Epidemiology, Inc. *American Journal of Infection Control, 24*, 313–342

Schroter-Morasch, H., Bartolome, G., Troppmann, N., & Ziegler, W. (1999). Values and Limitation of Pharyngolaryngoscopy (Transnasal, Transoral) in Patients with Dysphagia. *Folia Phoniatrica Logop, 51*, 172–182

Smith, C.H., Logemann, J.A., Colangelo, L.A., Rademaker, A.W., & Pauloski, B.R. (1999). Incidence and Patient Characteristics Associated with Silent Aspiration in the Acute Care Setting. *Dysphagia, 14*, 1–7

Staffel, J.G., Weissler, M.C., Tyler, E.P., & Drake, A.F. (1991). The Prevention of Postoperative Stridor and Laryngospasm with Topical Lidocaine. *Archives of Otolaryngology–Head and Neck Surgery, 117*, 1123–1128

Van Lieshout, J.J., Weiling, W., Karemaker, J.M., et al. (1991). The Vasovagal Response. *Clinical Science, 81*, 575–586

Willging, J.P., et al. (1996). Fiberoptic Endoscopic Evaluation of Swallowing in Children: A Preliminary Report of 100 Procedures. *Dysphagia, 11*, 162

Willging, J.P., et al. (1998). Lack of Effect of Fiberoptic Endoscope Passage on Swallowing Function in Children. *Dysphagia, 13*, 131

Wu, C.F., et al. (1997). Evaluation of Swallowing Safety with Fiberoptic Endoscope: Comparison with Videofluoroscopic Technique. *Laryngoscope, 107*, 396–401

11

Voice Disorders

Barbara H. Jacobson, Joseph C. Stemple, Leslie E. Glaze,
Bernice K. Klaben, and Michael Karnell

✦ **Principles of Diagnosis and Management**
✦ **Diagnostic and Management Issues for Specific Voice Disorders**

Knowledge of laryngeal anatomy and physiology is critical to the practice of medical speech–language pathology (American Speech-Language-Hearing Association, 2004b). Diseases and disorders that affect communication and swallowing in general often impact laryngeal functioning. In addition, surgical and medical procedures (e.g., thyroidectomy, intubation for respiratory failure) can result in detrimental effects on voice production through direct injury to laryngeal structures or through damage to peripheral nerves. The diagnosis and management of voice disorders rely heavily on a familiarity with the fields of otolaryngology, neurology, pulmonary medicine, gastroenterology, and surgical specialties (thoracic surgery, general surgery, and neurosurgery). Physicians in these specialties refer patients to speech–language pathologists with questions regarding confirmation of the voice disorder, description of the dysphonia, prognosis for improvement with voice therapy (either alone or combined with other treatment modalities), subsequent coordinated management, and, finally, behavioral therapy for the disorder. Practice guidelines in speech–language pathology state that patients with suspected voice disorders cannot be treated without an otolaryngologic examination (American Speech-Language-Hearing Association, 2004a). Laryngeal cancer and airway compromise may present as hoarseness. Due to the life-threatening nature of these conditions, a laryngoscopic exam must be performed by an otolaryngologist before beginning any treatment program for a patient with a voice disorder.

This chapter presents a broad overview of voice pathology practice in the medical setting. We discuss general principles relating to the diagnosis and management of voice disorders, and specific diagnostic and treatment issues for various classes of voice disorders. For more information about the diagnosis and management of voice disorders, several texts provide excellent coverage of this topic (Andrews, 1999; Aronson, 1990; Case, 1996; Colton, Casper, & Leonard, 2005; Morrison & Rammage, 1994; Stemple, Glaze, & Klaben, 2000). Also, the reader is referred to Chapters 12, 13, 21, and 22 for other relevant discussion.

✦ Principles of Diagnosis and Management

This section discusses general issues related to the diagnosis and management of voice disorders. Until the early 1980s, the practice of voice pathology relied heavily on auditory perceptual judgments of voice production for the differential diagnosis of dysphonias. However, in the past 25 years, clinical voice laboratories have emerged, and current practice in voice pathology relies on the objective analysis of voice production to complement perceptual analysis. This shift to more technology-based practice has placed increased demands on voice pathologists to be knowledgeable about instrumental measures and their application to diagnosis and treatment. Many clinicians use endoscopy and computer-based programs as treatment modalities to supplement traditional voice therapy. It is expected that this trend will continue, and competencies developed by American Speech-Language-Hearing Association (ASHA) reflect this (American Speech-Language-Hearing Association, 2004b).

Diagnosis

The aims of the diagnostic process for voice disorders are not so very different from those in other areas of specialization in speech–language pathology. Ultimately, the goal of assessment in medical speech–language pathology is to answer the question proposed by the referring physician. Steps in this process include establishing an etiology, identifying factors contributing to the disorder, creating a hierarchy of those factors in order of significance, estimating the severity of the disorder (from the clinician and patient perspectives), determining a treatment approach, identifying outcomes measures that will support treatment effectiveness, establishing prognosis, and determining other appropriate referrals. The tools that speech–language pathologists use for the diagnosis of

Table 11–1 Etiologies Associated with Various Types of Voice Disorders

Type of Voice Disorder	Possible Etiologies
Functional (nodules, polyps, cysts, edema, musculoskeletal tension, Reinke's edema, contact ulcer, granuloma)	Voice production techniques (misuse) Voice use/hygiene (abuse, overuse)
Atypical (psychogenic) (dysphonia/aphonia in presence of normal-appearing larynx, musculoskeletal tension)	Conversion event Psychiatric illness Nonspecific
Neurogenic (paresis, paralysis, myoclonus, spasmodic dysphonia, tremor, apraxia)	Upper motor neuron: amyotrophic lateral sclerosis (ALS), cortical/subcortical stroke, multiple sclerosis (MS)
	Lower motor neuron: direct damage to recurrent laryngeal nerve/superior laryngeal nerve, idiopathic (unknown etiology); brainstem stroke, MS, ALS, neurofibromatosis
	Extrapyramidal: Parkinson's disease (PD)
	Huntington's chorea (HC), MS
	Cerebellar: stroke, MS, degeneration
	Myoneural junction/muscle: myasthenia gravis, polymyositis, muscular dystrophy
	Traumatic brain injury (multiple neurologic sites)
Local irritation/systematic effects (edema, Reinke's edema, granuloma)	Gastroesophageal reflux
	Drugs (corticosteroid inhalers, antihistamines)
	Irritative inhaled substance (cigarettes, environmental)
	Allergies
	Lupus, rheumatoid arthritis
	Upper respiratory infection
	Menopause
	Sarcoidosis
	Intubation
Neoplastic (benign: papilloma, amyloid deposit; malignant)	Carcinoma (usually squamous cell)
	Papillomatosis
	Leukoplakia/dysplasia
	Amyloidosis

voice disorders are the history of the disorder, auditory perceptual analysis, instrumental measures, and descriptive scales of severity. **Table 11–1** lists the types of voice disorders and the etiologies that are associated with them.

Obtaining the History

Obtaining the history is one of the most important steps in the evaluation process for voice disorders. In neurogenic communication disorders, testing determines the nature of the disorder; in voice disorders, the history may provide most of the facts necessary to diagnose the dysphonia and determine the etiology. Information gathered during history taking often drives the remainder of the assessment and determines what direction it takes. Certain elements of the history are significant for establishing the etiology of the voice disorder. Factors that are important in differential diagnosis are the patient's description of the problem; onset (sudden versus gradual); character of the dysphonia (consistent versus variable); voice use patterns (at work, during leisure, at school); other associated events and co-occurring illnesses at the time of the onset of the dysphonia; and occurrence of the dysphonia (lifelong versus isolated event). Information regarding medical and surgical history, medications (including over-the-counter and illicit drugs, vitamin supplements), hydration, caffeine intake,

smoking and alcohol use, and history of psychological intervention are important. A review of the medical history with attention to the types of prior illnesses (e.g., back pain, chronic headaches) may be helpful in establishing a history of somatization. Finally, work and social histories help to establish patients' personality style and their manner of coping with daily stresses.

Auditory Perceptual Analysis

Ear judgments of voice quality have been used for many years in the diagnosis of voice disorders. Clinicians rely on auditory perceptual assessments of voice production for the monitoring of voice disorders. The experienced clinician has developed the listening skills required to discriminate voice characteristics. However, as studies have shown, a great deal of intrajudge and interjudge variability may preclude development of a reasonable listening instrument for the perceptual judgment of voice (Bassich & Ludlow, 1986; Gerratt, Kreiman, Antonanzas-Barroso, & Berke, 1993; Kreiman, Gerratt, Kempster, Erman, & Berke, 1993; Shrivastav, Sapienza, & Nandur, 2005). The presence of such variability means that the clinicians at a hospital or clinic should train themselves to judge auditory perceptual parameters of voice (and speech production and visual perceptual parameters, for that matter) similarly. This is accomplished

Table 11–2   Tasks that Can Be Used for Auditory Perceptual Analysis

Task	Objective	Expected Behavior
Sustained vowel	Judge voice quality, glottal competence s/z	Duration = 18–20 sec
Sustained /s/ and /z/	ratio: estimate glottal efficiency	1.4 or less
Singing up the musical scale	Estimate speaking pitch range	16 notes (2 octaves)
Soft–loud voice production	Assess ability to vary loudness and produce a shout	Appropriate shout; adequate loudness, variation
Oral reading: standard passage	Compare to sustained vowel/free conversation	Variations in pitch/loudness; adequate replenishing breaths
Free conversation	Compare to sustained vowel/oral reading; assess effects of emotion on voice	As above for oral reading (with more inflection); voice production is consistent
Coughing, throat clearing, laughter	Assess nonspeech vocal fold behavior	Sharp glottal coup
Specific words/sentences; varying loudness and pitch	Elicit hard glottal attack, adductor/abductor spasm, tremor, seek variations in voice disorder	Absence of symptoms

through listening to anchoring tapes that are periodically reviewed by the clinicians to realign internal listening standards and through reliability sessions in which the clinicians reach consensus on judging vocal parameters.

The collection of information for perceptual analysis usually consists of two portions: a controlled elicited task section and free conversation. The tasks are designed for the analysis of voice quality (hoarse/rough, hoarse/breathy, strained/strangled, breathiness, aphonia, pitch breaks), pitch appropriateness and range, and loudness appropriateness and range. An s/z ratio (for an estimation of the relationship between lung volumes available for speech and glottic competence) can be calculated. To identify specific abusive voice production behaviors, spasm, and tremor, ask the patient to repeat target words or sentences (e.g., tasks such as vowel-initial sentences, voiced/voiceless contrast sentences, and voiced continuant sentences). **Table 11–2** lists some tasks that can be used in a protocol for perceptual analysis. Rating scales for perceptual evaluation of voice include the GRBAS scale as described by Hirano (1981) and CAPE-V (American Speech-Language-Hearing Association Division 3: Voice and Voice Disorders, 2002).

The GRBAS derives its name from the acronym for its five scales: grade (degree of hoarseness), rough (irregularity heard in vocal fold vibration—frequency or amplitude), breathy (breathiness or air turbulence), asthenic (weakness and/or decreased loudness), and strained (tight voice quality related to perceived hyperfunction). Each of these parameters is rated along a four-point scale: 0, normal; 1, slight; 2, moderate; and 3, extreme. This scale has been used internationally; however, there is no recognized standardization for general use.

The Consensus Auditory-Perceptual Evaluation of Voice (CAPE-V) is an instrument for the perceptual evaluation of the severity of voice quality. Six vocal attributes are rated along a 10-cm linear analogue scale: overall severity (global impression of voice quality), roughness (irregularity in voice), breathiness (air escapage in voice), strain (perceived hyperfunction in voice production), pitch (relative deviation from normal for the person's age, gender, etc.), and loudness (relative deviation from normal for person's age, gender, etc). For each attribute, "consistent" or "intermittent" can be noted. In addition, there are two blank scales available for use for attributes such as voice break and aphonia. The authors developed a protocol for collecting a voice sample for perceptual

rating. They also emphasized the importance of standardizing voice collection techniques for all persons. The recommended tasks include sustained vowel production (/i/ and /a/), reading of six prescribed sentences, and at least 20 seconds of running spontaneous speech.

Assessing Severity

The severity of a voice disorder is relative to the perspective of the speech–language pathologist and the patient. Studies comparing clinicians' and patients' ratings of voice disorder severity and impact on daily functioning typically demonstrate a disparity in the perceptions of these two groups (Jacobson, Bush, & Grywalski, 1996; Llewellyn-Thomas, Sutherland, Hogg, Ciampi, Harwood, Keane, Till, & Boyd, 1984; Murry, Medrado, Hogikyan, & Aviv, 2004). Intuitively, this makes sense. Many factors contribute to how patients evaluate the effects of dysphonia on their lives. A person who is retired, lives alone, and has few social contacts may feel less handicapped by vocal fold immobility than another individual who has a more active social life and increased speaking demands. Perceptions of severity may even change as a patient moves through the continuum of care. For example, a patient who developed granulomas secondary to prolonged intubation for respiratory failure may report less handicap from dysphonia immediately after extubation due to pressing concerns regarding her unstable medical status. However, as her condition improves and she moves from the intensive care unit to a step-down unit to a regular medical floor, she may perceive her voice disorder as more severe as she attempts to communicate with family, friends, and medical staff.

Measures of quality of life have gained recent prominence in the drive to collect relevant data for assessing treatment outcomes. Some standardized and nonstandardized tools are available for voice disorders. Llewellyn-Thomas et al. (1984) developed a series of scales for the assessment of the effects of radiation therapy on voice and daily functioning in laryngeal cancer patients. Patients judged their ability to use their voices in work and social situations as well as the quality of their voices. Smith, Verdolini, Gray, Nichols, Lemke, Barkmeier, Dove, and Hoffman (1994) developed a questionnaire that collected information from patients regarding the functional impact of

Table 11–3 Instrumental Measures in the Voice Laboratory

Technique	Information	Equipment and Function
Acoustic recording and analysis	Fundamental frequency intensity Signal/harmonics-to-noise ratio	Microphone, playback speakers
		High-quality audio recording system
	Perturbation measures	Computer capabilities: recording, filtering, analog/digital/analog conversion
	Spectral features	
	Voice range profile	Data storage, and retrieval
		Acoustic analysis software
		Sound spectrogram
Aerodynamic measurement	Airflow rate and volume	Oral-nasal airflow mask
	Subglottal (intraoral) pressure	Oral sensing tube
	Laryngeal resistance	Pneumotachometer or warm wire anemometer
	Phonation threshold pressure	
Stroboscopic imaging of the larynx	Gross structure	Endoscopes (rigid, flexible)
	Gross movements	Stroboscopic light generator, audio and contact microphones
	Vibratory characteristics	Camera pack, lens, coupling devices
		Computer, monitor, color printer (external server)
Electroglottography (EGG)	Vocal fold contact area	Electroglottograph
Electromyography (EMG)	Muscle activity	Electromyography recorder

voice disorder on aspects of their lives. Information on employment, symptoms, risk factors, and family history was also elicited. In this study, significant effects were reported for work activities and social interaction for older patients. Jacobson, Johnson, Grywalski, Silbergleit, Jacobson, Benninger, and Newman (1997) developed the Voice Handicap Index (VHI), which is an instrument for assessing patient self-perceived handicap. It is a 30-item scale with three subscales: physical, emotional, and functional. A patient's total scale score must change by 18 points (in either direction) to demonstrate a change in self-perceived handicap that is not related to random variation. Hogikyan and Sethuraman (1999) developed the 10-item Voice-Related Quality of Life (V-RQOL) scale to measure similar aspects of self-reported quality of life changes with voice disorders. The further development of sensitive, reliable, and valid tools for assessing quality of life and the effects of medical, surgical, and behavioral interventions is required not only to understand patients' perception of their voice disorder, but also to respond to third-party payer demands for demonstrated treatment effectiveness.

The information obtained from the history and auditory perceptual analysis prepares the clinician for expected findings during instrumental voice analysis. Hypotheses formed during this initial phase can be tested and compared with acoustic, aerodynamic, and videostroboscopic findings.

The Clinical Voice Laboratory

The data generated by instrumental measures of voice constitute the first step in the objective description of voice quality. Knowledge of anatomy and physiology of the larynx and the mechanics of voice production can be examined indirectly through the use of instrumental vocal function measures, including acoustic analysis, aerodynamic measurement, movement tracings, and laryngeal imaging. Today, the clinical voice pathologist can employ several instrumental tools for assessment, treatment monitoring, and direct biofeedback of voice

production (**Table 11–3**). This complementary information improves understanding of the capabilities in normal and professional speakers and the voice production limits of disordered patients.

The clinical applications of these instruments can be directed at several purposes, including pathology detection, assessment of severity, differential diagnosis of a voice problem, and as a primary treatment tool. Objective measures of both vocal function and observation of the laryngeal image can be used by the voice pathologist to display, instruct, motivate, and justify treatment needs. Instrumental feedback may assist with achieving target behaviors. Repeated pre- and posttest measurements may reinforce the patient's progress. Finally, information about the vocal pathology offers an illustration or documentation of the pathology that may be more convincing than perceptual judgments of voice quality alone.

The user must always recognize that all noninvasive voice laboratory measurements are indirect estimates of various aspects of vocal function. One might make inferences about voice quality or laryngeal status using these measures. The only direct measure of vocal function is percutaneous electromyography. This invasive procedure requires collaboration with an otolaryngologist or neurologist in the clinical setting. With this in mind, the levels of observation that are represented by various measurement tools also dictate the limits of our interpretation of data (Titze, 1991a).

Acoustic Measurements

Acoustic measures of voice production provide objective and noninvasive measures of vocal function. Increasingly, these measures are available at an affordable cost, and voice pathologists find them a convenient indirect measure to document voice status across time. **Fig. 11–1** shows an acoustic analysis system for recording, storing, and analyzing the speech signal. Acoustic analysis routines are written based on assumptions of a nearly periodic, stable sound source, and recording protocols

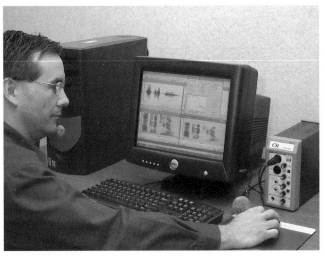

Figure 11–1 Acoustic analysis system. (Courtesy of KayPENTAX.)

Table 11–5 Suggested Protocol for Acoustic Analysis

Task	Measure
Sustained vowel (three trials each)	Fundamental frequency (Hz)
Comfort pitch	Jitter (%, msec)
High pitch (excluding falsetto)	Shimmer (dB)
Low pitch (excluding glottal fry)	Harmonics-to-noise ratio
Glissando (vowel glide from lowest point [f$_1$] in pitch range to highest point [f$_2$]	Semitone range [formula 5 [log (f$_2$/f$_1$) × 39.86]]
Soft to loud voice (count from 1 to 5)	Lowest intensity (dB)
	Highest intensity (dB)
Recite passage	Speaking fundamental frequency
	Habitual intensity (dB)
Conversation	Speaking fundamental frequency

must accommodate this underlying principle. A sustained or extracted vowel portion must be of sufficient length to preserve the validity of acoustic measurement (Karnell, 1991). If the pathologic sound source is aphonic (e.g., as in vocal fold paralysis) or so irregular (e.g., spasmodic dysphonia) that the patient cannot produce a sustained vowel, then acoustic analysis cannot be used with confidence for that speaker.

However, progress has been made toward recommendations on agreed guidelines for valid acoustic analysis. Acoustic signals may be classified into three types, according to the periodicity and stability of the sound source. **Table 11–4** summarizes the three signal types and the recommended analysis schemes. A full description of the summary recommendations is available from the National Center for Voice and Speech (NCVS) (Titze, 1995). Variations in fundamental frequency, intensity, and vowel selection affect the resulting acoustic measures (Glaze, Bless, & Susser, 1990; Horii, 1982; Orlikoff & Kahane, 1991). The number of trials must be adequate to represent the speech behavior. The voice pathologist must observe the patient's production carefully to elicit the most representative production. Test-retest reliability has also been a concern for users of acoustic analysis data. There is an inherent amount of intrasubject variability in all speech and voice productions. To use acoustic measures for pre- and posttreatment comparison, it is critical to exact a stable baseline measure. **Table 11–5** displays a sample recording protocol for acoustic measures.

Table 11–4 National Center for Voice and Speech Classification of Voice Signals

	Signal Quality	Acoustic/ Perceptual Measure
Type 1	Nearly periodic	Perturbation analysis
Type 2	Strong modulations (vibrato, tremor), intermittency (glottal fry, voice breaks)	Visual display (e.g., spectrogram); perturbation unreliable
Type 3	Chaotic or random	Perceptual judgments of voice quality; acoustic analysis unreliable

Fundamental Frequency   Once the pitch period (T) is detected, then fundamental frequency (F$_0$) can be calculated from the reciprocal (F$_0$ = 1/T). Fundamental frequency is the rate of vibration of the vocal folds, and is expressed in hertz (Hz), or cycles per second. Fundamental frequency is the acoustic measure of an audioperceptual correlate—pitch. The mean fundamental frequency can be measured during sustained vowels or extracted from connected speech. Variation in fundamental frequency during connected speech can be used to reflect changes in intonation. Fundamental frequency range, also called phonational range, measures the highest and lowest pitch a patient can produce. The numerical values of fundamental frequency are nonlinear. For example, the pitch difference between 200 and 400 Hz is far greater than the perceptual difference between 600 and 800 Hz. Therefore, the top and bottom frequencies measured in phonational range can be normalized on the musical scale and expressed as several notes, or semitones (Hirano, 1981).

Perturbation Measures   There are many fine waveform analysis routines, but most acoustic analysis programs offer measures of voice perturbation. Perturbation is defined as the cycle-to-cycle variability in a signal, and two common expressions of this term are jitter (frequency perturbation) and shimmer (amplitude perturbation). There is a range of mathematical calculations for these terms, which may vary based on three general parameters (Baken, 1987; Orlikoff & Baken, 1993):

1. Length of the analysis window: short- versus long-term averages

2. Absolute or relative measurement units: ratio or percentage

3. Statistical expression: central tendency (e.g., mean jitter) or variability (e.g., coefficient of variation of frequency)

Technical capabilities continue to improve, and optimal recording standards and equipment specifications may lead to increased stability and validity of acoustic measures (Titze, 1993; Titze, Horii, & Scherer, 1987; Titze & Winholtz, 1993).

Harmonics-to-Noise Ratio   Acoustic analysis programs often produce a ratio measure of the energy in the voice signal over the noise energy in the voice signal. Greater signal or harmonic energy in the voice is thought to reflect better voice quality. Large noise energy (random aperiodicity in the voice signal) represents more abnormal vocal function (Colton et al., 2005; Milenkovic, 1987).

Intensity Vocal intensity (I_0) is the acoustic correlate of another perceptual attribute, loudness. It is referenced to sound pressure level (SPL) and measured on the logarithmic decibel (dB) scale. Both mean intensity and intensity range (maximum and minimum) are useful measures of vocal function. Intensity measurements can be made with several different instruments, including sound-level meters, acoustic analysis programs, and some aerodynamic measurement devices. However, intensity measures are subject to several artifacts, including influence of ambient or background noise, inconsistencies in mouth to microphone distance, and variations with changes in speech task, vowel production, or fundamental frequency. A standard, well-monitored elicitation protocol helps minimize the potential sources of error in intensity measures.

Phonetogram The phonetogram, also known as the voice range profile (VRP) or the physiologic frequency range of phonation (PFRP) has been used by teachers of voice and phoniatricians (a term used outside the United States for physicians who treat voice disorders) for many years and has gained attention for its wide application to functional changes in voice production. In a systematic progression from lowest to highest pitch, the patient produces a frequency range at lowest and highest intensity levels. The resulting plot is an ellipse-shaped frequency/intensity profile, and its dimensions are expressed in semitones. This comprehensive assessment is a useful measure for before and after treatment and for long-term monitor of vocal range development in professional voice users (Bless, 1991; Sulter, Wit, Schutte, & Miller, 1994; Titze, 1992).

Spectral Analysis The sound spectrogram displays the glottal sound source and filtering characteristics of the speech signal across time. Both formant frequency energy (vocal tract resonation) and noise components (aperiodicity, transient or turbulent noise) of speech production are presented in a three-dimensional scale. The horizontal axis is time. The vertical axis is frequency, with the lowest energy band representing the fundamental, and formant trajectories above. A third scale is the darkness or gray scale (or color difference) that represents intensity change. Spectrogram analysis can provide an estimate of the harmonic-to-noise ratio of a speech production. Another form of spectral analysis is the line spectrum, which plots all harmonic energies at a single time point.

Frequency is plotted on the horizontal axis and amplitude on the vertical axis. Advanced mathematical routines, such as fast Fourier transform (FFT) and linear predictive coding (LPC), have been applied to spectral analysis to identify formant characteristics (Baken, 1987; Kent & Read, 2002). For voice pathologists, spectral analysis is useful in assessing the interaction between the sound source and vocal tract (supraglottic) influences.

Aerodynamic Measurements

Aerodynamic measurements are interpreted as a reflection of the valving activity of the larynx, representing both vocal fold configuration and movement, structure, and function (Schutte,

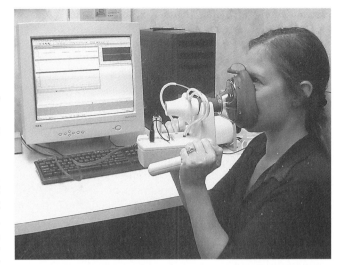

Figure 11–2 Aerodynamic analysis system. (Courtesy of KayPENTAX.)

1992). **Fig. 11–2** displays an aerodynamic recording system for measurement of airflow and pressure during speech production. Air flow and pressure can be measured under stable and transient speech productions. Average airflow rate or flow volume during sustained productions would reflect long-term or average aerodynamic measures. Momentary changes in oral pressure measured during production of plosive or fricative consonants are examples of transient or short-term aerodynamic measures (Miller & Daniloff, 1993; Scherer, 1991). Derived measures, such as laryngeal resistance or glottal power, integrate pressure and flow in a single measure (Hirano, 1981; Hoit & Hixon, 1992; Melcon, Hoit, & Hixon, 1989).

Like all instrumental measures, aerodynamic assessment must be observed carefully to avoid equipment or task artifact. Airflow masks, oral pressure sensing tubes, and oral coupling tubes require an airtight seal with the face or lips. The examiner must ensure patient compliance and comfort to elicit as natural a speech production as possible. Multiple trials are always useful for securing a stable baseline. Finally, the validity of aerodynamic measures should be verified by conducting a standard calibration routine prior to each examination session. **Table 11–6** displays a sample aerodynamic recording protocol.

Table 11–6 Suggested Protocol for Aerodynamic Analysis

Task	Measure
Deep inhalation/slow exhalation (two trials)	Estimated vital capacity/flow volume
Deep inhalation/fast exhalation (two trials)	Forced vital capacity
Sustained vowel (three trials each)	Phonation volume
Comfort pitch	Airflow rate
Highest sustainable pitch (excluding falsetto)	Peak flow rate
Lowest sustainable pitch (excluding glottal fry)	Phonation time
/ipipipipi/ (on one exhalation)	Subglottal pressure
	Glottal resistance
	Glottal efficiency
	Glottal power

Flow Measurement   There are two basic measurements of airflow used in speech production: flow volume and flow rate. Volume is the total amount of flow used during a certain production, such as a maximum phonation time. Volume is generally measured in liter or milliliter units. The spirometer is a respiratory measurement device that records volume measures. Two forms of this instrument are available: wet and dry spirometers. The wet spirometer has two chambers with known volumes of air and water contained within. As the patient blows air into the upper chamber, the volume of water displaced by the flow is measured directly. The dry spirometer utilizes a turbine mechanism. As air passes across the turbine, the number of rotations is calibrated with specific volume amount (Baken, 1987; Colton et al., 2005).

The measurement of airflow rate is somewhat less direct, and a range of devices and techniques are available. The most common airflow device is the pneumotachograph, which uses the principle of differential pressure across a known resistance to estimate flow rate. A pneumotachograph is essentially a metal tube, with a mechanical resistance (usually a wire mesh screen or a series of small tubes) inside. As airflow is blown through the tube and its resistance, differential pressures are measured at sites directly upstream and downstream to the resistance and flow is calculated using the differential pressure divided by the resistance. The amount of flow divided over the amount of time equals flow rate. A second device used to measure airflow is the warm wire anemometer. When flow passes over a warm wire within this instrument, the wire is cooled, changing the electrical resistance of the wire with the change in temperature. The change in resistance in the wire is proportional to the flow, and flow rate can be calculated from that change (Baken, 1987; Miller & Daniloff, 1993).

Subglottal Air Pressure Measurement   Pressure is defined as the force per unit area, acting perpendicular to the area. In voice production, respiratory (subglottal) pressure acts as a force building up below the adducted vocal folds, rising until the folds open and are set into oscillation. Subglottal air pressure is essentially the power supply, and variables such as vocal fold stiffness, hyperfunctional compression, and incomplete glottic closure influence the amount of subglottal effort needed to initiate phonation. Thus, voice pathologists use measures of subglottal pressure as an indicator of the valving characteristics of the vocal folds.

Estimating Subglottal Pressure   Subglottal pressure can only be measured directly through an invasive procedure that requires a needle puncture into the tracheal space directly below the vocal folds. A noninvasive, indirect estimate of subglottal pressure has been used clinically by measuring the intraoral pressure during production of an unvoiced plosive consonant. This pressure is an accurate estimate of the subglottal pressure only under the following assumptions:

1. The oral plosive constriction creates a momentary airtight seal, which provides a continuous opening from the lungs to the lips (assuming the velum is closed, or nares are pinched to avoid nasal leak).
2. The vocal folds are open so that the oral pressure produced in the plosive production is analogous with the respiratory effort that would be available as driving pressure to set the vocal folds in oscillation (Netsell, 1969).

Subglottic pressure is estimated from repeated production of an unvoiced plosive + vowel syllable (e.g., /pi/). An oral tube is placed between the closed lips and connected to a pressure transducer. The oral catheter must be placed carefully in the mouth, sealed by the lips, and not occluded by the tongue. The length, diameter, and angle of the tube can influence the pressure measurement (Baken, 1987). The peak intraoral pressure recorded during the plosive production is considered to equal the tracheal pressure.

Phonation Threshold Pressure   Titze (1991b, 1994) defines phonation threshold pressure as the minimal pressure required to set the vocal folds into oscillation. The measure has been estimated indirectly using intraoral pressures described above, measured at the exact moment of voice onset for barely audible phonation (Verdonlini-Marston, Titze, & Drucker, 1990). In general terms, phonation threshold pressure can be interpreted as a measure of the effort needed to begin phonation. Because speakers with vocal pathologies frequently report greater effort in "turning the voice on," this new measure may prove highly useful for assessing effects of treatment or phonosurgical results.

Laryngeal Resistance   Derived measures entail assessing the pressure and flow in a ratio or product. Laryngeal resistance is the quotient of peak intraoral pressure (estimated from production of an unvoiced plosive) divided by the peak flow rate (measured from production of a vowel) as produced in a repeated train of a consonant + vowel syllable (Smitheran & Hixon, 1981). This measurement is intended to reflect the overall resistance of the glottis and, by extension, serve as an estimate of the valving characteristic, whether too tight (hyperfunctional), too loose (hypofunctional), or normal (Hoit & Hixon, 1992; Melcon, Hoit, & Hixon, 1989). Unfortunately, derived measures pose some limits to interpretability. The magnitude of the derived value (e.g., high laryngeal resistance) is not meaningful without examining the separate contributions of pressure and flow. For example, a measure of increased laryngeal resistance values might be attributable to excessive subglottal pressure, insufficient transglottal flow, or both.

Other Physiologic Measures of Function

Inverse Filter   Any signal measured at the mouth is a product of two components: the glottal sound source and the resonance characteristic from the vocal tract. Inverse filtering is a technique that theoretically isolates these two components; the supraglottic or vocal tract influence is removed, leaving intact the glottal waveform only. Inverse filtering has been applied to both acoustic waveforms and airflow measurements. The pattern of the inverse filtered waveform can be described in terms of opening and closing slopes, speed and open quotients, and waveform minima and peaks (Colton et al., 2005; Fritzell, 1992). One limit to the inverse filter process is the imprecise estimation of vowel format frequencies and vocal tract area functions for the individual speaker (Titze, 1994).

Electroglottography   Electroglottography (EGG) is a noninvasive technique that uses electrical current passing through the neck to measure vocal fold contact across time. **Fig. 11–3** shows a typical electroglottograph. Two electrodes are placed on either side of the thyroid alae, with a small electrical current passing through as the vocal folds vibrate. Tissue conducts the current better than air, so the resistance increases

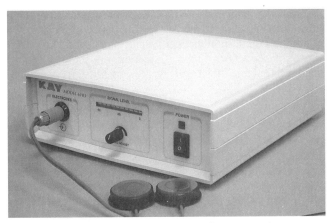

Figure 11–3 Electroglottograph. (Courtesy of KayPENTAX.)

when the vocal folds are opening and decreases during the closing phase. The EGG waveform displays this variable resistance and serves as an analogue of vocal fold opening and closing gestures during vibration, with peaks and troughs representing maximum points of abduction and adduction (Childers, Alsaka, Hicks, & Moore, 1987). The technique is not without artifact, however, because variations in tissue thickness, electrode placement, mucous interference, and laryngeal movements can produce error in this measure (Colton & Contour, 1990). Nonetheless, EGG has been used in combination with other physiologic measures of vocal function for cross-validation through simultaneous measurement. A most useful application was suggested by Karnell (1989), who synchronized an EGG signal with stroboscopy flash pulses to offer a real-time monitor of the vibratory phase points across the stroboscopic image.

Electromyography Electromyography (EMG) is a direct measure of laryngeal function and, as an invasive procedure, must be performed clinically by a neurologist or otolaryngologist. Electrodes are inserted percutaneously (through the neck) into specific laryngeal muscles, and the pattern of electrical activity is studied. The electrical signals recorded from the muscles are interpreted as normal or pathologic based on four basic features: timing (onset and offset) of muscle activity, and the pattern, number, and amplitude of muscle action potentials. The widest application of laryngeal EMG is for diagnosis and prognosis in vocal fold neuropathy, including paralysis, dystonia, and other neuromuscular disorders, and for discriminating vocal fold paralysis from mechanical fixation of the cricoarytenoid joint. Percutaneous EMG is used to identify the correct site of Botox injection for treatment of spasmodic dysphonia (Bless, 1991; Harris, 1981; Hirose, 1986; Karnell, 1989; Ludlow, 1991).

Laryngeal Imaging Laryngovideostroboscopy (LVS) has become a critical part of the evaluation process for speech–language pathologist since its inception and introduction into more common use in the 1980s. Whether it is performed by an otolaryngologist or speech–language pathologist, the dynamics of vocal fold vibration observed through LVS provide more informed decisions about the appropriateness of certain treatment approaches. LVS with its heightened image allows the clinician to determine the character of a particular lesion, e.g., edema versus cyst, pliant versus more chronic nodule, etc. With this information, a more accurate prognosis is possible. For an extended discussion of LVS, the reader is directed to texts by Karnell (1994) and Hirano and Bless (1993).

A rigid oral endoscope (70 or 90 degrees) is preferable for optimal image quality. Unfortunately, /i/ is the only vowel that allows for adequate visualization of the larynx and surrounding structures. However, vocal fold movement in certain voice disorders is better observed using a flexible endoscope. These include vocal fold immobility, spasmodic dysphonia, and paradoxical vocal fold movement (PVFM). Also, for any instance of a voice or speech disorder, in which connected speech should be observed, flexible endoscopy allows for a better view of laryngeal dynamics. For example, singers often complain of difficulty in particular sections of their vocal range. Flexible endoscopy gives the singer an opportunity to use relatively natural mouth and neck posture during singing while the clinician notes any abnormality in laryngeal area muscle tension, laryngeal closure, etc. With advances in nasoendoscope design, optic distortion can be avoided by the use of distal chip cameras—cameras that are located at the scope tip. Nasoendoscopy is also quite useful in education and treatment as a biofeedback technique. This is particularly the case in PVFM.

Several parameters of vocal fold appearance and motion are noted during the exam. These include indication of lesion(s) and location, glottal closure pattern, activity of supraglottic structures in lateral and anterior/posterior planes during phonation, vibratory symmetry, periodicity, vibratory amplitude, mucosal wave, vertical phase, and relative comparison of the open and closed phases of vibration.

There are several components needed to perform LVS and acquire images for further analysis. Basic elements include an endoscope, camera, light source, stroboscopy unit (which can be combined with the light source), digital recording system (e.g., DVD, videotape, computer), and viewing screen (e.g., LED, TV monitor, flat panel). Although hardcopies of exams on videotape or DVD have been common in the past, several manufacturers have developed technologies for capturing digital images and storing examinations to a server (e.g., Image Stream Medical, Littleton, MA; KayPENTAX, Lincoln Park, NJ) (**Figs. 11–4** and **11–5**). In addition, Image Stream Medical has developed a videoediting program that facilitates the direct production of edited examinations onto CD and into PowerPoint presentations.

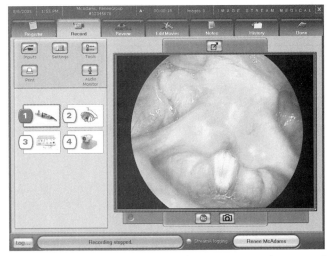

Figure 11–4 Image capture system with remote storage. (Courtesy of Image Stream Medical.)

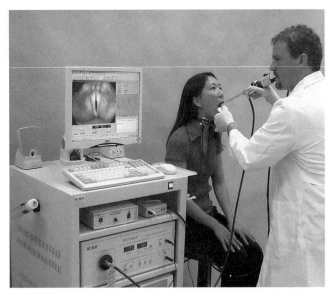

Figure 11–5 Laryngovideostroboscopy system. (Courtesy of KayPENTAX.)

It is anticipated that image manipulation and transmission over the Internet will become more common features in the future.

Normative Data

The number of instrumental measures of voice has expanded greatly over the past decades. Acoustic, aerodynamic, imaging, and physiologic measures of vocal function have been enhanced by better recording devices, signal processing techniques, and analysis routines. Voice pathologists have recognized the clinical applications of these measurement tools to integrate instrumental measurements in the diagnosis and treatment of voice-disordered patients. But interpretation must be done with care and users must be knowledgeable about the risks of artifact and error to ensure valid application of these measures. Some normative data are available for acoustic and aerodynamic analysis (Bless, Glaze, Biever-Lowery, Campos, & Peppard, 1993; Colton et al., 2005; Glaze, Bless, Milenkovic, et al., 1988; Glaze et al., 1990; Holmberg, Hillman, & Perkell, 1988, 1989). Clinicians who use instrumental analysis in their practice are encouraged to collect data on normal voice production with their equipment using their standardized protocols. As investigation into valid, reliable, and meaningful instrumental measures evolves, progress will continue in determining the markers of normal voice production.

Other Assessment Components

An oral-peripheral examination should always be a part of a voice evaluation. A thorough assessment includes observation of structures at rest and during speech and nonspeech movements. An evaluation of laryngeal area muscle tension is an integral part of the evaluation. Using Aronson's (1990) technique for palpating suprathyroid, thyroid, and infrathyroid structures (especially thyrohyoid space), judgments about resting muscle tension and the extent of movement on contraction when phonating can be made. In addition, base of tongue and jaw tension should also be assessed. Other important elements include informal assessments of speech, language, and cognition; hearing screening; and informal screening for dysphagia. Some

patients with vocal fold paralysis, laryngeal cancer, and neuromuscular disease are at risk for dysphagia, and any symptoms should be noted. In addition, patients with musculoskeletal tension dysphonia can report a globus (lump in the throat) sensation that may affect their swallowing function.

Principles of Treatment

The treatment of voice disorders has traveled the historical path from elocution-based treatments and public speaking applications to more specific physiologic approaches to voice therapy. The earliest speech–language pathology texts that discussed therapy for voice disorders described behavioral voice use changes that were meant to develop improved vocal habits as well as some specific methods of modifying improper vocal components such as breathing, posture, pitch, and loudness (West, Kennedy, & Carr, 1937; Van Riper, 1939).

Boone (1971) was perhaps the first to compile a collection of voice care ideas and formulate a philosophy or orientation of voice treatment that was called symptomatic voice therapy. The focus of symptomatic voice therapy was and remains the modification of deviant vocal symptoms identified by the voice pathologist during the diagnostic voice evaluation. These symptoms may be breathiness, low pitch, glottal fry phonation, the use of hard glottal attacks, and so on. Symptomatic voice therapy is based on the premise that most voice disorders are caused by the functional misuse or abuse of the voice components including pitch, loudness, respiration, phonation, and rate. When identified through the diagnostic process, the misuses are eliminated or reduced through various voice therapy techniques. To this end, Boone (1971) described 20 therapy techniques that he called "voice facilitating techniques." These techniques were developed to modify the inappropriate vocal symptoms; thus the term *symptomatic voice therapy*. The symptomatic approach to voice care continues today as described in detail by Boone, McFarlane, and Von Berg (2005).

Aronson (1990) suggested that voice therapy often focuses on identification and modification of the emotional and psychosocial disturbances associated with the onset and maintenance of the voice problem. This psychogenic voice therapy orientation is based on the assumption of underlying emotional causes for the voice disturbance. When these causes are resolved, a resolution of the voice disorder also occurs. Aronson (1990), Case (1996), Colton et al. (2005), and Stemple et al (2000) further discussed the need for determining the emotional dynamics of the voice disturbance from the perspectives of emotions as a cause of voice disorders, and voice disorders being the cause of emotional disequilibrium.

Stemple (2000) suggested an etiologic voice therapy orientation based on the reasonable assumption that there is always a cause for the presence of the voice disorder. If that cause (or causes) can be identified, then appropriate treatments can be devised for modifying or eliminating those causes. Once modified, the voice production has the opportunity to improve or return to normal. During the diagnostic evaluation, much effort is focused on identifying the direct and indirect causes of the voice disorder. Once the etiologic factors are treated, the vocal symptoms often improve without direct manipulation of the voice components. Direct symptom modification (i.e., raising the pitch, reducing breathiness, and so on) is reserved for situations where the inappropriate use of a voice component is found to be the primary etiologic factor. Etiologic voice therapy assumes that, once identified, the cause of the voice disorder can be modified or eliminated leading to improved voice production.

A physiologic voice therapy orientation is composed of holistic voice therapies devised to alter or modify the physiology of the vocal mechanism (Stemple et al., 2000). Normal voice production depends on a balance among respiratory airflow; laryngeal muscular strength, tone, balance, coordination, and stamina; and coordination among these and the supraglottic resonatory structures. Any disturbance in the physiologic balance of these three vocal subsystems may lead to a voice disturbance. Physiologic voice therapy strives to balance the physiology of voice production through direct physical exercise and manipulations of the laryngeal, respiratory, and resonatory systems. Examples of these physiologic therapies include the holistic approaches known as vocal function exercises (Stemple, 2000), resonant voice therapy (Verdolini-Marston, Burke, Lessac, Glaze, & Caldwell, 1995), and the accent method (Smith & Thyme, 1978). In addition, special care is taken to account for the health of the vocal fold cover. This care may be related to proper mucosal hydration, attention to voice abuse reduction, or antireflux regimens as examples.

An eclectic voice therapy orientation is the combination of any and all of the other orientations of voice therapy. Successful voice therapy is dependent on the voice pathologist using all of the therapy techniques that seem appropriate for individual patients. Many patients may share the same diagnosis; however, the etiologies and personalities, vocal needs, and emotional reactions to their voice problems may be very different. Because of these differences, the same pathologies may require very different management approaches (Stemple et al., 2000). Utilizing a case study, let us examine a typical patient with a voice disorder from the perspective of each voice therapy orientation.

Case One

A 32-year-old woman was diagnosed by the laryngologist as having small bilateral vocal fold nodules. She was referred for a voice evaluation and a voice therapy program.

History of the Problem

The patient was referred to the otolaryngologist by her internist because, during a regular physical examination, the patient complained of intermittent hoarseness, voice fatigue, loss of the upper part of her singing voice, and occasional aching in her throat. She reported that her voice quality was a little worse in the morning, cleared somewhat as the day progressed, and then worsened again by evening. The overall frequency and severity of the problem had increased over the past 6 months.

Medical History

The patient reported undergoing a tonsillectomy and appendectomy as a teenager. In addition to the surgeries, she was hospitalized for anorexia and bulimia on two different occasions. The last hospitalization lasted for 3 weeks and occurred 18 months prior to the evaluation. The patient continues to be treated for the eating disorder with bimonthly counseling and for mild depression with medication. Chronic medical conditions included asthma and frequent bronchitis, as well as airborne allergies. The patient also complained of heartburn. Daily medications were taken for depression, inhalers and steroids for asthma, antihistamines for allergies, and over-the-counter antacids. The patient also admitted to smoking about 10 cigarettes per day for the past 10 years. Her liquid intake was poor, consisting of approximately three cups of caffeinated coffee and four cans of caffeinated soda per day. Chronic throat clearing was noted throughout the evaluation. The patient indicated that on a day-to-day basis she felt only "fair" due to stress, fatigue, and frequent headaches caused by her allergies.

Social History

The patient was married for 10 years, but had been separated from her husband for 3 months, causing much stress and tension. She had three daughters ages 9, 7, and 4. The middle child was suspected of having a significant learning and behavioral disorder that contributed to the daily stress. The patient was not reluctant to talk about her depression and indicated that her unhappy marriage, the problem with her child, and her own poor self-concept were the major contributors to her emotional problems. The problems were now compounded by the pending divorce.

The patient had been employed for 6 years by an automobile factory that made plastic dashboards. Her job was in the molding room where the plastic was heated and molded in large machines. The molding process created fumes and vapors that apparently caused the patient much coughing during the day. In addition, the machines were noisy, requiring the workers to talk loudly to be heard. Most talking on the job was social among eight people who worked in the large, well-ventilated room.

Nonwork activities included mothering her children, which entailed harsh voice use, talking on the telephone with her sister, and singing soprano in the church choir. Her singing was currently curtailed because of the voice problem.

Oral-Peripheral Examination

The structure and function of the oral mechanism appeared to be well within normal limits for speech and voice production. The laryngeal sensations of dryness and occasional thickness were reported by the patient. Laryngeal area muscle tension and neck tension were demonstrated by the patient.

Voice Evaluation

The patient's voice quality was described as mild to moderately dysphonic, characterized by low pitch, inappropriate loudness, and husky dry hoarseness.

Respiration: s/z = 25 second/10 second; Patient demonstrated a thoracic, supportive breathing pattern. She tended to speak on residual air, especially toward the end of phrases.

Phonation: Breathiness and glottal attacks were noted during conversational voice. Occasional glottal fry was noted toward the end of phrases.

Resonation: Voice was produced with an elevated larynx and retracted tongue.

Pitch: Patient demonstrated an unusually low pitch conversationally.

Loudness: Patient spoke unusually loud for the speaking situation.

Rate: Normal

Acoustic measures and aerodynamic analysis revealed the following:

Fundamental frequency = 165 Hz

Frequency range = 140 to 480 Hz (21.3 semitones)

Jitter percent: sustained vowels = 0.56

Shimmer dB: sustained vowels = 0.67

Intensity (habitual) = 76 dB; airflow volume = 3200 mL

Airflow rate = 252 mL/sec, modal pitch

Phonation time = 12.7 second

Subglottic air pressure = 8.6 cm H_2O

Laryngeal videostroboscopic observation revealed moderate-sized bilateral vocal fold nodules. Glottic closure was hourglass with a mild ventricular fold compression. The amplitude of vibration and the mucosal wave were moderately decreased bilaterally. The open phase of the vibratory cycle was mild to moderately dominant, whereas the symmetry of vibration was irregular by 50%. In short, the patient demonstrated a stiff, out-of-phase vocal fold vibration.

Impressions

The patient presented with a voice disorder secondary to these possible etiologic factors:

✦ Long-term cigarette smoking

✦ Harsh employment environment in terms of fumes and talking over noise

✦ Poor hydration and large caffeine intake

✦ Frequent regurgitation

✦ Possible gastroesophageal reflux disease (GERD)

✦ Asthma and frequent bronchitis

✦ Airborne allergies

✦ Prescription medications causing mucosal drying

✦ Frequent coughing and throat clearing

✦ Emotional instability

✦ Shouting at her children

✦ Talking too loudly in general conversation

✦ Using a low pitch

✦ Laryngeal area muscle tension

Recommendations

Symptomatic Voice Therapy   General focus would use facilitating techniques to:

1. Raise pitch
2. Reduce loudness
3. Reduce laryngeal area tension and effort

This direct symptom modification would follow an explanation of the problem and would run concurrently with modification of the vocally abusive behaviors including:

1. Smoking
2. Caffeine intake
3. Coughing and throat clearing
4. Shouting at her children

Psychogenic Voice Therapy   General focus would explore the psychodynamics of the voice disorder. This exploration would include:

1. Detailed patient interview to determine the cause and effects of stress, tension, and depression
2. Determination of the exact relationship of emotional problems and voice problem
3. Counseling the patient about the effects of emotions on voice problems
4. Reduction of musculoskeletal tension caused by emotional upheaval
5. Support of ongoing psychological counseling.

Secondary focus would deal with modification/elimination of the abusive behaviors including:

1. Smoking
2. Caffeine intake
3. Coughing and throat clearing

Inappropriate use of pitch and loudness would most likely be viewed as obvious symptoms of the voice problem. As the psychodynamics improve, the voice symptoms would be expected to improve.

Etiologic Voice Therapy   The general focus would be on identifying the primary and secondary causes of the voice disorder and then to modify or eliminate these causes. The primary causes would include:

1. Smoking
2. Laryngeal dehydration from poor hydration, caffeine intake, and drugs
3. Voice abuse such as talking loudly over noise at work, shouting at her children, coughing, and throat clearing
4. Inhalation of plastic fumes

Secondary causes that may be more the result of the problem as opposed to a cause include:

1. Laryngeal area muscle tension due to increased mass and stiffness
2. Low pitch due to increased mass
3. Increased loudness due to effort to force stiff, heavy folds to vibrate

Therapy would focus on modification or elimination of the primary etiologic factors. The patient would be supported in her effort to stop smoking, encouraged to begin a hydration program and reduce caffeine intake, given vocal hygiene counseling in an effort to reduce the vocally abusive habits, and encouraged to wear a mask to filter her breathing at work. The secondary causes of tension—low pitch and increased loudness—would be expected to spontaneously improve as the primary causes were modified and the vocal fold condition improved.

Physiologic Voice Therapy General focus would be to evaluate the present physiologic condition of the patient's voice production and develop direct physical exercises or manipulations to improve that condition. This patient demonstrated increased mass and stiffness of the vocal folds that changed the physical dynamics of vocal fold vibration. Indeed, she was required to build greater subglottic air pressure to initiate and maintain vibration that required a high airflow rate. This increased pressure caused her to speak too loudly in conversation. She also attempted to overcome these problems by making physical adjustments such as increasing supraglottic tension in an effort to maintain her voice. When added to the mucosal and muscular stiffness, vocal hyperfunction was the result. The management program would therefore include:

1. Vocal function exercises designed to restrengthen and balance the laryngeal musculature and balance airflow to muscular activity and improve supraglottic placement of the tone
2. Hydration program and decrease in caffeinated products to improve the mucous membrane of the vocal folds
3. Discussion of medications with the patient's physician
4. Elimination of habit coughing and throat clearing
5. Vocal hygiene counseling for elimination of direct voice abuse

Eclectic Voice Therapy In the review of these orientations it is obvious that each management approach has certain strengths as well as inherent weaknesses. Patients may best be treated with the understanding and use of all these orientations. Therefore, eclectic voice therapy is the treatment of choice with any voice-disordered patient. This patient would best be served when the management plan included:

1. Symptom modification
2. Elimination/modification of the causes
3. Attention to the psychodynamics of the problem
4. Direct physiologic exercise and attention to the mucosal covering of the vocal folds.

✦ Diagnostic and Management Issues for Specific Voice Disorders

Functional Voice Disorders

This classification of voice disorders includes those that result from abuse, misuse, or overuse of the voice. Inappropriate voice production can cause vocal nodules, vocal polyps, Reinke's edema, vocal cysts, contact ulcers, and granulomas. (See Chapter 22 for a discussion of the pathophysiology of these lesions.) In clinical practice, these are the most common pathologies seen (Herrington-Hall, Lee, Stemple, Niemi, & McHone, 1988). In the past, speech–language pathologists and otolaryngologists have used the term *functional* to refer to disorders that were psychogenic in nature. For the purposes of this chapter, we use this term to refer to voice disorders that result when patients (1) generate voice in a way that disrupts the balance among respiration, phonation, and resonation necessary for efficient voice production (including increased musculoskeletal tension); and (2) use abusive voice behaviors (yelling, throat clearing, etc.).

Vocal Nodules

Vocal nodules are the most common of the structural lesions causing dysphonia. They may be categorized as acute or chronic. Videostroboscopy is often required to distinguish between these two types. Prognosis is excellent for elimination of nodules with voice therapy for nodules that are acute in nature (i.e., softened, more pliant). For hardened, chronic nodules, the outcome with voice therapy alone is somewhat uncertain. Murry and Woodson (1992) compared various management paradigms for patients with vocal nodules (voice therapy alone, surgery alone, and surgery and voice therapy) and found that improvements in voice were achieved with all three models. The type of nodule (chronic versus acute) was not a variable in this study. The authors discussed the need to consider the potential risks of surgery (disturbance of the cover of the vocal fold) and its cost balanced with its benefits when compared with voice therapy.

Vocal Polyps

A polyp generally presents as a unilateral lesion. This mass can be quite large, and when it involves the entire extent of the vocal fold it is considered to be Reinke's space edema or polypoid degeneration. The lesion can also be supra- or infraglottic. On occasion, a reactive nodule presents at the corresponding area on the opposite vocal fold. Polyps are most often treated surgically with postoperative voice therapy (Colton et al., 2005). However, there may be a place for preoperative voice therapy in eliminating reactionary edema around the site of the polyp, thereby clearing the surgical field for the surgeon. Although polyps can result from a single event of yelling or shouting, rather than from chronic voice abuse, voice therapy may still be required to return voice production to its premorbid state. Smoking is a significant etiology for polypoid degeneration, and patients must be counseled regarding the probable return of polyps if they continue to smoke.

Vocal Fold Cysts

Cysts (epidermoid or mucous retention) also usually appear as a unilateral lesion. As with polyps, there may be a reactive swelling or nodule on the vocal fold opposite the cyst. Often these masses are long-standing and in some cases asymptomatic. Videostroboscopy plays an important role in differentiating cysts from nodules (when there is a reactive nodule to the cyst). Elimination of vocal cysts is best achieved with surgery. Voice therapy is indicated preoperatively to reduce edema, if necessary. Postoperatively, voice therapy can lessen the effects of any voice use behaviors that may have contributed to the development of the cyst and restore the voice to its premorbid state.

Contact Ulcers and Granulomas

Contact ulcers and granulomas occur at the posterior commissure and vocal processes. Both lesions have been considered to occur from "aggressive" speaking styles that cause increased pressure and irritation at the vocal processes (Boone, 1971). They are often seen as a result of intubation. However, although the manner of voice production may be implicated in the development of either type of lesion, GERD appears to be the likely culprit in patients without intubation (Koufman, 1991; Koufman, Amin, & Panetti, 2000). Granulomas can recur and a partnership between the speech–language pathologist and otolaryngologist is crucial in their treatment.

Musculoskeletal Tension Dysphonia

Musculoskeletal tension dysphonia (MTD), also referred to as muscular tension dysphonia, arises from the misuse of extrinsic and intrinsic laryngeal muscles to produce voice. Often the larynx is virtually immobile in the neck, and patients can withdraw in pain when the thyroid cartilage and thyrohyoid space are palpated. Patients with MTD may also complain of a globus sensation at rest or during swallowing. Characteristic vocal fold appearances are associated with MTD. Morrison and Rammage (1994) discussed the typical presentations of this disorder. They stated that MTD can occur as either a primary (as a result of psychological stressors) or secondary (as the result of organic disease) disorder. Management of laryngeal area muscle tension is indicated for all patients who present with significant tension and pain at the larynx. Roy and Leeper (1993) presented results of a study in which manual tension reduction (Aronson, 1990) was used to reduce dysphonia. Seventeen patients with MTD (and normal-appearing vocal folds) who underwent therapy demonstrated improvement in auditory perceptual and acoustic measures after therapy. Further work in this area has demonstrated the efficacy of direct manipulation of the larynx in establishing more normal voice production (Roy, Ford, & Bless, 1996; Roy, Bless, Heisey, & Ford, 1997). Therapeutic massage (by a licensed or certified massage therapist) may help reduce overall body tension.

Atypical (Psychogenic) Voice Disorders

Although the majority of voice disorders seen by the voice pathologist involve some form of voice misuse or abuse, challenging, atypical disorders associated with personality and/or emotional disorders also exist. The major types of laryngeal pathologies caused by personality conflicts are conversion aphonia, conversion dysphonia, and mutational falsetto. The management plans for these pathologies include four major stages. The first stage is the medical evaluation. As with all voice disorders, it is essential that the presence of organic pathology be ruled out prior to the initiation of therapy. The report of normal laryngeal structures also confirms the diagnosis of a personality-related disorder in the presence of inappropriate and often unusual vocal symptoms.

The second stage is the diagnostic voice evaluation. During the evaluation, the voice pathologist, through a detailed psychosocial interview, develops the history of the pathology and ascertains how the patient functions socially and physically within the environment. An impression of the patient's personality evolves. The diagnostic time is also used to prepare the patient for vocal change. This is accomplished by explaining to the patient how the vocal mechanism works and describing what is happening physiologically within the larynx to create the present voice. Although no attempt is yet made to explain why this is occurring, the physiologic description provides the patient with a rationale for the vocal problems.

The third stage is the direct manipulation of the voice. The type of manipulation varies, depending on the phonation abilities demonstrated by the patient. Vocal manipulation most often begins during the diagnostic evaluation. The expected result is a dramatic change in the voice toward normal phonation. Greene (1972) and Boone (1971) both reported that these patients often attain normal voicing during the first treatment session. This has also been our experience.

The fourth stage involves counseling to determine why the disorder was present. The conversion voice disorders occur in patients who have undergone some physical or emotional trauma. It is the patient's subconscious effort to escape the unpleasant situation or the memory of the situation that promotes the reaction. Once normal voicing has been achieved, it is a natural transition to begin examining why the problem existed. By this time the voice pathologist has gained excellent trust and rapport with the patient. With interview questions that are structured in a nonthreatening manner, the voice pathologist can usually determine the cause of the problem. Patients frequently volunteer the necessary information, which often opens a floodgate of emotion.

Once the cause or causes have been identified and discussed, the voice pathologist needs to determine if further professional counseling is advisable. If so, the appropriate referral should be discussed with the patient and made with the patient's consent. Let us now examine each personality-related laryngeal pathology.

Conversion Aphonia

Conversion voice disorders, called hysteric, hysterical, nervous, functional, and psychosomatic aphonia, have long been discussed in medical journals. Many treatments have been advocated in the literature. Russell (1864) suggested that hysteric aphonia was a mental or moral ailment that required moral treatment. The method of cure was "to rouse the will, and thus rid the body of its thousand morbid things." Ward (1877) advocated the application of an astringent to the vocal folds along with simultaneous electric shock. The pain of both procedures would influence the patient to talk. Goss (1878), Ingals (1890), and Bach (1890) also utilized painful "remedies" such as bitter tonics, iron, quinine, arsenic, and strychnine. Techniques advocated today are certainly less radical but no less imaginative. Let us examine three of these strategies.

Strategy 1 By the time patients with conversion aphonia are referred to the voice pathologist, they are often truly seeking relief from the disorder and are subconsciously ready for change. Often, the event that precipitated the need for the conversion reaction has passed. Some patients may continue to receive secondary gains from the disorder and resist all therapeutic modifications, but the majority will respond quickly to direct voice therapy.

Following the interview period of the diagnostic evaluation, the voice pathologist presents a physiologic description of the vocal mechanism, utilizing simple line drawings, video prints, or actual video of the vocal folds. This demonstrates how the adductor muscles are not pulling the vocal folds together, causing the voice to be whispered. With this visual approach, the voice pathologist has given the patient a nonthreatening, reasonable explanation as to why phonation is not occurring. No comment is yet made regarding the patient's inherent ability to phonate. In fact, the "blame" for lack of phonation has been removed from the patient and placed squarely on the faulty laryngeal mechanism.

Traditional therapy approaches then examine the patient's ability to phonate during nonspeech phonatory behaviors such as coughing, throat clearing, laughing, crying, sighing, audible yawning, and gargling. When phonation is identified in one of these behaviors, it is then shaped into vowel sounds, nonsense syllables, words, and short phrases. The voice pathologist must demonstrate much patience at this time. Most patients have not phonated for several weeks or even years. It is possible to proceed too quickly and frightening the patient away from phonation. But once good, consistent phonation is established under practice conditions, the voice pathologist begins to gently insist that it be used during the therapy conversations.

Strategy 2   Another therapy technique utilizes the falsetto voice. The patient again is instructed in the physiology of the laryngeal mechanism and how it relates to the vocal difficulties. It is explained that we are going to manipulate the vocal mechanism in a manner that will force the muscles to pull the vocal folds together. The voice pathologist then produces the falsetto tone on the sound /aɪ/. The patient is told in a matter-of-fact manner that everyone can produce this tone, even those who are having vocal difficulties. The falsetto is again demonstrated by the voice pathologist, and the patient is instructed to produce the same sound. Some patients initially resist the falsetto production, but in our experience, with a little coaching, the majority of patients eventually produce the tone. The falsetto is then stabilized briefly on vowels. Alternatively, a "puppy cry" on the sound /m/ can be used to achieve a high-pitched phonation.

It is explained to the patient that we are going to use the muscle tension created by producing the falsetto tone to force the vocal folds to pull together normally. The patient is then given a list of two-syllable phrases and asked to recite them in the falsetto voice. During this exercise, the patient is constantly encouraged to speak swiftly and loudly. After the voice stabilizes in a relatively strong falsetto, the patient is halted and asked to match the clinician singing down the scale about three to four notes from the original falsetto tone. The patient is then asked to continue reciting the phrases at this new pitch level. The same procedure is repeated two or three more times until the patient is fairly closely approximating a normal pitch level. The patient is continually encouraged to produce these phrases louder and faster until eventually the voice "breaks" into normal phonation.

Occasionally, the patient approximates normal phonation but then hesitates as if somewhat reluctant to produce normal voice. When this occurs, the patient is instructed to "drop way down" and produce a guttural voice quality while reciting the phrases. This will "produce more tension." After a few minutes, the patient is taken back to the falsetto voice with the break into normal phonation usually occurring soon after.

Strategy 3   Another technique that we have found useful is the use of direct visual feedback using laryngeal videoendoscopy. While the patient is being scoped, either with rigid or flexible endoscopes, an explanation is given related to the positioning of the vocal folds and how that positioning relates to the present vocal problem. The patient is able to monitor the video over the voice pathologist's shoulder. The patient is

then instructed in various manipulations of the vocal folds such as deep breathing, light throat clearing, and attempts to produce tones of various loudness levels and pitches. We have had surprising success in the quick return of normal voicing using this procedure.

It is extremely important that the voice pathologist be patient when utilizing any of these techniques. The normal time frame from aphonia to normal voice is approximately 30 to 45 minutes. These techniques work for the following reasons:

1. The patient is ready for change.
2. The voice pathologist has given a reasonable explanation for why the voice is gone.
3. The voice pathologist has demonstrated confidence in the therapeutic techniques.

Following return of voice, it is necessary to explore the actual cause of the conversion reaction. It is desirable to do this in a direct manner by suggesting to the patient that stress may very often contribute to this lack of vocal fold closure. By this time the patient has developed strong confidence in the voice pathologist and often freely provides information related to psychosocial problems that may be related to the development of the conversion reaction. Appropriate counseling or referrals may then be accomplished.

Conversion Dysphonia

Aphonia is the most common conversion voice disorder, but many other vocal symptoms with varying degrees of dysphonia may occur as conversion voice disorders. The voice pathologist recognizes these vocal symptoms as a conversion disorder when the medical exam yields normal appearing vocal folds; when the history of the problem yields limited reason for the occurrence of a voice disorder; with the recognition of an atypical voice quality when compared with "normal" dysphonias; and in the patient's ability to produce normal phonation while producing nonspeech vocal behaviors.

Treatment for conversion dysphonia follows the same approach as that suggested for the aphonic patient. It is important to note that some very bizarre-sounding dysphonias can occur. Seldom, however, can a conversion voice disorder patient create a vocalization that the voice pathologist cannot also produce. True hoarseness is difficult to imitate. A helpful aid in determining exactly how the patient is producing voice and for confirming the conversion disorder diagnosis is to imitate the vocal behavior.

Functional Falsetto

Functional falsetto is the production of the preadolescent voice in the postadolescent male. The falsetto voice often draws unwanted attention to the postpubescent, physically mature patient. Whatever the reason for the development of this voicing behavior, most patients are ready and willing to modify the voice with direct therapy.

Treatment Strategies   Several therapy techniques are used to modify mutational falsetto voices. The first step of any technique is to offer the patient a reasonable explanation for the vocal difficulty. We often describe to patients how the vocal folds rapidly grow during puberty, causing an awkwardness in how the vocal muscles work. This awkwardness causes the muscles to "pull" inappropriately, not permitting a deeper voice to be produced. The exercises used are designed to encourage the appropriate "pull." The second step is to utilize direct vocal manipulation. The following procedure is recommended:

1. Ask the patient to produce a hard glottal attack (HGA) on a vowel. Demonstrate how the vowel should be produced with effort closure. When the glottal attack is produced correctly, the pitch will break into the normal lower register, as the falsetto positioning for the HGA cannot initiate this form of effort closure. If the pitch does not break, grasp the larynx with your thumb and index finger and hold it in a lowered position in the neck as the vowel is being produced. If, after several trials, this fails to elicit the desired sound, depress the tongue with a tongue depressor, again as the patient produces the glottal attack.

2. When the lower pitch is produced, identify it immediately as the appropriate voice sound. Have the patient repeat it several times using the glottal attack. Then produce several different vowel sounds while attempting to reduce and then extinguish the effort of the glottal attack. Stabilize the normal voice on vowel prolongations.

3. Immediately move from vowels into words and phrases while maintaining the lower voice register. Attempt to expand the phrases through paragraph reading and into conversational speech during the initial therapy session.

Using this approach, the voice change is expected to be sudden and the progress of therapy rapid. The best way of accomplishing this sudden improvement is for the voice pathologist to be aggressive with the therapy approach. It must be remembered that the voice is new to the patient. His auditory feedback system does not yet identify the new voice as belonging to him. Initially, the voice may want to shift back into the falsetto. Positive encouragement may be necessary. Follow-up sessions may be utilized to stabilize the new voice.

Most patients are somewhat excited by and proud of the new voice, but some are embarrassed by the sudden voice quality change. When the latter is the case, the patient may require a gradual desensitization program as a part of the stabilization process. A desensitization program involves establishing with the patient a personal hierarchy of communication experiences from the least difficult to the most difficult speaking situation. A typical hierarchy may include:

1. Talking to strangers in a fast-food restaurant or a store
2. Talking to family members
3. Talking to selected friends
4. Talking in the classroom

Neurogenic Voice Disorders

Voice production is affected in many neurologic diseases and disorders. This section describes the salient features of voice in these disorders and briefly reviews treatment approaches. When discussing the differential diagnosis of neurogenic voice disorders, it is helpful to categorize them in terms of upper motor neuron, lower motor neuron (including peripheral nerve), extrapyramidal, cerebellar, and myoneural junction and muscle disorder etiologies. The diagnosis of these voice disorders relies on a careful examination of the patient's med-

ical history (including radiologic exams), family history, and extent and course of symptoms. Some neurologic disease [e.g., amyotrophic lateral sclerosis (ALS)] may present initially as change in voice, and the speech–language pathologist can provide important information for eventual diagnosis. A referral to a neurologist may be indicated when you observe (or patients describe) any weakness in their extremities, fasciculations (twitching) in muscles, loss of sensation, or gait disturbances that are not explained by previous medical history.

Upper Motor Neuron Disorders

Relevant neurologic disorders that result from upper motor neuron (UMN) disturbance are cortical and subcortical strokes, pseudobulbar/supranuclear palsy, and some presentations of ALS and multiple sclerosis (MS). The most obvious vocal characteristic is harshness and/or hoarseness with a spastic component. Patients with dominant hemisphere strokes (in Broca's area) can exhibit phonatory apraxia. They are unable to initiate phonation or other nonspeech laryngeal behavior (coughing, clearing throat) volitionally. Typically, this is a transitory finding and patients quickly recover and the apraxia evolves into a verbal or nonverbal apraxia. Occasionally, patients complain of a gradual onset of hoarseness that, on careful listening, appears to be spastic and strained in nature. This may be the first sign of a bulbar presentation of ALS. In addition, Silbergleit (1993) has shown that ALS patients with perceptually normal voices demonstrate abnormal acoustic measures when compared with normal age- and sex-matched subjects.

Treatment for patients with voice disorders related to UMN disorders is directed toward improving the functioning of all systems involved in voice production. For patients with ALS, exercise is not indicated. These patients eventually require augmentative communication systems. Amplification systems may be of use for patients who have relatively intact speech, but are unable to produce adequate loudness. In general, the primary goal of treatment is to help the patient produce a more relaxed phonation, particularly in coordination with appropriate respiratory support for voice. Positional alterations (lying down, sitting in a reclined chair) can be helpful to facilitate this.

Lower Motor Neuron Disorders

For our purposes, this category of voice disorders includes those that result from damage or disorders in the brainstem and peripheral nerves. Dysphonia may be absent or minimal if the vocal fold is paretic and there is good compensation from the intact vocal fold. The salient auditory perceptual characteristics of vocal fold immobility are breathiness, hoarse/breathy quality, and diplophonia. Inspiratory stridor can signal the possibility of bilateral recurrent laryngeal nerve damage. In unilateral vocal fold immobility due to recurrent laryngeal nerve damage, patients often use a higher than normal habitual pitch. This occurs because the cricothyroid muscle is still intact on that side and can still assist in vocal fold adduction. When either one or both vocal folds are paralyzed in the abducted position (adductor paralysis), then the risk of dysphagia exists. Vocal fold appearance can assist in the determination of the site of the lesion (**Table 11–7**). Patients with ALS can have lower motor neuron damage as can patients with MS. For

Table 11–7 Vocal Fold and Palatal Appearance as a Result of Brainstem or Peripheral Nerve Damage

Site of Lesion	Unilateral Damage	Bilateral Damage
Above the level of origins of pharyngeal, superior laryngeal, and recurrent laryngeal branches of the vagus	Ipsilesional vocal fold remains in abducted position on phonation; decreased palatal elevation on the same side	Both vocal folds are fixed in abducted position on phonation; decreased palatal elevation bilaterally
Below the origin of the pharyngeal branch and above origins of superior laryngeal and recurrent laryngeal branches	Vocal folds appear as above; no effect on palatal elevation	Vocal folds appear as above; palatal elevation is normal
Superior laryngeal nerve	Vocal fold adduction occurs, but there is tilt of anterior commissure and epiglottis away from the side of the lesion; palatal elevation is normal	Bowed vocal folds with overhanging epiglottis; no effect on palatal elevation
Recurrent laryngeal nerve	Ipsilesional vocal fold fixed in paramedian position; palatal elevation is normal	Both vocal folds fixed in paramedian position; no effect on palatal elevation

From Aronson, A. (1990). *Clinical Voice Disorders,* 3rd ed. New York: Thieme.

patients with hemiparesis or bilateral weakness, upper torso support through the use of abdominal paddles or bracing may help to improve respiratory support for the voice.

Otolaryngologists usually delay any surgical intervention (vocal fold augmentation or medialization) until 6 months to 1 year after the onset of vocal fold immobility. Use of temporary vocal fold augmentation (e.g., fat, collagen) may be used to achieve voice and manage dysphagia. Voice therapy is indicated to speed the development of overadduction by the normal vocal fold and to minimize maladaptive phonatory behaviors (e.g., muscular tension, ventricular fold adduction). (See Chapter 22 for a further discussion of the management of vocal fold immobility.)

Extrapyramidal Disorders

Disorders considered extrapyramidal in nature include Parkinson's disease (PD) and Huntington's chorea (HC), among others. Essential voice tremor is generally thought to be caused by extrapyramidal damage. PD is the most common disorder in this group. Patients with PD have "hypokinetic" dysarthria, and voice production is characterized by mono-pitch, reduced loudness, and low pitch (Darley, Aronson, & Brown, 1975). Patients with HC have "hyperkinetic" dysarthria, and voice is strained and monopitch in quality (Aronson, 1990).

Ramig, Pawlas, and Countryman (1995) have developed a treatment program for patients with PD. This approach capitalizes on the ability of patients to use voluntary control of loudness and pitch to improve overall speech production. Studies have demonstrated direct effects on instrumental measures (Ramig & Dromey, 1996; Smith, Ramig, Dromey, Perez, & Samandari, 1995) as well as maintained effects over time (Ramig, L.O., Sapir, S., Countryman, Pawlas, O'Brien, Hoehn, & Thompson, 2001).

Cerebellar Disorders

Damage to the cerebellum through degeneration or stroke results in voice that may be hoarse with fluctuations in loudness and pitch. Movements of the vocal folds and respiratory system are incoordinate. Treatment is designed to improve the timing of the onset of phonation with respiratory support.

Spasmodic Dysphonia

Spasmodic dysphonia (SD), as described in Chapter 22, is considered a neurogenic voice disorder of uncertain etiology. Spasmodic dysphonia is not a disease, nor is it associated with one specific neurologic disease. Blitzer, Lovelace, Brin, Fahn, and Fink (1985) describe SD as a dystonia (an excess of normal movement); this argues for its inclusion as an extrapyramidal disorder. SD is classified into adductor (AD), abductor (AB), and mixed types. In some patients, there is a familial history of other dystonias (e.g., blepharospasm, stuttering). Flexible nasoendoscopy is the preferred imaging technique for diagnosis because AD and AB spasms may disappear during the sustained phonation required for visualization under rigid endoscopy. Tremor also may be perceived at high sustained pitch. Atypical (psychogenic) voice disorders can present as SD and discriminating the two can be difficult (Roy, Gouse, Mauszycki, Merrill, & Smith, 2005).

Many patients obtain symptomatic relief with Botox injections. However, not all choose to undergo this treatment, and voice therapy may help them to reduce some behaviors they have developed as a result of the muscular effort necessary to produce voice. Murry and Woodson (1995) found that voice therapy that occurred after injections of Botox was effective in prolonging the amount of time between injections for patients with AD SD.

Myoneural Junction and Muscle Disorders

Myasthenia gravis (MG), polymyositis, and oculopharyngeal dystrophy are examples of diseases characterized by disturbances of the myoneural junction (e.g., MG) or muscle (e.g., polymyositis). Voice symptoms are related to the site of damage. For patients with MG, progressive hypophonia occurs with use. Patients with a description of rapid vocal fatigue are assessed by using a counting task (up to 100 and beyond). Gradual deterioration of the voice is apparent with increased duration of counting. Treatment is usually symptomatic.

Case Two

A 62-year-old man was referred by an otolaryngologist for assessment of voice. His primary complaint was hoarseness for the past 6 months. The otolaryngologist stated that the laryngoscopic exam was normal.

History of the Problem

The patient noticed the onset of hoarseness approximately 6 months ago. It was not associated with an upper respiratory infection or surgery. He had not noticed any worsening of his hoarseness, but his daughter, who lived out of state, had told him that she thought it was worse. His voice was bad in the morning, better throughout the day, but worsened at night, especially with fatigue. The patient described some difficulty in producing sufficient loudness in noise (e.g., restaurants, noisy parties). He noted that he had occasional difficulty swallowing dry foods (e.g., crackers, bread). The patient drank six glasses of water daily. Alcohol intake was rare (less than one time per month). He drank decaffeinated coffee and noncaffeinated soda.

Medical History

There was no recent history of surgery. The patient had a history of hypertension, osteoarthritis, and seasonal allergies. There were no complaints associated with GERD. Current medications included Cardizem, an over-the-counter antihistamine, and ibuprofen. There was no prior smoking history.

Social History

The patient was married and lived with his wife. He was a retired auto factory worker. Leisure activities included gardening, reading, and a monthly social club. He described his speaking demands in these activities as moderate.

Oral-Peripheral Exam

Facial symmetry was present. Strength and force against resistance was within normal limits for jaw, lips, and tongue. There were questionable fasciculations in the tongue. Gag reflex was present bilaterally. Palatal elevation was symmetric, but appeared slow. The patient noted occasional thick secretions. There was no laryngeal area muscle tension.

Voice Evaluation

Voice quality was mildly dysphonic and was characterized by low pitch and hoarse/rough quality.

Respiration: s/z ratio = 20/18 second (1.11). Breathing pattern was thoracic. The patient used adequate replenishing breaths during conversation.

Phonation: Occasional strained voice was heard throughout the assessment, especially at the end of a phrase. There was a slight rough quality to the voice.

Resonation: Within normal limits

Pitch: Habitual pitch was low. Pitch variability during conversation was somewhat reduced.

Loudness: Within normal limits in conversation. Vocal fold compression was reduced on the shout.

Rate: Within normal limits

Abuses

No hard glottal attacks were apparent during this assessment. The patient reported no chronic throat clearing, coughing, or yelling and shouting. Acoustic and aerodynamic measures were as follows:

Fundamental frequency = 100 Hz

Frequency range = 90 to 225 Hz (15.8 semitones)

Jitter = 0.33 msec

Shimmer = 5.67%

Intensity (habitual) = 68 dB

Airflow volume = 3000 mL

Airflow rate = 196 mL/sec, habitual pitch

Phonation time = 14 second

Subglottic air pressure = 6 cm H_2O

Laryngeal videostroboscopy revealed no obvious laryngeal pathology. Glottic closure pattern was complete. Vocal fold adduction and abduction appeared symmetric but slightly sluggish, especially during repetitive /i/ production. Vibratory amplitude of both vocal folds was diminished. Vibratory symmetry was irregular by 25%.

Impressions

The patient presented with a mild dysphonia of an uncertain etiology. Vocal hygiene and voice production appeared to be within normal limits. There was no history of a precipitating respiratory infection or surgery. The presence of questionable tongue fasciculations combined with diminished speed and briskness of movement of both vocal folds pointed toward a possible neurologic etiology.

Recommendations

1. Refer to neurology for assessment.
2. Postpone voice therapy until definitive diagnosis.
3. Consider videofluoroscopic swallowing evaluation.

Full neurologic examination revealed that the patient was in the early stages of ALS, with a bulbar presentation. The patient was followed in an interdisciplinary ALS clinic, and appropriate speech pathology interventions occurred as needed (education, swallowing assessment, augmentative communication). No voice therapy was recommended for this patient after diagnosis, but education regarding optimal voice use helped him to preserve his voice and speech as long as possible.

Neoplastic Lesions

Vocal fold masses that fall into this category are differentiated from functional voice disorders because they arise from disease processes. Patients may develop secondary poor voice production behaviors as a means of compensating for lesions. Otolaryngologists provide the primary management for these patients. The most common malignant tumor is carcinoma (usually squamous cell). Leukoplakia and dysplasia are considered precancerous conditions and patients are closely monitored by the otolaryngologist. Benign lesions included in this group are papillomas and amyloid masses. Voice therapy is generally secondary to surgical or medical management. Intervention occurs after medical or surgical procedures.

Papilloma is commonly treated by surgical removal of the lesions. However, studies have been initiated to investigate the use of other treatment modalities. For example, photodynamic therapy (PDT) has been used for patients with recurrent papilloma. In PDT, patients receive an injection of a photosensitive drug. This drug is eventually shed from the body but retained longer in abnormal cells and in the skin. A laser light source is directed toward the abnormal cells (tumor or papilloma). In essence, the drug enhances the sensitivity of the mass to light and the tumor begins to reduce in size. Patients who undergo this therapy are extremely light-sensitive for approximately 30 days after receiving the drug and are counseled to stay out of the sun. Patients with papilloma who are undergoing this procedure have removal or debulking of the papilloma at the time of the drug injection and light exposure. Postsurgically, voice therapy is useful for helping patients to achieve the best voice possible with their existing laryngeal condition. Antiviral therapy (e.g., α-interferon) is also used to treat laryngeal papillomatosis (Aaltonen, Rihkanen, & Vaheri, 2002).

Paradoxical Vocal Fold Movement

Paradoxical vocal fold movement is characterized by wheezing or inspiratory stridor due to inappropriate closure of the true vocal folds throughout the respiratory cycle. This adductory vocal fold movement produces respiratory airway obstruction that may be intermittent or continuous, ranging from mild to severe episodes depending on the degree of uncontrolled glottal closure during inhalation. Individuals with this disorder demonstrate normal vocal fold movement during sustained phonation and speech. During an episode, they may often have normal inhalations between phrases while speaking. During a normal respiration cycle, the true vocal folds abduct (**Fig. 11–6**) with inhalation and partially adduct with exhalation. This physiologic cycle allows unimpeded movement of air into the lungs during inspiration and helps maintain alveolar patency by providing positive airway pressure during expiration. There are many synonyms in the medical litera-

Table 11–8 Medical Descriptors for Paradoxical Vocal Fold Movement

Atypical Asthma	Laryngeal Stridor
Emotional laryngeal wheezing	Munchausen's stridor
Emotional laryngospasms	Nonorganic airway obstruction
Episodic laryngeal dyskinesia	Paradoxical vocal cord dysfunction
Factitious asthma	Pseudoasthma
Functional laryngeal obstruction	Psychogenic stridor
Functional upper airway obstruction	Psychosomatic stridor
Hysterical stridor	Variable vocal cord dysfunction
Laryngeal asthma	Vocal cord dysfunction
Laryngeal dyskinesia	Upper airway obstruction
Laryngeal spasm	

ture used to reference paradoxical vocal fold movement (**Table 11–8**).

The nature of the onset of paradoxical vocal fold movement is not well understood and the incidence is unknown. Onset has been reported in individuals from ages 3 to 82, with greater frequency in the second to fourth decades. A female predominance is also suggested among the adult cases. Participation in competitive sports or strenuous physical activity or family/individual expectations toward high achievement is also reported with younger individuals.

Predisposing and precipitating factors of paradoxical vocal fold movement have been reported to occur in several different categories: (1) associated with or masquerading as asthma (Brown, Merritt, & Evans, 1988; Christopher, Wood, Eckert, Blager, Raney, & Souhrada, 1983; Hayes, Nolan, Brennan, & FitzGerald, 1993; Martin, Blager, Gay, et al., 1987; Newman & Dubester, 1994); (2) exercise-induced stridor or wheezing (Brugman & Simons, 1998; Hurbis & Schild, 1991; Kivity, Bibi, Schwarz, Greif, Topilsky, & Tabachnick, 1986; Koester & Amundson, 2002; Lakin, Metzger, & Haughey, 1984; Landwehr, Wood, Blager & Milgrom, 1996; McFadden & Zawadski, 1996; Morris, Deal, Bean, Grbach & Morgan, 1999; Rice, Bierman, Shapiro, Rurukawa, & Pierson, 1985; Rupp, 1996); (3) as a focal laryngeal dystonia, or part of Gerhardt's syndrome (Marion, Klap, Perrin, & Cohen, 1992); (4) psychogenic (Cormier, Camus, and Desmeules, 1980; Sim, McClean, Lee, et al., 1990; Skinner & Bradley, 1989); (5) drug-induced laryngeal dystonic reactions; and (6) associated with gastroesophageal reflux (Maceri & Zim, 2001; Powell, Karanfilov, Beechler, Treole, Trudeau, & Forrest, 2000; Koek & Pi, 1989).

The diagnosis of paradoxical vocal fold movement is one of exclusion. Individuals with paradoxical vocal fold movement often present with acute respiratory distress requiring emergency medical treatment. The differential diagnosis of an acute episode of airway obstruction in an adult includes allergic reaction, foreign-body obstruction, infection, aspiration, vocal fold paresis or paralysis, laryngeal trauma or abnormality, and mass lesion. Although each case is managed individually, a trained multidisciplinary team consisting of specialists from the pulmonary, otolaryngology, psychiatry, gastroenterology, and speech–language pathology disciplines can accurately diagnose and facilitate the cessation of the paradoxical vocal fold episodes.

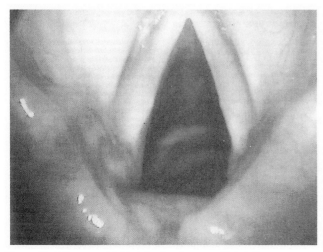

Figure 11–6 True vocal fold abduction in normal inhalation.

Medical testing may include assessment of pulmonary flow volume loops, arterial blood gases, bronchial challenge testing (methacholine/histamine challenge), and chest x-rays. Brugman and Newman (1993) have stated that the gold standard for paradoxical vocal fold movement diagnosis is transnasal fiberoptic laryngoscopy during an acute attack. During a paradoxical episode of inspiratory stridor, a diamond-shaped posterior glottal chink or ventricular fold compression with vocal fold adduction is observed (**Fig. 11–7**). With direct observation of the true vocal folds, Koufman (1994) reported certain tasks such as phonating the vowel /i/ and sniffing, in rapid alternating succession, counting rapidly and loudly, and nonspeech tasks of coughing, panting, and throat clearing may reveal a pattern of vocal fold adductory and abductory movement consistent with paradoxical movement.

Treatment intervention to reduce or eliminate episodes includes psychiatric, pharmacologic, and behavioral approaches. Over the years, several therapeutic interventions have been

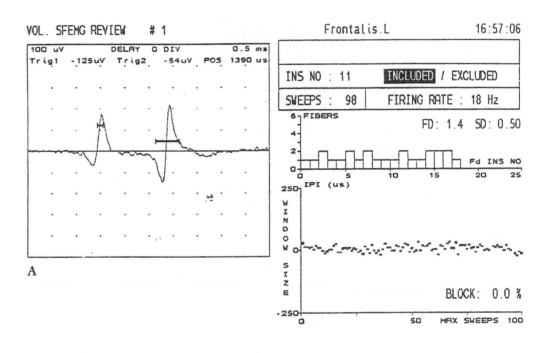

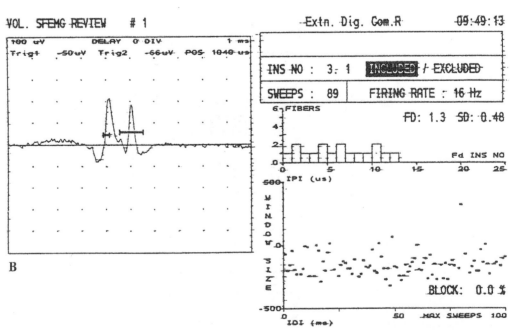

Figure 11–7 (A) Normal single-fiber electromyography (SFEMG) from the frontalis muscle. The two spikes represent the potentials from two individual muscle fibers of the same motor unit. The bold horizontal lines crossing the potentials above the baseline represent "triggers" (voltage thresholds for the computer program to recognize) for the display of the potential and the calculation of when the second spike fires relative to the first. From the IPI (interpotential interval) seen in the graph in the lower right, a calculation is made of the "jitter," or variability between the firing of the first and second muscle fibers. Most of this variability results from neuromuscular transmission. In this case the jitter was 11 microseconds, (normal < 45 μsec). **(B)** This abnormal SFEMG from a patient with MG demonstrated jitter of 99 μsec.

Table 11–9 Therapeutic Interventions for Paradoxical Vocal
Fold Movement

Adrenal corticosteroids	Biofeedback techniques
Hydrocortisone	Breathing exercises
Beclomethasone	Bilateral laryngeal nerve block
Antianxiety agents	Continuous positive airway pressure (CPAP)
Diazepam	Helium-oxygen mixture
Anticholinesterase agents	Humidified air
Edrophonium	Intubation
Antihistamines	Intermittent positive pressure ventilation
Diphenhydramine	Oxygen
Hydroxyzine	Placebo therapy
Antipsychotic agents	Psychotherapy
Chlorpromazine	Relaxation techniques
β_2–agonists	Right phrenic nerve transplant
Calcium antagonists	Voice therapy
Nifedipine	Self-hypnosis
H1-receptor antagonists	Tracheostomy
Cromolyn sodium	Visual feedback
H2-receptor antagonists	
Cimetidine	
Ranitidine	
Nebulized β-adrenergic agents	
Nonnarcotic analgesics	
Acetaminophen	
Orphan drug	
Botulinum toxin	
Parasympathetic antagonists	
Atropine	
Proton pump inhibitor	
Omeprazole	
Sympathomimetic (adrenergic) agents	
Ephedrine	
Epinephrine	
Inhaled albuterol	
Isoproterenol	
Tricyclic antidepressants	
Amitriptyline	
Desipramine	
Xanthine derivatives	
Aminophylline	
Theophylline	

prescribed in an attempt to treat this disorder (**Table 11–9**). These fall into the categories of psychiatric, pharmacologic, and behavioral management. Psychiatric intervention in the form of psychotherapy using methods of relaxation and supportive therapy (Caraon & O'Toole, 1991; Gavin, Wamboldt, Brugman, Roesler & Wamboldt, 1998; Kissoon, Kronick, & Frewen, 1988; Selner, Staudenmayer, Koepke, Harvey, & Christopher, 1987) has been effective when emotional or psychological issues and

family dynamics have been involved. Pharmacologic interventions including bronchodilators have been used in an attempt to relieve symptoms (Barnes, Grob, Lachman, Marsh, & Loughlin, 1986; Corren & Newman, 1992); however, success depends on the etiology of the disorder. Loughlin and Koufman (1996) reported on 12 adult patients who presented with episodic stridor or laryngospasms related to eating or in some cases, awakened from a sound sleep. Laryngeal examinations revealed signs of gastroesophageal reflux that included laryngeal erythema, arytenoid and interarytenoid edema and erythema, and Reinke's edema. Abnormal results from 24-hour, double-probe pH monitoring were found in 10 of the 12 patients. It was reported that all patients had cessation of the laryngospasms within 1 to 4 months following an antireflux regimen consisting of dietary and lifestyle modifications and the administration of oral omeprazole. Symptoms are not routinely controlled with pharmacologic agents when the episodes are functional or psychogenic in origin (Ophir, Katz, Tavori, & Aladjem, 1990; Patterson, Schatz, & Horton, 1974).

Speech therapy alone or in combination with other treatment interventions has proven to be successful in the reduction or elimination of paroxysms of wheezing, stridor, and dyspnea. Martin et al (1987) have presented a nonthreatening treatment approach that facilitates laryngeal relaxation by maintaining continuous airflow through the glottis utilizing diaphragmatic breathing. Through therapy focusing on self-awareness, the individual is encouraged to become aware of sensations of heightened laryngeal and respiratory tension during an episode in comparison to laryngeal sensations when voluntary control is exercised. Therapy techniques include relaxation exercises to relax the oropharyngeal and upper body musculature, utilizing diaphragmatic breathing without laryngeal constriction or tension, and focusing on prolonged exhalation. Individuals are encouraged to practice therapy techniques daily and to use the techniques at the first sign of laryngeal tightness or stridor (Newsham, Klaben, Miller, & Saunders, 2002).

Case Three

An 18-year-old female college athlete, who was awarded a full scholarship to play basketball, was diagnosed by a pulmonologist as having inspiratory stridor during exercise. Her symptoms of noisy, labored breathing occurred during rigorous exercise workouts, especially when doing consecutive sprints and playing in the basketball games.

History

Past medical history was positive for mild tuberculosis when she was 8 years old that was treated successfully without sequelae. She was never restricted in any physical activities on the basis of her heart or lungs. While in high school she played basketball as a forward/center and graduated as one of the highest average rebounders per game in the state. She also ran track and competed in the district finals in hurdles. During her freshman year in college and approximately 4 months into basketball season, she reported dyspnea after wind sprints and during basketball practice. She was evaluated by a pulmonologist and diagnosed with exercise-induced asthma. Her symptoms continued throughout the basketball season. She was only able to exert herself maximally for about 5 minutes before she would experience dyspnea. During her freshman season, several different medications were tried, including Azmacort, Albuterol, Serevent, Ventolin, AeroBid, Proventil, Medrol dose pack, and Pepcid. Minimal improvement of her symptoms was noted. After the season was completed, the respiratory symptoms disappeared.

When practice resumed in the fall of her sophomore year, the symptoms resumed and were exacerbated with almost any form of exercise. The athletic trainer stated that her noisy breathing was so loud that it echoed in the gymnasium. After running just one sprint, the trainer reported that her breathing would get progressively louder, with wheezing and air hunger, forcing her to stop and bend over. The wheezing would last up to several minutes before subsiding. The patient reported no relief from the bronchial dilators. She subsequently was evaluated by another pulmonologist who prescribed a thallium stress test. The results of this examination and spirometry were normal. The pulmonologist, on listening to a recorded sample of an episode, suspected a vocal cord dysfunction syndrome. The patient was then referred to an otolaryngologist who then referred her to our voice clinic.

Evaluation

A thorough case history was taken and a videolaryngoscopy examination was completed. This patient was unable to spontaneously reproduce the sound that was made during the acute episodes. She described the acute attack as not being able to get enough air, shortness of breath, tightness in the throat and upper chest, and a feeling of her throat closing. During the videolaryngoscopy examination the patient was able to view her own exam on a monitor. She was requested to adduct the true vocal folds while inhaling and produce inspiratory stridor. She reported that this was the exact sensation of "not being able to breathe in, to get air" that she felt during an episode.

In the case history, the patient reported that she felt an extreme amount of pressure from her father and coach to play basketball. These episodes were emotionally upsetting to her and she was scared that she would be redshirted for the season. She stated that she just didn't know what else to do because the bronchodilators were not effective.

Treatment

Therapy was initiated utilizing the treatment approach suggested by Martin et al. (1987). This patient was taught to inhale or sniff in through the nose and gently exhale through the mouth. It was also recommended to prolong exhalation through pursed lips or by saying a soft /s/ or /f/. Attention was given to abdominal expansion during inhalation and relaxation during exhalation by placing her hand on the abdomen. In addition, visual imaging techniques were taught as a method of keeping the glottis open during rapid breathing. These included visualizing the throat being as wide open as a

baseball during inhalation and picturing her vocal folds in complete abduction during inhalation as was seen on the videolaryngoscopy examination. Other techniques were used to help her gain control over fast breathing. She was taught to inhale and exhale with an open jaw and relaxed tongue using diaphragmatic breathing. During an episode she was coached to sniff in through the nose and count aloud on exhalation. She was encouraged to remain upright, walking around instead of bending over, and stopping all activity.

The patient's athletic trainer was present for all therapy sessions. He then served as her coach outside the therapy setting especially during basketball practices. Eleven basketball drills were identified that presented difficulty for this patient. For each practice, the trainer was asked to keep a log of her respiratory episodes with each drill. At the end of each practice, the patient was able to review the number of drills partially or totally completed, total number of seconds/minutes spent in recovering from the episodes, number of seconds/minutes each episode lasted, and total number of minutes of actual practice. Videotapes of her practices were also reviewed with the athletic trainer, speech–language pathologist, and patient. The speech–language pathologist also observed the patient during selected basketball practices and games. The patient was followed over a 4-month period. During that time the bronchodilators were gradually reduced and then eliminated. Toward the end of the basketball season, she was able to complete all practice drills and played in competitive games without incident.

✦ Conclusion

In the field of medical speech–language pathology, laryngeal function is heavily integrated into considerations of diagnosis and treatment for a variety of communication and swallowing disorders. Disturbances in phonation can occur in many neurologic diseases and disorders. Medical and surgical management places patients at risk for the development of iatrogenic laryngeal pathologies such as granuloma (from intubation) and edema (drug-induced effects). The speech–language pathologist must be alert to these possible etiologies for dysphonia and aphonia. In addition, atypical voice disorders (including paradoxical vocal fold movement) may occur as reactions to illness or medical treatment as well as to life events.

Although speech–language pathologists continue to rely on auditory perceptual analysis for a portion of diagnosis and treatment monitoring, the availability of instrumentation and technology for laryngeal imaging and analysis has altered the scope of practice. The competencies required for providing service to patients have expanded and have shifted this subspecialty to a more medical focus than in the past. The topics covered in this chapter indicate the extent of knowledge needed to function as a consultant to physicians and as a provider of voice therapy based on a solid foundation of laryngeal physiology.

Study Questions

1. Describe the physiology of paradoxical vocal fold movement.
2. Explain the various symptoms of atypical voice disorders.
3. Discuss basic instrumentation and its function as used in the evaluation of voice.
4. What are the limitations of instrumental voice assessment?
5. What are the steps in the diagnostic process in voice disorders?
6. Specify the vocal pathologies in which voice therapy is a primary treatment option.

7. Prepare a checklist that a speech–language pathologist might use for educating a patient who has a voice disorder.

8. Discuss the various emphases in the following approaches to voice disorders

    A. Symptomatic therapy

    B. Etiologic therapy

    C. Physiologic therapy

    D. Eclectic therapy

    E. Psychogenic therapy

9. How is voice therapy of use in the management of spasmodic dysphonia?

10. Describe the voice symptoms in the following neurologic diseases:

    A. Amyotrophic lateral sclerosis (ALS)

    B. Multiple sclerosis (MS)

    C. Parkinson's disease (PD)

    D. Myasthenia gravis (MG)

    E. Pseudobulbar palsy

    F. Brainstem stroke

    G. Neurofibromatosis

    H. Cerebellar degeneration

References

Aaltonen, L.M., Rihkanen, H., & Vaheria, A. (2002). Human Papillomavirus in Larynx. *Laryngoscope, 112,* 700–707

American Speech-Language-Hearing Association. (2004a). *Knowledge and Skills for Speech–Language Pathologists with Respect to Vocal Tract Visualization and Imaging.* Rockville, MD: Author

American Speech-Language-Hearing Association. (2004b). Voice Assessment. In: *Preferred Practice Pattern for the Profession of Speech-Language.* Rockville, MD: American Speech-Language-Hearing Association

American Speech-Language-Hearing Association Division 3: Voice and Voice Disorders. (2002). *Consensus Auditory-Perceptual Evaluation of Voice (CAPE-V).* Rockville, MD: American Speech-Language-Hearing Association

Andrews, M.L. (1999). *Manual of Voice Treatment: Pediatrics Through Geriatrics.* Clifton Park, NY: Thomson Delmar Learning

Aronson, A. (1990). *Clinical Voice Disorders: An Interdisciplinary Approach,* 3rd ed. New York: Thieme.

Bach, J. (1890). Hysterical Aphonia. *Medical News-Philadelphia, 57,* 263–264

Baken, R.J. (1987). *Clinical Measurement of Speech and Voice.* Boston: College-Hill Press

Barnes, S., Grob, C., Lachman, B., Marsh, B., & Loughlin, G. (1986). Psychogenic Upper Airway Obstruction Presenting as Refectory Wheezing. *Journal of Pediatrics, 109,* 1067–1070

Bassich, C.J., & Ludlow, C.L. (1986). The Use of Perceptual Methods by New Clinicians for Assessing Voice Quality. *Journal of Speech and Hearing Disorders, 51,* 125–133.

Bless, D.M. (1991). Assessment of Laryngeal Function. In: C.N. Ford & D.M. Bless (Eds.), *Phonosurgery* (pp. 91–122). New York: Raven Press

Bless, D.M., Glaze, L.E., Biever-Lowery, D.M., Campos, G., & Peppard, R. (1993). Stroboscopic, Acoustic, Aerodynamic, and Perceptual Attributes of Voice Production in Normal Speaking Adults. In: I.R. Titze (Ed.), *Progress Report 4* (pp. 121–134). Iowa City: National Center for Voice and Speech

Blitzer, A., Lovelace, R.E., Brin, M.F., Fahn, S., & Fink, M.E. (1985). Electromyographic Findings in Focal Laryngeal Dystonia (Spastic Dysphonia). *Annals of Otology, Rhinology, and Laryngology, 94,* 591–594

Boone, D. (1971). *The Voice and Voice Therapy.* Englewood Cliffs, NJ: Prentice-Hall

Boone, D. R., McFarlane S. C., & Von Berg, S.L. (2005). *The Voice and Voice Therapy,* 7th ed. Boston: Allyn & Bacon

Brown, T., Merritt, W., & Evans, D. (1988). Psychogenic Vocal Cord Dysfunction Masquerading as Asthma. *Journal of Nervous and Mental Disease, 176,* 308–310

Brugman, S., & Newman, K. (1993). Vocal Cord Dysfunction. *Medicine/Science Update, 11,* 1–5

Brugman, S.M., & Simons, S.M. (1998). Vocal Cord Dysfunction: Don't Mistake It for Asthma. *Physician Sportsmedicine, 26,* 63–85

Caraon, P., & O'Toole, C. (1991). Vocal Cord Dysfunction Presenting as Asthma. *Irish Medical Journal, 84,* 98–99

Case, J. (1996). *Clinical Management of Voice Disorders,* 3rd ed. Austin, TX: Pro-Ed

Childers, D.G., Alsaka, Y.A., Hicks, D.M., Moore, G.P. (1987). Vocal Fold Vibrations: An EGG Model. In: T. Baer, C. Sasaki, & K. Harris (Eds.), *Laryngeal Function in Phonation and Respiration* (pp. 181–202). Boston: College-Hill Press

Christopher, K., Wood, R., Eckert, R., Blager, F., Raney, R., & Souhrada, J. (1983). Vocal-Cord Dysfunction Presenting as Asthma. *New England Journal of Medicine, 308,* 1566–1570

Colton, R., Casper, J., & Leonard, R. (2005). *Understanding Voice Problems: A Physiological Perspective for Diagnosis and Treatment,* 3rd ed. Baltimore: Lippincott Williams & Wilkins

Colton, R.H., & Contour, E.G. (1990). Problems and Pitfalls of Electroglottography. *Journal of Voice, 4,* 10–24

Cormier, Y., Camus, P., & Desmeules, M. (1980). Non-Organic Acute Upper Airway Obstruction: Description and a Diagnostic Approach. *American Review of Respiratory Disease, 121,* 147–150.

Corren, J., & Newman, K. (1992). Vocal Cord Dysfunction Mimicking Bronchial Asthma. *Postgraduate Medicine, 92,* 153–156

Darley, F.L., Aronson, A.E., & Brown, J.R. (1975). *Motor Speech Disorders.* Philadelphia: W.B. Saunders

Fritzell, B. (1992). Inverse Filtering. *Journal of Voice, 6,* 111–114

Gavin, L.A., Wamboldt, M., Brugman, S., Roesler, T.A., & Wamboldt, F. (1998). Psychological and Family Characteristics of Adolescents with Vocal Cord Dysfunction. *Journal of Asthma, 35,* 409–417

Gerratt, B., Kreiman, J., Antonanzas-Barroso, N., & Berke, G.S. (1993). Comparing Internal and External Standards in Voice Quality Judgments. *Journal of Speech and Hearing Research, 36,* 14–20

Glaze, L.E., Bless, D.M., Milenkovic, P.H., et al. (1988). Acoustic Characteristics of Children's Voice. *Journal of Voice, 2,* 312–319

Glaze, L.E., Bless, D.M., & Susser, R.D. (1990). Acoustic Analysis of Vowel and Loudness Differences in Children's Voice. *Journal of Voice, 4,* 37–44

Goss, F. (1878). Hysterical Aphonia. *Boston Medical and Surgical Journal, 99,* 215–222

Greene, M. (1972). *The Voice and Its Disorders,* 3rd ed. Philadelphia: J.P. Lippincott

Harris, K. (1981). Electromyography as a Technique for Laryngeal Investigation. *ASHA Reports, 11,* 70–87

Hayes, J., Nolan, M., Brennan, N., & FitzGerald, M. (1993). Three Cases of Paradoxical Vocal Cord Adduction Followed Up Over a 10-Year Period. *Chest, 104,* 678–680

Herrington-Hall, B., Lee, L., Stemple, J., Niemi, K.R., & McHone, M.M. (1988). Description of Laryngeal Pathologies by Age, Sex, Occupation in a Treatment Seeking Sample. *Journal of Speech and Hearing Disorders, 53,* 57–65

Hirano, M. (1981). *Clinical Examination of Voice.* New York: Springer-Verlag

Hirano, M., & Bless, D.M. (1993). *Videostroboscopic Examination of the Larynx.* San Diego: Singular Publishing

Hirose, H. (1986). Electromyography of the Laryngeal and Pharyngeal Muscles. In: C.W. Cummings, J.M. Frederickson, L.A Harker, C. Krause, D. Schuller & M.A. Richardson (Eds.), *Otolaryngology-Head and Neck Surgery* (pp. 1823–1828). St. Louis: Mosby

Hogikyan, N.D., & Sethuraman, G. (1999). Validation of an Instrument to Measure Voice-Related Quality of Life (V-RQOL). *Journal of Voice, 13,* 557–569

Hoit, J.D., & Hixon, T.J. (1992). Age and Laryngeal Airway Resistance During Vowel Production in Women. *Journal of Speech and Hearing Research, 35,* 309–313

Holmberg, E.B., Hillman, R.E., & Perkell, J.S. (1988) Glottal Airflow and Transglottal Air Pressure Measurements for Male and Female Speakers in Soft, Normal, and Loud Voice. *Journal of the Acoustical Society of America, 84,* 511–529

Holmberg, E.B., Hillman, R.E., & Perkell, J.S. (1989) Glottal Airflow and Transglottal Air Pressure Measurements for Male and Female Speakers in Low, Normal and High Pitch. *Journal of Voice, 3,* 294–305

Horii, Y.(1982). Jitter and Shimmer Differences Among Sustained Vowel Phonations. *Journal of Speech and Hearing Research, 25,* 12–14

Hurbis, C., & Schild, J. (1991). Laryngeal Changes During Exercise and Exercise-Induced Asthma. *Annals of Otology, Rhinology, and Laryngology, 100,* 34–37

Ingals, E. (1890). Hysterical Aphonia, or Paralysis of the Lateral Crico-Ary-tenoid Muscles. *Journal of the American Medical Association, 15,* 92–95

Jacobson, B., Bush, C., & Grywalski, C. (1996). Voice Handicap Index (VHI) and Clinicians' Perceptual Judgments: A Comparison. Presented at ASHA Convention, Seattle, WA

Jacobson, B.H., Johnson, A., Grywalski, C., Silbergleit, A., Jacobson, G., Benninger, M.S., Newman, C.W. (1997). The Voice Handicap Index (VHI): Development and Validation. *American Journal of Speech–language Pathology, 6,* 66–70

Karnell, M.P. (1989). Synchronized Videostroboscopy and Electroglottography. *Journal of Voice, 3,* 68–75

Karnell, M.P. (1991). Laryngeal Perturbation Analysis: Minimum Length of Analysis Window. *Journal of Speech and Hearing Research, 34,* 544–548

Karnell, M.P. (1994). *Videoendoscopy—From Velopharynx to Larynx.* San Diego: Singular Publishing

Kent, R.D., & Read, C. (2001). *The Acoustic Analysis of Speech,* 2nd ed. Clifton Park, NY: Thomson Learning

Kissoon, N., Kronick, J., & Frewen, T. (1988). Psychogenic Upper Airway Obstruction. *Pediatrics, 81,* 714–717

Kivity, S., Bibi, H., Schwarz, Y., Greif, Y., Topilsky, M., & Tabachnick, E. (1986). Variable Vocal Cord Dysfunction Presenting as Wheezing and Exercise-Induced Asthma. *Journal of Asthma, 23,* 241–244

Koek, R., & Pi, E. (1989). Acute Laryngeal Dystonic Reactions to Neuroleptics. *Psychosomatics, 30,* 359–364

Koester, M.C., & Amundson, C.L. (2002). Seeing the Forest Through the Wheeze: A Case-Study Approach to Diagnosing Paradoxical Vocal-Cord Dysfunction. *Journal of Athletic Training, 37,* 320–324

Koufman, J.A. (1991). The Otolaryngologic Manifestations of Gastroesophageal Reflux Disease (GERD): A Clinical Investigation of 225 Patients Using Ambulatory 24–Hour pH Monitoring and an Experimental Investigation of the Role of Acid and Pepsin in the Development of Laryngeal Injury. *Laryngoscope, 101,* 1–78

Koufman, J. (1994). Paradoxical Vocal Cord Movement. *Visible Voice, 3,* 49–53, 70–71

Koufman, J.A., Amin, M.R., & Panetti, M. (2000). Prevalence of Reflux in 113 Consecutive Patients with Laryngeal and Voice Disorders. *Otolaryngology Head and Neck Surgery, 123,* 385–388

Kreiman, J., Gerratt, B.R., Kempster, G.B., Erman, A., & Berke, G.S. (1993). Perceptual Evaluation of Voice Quality: Review, Tutorial, and a Framework for Future Research. *Journal of Speech and Hearing Res, 36,* 21–40

Lakin, R., Metzger, W., & Haughey, B. (1984). Upper Airway Obstruction Presenting as Exercise Induced Asthma. *Chest, 86,* 499–501

Landwehr, L.P., Wood, R.P., Blager, F.B., & Milgrom, H. (1996). Vocal Cord Dysfunction Mimicking Exercise-Induced Bronchospasm in Adolescents. *Pediatrics, 98,* 971–974

Llewellyn-Thomas, H.A., Sutherland, H.J., Hogg, S.A., Ciampi, A., Harwood, A.R., Keane, T.J., Till, J.E., & Boyd, N.F. (1984). Linear Analogue Self-Assessment of Voice Quality in Laryngeal Cancer. *Journal of Chronic Disease, 37,* 917–924

Loughlin, C., & Koufman, J. (1996). Paroxysmal Laryngospasm Secondary to Gastroesophageal Reflux. *Laryngoscope, 106,* 1502–1505

Ludlow, C.L. (1991). Neurophysiological Assessment of Patients with Vocal Motor Control Disorders. In: *Assessment of Speech and Voice Production: Research and Clinical Applications* (pp. 161–171). Bethesda, MD: National Institute on Deafness and Other Communicative Disorders

Maceri, D.R., & Zim, S. (2001). Laryngospasm: An Atypical Manifestation of Severe Gastroesophageal Reflux Disease. *Laryngoscope, 111,* 1976–1979

Marion, M.H., Klap, P., Perrin, A., & Cohen, M. (1992). Stridor and Focal Laryngeal Dystonia. *Lancet, 339,* 457–458

Martin, R., Blager, F., Gay, M., et al. (1987). Paradoxical Vocal Cord Motion in Presumed Asthmatics. *Seminars in Respiratory Medicine, 8,* 332–337

McFadden, E.R., & Zawadski, D.K. (1996). Vocal Cord Dysfunction Masquerading as Exercise-Induced Asthma: A Physiologic Cause for "Choking" During Athletic Activities. *American Journal of Respiratory Critical Care Medicine, 153,* 942–947

Melcon, M., Hoit, J.D., & Hixon, T.J. (1989). Age and Laryngeal Airway Resistance During Vowel Production. *Journal of Speech and Hearing Disorders, 54,* 282–286

Milenkovic, P.H. (1987). Least Mean Squares and Measures of Voice Perturbation. *Journal of Speech and Hearing Research, 30,* 529–538

Miller, C.J., & Daniloff, R. (1993). Airflow Measurements: Theory and Utility of Findings. *Journal of Voice, 7,* 38–46

Morris, M.J., Deal, L.E., Bean, D.R., Grbach, V.X., & Morgan, J.A. (1999). Vocal Cord Dysfunction in Patients with Exertional Dyspnea. *Chest, 116,* 1676–1682

Morrison, M., & Rammage, L. (1994). *The Management of Voice Disorders.* San Diego: Singular

Murry, T., Medrado, R., Hogikyan, N.D., & Aviv, J.E. (2004). The Relationship Between Ratings of Voice Quality and Quality of Life Measures. *Journal of Voice, 18,* 183–192

Murry, T., & Woodson, G.E. (1992). A Comparison of Three Methods for the Management of Vocal Fold Nodules. *Journal of Voice, 3,* 271–276

Murry, T., & Woodson, G.E. (1995). Combined-Modality Treatment of Adductor Spasmodic Dysphonia with Botulinum Toxin and Voice Therapy. *Journal of Voice, 9,* 460–465

Netsell, R. (1969). Subglottal and Intraoral Air Pressures During Intervocalic Contrast of /t/ and /d/. *Phonetica, 20,* 68–73

Newman, K., & Dubester, S. (1994). Vocal Cord Dysfunction: Masquerader of Asthma. *Seminars in Respiratory and Critical Care Medicine, 15,* 161–167

Newsham, K.R., Klaben, B.G., Miller, V.J., & Saunders, J.E. (2002) Paradoxical Vocal-Cord Dysfunction: Management in Athletes. *Journal of Athletic Training, 37,* 325–328

Ophir, D., Katz, Y., Tavori, I., & Aladjem, M. (1990). Functional Upper Airway Obstruction in Adolescents. *Archives of Otolaryngology Head and Neck Surgery, 116,* 1208–1209

Orlikoff, R.F., & Baken, R.J. (1993). *Clinical Voice and Speech Measurement.* San Diego: Singular

Orlikoff, R.F., & Kahane, J.C. (1991). Influence of Mean Sound Pressure Level on Jitter and Shimmer Measures. *Journal of Voice, 5,*113–119

Patterson, R., Schatz, M., & Horton, M. (1974). Munchausen's Stridor: Non-Organic Laryngeal Obstruction. *Clinical Allergy, 4,* 307–310

Powell, D.M., Karanfilov, B.I., Beechler, K.B., Treole, K., Trudeau, M.D., Forrest, L.A. (2000). Paradoxical Vocal Cord Dysfunction in Juveniles. *Archives of Otolaryngology Head and Neck Surgery, 126,* 29–34

Ramig, L.O., & Dromey, C. (1996). Aerodynamic Mechanisms Underlying Treatment Related Changes in SPL in Patients with Parkinson Disease. *Journal of Speech and Hearing Research, 39,* 798–807

Ramig, L., Pawlas, A., & Countryman, S. (1995). *The Lee Silverman Voice Treatment (LSVT): A Practical Guide to Treating the Voice and Speech Disorders in Parkinson Disease.* Iowa City, IA: National Center for Voice and Speech

Ramig, L.O., Sapir, S., Countryman, S., Pawlas, A., O'Brien, C., Hoehn, M., & Thompson, L.I. (2001). Intensive voice treatment (LSVT) for patients with Parkinson's disease: a 2-year follow-up. *Journal of Neurology, Neurosurgery, and Psychiatry, 71,* 493–498

Rice, S.G., Bierman, C.W., Shapiro, G.G., Rurukawa, C.T., & Pierson, W.E. (1985). Identification of Exercise-Induced Asthma Among Intercollegiate Athletes. *Annals of Allergy, 55,* 790–793

Roy, N., Bless, D.M., Heisey, D., & Ford, C.N. (1997). Manual Circumlaryngeal Therapy for Functional Dysphonia: An Evaluation of Short- and Long-Term Treatment Outcomes. *Journal of Voice, 11,* 321–331

Roy, N., Ford, C.N., & Bless, D.M. (1996). Muscle Tension Dysphonia and Spasmodic Dysphonia: The Role of Manual Laryngeal Tension Reduction in Diagnosis and Management. *Annals of Otology, Rhinology, Laryngology, 105,* 851–856

Roy, N., Gouse, M., Mauszycki, S.C., Merrill, R.M., & Smith, M.E. (2005). Task specificity in adductor spasmodic dysphonia versus muscle tension dysphonia. *Laryngoscope, 115,* 311–316

Roy, N., Leeper, H.A. (1993). Effects of the Manual Laryngeal Musculoskeletal Tension Reduction Technique as a Treatment for Functional Voice Disorders: Perceptual and Acoustic Measures. *Journal of Voice, 7,* 242–249

Rupp, N.T. (1996). Diagnosis and Management of Exercise-Induced Asthma. *Physician Sportsmedicine, 24,* 77–87

Russell, J. (1864). A Case of Hysterical Aphonia. *British Medical Journal, 8,* 619–621

Scherer, R.C. (1991). Aerodynamic Assessment in Voice Production. In: *Assessment of Speech and Voice Production: Research and Clinical Applications* (pp. 42–49). Bethesda, MD: National Institute on Deafness and Other Communicative Disorders

Schutte[p47], H.K. (1992). Integrated Aerodynamic Measurements. *Journal of Voice, 6,* 127–134

Selner, J., Staudenmayer, H., Koepke, J., Harvey, R., & Christopher, K. (1987). Vocal Cord Dysfunction: The Importance of Psychologic Factors and Provocation Challenge Testing. *Journal of Allergy and Clinical Immunology, 79,* 726–733

Sette L., Pajno-Ferrara, F., Mocella, S., Portuese, A., & Boner, A.L. (1993). Vocal Cord Dysfunction in an Asthmatic Child: Case Report. *Journal of Asthma, 30,* 407–412

Shrivastav, R., Sapienza, C.M., & Nandur, V. (2005). Application of Psychometric Theory to the Measurement of Voice Quality Using Rating Scales. *Journal of Speech, Language, and Hearing Research, 48,* 323–335

Silbergleit, A.K. (1993). Acoustic Analysis of Voice in Amyotrophic Lateral Sclerosis. Unpublished doctoral dissertation. Detroit, MI: Wayne State University

Sim, T., McClean, S., Lee, J., Naranjo, M.S., & Grant, J.A. (1990). Functional Laryngeal Obstruction: A Somatization Disorder. *American Journal of Medicine, 88,* 293–295

Skinner, D., & Bradley, P. (1989). Psychogenic Stridor. *Journal of Laryngology and Otology, 103,* 383–385

Smith, E., Verdolini, K., Gray, S., Nichols, S., Lemke, J., Barkmeier, J., Dove, H. & Hoffman, H. (1994). Effects of Voice Disorders on Quality of Life. *NCVS Status Progress Report, 7,* 1–17

Smith, M.E., Ramig, L.O., Dromey, C., Perez, K.S., & Samandari, R. (1995). Intensive Voice Treatment in Parkinson's Disease: Laryngostroboscopic Findings. *Journal of Voice, 9,* 453–459

Smith, S., & Thyme, K. (1978). *Accent Metoden: Special Paedagogisk Forlag A-S.* Denmark: Herning

Smitheran, J., & Hixon, T.J. (1981). A Clinical Method for Estimating Laryngeal Airway Resistance During Vowel Production. *Journal of Speech and Hearing Disorders, 46,* 138–146

Stemple, J. (2000). *Voice Therapy: Clinical Case Studies,* 2nd ed. San Diego: Singular

Stemple, J., Glaze, L., & Klaben, B.G. (2000). *Clinical Voice Pathology: Theory and Management,* 3rd ed. San Diego: Singular

Sulter, A.M., Wit, H.P., Schutte, H.K., & Miller, D.G. (1994). A Structured Approach to Voice Range Profile (Phonetogram) Analysis. *Journal of Speech and Hearing Research, 37,* 1076–1085

Titze, I.R. (1991a). Measurements for Assessment of Voice Disorders. In: *Assessment of Speech and Voice Production: Research and Clinical Applications* (pp. 42–49). Bethesda, MD: National Institute on Deafness and Other Communicative Disorders

Titze, I.R. (1991b). Phonation Threshold Pressure: A Missing Link for Glottal Aerodynamics. In: I.R. Titze (Ed.), *Progress Report 1* (pp. 1–14). Iowa City, IA: National Center for Voice and Speech

Titze, I.R. (1992). Acoustic Interpretation of the Voice-Range Profile (Phonetogram). *Journal of Speech and Hearing Research, 35,* 21–35

Titze, I.R. (1993). Towards Standards in Acoustic Analysis of Voice. In: I.R. Titze (Ed.), *Progress Report 4* (pp. 271–280). Iowa City, IA: National Center for Voice and Speech

Titze, I.R. (1994). *Principles of Voice Production.* Englewood Cliffs, NJ: Prentice-Hall

Titze, I.R. (1995). *Summary Statement of the Workshop on Acoustic Voice Analysis.* Iowa City, IA: National Center for Voice and Speech

Titze, I.R., Horii, Y., & Scherer, R.C. (1987). Some Technical Considerations in Voice Perturbation Measurements. *Journal of Speech and Hearing Research, 30,* 252–260.

Titze, I.R., & Winholtz, W.S. (1993). Effect of Microphone Type and Placement on Voice Perturbation Measurements. *Journal of Speech and Hearing Research, 36,* 1177–1190

Van Riper, C. (1939). *Speech Correction Principles and Methods.* Englewood Cliffs, NJ: Prentice-Hall

Verdolini-Marston, K., Burke, M., Lessac, A., Glaze, L., & Caldwell, E.A. (1995). Preliminary Study of Two Methods of Treatment for Laryngeal Nodules. *Journal of Voice, 9,* 74–85

Verdolini-Marston, K., Titze, I.R., & Drucker, D.G. (1990). Changes in Phonation Threshold Pressure with Induced Conditions of Hydration. *Journal of Voice, 4,* 142–151

Ward, W. (1877). Hysterical Aphonia. *Chicago Medical Journal Examiner, 34,* 495–505

West, R., Kennedy, L., & Carr, A. (1937). *The Rehabilitation of Speech.* New York: Harper and Brothers

12

Rehabilitation of the Head and Neck Cancer Patients

Michael S. Benninger, Cynthia Grywalski, and Debra Phyland

✦ Anatomic Regions of the Head and Neck

✦ Tissue Changes in Head and Neck Cancer

✦ Head and Neck Tumor Sites and Symptoms

✦ Diagnosis of Head and Neck Cancer

✦ Clinical Tumor Classification

✦ Medical and Surgical Management of Head and Neck Cancers

✦ Multidisciplinary Management

✦ Timing of Speech–Language Pathology Service

✦ Management of Speech Following Head and Neck Cancer Treatment

✦ Swallowing Changes After Head and Neck Cancer Treatment

✦ Case Studies

Cancer is second only to heart disease as the major cause of death in the United States, accounting for about 22% of all deaths (Silverberg & Lubera, 1988). Head and neck cancers account for about 10% of all cancers and 5% of all cancer deaths, if skin cancers are included. The American Cancer Society (2002) estimated that there were 37,800 newly diagnosed cases of oral cavity, pharyngeal, and laryngeal cancers in the United States during 2002, and an estimated 11,100 deaths resulted from these cancers. Using these estimates, oral cavity, pharyngeal, and laryngeal cancers accounted for 3% of all newly diagnosed cancers and 2% of all deaths from cancer. Although these percentages may not seem staggering, the effects of head and neck cancers are often pronounced, interfering with an individual's physical, psychological, and social well-being. These diseases and the treatment regimen used to try to cure them can drastically alter basic life functions. For this reason, head and neck cancer patients require management from several medical and nonmedical perspectives.

Head and neck cancers afflict more men than women, although incidence and mortality rates for women have increased over the past 30 years (American Cancer Society, 2002). This increase has coincided with increases in the number of women who use tobacco, a known risk factor for head and neck cancers. Incidence and mortality rates for some head

and neck cancers are higher for African Americans, possibly related to differences in nutrition or socioeconomic factors that interfere with early detection and improved survival. Incidence rates for specific cancer sites within the head and neck vary with geography. For example, oral cavity and oropharyngeal cancers account for almost half of all cancers in the East and Far East (Johns & Papel, 1987). The incidence of nasopharyngeal carcinoma in the people of Kwang Tung Province in China is 25 times higher than it is in Whites (Decker & Goldstein, 1982). Environmental, cultural, ethnic, and genetic conditions are likely explanations for the relationship between the predominance of a particular head and neck cancer site and geographic location.

Speech–language pathologists become involved in the therapeutic regimen for head and neck cancer patients because one or more of the basic speech subsystems (respiration, phonation, resonation, and articulation) or swallowing may be affected by the cancer treatment to varying degrees. Head and neck tumors are challenging to manage from a medical standpoint because of the complexity, compactness, and important functions of head and neck structures. Head and neck cancers may invade any of the organs or air-filled spaces that form the upper aerodigestive tract, from the base of the skull superiorly to the trachea inferiorly, and from the tip of the nose anteriorly to the pharyngeal wall posteriorly. When surgical removal of a head and neck tumor is undertaken, it can be difficult to maintain negative (noncancerous) margins because structures are close in proximity. Surgical resection of the tumor often involves removal of more than the tumor resulting in resection of important host structures. These tumors may seriously interfere with basic human functions, such as breathing, swallowing, and speaking. Treatment of these tumors may result in permanent physical alterations and drastic lifestyle changes. Speech–language pathologists must predicate their plans for rehabilitation of these patients with sound knowledge of normal head and neck anatomy and physiology. They must understand the functional consequences that result from alterations in head and neck structures. They need to maintain current knowledge of medical treatments for head and neck cancer. They must seek and exchange information with other medical specialists who care for this group of patients. Above all, they must apply the information they have gathered to effectively manage their patients' communication and swallowing problems, recognizing that each patient's responses to the cancer, its treatment, and the subsequent rehabilitation course are unique. **Appendix 12–1** lists the competencies that speech–language pathologists need for working with head and neck cancer patients.

This chapter presents a framework for provision of speech–language pathology services to head and neck cancer patients. We provide a general description of the anatomic subdivisions of the mucosal surfaces that line the head and neck, common tumor sites and symptoms for each anatomic subdivision, diagnostic procedures for head and neck cancers, medical treatment options, guidelines for the timing of speech and swallowing intervention, alterations in speech and swallowing following head and neck cancer treatment, and management procedures. The information in this chapter is primarily intended to assist speech–language pathologists who are preparing to work with head and neck cancer patients in a medical setting by offering basic information and practical guidelines. The framework for rehabilitation presented in this chapter emphasizes the health care team approach because treatment for head and neck cancer patients is multifaceted and requires information from many different medical and nonmedical perspectives.

✦ Anatomic Regions of the Head and Neck

The most common cancer of the head and neck is squamous cell carcinoma, which may involve any of the mucosal surfaces of the upper aerodigestive tract. Tumors that form on these mucosal surfaces can have an impact on speech and swallowing. Our discussion of head and neck anatomy focuses on these internal structures, where tumors are frequently found. It is helpful to conceptualize the internal head and neck region as four distinct compartments with landmark structures and air-filled spaces that can be found in each one, keeping in mind that tumors frequently do not contain themselves inside these somewhat arbitrarily determined compartments. The following description of head and neck anatomy is general at best. Readers who want more thorough descriptions are referred to sources that emphasize the anatomy of the speech and swallowing mechanisms, such as Zemlin (1988).

The four major intrinsic cavities of the head and neck region are the nasal cavity, the oral cavity (including lips, cheeks, and

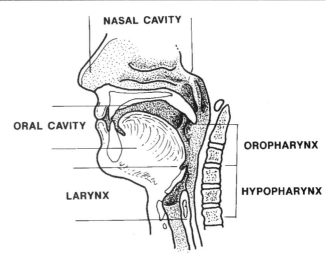

Figure 12–1 The four internal compartments of the head and neck.

buccal spaces), the pharyngeal cavity, and the laryngeal cavity (**Fig. 12–1**). The framework for these cavities is bony and cartilaginous. Muscles and connective tissues attach to the framework, and all is covered with a lining of moist mucosa. The structures and air spaces located in each cavity help to define the anatomic boundaries.

The Nasal Cavity

The nasal cavity serves as a passage for air and is divided medially by the nasal septum into somewhat symmetrical chambers. The anterior nares (nostrils) connect the nasal cavity with the external environment. The posterior nares (choanae) connect the nasal cavity to the nasopharynx. Other important structures to be noted in the nasal cavity are the superior, middle, and inferior nasal turbinates. These tissue masses serve to heat, moisten, and filter nasally inhaled air. The sinuses and the lacrimal (tear) system drain into the nose by way of several ostia that drain into the middle and inferior turbinate meatus. Cranial nerve I (olfactory) innervates the upper portion of the nose.

The Oral Cavity

The oral cavity is the mouth, which contains several structures necessary for speech and swallowing. It is bounded anteriorly by the lips, laterally by the buccal (cheek) spaces, posterolaterally by the anterior faucial pillars, superiorly by the juncture of the hard and soft palates, and inferiorly by the floor of the mouth, with its mobile anterior two thirds of the tongue. Important structures in the oral cavity are the lips, teeth, gums, buccal mucosa, upper alveolar ridge, lower alveolar ridge, retromolar gingiva (retromolar trigone), floor of the mouth, sublingual salivary gland and ducts, hard palate, and freely mobile portion (anterior and middle third portions) of the tongue.

The Pharynx

The pharynx is a tube-shaped cavity made up primarily of connective tissue superiorly and muscle tissue inferiorly. It allows the passage of air and food. In adults, the superior border of the pharynx is at the level of the base of the skull, and the inferior border is at the level of the cricoid cartilage and the sixth cervical vertebra. The pharynx is divided into three sections: the nasopharynx, the oropharynx, and the hypopharynx. The nasopharynx connects superiorly with portions of the sphenoid and occipital bones of the skull. On its lateral walls are the openings to the eustachian tubes, which communicate with the tympanic cavities bilaterally. The soft palate is the inferior border of the nasopharynx as well as the superior border of the oropharynx. The oropharynx extends inferiorly to the level of the hyoid bone, and connects with the oral cavity anteriorly at the anterior faucial pillars. The oropharynx contains the posterior third portion of the tongue, or tongue base, and the palatine tonsils. Contiguous with the oropharynx is the hypopharynx, with its superior border at the level of the hyoid bone. Its inferior border is the pharyngoesophageal segment, a sphincter of muscle that marks the bottom of the pharynx and the top of the esophagus. Laterally, the hypopharynx shares margins with the larynx at the pyriform sinuses, although the medial walls of the pyriform sinuses are considered part of the larynx.

The Larynx

The intrinsic larynx is the fourth major head and neck cavity. It is suspended superiorly from the U-shaped hyoid bone by accessory laryngeal muscles. The hyoid bone can be considered a part of the larynx because it is an important attachment site, although it is also considered a lingual bone because several lingual muscles attach to it (Citardi, Gracco, & Sasaki, 1995). The larynx extends from the epiglottis and valleculae superiorly to the lower border of the cricoid cartilage inferiorly. The valleculae are bilateral grooves formed by the tongue base and epiglottis that act as holding tanks for material about to be swallowed and channel it away from the laryngeal inlet. Like the pharynx, the larynx is divided into three distinct anatomic sections: the supraglottic larynx, the glottic larynx, and the subglottic larynx. The supraglottic larynx contains the epiglottis (lingual and laryngeal aspects), ventricular folds (false vocal folds), the superior portions of the arytenoid cartilages, and the aryepiglottic folds. The glottic larynx runs the horizontal length of the true vocal folds from the anterior commissure, where the vocal folds have a common attachment to the inner angle of the thyroid cartilage, to the posterior commissure, where each fold attaches to its respective arytenoid cartilage at the vocal process. The superior border of the glottic larynx is the laryngeal ventricle, which is the space that separates the false and true vocal folds. The inferior border of the glottic larynx, marked at 1 cm below the free medial margins of the true vocal folds, is the superior border of the subglottic larynx. The lower margin of the cricoid cartilage is the inferior boundary of the subglottic larynx, where the trachea begins.

Neural, Vascular, and Lymphatic Systems

It is important to keep in mind that the head and neck region contains bone, cartilage, and neural, vascular, and lymphatic networks that can become involved directly or indirectly in the neoplastic disease process. Cranial nerves V (trigeminal), VII (facial), IX (glossopharyngeal), X (vagus), XI (spinal accessory), and XII (hypoglossal) have sensory and motor branches coursing through the head and neck that could be disturbed by perineural invasion of the tumor or its subsequent treatment.

The function of lymphatics is to return water and protein to the blood from interstitial fluid (Anthony & Koldhoff, 1975). Lymphatic vessels and nodes are well represented in the head and neck. Regional lymph node status is one of the components of head and neck tumor classification and staging [the "N" in the tumor, node, metastasis (TNM) classification system]. Lymph is a clear, watery fluid that flows through lymphatic vessels and one or more lymph nodes before leaving the neck by way of the thoracic duct or the right lymphatic ducts. Passage of lymph through more than one lymph node may explain tumor spread in this region, as lymph from an area of tumor travels through several head and neck lymph nodes before leaving the area. The system of lymphatic drainage in the head and neck is relatively closed off from the rest of the body, and provides probable explanations for the local containment of tumor spread frequently seen in this region (Cachin, 1989). Lymphatic representation is much more limited and confined in the intrinsic structures of the larynx than it is in external laryngeal structures, resulting in mechanisms of metastasis that are more limited and confined as well (Doyle, 1994). More extensive nodal involvement indicates less favorable prognosis (Barnes, 1989; Richard, Sancho-Garnier, & Micheau, 1987).

✦ Tissue Changes in Head and Neck Cancer

The four major internal cavities of the head and neck form a contiguous tract for air and food, called the upper aerodigestive tract. A mucous membrane consisting of stratified squamous epithelium lines the oral cavity, oropharynx, hypopharynx, and glottic larynx; the nasal cavity, supraglottic larynx, and subglottic larynx have ciliated columnar epithelium; and the nasopharynx has mixed mucosa (Cachin, 1989). There are several histologic changes that can occur in these membranous linings. Some of these changes result in benign growths, such as nodules, polyps, and cysts. Some cellular changes indicate a precancerous state. *Leukoplakia* is a term that describes a "white patch" of abnormal growth and signifies changes in the normal mucosa, some of which may be premalignant. *Atypia, metaplasia, dysplasia,* and *hyperplasia* are other terms used to describe cellular changes in normal mucosa that may be precancerous. In the head and neck, squamous cell carcinoma is by far the most common type of malignancy, and the one discussed in this chapter. It is found in over 90% of all laryngeal cancers (Tucker, 1993). Adenocarcinomas (malignant tumors originating in accessory salivary and mucous gland epithelium) and sarcomas (malignant tumors originating in bone, cartilage, muscle, or connective tissue) occur much less frequently in the head and neck. The earliest detectable malignant change in the squamous epithelium is called carcinoma in situ. The cellular changes associated with carcinoma in situ are restricted to the thickness of the epithelium, and do not invade the basement membrane or other tissue layers (Bauer, 1974). More invasive cellular changes are systematically classified and staged, as explained below.

Almost all malignant cellular changes in the head and neck are reactions to chronic irritation, and most of this irritation is associated with common carcinogenic agents, principally tobacco (including smokeless) and alcohol. Gastroesophageal reflux has been studied as a comorbid condition for some cancers, particularly cancer of the larynx (Koufman & Burke, 1996). Poor oral hygiene has also been studied for its role in oral cavity cancers (Decker & Goldstein, 1982). There has been research interest in the area of cancer genetics that may help to identify individuals who are more likely to develop head and neck cancers or have a worse prognosis. Loss or inactivation of certain tumor suppressor genes has been found in patients with squamous cell carcinoma of the head and neck, and this loss has been related to poor patient survival (Pearlstein, Benninger, Worsham, et al, 1997).

✦ Head and Neck Tumor Sites and Symptoms

The site and size of the tumor determine the constellation of symptoms that patients with head and neck cancer experience (Benninger, 1992b). The universal symptoms of pain, bleeding, and a nonhealing sore or ulcer are common. Otalgia, or ear pain, is often reported, but this is more often a referred pain from tumors in the oral cavity, pharynx, larynx, or trachea than from an ear tumor. A lump or thickening on the neck or in the mouth is reported by patients, as is difficulty in chewing, swallowing, and moving the tongue or jaw.

Less than 1% of all malignancies are carcinomas of the nasal and paranasal areas (Bush & Bagshaw, 1982; Sisson, Toriumi, & Atiyah, 1989). Patients with nasal cavity tumors do not typically work with a speech–language pathologist because speech and swallowing dysfunction are atypical. Large, obstructive tumors in the nasal or nasopharyngeal cavity certainly could cause hyponasal resonance, but a more critical symptom is blockage of nasal airflow, and this requires medical management.

Common tumor sites in the oral cavity are the anterior floor of the mouth, the lateral floor of the mouth, the mobile portion of the tongue, and the hard palate. Oral cavity cancers appear as lumps in the mouth or ulcers that do not heal. They may become irritated and bleed during chewing or denture use. Patients may report that they have been eating softer diets to ease mouth pain.

The tonsil, base of tongue, and soft palate are common sites for tumors in the oropharynx. Tumors here are often asymptomatic in the early stages, and as a result they are associated with increased metastatic rates, treatment failures, and mortality rates. Sixty percent of tonsil or base of tongue tumors metastasize regionally (Lee, 1987). An external neck mass may be the initial symptom from any head and neck tumor, although it is more common in nasopharyngeal, oropharyngeal, and hypopharyngeal cancers. Another common symptom with pharyngeal tumors is ear pain. This is a referred pain from the tumor site to the ear mediated by cranial nerves VII, IX, or X. Dysphagia and odynophagia (painful swallowing) are common complaints. Hoarseness is present only in fairly advanced hypopharyngeal cancers. A gradually worsening sore throat is a typical symptom of oropharyngeal tumors.

Early nasopharyngeal tumors may produce mild nasal obstruction and posterior nasal drainage, but patients can often ignore these symptoms because they are common occurrences in general. The two most commonly presenting symptoms of nasopharyngeal tumors are serous otitis media from Eustachian tube obstruction and a neck mass. As these tumors advance, worsening nasal obstruction and epistaxis (nose bleeding) may occur.

Tumors in the supraglottic larynx are primarily found on the epiglottis, the aryepiglottic fold, or the false vocal fold. Tumors in the glottic larynx are typically on the vocal folds. These structures form the three levels of sphincteric airway protection during swallowing (Logemann, 1983). When supraglottic tumors are surgically excised, the supraglottic laryngectomy patient is left with only the true vocal folds for airway protection, and this may cause serious swallowing problems. Fortunately, most patients can eat and swallow in a satisfactory manner following supraglottic laryngectomy with appropriate swallowing therapy. Early cancerous lesions on the true vocal folds cause persistent hoarseness or a breathy voice, and concern about voice changes usually brings patients to the otolaryngologist. Other symptoms of laryngeal cancer that are reported in the course of the disease are scratchy throat, dysphagia, odynophagia (painful swallowing), hemoptysis (spitting up blood), chronic cough, and otalgia (ear pain). Dyspnea (breathing difficulty), stridor (noisy inhalation), and halitosis (foul-smelling breath) are generally late-appearing symptoms, indicative of airway obstruction and tissue necrosis. Isolated subglottic tumors are rare, but the subglottis may be the site of tumor extension.

Systemic (entire body) symptoms are uncommon in patients with squamous cell carcinoma of the head and neck, except in advanced disease when weight loss and general feelings of malaise and fatigue occur. Halitosis is common in many patients with head and neck cancers, particularly in those who consume alcohol excessively. Because most of these patients have had a long history of tobacco exposure, it is not unlikely that they will have sequelae of such exposure, such as chronic obstructive pulmonary disease, emphysema, hypertension, or even lung cancer. Cognitive decline, particularly short-term memory deficit, may also be present in these patients, particularly those with a history of heavy alcohol consumption (Logemann, 1983). These other medical conditions should be considered when planning treatment. For example, a supraglottic laryngectomy for removal of an epiglottic tumor may be contraindicated if the patient also has severe pulmonary disease and cannot risk compromised swallowing.

Patients with any of the symptoms discussed above may find their way to a speech–language pathologist for evaluation of speech, voice, and/or swallowing before a medical exam has taken place. Because a malignant tumor may be the cause of patients' symptoms, referral to an otorhinolaryngologist is necessary. Delays in diagnosis and treatment can be avoided by the astute clinician who recognizes the importance of the physical exam in the expedient identification and treatment of head and neck cancers.

✦ Diagnosis of Head and Neck Cancer

Obtaining the History

Patients who are experiencing physical or functional changes of head and neck structures are frequently referred to an otorhinolaryngologist. Clinical assessment comprises a medical history and a physical exam, which then may lead to further testing, such as computed tomography (CT), magnetic resonance imaging (MRI), blood sampling, and tissue biopsy procedures. A thorough history of presenting symptoms is most essential in the evaluation of patients with head and neck cancers. Risk factors associated with development of carcinoma need to be identified, particularly remote and current exposure to tobacco and alcohol. Other important areas of questioning pertain to previous medical or surgical problems, current use of medications, and the course of symptom progression. It would be remiss if history taking did not include assessment of the patient's psychosocial and cognitive status because this provides information about likely coping abilities and available support from family and friends if medical or surgical management is undertaken.

The Physical Exam

Once a complete history has been obtained, the physical exam is undertaken to palpate areas of the head and neck, including lymph node areas on the neck, and visually inspect the skin, scalp, and mucosal surfaces of the ears, nose, oral cavity, pharynx, and larynx. Indirect exams with a light, a head mirror, and a small angled laryngeal mirror placed strategically in the oropharynx are used to look at the nasopharynx, hypopharynx, and larynx. If a patient's strong gag prohibits indirect examination of the larynx, a topical anesthetic may be used to numb the oropharynx or it may be necessary to transnasally pass a flexible fiberoptic endoscope, an instrument made up of long, very thin cylinders, some of which illuminate the larynx and others that allow its viewing through an eyepiece. It may be necessary to assess the vibratory function of the vocal folds with laryngeal videostroboscopy. This exam simulates slow motion of vocal fold vibration by controlling the timing of light flashes on the larynx during phonation. With laryngeal videostroboscopy, the effects of vocal fold lesions on vibratory function can be determined. It may allow for identification of an adynamic segment of the vocal fold, such as an area of leukoplakia that may suggest early invasion of a lesion (Hirano, Hirade, & Kawasaki, 1985). Exams with the flexible fiberoptic endoscope and laryngeal stroboscope allow for videotaped documentation and tracking of the tumor throughout the course of treatment. Videotaped exams also make it possible to present and discuss a case at a tumor board conference. The composition and function of a multidisciplinary tumor board for head and neck cancer are discussed later in the chapter.

For optimal direct viewing of the larynx and pharynx, a direct pharyngoscopy/laryngoscopy is frequently performed. This procedure is the key to accurate diagnosis and staging of the disease. It is generally not a procedure done in the clinic, but one performed in the operating room with the patient under general anesthesia. Bastian, Collins, Kaniff, and Matz (1989) described a clinic procedure using a flexible laryngoscope and adequate anesthesia to appropriately stage the tumor and obtain biopsies, obviating the need for general anesthesia in the operating room. At the time of the direct pharyngoscopy/laryngoscopy, a tissue biopsy is usually obtained and sent to a pathology laboratory for confirmation of malignancy. This procedure can also be used to identify a possible second primary tumor. Individuals with a tumor in the head and neck have a 7% chance of having a second tumor somewhere else in the aerodigestive tract (Benninger, Enrique, & Nichols, 1993). This could be in the pharynx, larynx, lungs, or esophagus.

The chance of patients' having a second primary tumor has made some medical practitioners advocate the use of triple

endoscopy (direct bronchoscopy, esophagoscopy, and pharyngoscopy/laryngoscopy) for all patients with an index squamous cell carcinoma (tumor responsible for the patient's symptoms), but this is not always necessary. Direct pharyngoscopy/laryngoscopy is the usual procedure for the evaluation and staging of most head and neck cancer patients, and bronchoscopy and esophagoscopy may be reserved for patients who report symptoms that would suggest pulmonary or esophageal involvement (Benninger et al, 1993; Benninger, Shariff, Blazoff, 2001).

Noninvasive imaging techniques are also used to gather diagnostic information, particularly in the detection of metastatic disease. The two most common techniques used with head and neck cancers are CT scanning and MRI. A CT scan provides a series of x-ray views in slices of the head and neck. MRI uses radio waves traveling through a magnetic field to make detailed images of head and neck structures. These tests have functional prediagnostic applications and provide important information about tumor features, but the clinical and operative examinations are the primary information sources used to stage the disease.

✦ Clinical Tumor Classification

Squamous cell carcinomas of the head and neck are clinically classified based on the findings from the physical exam and any other procedures that were administered prior to the initiation of treatment, such as endoscopy, fine-needle aspiration biopsy, CT scanning, MRI, chest films, and blood chemistry tests. Clinical staging follows the American Joint Commission for Cancer Staging and is commonly referred to as the TNM system (Robins, 2001). The T assesses the size or anatomic extent of the primary tumor and is followed by either "IS," which abbreviate "in situ," or a number ranging from 0 to 4. A T_0 classification is reported when there is no tumor; a T_{IS} lesion is reported when the tumor is a carcinoma in situ, the earliest identifiable neoplasm; and T_1, T_2, T_3, and T_4 lesions are reported based on gradually increasing tumor size, with a T_1 lesion smaller than a T_4 lesion.

The next part of the classification system, the N, is used to report the number, size, and location of local lymph nodes that have become involved in the disease process by way of a number ranging from 0 to 3. An N_0 is reported when no regional lymph node involvement is found; an N_3 represents a metastasis in a lymph node more than 6 cm in greatest dimension. This classification describes lymph node metastasis to the neck only, and is dependent only on the neck disease and not on the size of the primary tumor. In addition, lymph node metastasis is usually described by the location of the nodes in the neck, using the following neck divisions: submental and submaxillary triangle nodes; high, middle, and low jugular chain nodes; posterior triangle nodes; and peritracheal nodes (Spector, 1987).

The final classification marker, the M, is used to describe metastasis (spread) of the tumor to distant body regions. Except for a classification of M_X, which is reported when distant metastasis cannot be assessed (an "X" after any of the tumor classification markers indicates an inability of that component to be assessed), this classification is basically binary, with M_0 indicating no distant metastasis and M_1 indicating that distant metastasis is present.

Distant metastases are uncommon in squamous cell carcinoma of the head and neck except in advanced or recurrent

Table 12–1 Staging of Head and Neck Carcinoma

Stage I	$T_1 N_0 M_0$
Stage II	$T_2 N_0 M_0$
Stage III	$T_3 N_0 M_0$ or $T_{1-3} N_1 M_0$
Stage IV	$T_4 N_{0-1} M_0$ or $T_{1-4} N_{2,3} M_0$ or any T, any N, M_1

disease, with the lungs being a common metastatic site. Because these patients usually have a history of chronic smoking, and pulmonary compromise is often present, a chest x-ray is recommended as part of the pretreatment workup.

Once the TNM classification markers have been assigned, they may be grouped into one of four stages, ranging from the earliest cancers that fall into the stage I category to those most advanced that are placed into the stage IV category (**Table 12–1**). These stages have substantial prognostic significance because the likelihood of treatment failure and worsening chance for survival are associated with each advancing stage.

✦ Medical and Surgical Management of Head and Neck Cancers

Surgery and radiation therapy are the most common treatment modalities for squamous cell carcinoma of the head and neck. Surgical excision may be done with microsurgical instruments or a microspot laser. Surgery and radiation therapy may be administered alone, in combination with each other, or in combination with other treatment modalities, depending on the nature, site(s), and extent of the disease, the current health status of the patient, and any previous treatment procedures. One of the side effects of radiation therapy, and perhaps chemotherapy, is significant change in glandular secretions with temporary or permanent decrease in salivation, resulting in dry mouth and throat, or xerostomia. Chemotherapy as the sole treatment for head and neck cancer has not shown an improvement over surgery and/or radiation therapy. However, in an attempt to reduce recurrence rates after standard therapy or in many cases to preserve important structures such as the larynx, chemotherapy is now being used in combination with radiation therapy and/or surgery, especially for advanced-stage tumors (Amrein, 1991). The combination of radiation therapy and chemotherapy is now being routinely offered to some patients with fairly advanced tumors, such as T_3 laryngeal cancers, as an organ-preserving alternative to surgical ablation (Department of Veterans Affairs Laryngeal Cancer Study Group, 1991). At this time, there is little evidence to support the use of chemotherapy as the sole treatment for squamous cell carcinoma of the head and neck other than for palliation; however, drug therapy may have promise for future cures. New directions in cancer treatment, such as biologic modifiers and immunotherapy, are being investigated and may well be used in future management of head and neck cancer (Alessi, Hutcherson, & Mickel, 1989; Jones & Weissler, 1990). One treatment option that may be considered in advanced, unresectable cancers is to "do nothing" from an aggressive medical standpoint, and such a decision should be made after carefully counseling the patient and family about the probable treatment outcomes. If this option is chosen, a hospice program could be considered.

Photodynamic therapy (PDT) is currently being studied for its effects on some forms of cancer, including the oropharynx and larynx. It involves the use of a light-sensitive drug that is retained by cancerous cells. Application of light then destroys these marked cells. Skin sensitivity to light is the major side effect of PDT, and the results of its effectiveness in head and neck cancers are not yet conclusive. Although there is some controversy related to preferred treatment protocols based on treatment results at specific medical centers, and all the treatment approaches cannot be addressed in this chapter, a summary of reasonable treatment options for head and neck squamous cell carcinoma follows.

Nasal Cancers

Nasal cancers are predominantly squamous cell carcinomas, basal cell carcinomas, or malignancies of glandular origins, such as adenocarcinomas. Because many nasal tumors originate on the skin of the nose and invade the nasal cavities by direct extension, surgical excision is usually the preferred option. Because of the complicated anatomy of this region, identification of free margins of resection is frequently difficult. Graded resections with intraoperative pathologic marginal control (Mohs' chemosurgery) have allowed for resections with improved reliability of complete tumor extirpation. Larger nasal tumors and those that involve the paranasal sinuses or palate require en bloc (whole) resections, which may significantly interfere with nasal breathing, balanced resonance, and swallowing. Vision may be affected by these tumors if orbital resection is required. Additional radiation therapy or chemotherapy is usually recommended following surgery. The cosmetic effects of nasal cancers and their treatments may be devastating to the patient, but deformities can often be corrected with further surgery or prosthetics.

Oral Cavity Tumors

Oral cavity tumors are usually treated by surgery alone, or surgery and radiation therapy combined. Key functional decisions in oral cavity tumors revolve around potential effects on chewing, swallowing, and articulation of speech, as well as cosmesis. Small cancers, such as a T_1 tumor of the anterior tongue, are usually amenable to surgical excision with wide margins. Because the tongue has limited barriers against tumor spread, larger tumors usually require postoperative radiation therapy. Surgical closure of an area where the tumor was excised can be done, at times, with tissue surrounding the lesion, and this is known as primary closure. T_3 or T_4 tumors often result in large defects of the tongue, the floor of the mouth, or mandible, and may require reconstruction with tissue from nearby body sites, such as regional myocutaneous flaps or skin grafts, and this is known as secondary closure. In these types of closures, the replaced tissue cannot provide the same function as the original tissue, and the patient will often have difficulty with swallowing and speech, sometimes severe and incapacitating. Free flaps from distant body parts can also be used for reconstruction, and there are certain donor sites especially well suited to repair large defects of the oral cavity, such as using the iliac bone from the pelvis or the radial forearm, along with some of the surrounding muscle to patch portions of the mandible. Flaps with neuronal networks can be placed at the site of the surgical defect and anastomosed to existing neuronal structures, in an attempt to restore motor and sensory function to the reconstructed area.

Nasopharyngeal and Oropharyngeal Cancers

Nasopharyngeal cancers may be treated with radiation therapy alone, although combining it with chemotherapy may provide better disease control. The trend has been to treat more with combined radiation and chemotherapy in the recent past. Small T_1 tumors may be amenable to surgical resection, although the difficulty with access to the nasopharynx and success of radiation has made surgery a rarely used option. However, salvage surgery is a possible option for those who have failed radiation therapy (Shu, Shiau, Chi, Yen, & Li, 1999).

The management of cancers of the oropharynx is somewhat controversial. Both radiation therapy and surgery have been advocated as primary modalities. The decision to treat with one or the other depends mostly on the nature of the tumor. The advantage of radiation therapy is that it is more likely to preserve important structures and, in turn, their functions. Furthermore, oropharyngeal tumors tend to be particularly radiosensitive, resulting in initially good response rates. The outcome of primary radiation therapy, with surgical salvage for failures, is comparable to surgery followed by postoperative radiation therapy. Surgery usually requires reconstructive techniques such as flaps for repair of surgical deficits, and difficulties with swallowing and speech are common in all but early tumors treated with surgery. Despite these problems, many patients can learn to function adequately. Stage IV tumors of the base of the tongue usually require a total glossectomy, which typically results in a profound compromise of speech and swallowing function in all but a few patients. Therefore, many medical practitioners have resorted to radiation therapy alone or combined radiation therapy with chemotherapy. It should be noted that multifraction radiation therapy can occasionally leave a patient with as much or more functional limitation as surgery. Specifically, tissue fibrosis and xerostomia can lead to significant functional compromise in speech and swallowing outcomes (Cooper, Fu, Marks, & Silverman, 1995).

Laryngeal Cancers

Patients with T_1 and T_2 cancers of the supraglottic larynx usually have successful disease control with either radiation therapy or surgery. Although partial supraglottic laryngectomy can be performed for some small cancers (such as a T_1 tumor of the epiglottis), larger tumors (such as a T_2 tumor of the false vocal fold) would typically require a formal supraglottic laryngectomy. Recently, laser excision of these larger supraglottic tumors has resulted in good local control with perhaps less morbidity. Surgery is more commonly performed for larger supraglottic tumors than use of radiation therapy.

A supraglottic laryngectomy may leave an individual with serious swallowing difficulties, although voice quality would tend to be quite good. One of the most important contributing factors to the swallowing difficulties is the removal of the epiglottis. During normal swallowing, the larynx elevates and moves forward, and the epiglottis covers the laryngeal introitus while directing the bolus (material to be swallowed) into lateral channels called the pyriform sinuses, providing protection from

aspiration. This protection is lost following supraglottic laryngectomy. The false vocal folds play an important role in preventing the egress of air from the lungs and are necessary for creating subglottic pressure, which also helps to prevent aspiration. When they are removed, as in a standard supraglottic laryngectomy, swallowing decompensates. Furthermore, these patients usually have temporary tracheostomies due to postsurgical swelling and airway obstruction, and the redirection of air through the tracheostomy tube also prevents adequate subglottic pressure. The tube holds the remaining laryngeal structures more tightly in the neck, limiting the upward and forward movement of the larynx during the swallow. It is sometimes difficult to swallow well until the tracheostomy tube has been plugged or preferably removed.

Most patients who have had supraglottic laryngectomies can learn to swallow by mouth using strategies that maximize preserved swallowing abilities. Some T_3 supraglottic cancers can be treated with extended supraglottic laryngectomies, although most T_3 and T_4 tumors require a total laryngectomy.

T_1 glottic cancers can be treated with radiation therapy or surgery, and there is some controversy over which modality is preferred. Survival with primary radiation therapy and surgical salvage of recurrent tumors is comparable to primary surgery and radiation salvage or further surgical salvage with either partial or total laryngectomy, and this survival rate has been reported as approximately 95% (Pellitteri, Kennedy, Vrobec, Beiler, & Hellstrom, 1991). Because results for these two modalities are similar, a key factor in determining preferred treatment is voice outcome. Subjective judgments of voice quality in patients who have undergone radiation therapy have been inconsistent (Llewellyn-Thomas, Sutherland, Hogg, Ciampi, Harwood, Keane, Till, & Boyd, 1984; Stoicheff, 1975; Stoicheff, Ciampi, Passi, & Fredrickson, 1983). Selected objective measures of postradiation voices have been outside the range of normal (Lehman, Bless, & Brandenburg, 1988). Radiation therapy is used in an attempt to control the tumor while preserving the most natural voice possible, although there have been perceptual voice abnormalities detected by a skilled listener 10 years after radiation therapy was used to treat patients with early glottic carcinoma (Morgan, Robinson, Marsh, & Bradley, 1988). Voice outcomes with T_1 tumors confined to one vocal fold and not involving the anterior commissure or the vocal process of the arytenoid were favorable whether treated with radiation or surgery (McGuirt, Blalock, Koufman, & Feehs, 1992). Larger T_1 and any T_2 tumors are preferentially treated by radiation initially. Continuation of smoking following treatment, larger tissue biopsies taken for diagnosis, and complications of treatment are the key factors associated with poor voice outcome and recurrence following radiation therapy for T_1 and T_2 glottic cancer (Benninger, Gillen, Thieme, Jacobson, & Dragovich, 1994). Larger T_2 cancers can be managed with partial laryngectomy or hemilaryngectomy, but less than optimal voice and swallowing outcomes would make this treatment modality less attractive than radiation therapy. Partial laryngectomy procedures, including hemilaryngectomy and supraglottic laryngectomy, are viable options in cases of radiation therapy failure, with high expectation of disease control and limited morbidity (Nichols & Mickelson, 1991).

T_3 glottic cancers have traditionally been treated with total laryngectomy, which is still considered the standard against which other treatments are compared. Swallowing is generally good after total laryngectomy, although problems do arise, and voice restoration with one of the alaryngeal voice modalities allows for functional communication. A combination of chemotherapy and radiation therapy has been offered to patients with T_3 glottic carcinomas, in an attempt to preserve the larynx, and the survival rate of these patients has been reported as comparable to the survival rate of patients who received only surgery (Pfister, Harrison, Strong, & Bosl, 1992; Shu et al, 1999). It is reasonable to offer a patient with a T_3 laryngeal cancer either primary surgery with a total laryngectomy or laryngeal preservation with combined chemotherapy and radiation therapy, reserving surgical salvage for recurrence. T_4 glottic tumors are best treated with total laryngectomy followed by radiation therapy.

Metastatic Neck Disease

Metastatic disease to nearby areas is common in squamous cell carcinoma of the head and neck, particularly in advanced disease. The likelihood of neck metastases depends on the site and stage of the tumor. Cancers of the tonsil, tongue, nasopharynx, and pyriform sinuses are particularly likely to have metastasized, even at the time of initial presentation of the tumor. Many of these tumors have nonpalpable metastases or occult (concealed) disease in the neck. If there is obvious disease involvement, or if the likelihood of occult disease is greater than 25 to 30%, a neck dissection to remove cancerous lymph nodes should be considered. There are different types of neck dissections. One is a radical neck dissection, which occurs when all cervical lymph nodes are surgically removed. With this type of dissection, the sternocleidomastoid muscle and spinal accessory nerve are cut, resulting in difficulty with head turning and shoulder raising. Another type of neck dissection is a modified radical neck dissection, which is less ablative and preserves some nonlymphatic structures that are removed in a radical neck dissection. A CT scan or an MRI of the neck can elucidate metastatic neck disease, often prior to the nodes being palpable. Occult disease or a single metastasis less than 2 cm in size can be managed with radiation therapy in most circumstances, although the presence of larger single nodes or multiple nodes usually requires surgery. On occasion, a patient will present with a metastatic lymph node and an unknown primary tumor. In such cases, random biopsies of the nasopharynx, tonsil, base of tongue, and pyriform sinuses may identify the index tumor.

The extent of lymph node metastases has been associated with prognosis. Larger lymph nodes, bilateral nodes, and multiple nodes result in higher nodal (N) staging and correspond to poorer prognosis, whereas solitary small (less than 3 cm) nodes correspond to a more favorable prognosis.

✦ Multidisciplinary Management

The Head and Neck Tumor Board

Many patients with head and neck cancer receive comprehensive care by a treatment and rehabilitation team. Although it is typically the otolaryngologist/surgeon who acts as the primary care coordinator, other medical specialists are needed to provide thorough management. A critical, and perhaps mandatory, forum for treatment planning and information exchange is a multidisciplinary head and neck tumor board

meeting. Frequency of meetings and composition of attendees most likely depends on the number of patients treated for head and neck cancers at a given medical center and the medical specialists available. At a minimum, an otolaryngologist (who may also be the surgeon), a radiation oncologist, and a medical oncologist are needed to delineate the medical treatment plan. Histologic and imaging information, provided by a pathologist and a radiologist respectively, assists in this endeavor. In addition, a maxillofacial surgeon or prosthodontist may add significantly to the efforts. However, tumor boards should encompass more than medical treatment specifications. Total rehabilitation cannot be achieved without a broader consideration of the person who has the cancer, and additional team members are beneficial.

One of the key individuals at a head and neck tumor board meeting is the cancer coordination nurse, nurse practitioner, or clinical nurse specialist. This individual ensures that all tests and evaluation results are available, coordinates treatment activities and scheduling with the patient and family, and provides for continuity of care and facilitation of treatment, particularly when this involves combined modalities (Benninger, 1992a). A social worker can help to coordinate care and a research nurse or assistant can help enroll patients in research studies that may be important in advancing medical knowledge for the future. As society becomes more familiar with nontraditional treatment options, such as massage, chiropractor, nutritional, vitamin, realignment therapy, etc., it may become worthwhile to have a complementary and alternative medical practitioner as a consultant to the group. Finally, given the critical role of smoking in the etiology of head and neck cancers, a smoking-cessation program should be available.

The Role of the Speech–language Pathologist

A speech–language pathologist is needed to provide information to the team about the swallowing and communication problems that are likely in a given patient, and the feasibility of voice restoration procedures. Any new approaches to voice restoration, speech and swallowing prosthetics, or swallowing rehabilitation can be presented in the context of discussing patients who might benefit from them. Patients in need of pretreatment evaluation and counseling can be identified at the tumor board meeting. It is helpful to have as thorough a description of the tumor and planned surgical resection as possible, perhaps even an illustration of tumor location and resection boundaries, to predict possible functional limitations. It is also important to know whether adjuvant radiotherapy or chemotherapy is planned. **Figure 12–2** shows a case presentation form and **Fig. 12–3** is a basic diagram of head and neck structures on which the surgeon may draw the tumor and the planned resection margins. Patients and their family members may meet the speech–language pathologist for the first time soon after the tumor board meeting, an important first step in establishing a sound clinical relationship that will continue well into the future at various levels. Discussions between tumor board members and patients following the tumor board meeting can easily overwhelm the patient, who may be hearing the diagnosis of cancer and the details of the planned treatment for the first time, so information bombardment should be avoided. It is more important for the speech–language pathologist to meet the patient and informally obtain a cursory

MULTIDISCIPLINARY HEAD AND NECK TUMOR CONFERENCE

NAME: DATE:

MRN: AGE:

REFERRED FROM: REFERRED TO:

PHMX: TOBACCO:

ALLERGY: ETOH:

MEDS: FAMILY HX:

History:

Physical:

Pathology:

Radiological Studies:

TUMOR SITE: T   N   M   STAGE

Treatment Alternatives:

1)

2)

3)

Treatment Planned:

Follow-up Studies/Referrals:

Protocol Alternatives:

Figure 12–2 A multidisciplinary head and neck tumor board data collection form.

idea of communication needs, ongoing speech, swallowing, and cognitive functioning. Pretreatment appointments can be rescheduled for another time prior to the initiation of the medical treatment, when patients will be more receptive to explanations about likely functional changes in speech and swallowing and what can be done about them.

There are other medical specialists who may not be directly involved with the decision-making process for medical management, but are called on to provide services during rehabilitation. Physical therapists may work with patients who have limited range of shoulder motion because the spinal accessory nerve was sacrificed in a radical neck dissection. Nutritionists, psychologists, psychiatrists, and vocational counselors are helpful referral sources, although they may not be regular members of the management team (Casper & Colton, 1993).

✦ Timing of the Speech–Language Pathology Service

The speech–language pathologist may become involved in a head and neck cancer case at any stage along the continuum of patient care, from prediagnosis to posttreatment rehabilitation. The timing of service provision along this continuum is an important consideration in optimal management of speech and swallowing. Intervention can be divided into three periods: pretreatment, immediate posttreatment, and extended posttreatment. Although the timing of service provision usually varies from patient to patient because of the specific circumstances in each case, there are some general guidelines for management issues related to speech and swallowing as they crop up along the medical course.

MULTIDISCIPLINARY HEAD AND NECK TUMOR CONFERENCE

NAME: MRN:

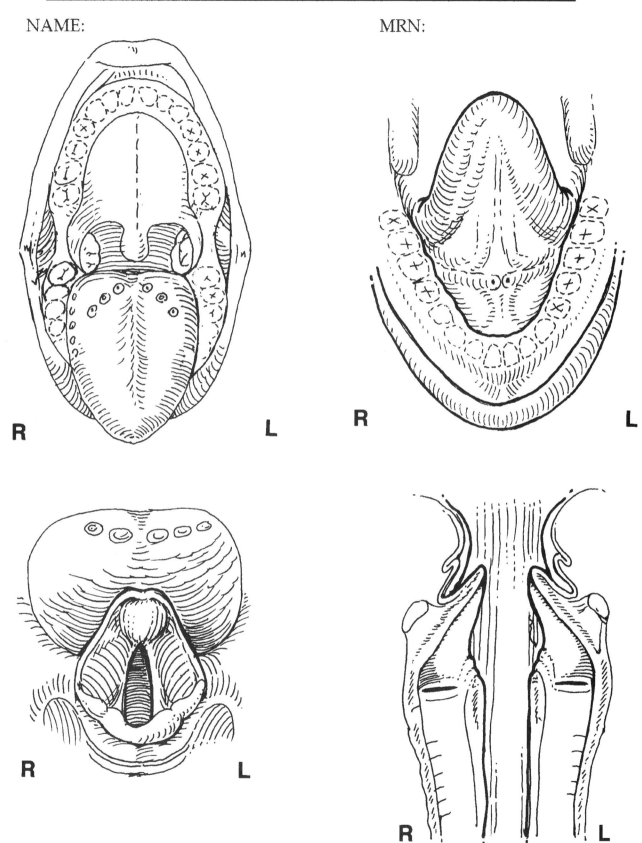

Figure 12–3 Diagram of head and neck structures for drawing surgical margins.

Pretreatment Intervention

Speech–language pathologists are involved most extensively with surgical head and neck patients, although they also are frequently involved in management of both the acute and chronic effects of radiation therapy on speech and swallowing. This discussion pertains to the surgery patient. Presurgical consultation is highly preferred. During this period, intervention is focused on speech, language, and swallowing assessments, patient and family education, and counseling. It would be ideal for the speech–language pathologist to see every patient soon after the diagnosis and treatment options have been given. Information about likely speech and swallowing changes related to specific treatments could then be used by the patient and family in the decision-making process. It is also useful for the speech–language pathologist to meet with the patient to assess the effects of the tumor on speech and swallowing before surgery. This information is important to the prediction of functional outcomes and can provide a baseline for postsurgical comparison (Groher, 1997; McKinstry & Perry, 2003).

If the initial meeting between the speech–language pathologist and the patient is at the time when the patient first hears the diagnosis and recommended treatment options, then getting a sense of the patient's reactions will assist in adjusting the timing of intervention procedures. Most individuals fear cancer. The issues paramount to patients who have just heard a diagnosis of head and neck cancer are the chance for cure and the effects treatment will have on their daily functioning and general well-being. The most opportune time to begin intervention may not be when the patient receives the diagnosis.

For some, pain management surpasses all other medical or personal considerations. Pain, either prior to or after treatment, can skew a patient's general perspective and limit receptiveness to intervention procedures that may at the time seem only remotely related. Initial provision of speech and swallowing services, even of something as seemingly tolerable as patient education, may have to wait until the patient's pain has been controlled. Family education may be a better intervention target at times when pain interferes with direct patient intervention. Postsurgical pain is usually not a lengthy interference in speech and swallowing intervention, but time is needed for surgical sutures to heal.

The speech–language pathologist should check with the surgeon for the most appropriate time to begin direct remediation procedures. Rigid adherence to guidelines for rehabilitation of speech and swallowing in head and neck cancer patients can be difficult because of the individual nature of each case. It is best to have broad goals for all patients, and step back frequently to look at the entire rehabilitation picture for each patient, making adjustments in specific speech and swallowing objectives as the patient's needs dictate. Some flexibility in the timing of information provision, communication retraining, and counseling will be necessary.

Preparation of the pretreatment session by the speech–language pathologist involves thorough review of the patient's medical record. The initial session should focus on exchange of information between the patient and the speech–language pathologist. A comfortable starting point is to have the patient tell the clinician what he or she has already been told about the diagnosis and planned treatment. This retelling can be a transition point for more specific discussion about likely changes in speech and swallowing. The course of rehabilitation should be described.

Following this, the patient may list concerns about rehabilitation by order of importance. Although speech–language pathologists address issues related to communication, speech, and swallowing, and these issues are often inextricably tied to the medical aspects of the patient's care, specific medical concerns should be addressed by the appropriate medical specialist.

The pretreatment session should include assessment of a patient's current communication and swallowing status, physical abilities to use alaryngeal methods of communication, and general cognitive function particularly for new learning, alertness, and attentiveness. Formal evaluation of overall speech intelligibility or conversational speech understandability should be undertaken using a standardized test such as the Fisherman Logemann Test of Articulation Competence or the Frenchay Test of Dysarthria (Enderby, 1983; McKinstry & Perry, 2003). The information yielded can help determine whether the pretreatment speech disorder reflects the site and extent of the tumor. It is also important in the prediction of functional outcomes of cancer management and in treatment planning. If appropriate, measures of aspects of communication other than impairment may also be undertaken. Specifically this may involve evaluation of the patient's current communication satisfaction and perception of limits on speech-related activity and social participation (World Health Organization, 2000). It is important to gain an understanding of the patients total communication needs and thereby embrace a holistic communication framework in presurgical assessment.

If surgery is the planned treatment and speech deficits are likely, it is a good idea to establish a reliable alternative method of communication that the patient can use during the immediate postsurgery period, such as writing, gesturing, mouthing words, or pointing to pictures on a communication board. **Appendix 12–2** is a checklist of discussion topics to be covered during a preoperative or immediate postoperative counseling session.

Postsurgical Intervention

The opportunity for pretreatment intervention is not always possible. The immediate posttreatment follow-up needs to begin with the information that would have been presented during the pretreatment sessions. Even if pretreatment intervention occurred, a review of information about the effects of the surgery on speech and swallowing should provide the patient with a basis for treatment. Anatomic and physiologic changes that have altered communication and swallowing should not be skimmed over because the patient's understanding of these changes assists with further explanations about various treatment approaches. For patients who have had surgery and an uncomplicated immediate postsurgical course, speech and swallowing rehabilitation can begin within a 2-week period following the surgery. The surgeon should indicate that surgical sutures can withstand movement before aggressive therapy begins. Recovery complications postpone direct rehabilitation efforts, but this may be an optimal time to provide the patient and family members with necessary information and support. Immediate postsurgical speech and swallowing assessment provides a measure of the amount of impairment, which gives an indication of the length of treatment. Speech may not be a functional communication mode, and assistive or alternative methods of communication must be practiced.

The immediate postsurgical period can be one of emotional upheaval because of diminished ability to communicate. In addition, patients have to deal with the physical and functional alterations as a result of the surgery. The emotional status of the patient can interfere with rehabilitation attempts. For example, total laryngectomy patients having difficulty accepting their loss of voice may be quite unmotivated during initial training of an electrolarynx. It is sometimes beneficial for patients to meet with a person who has had a similar type of surgery. Visitation should be arranged at the patient's request, however, because the amount of benefit is a function of readiness for rehabilitation. The immediate postsurgical treatment period should be the time when the patient is presented with the specific plan for speech and swallowing intervention.

Outpatient Speech–Language Pathology Services

The extended postsurgical treatment is the time when the "work" of rehabilitation gets done and the plan is put into action. Certainly patients requiring prosthetic devices, alaryngeal speech training, or specialized swallowing strategies will have extended rehabilitation courses. Patients who have been discharged from the hospital and who have returned to their typical living environment begin to experience the limitations in daily functioning that resulted from the surgery, including limitations in speaking and swallowing. The extended postsurgical period focuses on restoration of communication and swallowing to a degree that matches as closely as possible premorbid abilities. Motivation may wax and wane. In general, as healing proceeds and the patient begins to regain a level of lost function, motivation improves.

✦ Management of Speech Following Head and Neck Cancer Treatment

Radiation therapy and surgery are the most common treatments for head and neck cancer. These treatments are used separately, in combination, and with other forms of treatment. Radiation therapy and surgery for head and neck cancers result in relatively predictable patterns of functional deficits in speech and swallowing that can range from mild and transient to severe and chronic. These deficits are caused by tissue reactions and alterations in anatomic structures. Speech–language pathologists should have a clear understanding of likely problems in speech and swallowing following head and neck cancer treatment so that they can provide specific management techniques that restore normal function or retain functional levels as close to normal as possible. It is primarily the surgery patient who requires the most extensive speech and swallowing treatment. Resections of the tongue, mandible, palate, larynx, and pharynx result in relatively predictable speech and swallowing changes, which are the focus of this discussion.

Speech Changes and Their Management

Normal speech requires sensory and motor integration of respiration, phonation, articulation, and resonation. Treatment for head and neck tumors can alter one or more of these speech systems depending on the location and size of the tumor, the planned treatments, and the patient's ability to compensate for any treatment alterations. In general, smaller tumors require less ablative treatment and result in more preserved speech function, whereas larger tumors exact a higher functional cost. Unilateral tumors are generally not as limiting as bilateral disease. Some general predictions about alterations in speech can be given to patients prior to treatment, based on knowledge of tumor site, tumor size, and planned treatment, although patients' specific problems vary depending on their adaptability following treatment. Small tumors treated with radiation therapy alone or combined radiation therapy and surgery do not typically produce speech alterations. There are potential side effects associated with radiation therapy to the oral and oropharyngeal cavities, such as xerostomia (mucosal dryness), oral and pharyngeal mucosa inflammation, soft tissue and bone pain, and thicker consistency of saliva. These side effects usually do not interfere with speech production as much as swallowing, as will be discussed later in this chapter. Large tumors usually require extensive surgical resection, which will likely result in some degree of compromised speech.

Glossectomy

Speech deficits may occur following a glossectomy. This procedure removes part or all of the tongue. An appreciation of the tongue's function in normal articulation assists in understanding the compromising effects that glossectomy can have on speech. Many consonants and all vowel differentiations in English require execution of precise and rapidly coordinated movements and shape alterations by the tongue (Casper & Colton, 1993). The severity of the speech impairment is usually commensurate with the extent of tongue resection, the degree of limitation in tongue mobility, and the patient's ability to compensate by using intact remaining oral structures. For example, vowel differentiation in total glossectomy patients has been accomplished by widening and narrowing the pharynx (Weber, Ohlms, Bowman, Jacob, & Goepfert, 1991). Partial glossectomy patients have shown improvement in the acoustic signals for vowel distinctions by using tongue protrusion and increased jaw height (Hamlet, Patterson, & Fleming, 1992). Compensatory positions of the lips and jaw may become the targets of speech therapy following tongue surgery. Slower speaking rates, exaggerated articulatory movements, and sound approximations assist the glossectomy patient with clearer speech. Range of motion and strength exercises are also part of speech rehabilitation.

Although the tongue is the primary structure in the oral and oropharyngeal cavities on which speech intelligibility and naturalness depend, it is important to remember that other structures also contribute to these aspects. Tumors that require surgical alteration of these structures may have deleterious effects on speech. For example, resonance may be disturbed by palatectomy or pharyngectomy.

Application of Prosthetics

Maxillofacial prosthetics are used for anatomic, functional, or cosmetic restoration for acquired surgical defects in head and neck cancer patient (Schaff, 1984). Intraoral prostheses restore resected portions of the oral cavity. An obturator is an intraoral prosthesis that closes an opening. For example, palatal obturators may be helpful for patients who have had a maxillectomy. An extended denture may return speech to normal for patients who have had soft palate or pharyngeal surgery with subsequent impairment of velopharyngeal closure. Glossectomy patients can benefit from a maxillary prosthesis that lowers the hard palate and facilitates improved function of a tongue with restricted movement. Because intraoral prostheses depend on the teeth or a stable denture, it is important for patients to maintain optimal oral and dental care throughout the period of medical treatment.

Rehabilitation for Laryngeal Cancer

Treatments for laryngeal tumors interfere with phonation. Small laryngeal tumors may be treated with radiation therapy alone, or a combination of radiation therapy and surgery. Radiation therapy as the sole treatment for laryngeal cancer preserves laryngeal structures, but it can irritate, dry, and inflame vocal fold mucosa and lead to a period of increased hoarseness. This, in turn, may set up hyperfunctional voice production as a compensatory reaction in a patient. Voice therapy may benefit such a patient. The speech–language pathologist provides a behavioral modification program aimed at improving voice hygiene, and an exercise program aimed at reduction of adductory forces on the vocal folds, in an attempt to prevent worsening dysphonia and optimize voice quality during and following radiation therapy.

Large laryngeal tumors usually require removal of part or all of the larynx. Conservative procedures include hemilaryngectomy and supraglottic laryngectomy. Total laryngectomy is performed when laryngeal tumors are large enough to preclude safe surgical margins with more conservative approaches. A standard hemilaryngectomy implies a resection in the superior-inferior, or vertical, plane (Doyle, 1994). For this reason, it is also known as a vertical partial laryngectomy. A hemilaryngectomy leaves one side of the larynx intact and some tissue bulk on the operated side. Therefore, phonation is possible, although the voice is dysphonic. A standard supraglottic laryngectomy is a horizontal resection above the level of the true vocal folds. Voice tends to be good because both vocal folds are preserved, but swallowing is often severely compromised because this procedure removes the sphincteric protection of the false vocal folds and the epiglottis with the aryepiglottic folds (Logemann, 1983).

Total laryngectomy removes the entire larynx. The sound source for speech is no longer coupled to respiratory function from below or articulatory and resonatory function from above. Total laryngectomy results in sudden and complete loss of voice. Patients may incorrectly assume that whispering is still possible after total laryngectomy, and the disconnection of respiratory airflow and speech articulators needs to be explained to the patient when treatment options are discussed. In addition, information about methods of alaryngeal speech must be presented in an unbiased fashion. A dependable method of communication for the period immediately following surgery needs to be planned, such as writing, gestures, or picture boards. Ideally, all these concerns about communication should be brought up preoperatively so that the patients have an awareness of expected functional losses and a means of coping with them, albeit rudimentary. The types of questions patients ask about treatment-related changes in communication may indicate their level of responsiveness to

rehabilitation efforts, and can be used by the speech–language pathologist to gauge the flow of information.

Postoperative speech rehabilitation for the total laryngectomy patient usually begins a few days following the surgery, while the patent is still in the hospital. Clear and concise information about the anatomic and physiologic changes that resulted from the surgery and their effects on communication should be provided. There are published sources that contain essential information and helpful illustrations for new laryngectomy patients, such as Keith and Thomas (1996). This source and others can be handy references for laryngectomy patient to have as reinforcement of the information provided directly by the speech–language pathologist throughout the course of rehabilitation.

Alaryngeal Speech

Alaryngeal speech options are the primary focus of rehabilitation for the total laryngectomy patient. The three most common alaryngeal speech methods are the artificial larynx (or electrolarynx), esophageal speech, and tracheoesophageal speech. It is ultimately the patient who must make the decision as to which method or methods to use. Each method has advantages and disadvantages that prospective users and their listeners need to consider. The speech–language pathologist should present each method of alaryngeal speech in an unbiased fashion, recognizing that the best method of speech restoration for one patient may poorly suit another.

Artificial Larynges

There are many different types of artificial larynges, but each has as its primary action the deliverance of sound (usually a buzzing tone) to the oral cavity that can then be shaped into speech by the articulators. Speech–language pathologists should be familiar with these instruments and be able to provide demonstration of their use. These instruments may be grouped into four categories based on the manner of sound generation and the location on the body for sound conduction: electronic neck-type, electronic mouth-type, electronic interdental type, and pneumatic type (Salmon, 1994). The electronic neck-type and electronic mouth-type artificial larynxes are the most common of these devices. The electronic neck-type artificial larynx has battery-produced sound that is conducted to the oral cavity by way of the neck tissue against which the head of the device is placed. Neck tissue should be supple and local swelling should be minimal for optimal sound conduction, making the electronic neck-type artificial larynx less functional during the immediate postoperative period. The electronic mouth-type artificial larynx conducts battery produced sound to the oral cavity by way of a mouth tube. This tube remains in the oral cavity as speech is articulated. It is preferred during the immediate postoperative period, when neck-type devices cannot be used. The electronic interdental-type artificial larynx is designed to become a part of an upper denture. The battery-produced sound is activated by a hand-held control. This type of artificial larynx requires coordinated efforts from the patient's physician, speech–language pathologist, and dentist. Pneumatic devices produce sound by using air from a patient's stoma to vibrate an external rubber membrane. The sound is carried to the oral cavity by a mouth tube, which remains in place while speech is articulated. Pneumatic

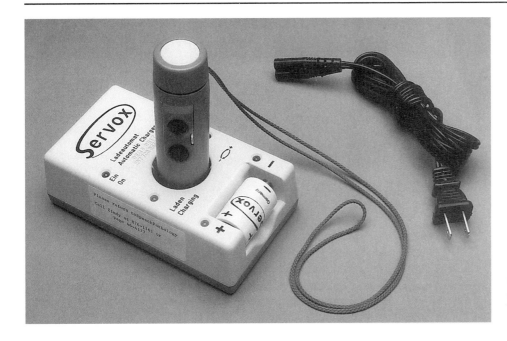

Figure 12–4 A Servox electrolarnyx, battery, and battery recharger. (Courtesy of Siemens Hearing Instruments, Inc., Prospect Heights, IL.)

devices are not as common as electronic devices. The various types of artificial larynges are pictured and described by Salmon (1994). An electrolarynx, battery, and battery charger are shown in **Fig. 12–4**.

Training in the use of an artificial larynx is part of the comprehensive speech rehabilitation program for total laryngectomy patients. Treatment goals often include care of the device, location of body placement for optimal sound conduction, timing of sound activation with speech, reduced speaking rate, and slightly exaggerated articulatory movements. Because the artificial larynx produces continuous sound at the push of a button, and the sound is maintained throughout the entire spoken utterance, strategies for normal phrasing and dealing with the inability to produce voice/voiceless contrasts are helpful. Advanced artificial larynx users can learn volume and pitch alterations to more closely approximate the linguistic components of normal speech, although this aspect of communication remains severely compromised. A patient may use an artificial larynx as a primary or secondary method for communication after comparing its advantages and disadvantages with the other alaryngeal methods of communication. Demonstration by a proficient artificial larynx speaker may assist the new laryngectomy patient with the decision regarding alaryngeal speech options.

Esophageal Speech

Esophageal speech is the second method of alaryngeal communication. There are two kinds of esophageal speech, inhalation and injection, both of which are based on esophageal insufflation. Air is either inhaled (inhalation) or injected (injection) into the hypopharynx. This air is then quickly expelled through a narrow sphincter of muscle fibers at the juncture of the hypopharynx and the esophagus [the pharyngoesophageal (PE) segment], which vibrates in response to the airflow and creates sound. Thus, sound is once again powered by an air supply that vibrates an internal body structure. However, the air supply that generates sound in esophageal speech comes

from air trapped within the oral and oropharyngeal cavities rather than the lungs, resulting in reduced air volumes and the need to frequently insufflate the PE segment for continuous speech. This reduced power source and the need to frequently replenish air results in salient perceptual features that distinguish esophageal speech from the other forms of alaryngeal speech (Robbins, 1984; Robbins, Fisher, Blom, & Singer, 1984). Esophageal speech using the injection method requires considerable training, and not every laryngectomy patient who tries esophageal speech is successful at it. However, some patients spontaneously develop esophageal speech using the inhalation mode without any training or effort (thereby attesting to the integrity of the PE segment for vibration) and may choose this method as their primary means of communication.

Major goals for communication rehabilitation with esophageal speech include optimal air intake methods, sound shaping, avoidance of stoma and air injection noise, and appropriate phrase lengths. It might be beneficial for a new laryngectomy patient who is considering esophageal speech to observe and listen to a proficient esophageal speaker.

Tracheoesophageal Speech

Tracheoesophageal speech is the third alaryngeal speech option. This option requires that a fistula be surgically created in the common wall of the posterior trachea and the anterior esophagus. A voice prosthesis is housed in this fistula, with its proximal end in the stoma and its distal end in the esophageal lumen. For voice restoration, pulmonary air ready for exhalation from the stoma is redirected through the voice prosthesis by stoma occlusion. The exhaled column of air travels through the voice prosthesis, enters the esophagus, and travels superiorly to vibrate the PE segment and create sound. The tracheoesophageal (TE) puncture procedure and voice prosthesis were introduced by Singer and Blom (1980). There have been modifications in voice prostheses since then, but the original concept of sound generation by rerouting pulmonary air through a valved voice prosthesis has remained the same. The idea of a

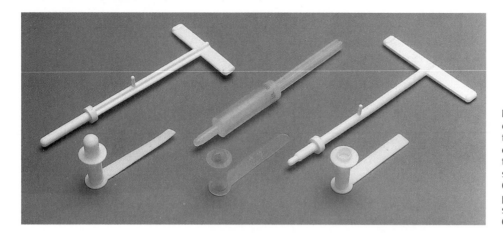

Figure 12–5 Examples of three tracheoesophageal voice prostheses. On the left is a Blom-Singer duckbill type of voice prosthesis with its inserter. In the center is a Bivona ultra-low pressure voice prosthesis with its inserter. On the right is a Blom-Singer low-pressure voice prosthesis with its inserter. (Courtesy of Blom-Singer, Carpinteria, CA.)

one-way valved voice prosthesis is important because the valve allows air to enter the esophagus but prohibits secretions and food in the esophagus from entering the trachea. Occlusion of the stoma is necessary to divert pulmonary air through the voice prosthesis. Finger closure is one method of stoma occlusion. Another method involves the use of an adjustable tracheostoma valve (Blom, Singer, & Hamaker, 1982). This valve is secured over the stoma and closes with exhalation for speech, eliminating the use of a hand to speak. Doyle (1994) has described TE speech procedures and provided photographs of various types of voice prostheses. **Figure 12–5** shows three types of TE voice prostheses. **Figures 12–6** and **12–7** show an indwelling type of voice prosthesis. The indwelling types remain in situ for long periods (6 to 12 months) and are inserted by a trained professional, whereas the others rely on regular (daily/weekly) self-maintenance and removal. Some patients use a heat and moisture exchanger (HME) system to improve secretion management (**Fig. 12–7**). The decision as to whether or not to opt for an in-dwelling type and which product to choose will be influenced by several variables such as cost, ability of patient or caregiver to manage and change the prosthesis, patient preference, and surgery-related factors (Delsupehe, Zink, Leiagere & Delaere, 1998).

Although TE speech is not the preferred alaryngeal speech option for every laryngectomy patient, it has become popular and widely used. Many patients undergo a TE puncture at the time of the total laryngectomy (a primary TE puncture) but it may be done as a separate procedure after the total laryngectomy (secondary TE puncture). There is controversy surrounding the timing of the TE puncture, in part because individual patient factors that are likely to influence success with either method have not been identified (Doyle, 1994).

Patient candidacy should be assessed by the speech–language pathologist, preferably before any decisions regarding alaryngeal speech restoration have been solidified. Candidacy criteria include patient motivation, functional visual acuity, functional manual dexterity, adequate pulmonary support for speech, mental stability, stoma integrity, and the ability to care for and use the voice prosthesis (Andrews, Mickel, Monahan, Hanson, & Ward, 1987). For the secondary TE puncture procedure, air insufflation of the esophagus is done by the speech–language pathologist prior to the puncture procedure to evaluate the vibratory capabilities of the PE segment. With some patients, results of esophageal air insufflation indicate that PE segment spasm, hypertonicity, or hypotonicity is interfering with sound production. Although this does not necessarily preclude a patient from acquiring TE speech, it indicates that further medical procedures or behavioral modifications aimed at optimizing the vibratory capabilities of the PE segment should be considered. For example,

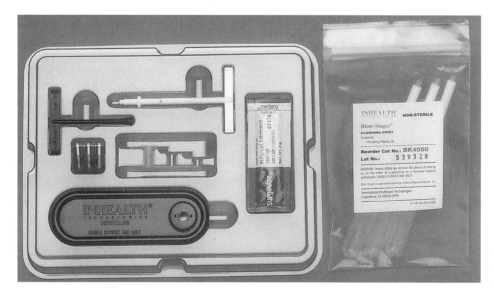

Figure 12–6 A Blom-Singer indwelling voice prosthesis kit with pipettes for in situ cleaning. (Courtesy of Blom-Singer, Carpinteria, CA.)

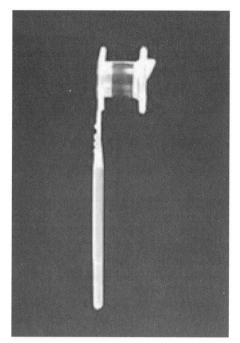

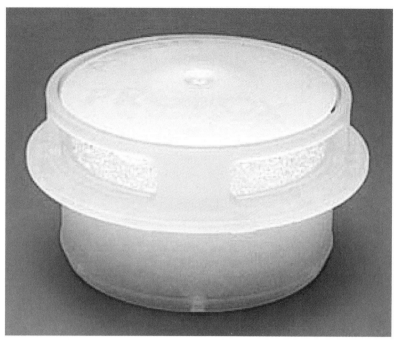

A

B

Figure 12–7 (A) A Provox 2 indwelling prosthesis. **(B)** Heat and moisture exchanger (HME). (Courtesy of ATOS Medical, Milwaukee, WI.)

botulinum toxin injection has recently been used for relaxation of the PE segment.

As with the other methods of alaryngeal speech restoration, the general rehabilitation goal for communication with TE speech is the most natural and intelligible speech possible. More specific goals include prosthesis fitting, insertion, removal, and care procedures, coordination of stoma occlusion, speech onset and sound generation, appropriate effort, optimal loudness, and phrasing. Patients considering the TE puncture and voice prosthesis would benefit from a visit by a TE speaker. In fact, it is a good idea to ask new laryngectomy patients if they would like a laryngectomy visitor to assist them in their rehabilitation efforts at any point along the course of recovery. It should be the patient's choice whether or not to meet with a laryngectomy visitor. Patients who participate in their medical care through decision making may be more likely to adapt to functional limitations over time.

Candidacy for a TE puncture may be influenced by the nature of the surgical procedure with laryngectomy, particularly whether free flaps have been used. Although free flaps can be used for vibratory segment reconstruction with some success, the patency of the segment is dependent on the type and nature of the reconstruction and can be evaluated with the air insufflation test (Haughey, Fredrickson, Sessions, & Fuller, 1995). Speech–language pathologists may assist patients in choosing a method or methods of alaryngeal speech by describing the features that differentiate each of the three methods. In addition, it may be beneficial for patients to speak with and observe alaryngeal speakers who are effective communicators.

Because of the compact nature of head and neck structures, there are times when multiple structures are involved in the excision of the tumor, each with its own effect on postsurgical speech abilities. Depending on the specific site of lesion, patients may have surgical excision of both the tongue and the larynx. Serious speech deficits result in patients who have total glossectomy with total laryngectomy. The loss of the tongue interferes with articulation and the loss of the larynx interferes with phonation. These patients require lengthy and creative rehabilitative efforts for resumption of some degree of functional communication, sometimes involving augmentative or assistive communication devices.

Respiratory Changes Requiring Speech Intervention

Compromised respiration may result from a tumor in any of the internal cavities of the head and neck. Breathing difficulty may gradually worsen as the tumor grows, eventually becoming an emergency situation that could require a tracheostomy. In addition, respiration may be compromised due to lung disease from a history of smoking, which is common in head and neck cancer patients. Swelling following surgical excision of a tumor in the head and neck may necessitate the need for a tracheostomy. Respiratory compromise is a medical management problem. Once an airway has been secured, respiratory support for speech can be assessed and addressed. Succinct explanations of the normal process of respiration and the specific changes in this process resulting from the tumor and its treatment should be given to tracheostomized patients. Patients with temporary tracheostomies may be assessed for appropriateness of a speaking valve to restore voice, and then trained in its use. Certainly patients who have had permanent rerouting of oral and nasal breathing to stoma breathing with total laryngectomies have to make pronounced speech adaptations, as was previously discussed. For these patients, exhaled air from the stoma can no longer be made audible because the vocal folds have been removed, and the air cannot be shaped by articulators because it bypasses them, unless a TE puncture is made to restore airflow through the oral cavity. Speech–language pathologists should plan to provide laryngectomy patients with information about the respiratory changes that result from the rerouted airway, and the effects that these changes have on speech. Many of these patients would benefit from seeing diagrams, drawings, and three-dimensional models. A discussion of common postsurgical problems related to stoma breathing might make the adjustment easier for patients. One of the most important topics for discussion should be keeping the stoma area clear of potential obstruction. Ways to deal with the increased amount and viscosity of mucus should be suggested, including adequate daily water intake, humidification of environmental air, and air filtration with stoma covers. Mucus expectoration from the stoma instead of the mouth should be discussed. Reduced ability to hold the breath at the level of the larynx may interfere with lifting heavy objects and other activities that require stabilization of the thoracic cavity, and this needs to be addressed. Reduction in smell and taste because of rerouted airflow needs to be explained. Finally, the total laryngectomy patient needs to consider some means of identification as a stoma or neck breather, because standard first aid procedures for artificial respiration (i.e., mouth-to-mouth resuscitation) would have to be modified for these patients.

✦ Swallowing Changes after Head and Neck Cancer Treatment

Normal swallowing, like normal speech, is a well-integrated motor and sensory activity involving structures in the oral, pharyngeal, and laryngeal cavities, as well as the esophagus. In the oral cavity, the teeth, tongue, hard palate, and mandible are involved in preparation of the bolus; the tongue then collects and squeezes it posteriorly to the oropharynx. The swallow response is elicited in the oropharynx and involves closure of the velopharynx, superior and anterior movements of the hyoid bone and larynx, laryngeal closure, tongue base movement toward a bulging pharyngeal wall, peristaltic pharyngeal waves, and relaxation of the cricopharyngeal muscle (McConnel, Pauloski, Logemann, Rademaker, Colangelo, Shedd, Carroll, Lewin, & Johnson, 1995).

Swallowing dysfunction can occur prior to treatment of head and neck cancer as a consequence of tumor infiltration or obstruction, so evaluation of the swallow pretreatment is prudent. After radiation therapy or surgery for head and neck tumors, difficulties at any point in the dynamic swallowing process can occur, and may range in severity from negligible and transient to severe and chronic, depending on the residual effects of the treatment and the compensatory abilities of the patient.

Effects of Radiation

Radiation therapy to the oral cavity and neck may result in inflammation and dryness of oral and pharyngeal mucosa, thickening and reduction of saliva, mouth and throat pain, changes in taste, and loss of appetite (Groher, 1997). These side effects may produce dysphagia that worsens as the treatment progresses and may remain for a period of time or even develop months or years after treatment has been completed. Radiation therapy may be used before or after surgical resection for a head and neck tumor, producing combinations of swallowing problems related to both of the medical treatments that were used. Swallowing strategies that may benefit these patients include reduction of bolus size, modification of diet consistencies, multiple swallows for each bolus, and use of foods with strong flavors.

Effects of Surgery

Surgical resections for head and neck cancer result in predictable patterns of dysphagia related to the specific anatomic or neurologic insult produced by the resection (Blom, Singer, & Hamaker, 1982). Swallowing problems may occur following tracheostomy, glossectomy, mandibulectomy, palatal resection, pharyngectomy, and laryngectomy. A tracheostomy procedure results in dysphagia because of decreased laryngeal elevation, poorly coordinated laryngeal closure, desensitization of the reflexive cough, and pooled secretions. Cuff inflation should not be considered a protection against aspiration in patients with a tracheostomy. Oral and oropharyngeal resections cause an assortment of dysphagic symptoms, depending on the surgery site and the method of reconstruction. Restricted mobility of the lips, tongue, mandible, soft palate, and pharynx and the use of closure techniques that fill in the surgical defect with nonfunctional tissue can interfere with swallowing in the oral preparatory, oral, and pharyngeal phases of swallowing. There may be interference with chewing, diminished bolus propulsion, reduced tongue pressure, premature spillage, slow oral transit, oral cavity residue, delayed elicitation of involuntary swallowing responses, reduced pharyngeal peristalsis, pharyngeal residue, and aspiration. Subtotal laryngeal resections remove structures that act as sphincteric protection during swallowing. For example, supraglottic laryngectomy removes the false vocal folds, epiglottis, and aryepiglottic folds, which leaves only the true vocal folds to protect the airway. Dysphagia after total laryngectomy may be related to alterations in the shape and function of the pharynx, benign pharyngeal or esophageal stricture, cricopharyngeal dysfunction, and effects of radiation therapy. Of course, tumor recurrence is a suspicion when there is a change in swallowing function.

The use of free flaps in the surgical repair of defects can have major implications for swallowing function, commonly affecting either the oral or pharyngeal phases of the swallow. Confounding factors such as bulkiness, tethering of structures, disruptions to mobility, and the development of postoperative fistulas can all complicate swallowing function and recovery (Galati & Johnson, 1999). Swallowing outcomes for these patients may also be poor because of the extent of the tumor necessitating reconstruction. The swallowing outcomes from primary closure versus reconstruction using free flaps are controversial (Logemann, 1990). An understanding of the surgical procedure and the nature of reconstruction is crucial to the prediction and interpretation of the resulting swallow function and to intervention planning. More recent attention to the improvement of function as well as structure in surgical reconstruction has achieved improved long-term swallowing outcomes.

Evaluation of Swallowing

Swallowing assessment for head and neck cancer patients usually includes a clinical examination, a radiologic study, and often a fiberoptic endoscopic evaluation of swallowing (FEES). The results of assessment should pinpoint the swallowing problems, determine the effects of compensatory or facilitating strategies, and guide treatment decisions. Some common swallowing strategies used with head and neck cancer patients are positional changes, consistency modifications, bolus size adjustments, bolus placement adjustments, effortful swallows, and double swallows (Kronenberger & Meyers, 1994; Logemann, 1990). Oral prostheses and specially designed feeding utensils may improve swallowing function for these patients, depending on the specific cause for the dysphagia. Swallowing is one of those routine physiologic functions that patients may expect to resume with minimal or no effort. This is not always the case with head and neck cancer patients. Patients need to be aware that restoration of optimal swallowing function usually requires diligent and extensive effort on their part and aggressive swallowing therapy on the part of the speech–language pathologist.

✦ Case Studies

Case One

A 56-year-old man who smoked one pack of cigarettes daily and drank alcohol a few times each week for 30 years presented with a 4-month history of hoarseness at his initial otolaryngologic exam. Results of an indirect laryngeal exam showed a right vocal fold mass resembling carcinoma that extended nearly the length of the fold but did not cross at the anterior commissure. This fold was mobile. The mass was classified as $T_1 N_0 M_0$ and stage I. Direct microlaryngoscopy and biopsy of the mass were done, and results of the pathology report showed squamous cell carcinoma. Radiation therapy was the recommended treatment. The patient had an initial voice evaluation prior to having radiation therapy. His voice was moderately dysphonic at that time and there were no swallowing complaints. Laryngeal videostroboscopy showed severely reduced mucosal wave and amplitude of the right fold. Voice hygiene instructions were given to the patient in an attempt to minimize voice problems during radiation therapy. These instructions included cessation of smoking, reduction of throat clearing, increased daily water consumption, and habitual use of a quiet voice with environmental adjustments to reduce the need for louder voice. Vocal quality was judged as improved when reevaluated 3 weeks after completion of radiation therapy. The patient was seen regularly by his otolaryngologist for the next few months. Laryngeal exams were negative during this postradiation period, but the vocal fold mucosa did not return to normal. Eight months after radiation therapy there was recurrence on the right vocal fold, and extension of the tumor to the anterior portion of the left vocal fold was found. An extended hemilaryngectomy that included all of the right side of the larynx and a significant portion of the left side of the larynx was done. The hyoid bone, arytenoids, and most of the epiglottis were preserved. The epiglottis was pulled inferiorly and used to fill in the anterior portion of the thyroid cartilage that was surgically removed. Tissue from the right false vocal fold was used in place of the excised right true vocal fold. A tracheostomy was done at the time of the surgery to prevent airway compromise related to swelling.

The patient was seen by the speech pathologist in the hospital 3 days following the surgery. An oral peripheral examination was done, but it was limited because surgical sutures could not be disturbed. Results of the oral peripheral examination showed reduced frequency of spontaneous swallow, delayed volitional swallow, pooled secretions in the oral cavity, drooling, and gurgly vocal quality. The patient was discharged from the hospital with tracheostomy and nasogastric tubes in place. He was not eating by mouth at the time of discharge, but he was handling his secretions and he had a productive cough. He had a videofluorographic study 2 weeks after surgery, which showed severe dysphagia with aspiration secondary to premature spillage from reduced size of valleculae and reduced constriction of reconstructed tissue at the level of the glottis. Intensive swallowing therapy was recommended. The focus of this therapy was the supraglottic swallow technique. Flexible fiberoptic endoscopy was used during therapy sessions to monitor swallowing proficiency and provide visual feedback to the patient about effortful swallow attempts. During that time, the tracheostomy tube was removed.

A repeat videofluorographic study was done after 4 weeks of swallowing therapy, showing improved constriction of the glottis. Swallow was safe for thick and solid consistencies with the supraglottic swallowing technique. Other swallowing recommendations included an upright feeding position, small bolus size, and multiple daily feedings. The nasogastric tube was removed once nutrition was maintained with oral intake. Swallowing was reassessed during the next month in the speech pathology clinic using flexible fiberoptic endoscopy. The patient slowly started to gain weight. He reported that he had tried drinking thin liquids at home. Thin liquids were then introduced in the clinic and swallowed without clinical signs of aspiration. The patient was instructed to watch for and report any symptoms of pulmonary problems during the course of swallowing rehabilitation, but these did not occur. Swallowing rehabilitation for this extended hemilaryngectomy patient consisted of two videofluorographic studies, two bedside swallowing assessments during his hospitalization period, and 2 months of swallowing therapy as an outpatient with flexible fiberoptic endoscopy to monitor progress.

Case Two

A 49-year-old woman had undergone a total laryngectomy, bilateral neck dissection, and primary tracheoesophageal puncture. Radiation therapy was planned following surgery. The speech–language pathology service was consulted postoperatively. The patient was seen 4 days after her surgery. She used writing as her primary method of communication during the immediate postoperative period. The speech–language pathologist discussed with the patient the speech changes that resulted from anatomic and physiologic changes related to the surgery. A brief explanation of voice rehabilitation methods was given. An electrolarynx was demonstrated by the clinician and tried by the patient. Sound conduction was poor with neck placement because of neck tissue swelling. Speech with cheek placement was fair. An oral adaptor was tried, but this did not improve speech intelligibility. During her stay in the hospital, the patient used a loaner electrolarynx and had daily speech therapy. Training with this device continued on an outpatient basis, after the patient's hospital discharge.

She was able to use neck placement 3 weeks after her surgery. She had a 6-week course of postoperative radiation therapy, which interfered with neck placement of the electrolarynx and compromised speech intelligibility. During that time, she developed skin irritation around her stoma and neck swelling. A stent was kept in her stoma to prevent closure during radiation therapy. These side effects of radiation therapy interfered with swallowing and fitting of a voice prosthesis. We discussed bolus consistency modifications for her to use during the remaining portion of her radiation treatment. We postponed voice prosthesis fitting until completion of radiation therapy.

Two weeks after she completed radiation therapy, the TE puncture was sized and a voice prosthesis was inserted. Voice quality was strained and there were breaks in sound production. Radiographic study of TE voice production showed hypertonicity of the upper esophageal segment, characterized by an anterior bulge of tissue at the level of the cricopharyngeal segment during voicing attempts. Treatment options included doing nothing, cricopharyngeal myotomy, or injection of botulinum toxin to the hypertonic muscles. The patient did not want another surgical procedure, so she decided to have the injection. Alaryngeal voice reassessment 1 week after the injection showed improvement in voice and speech intelligibility without breaks in sound. In addition, tightness during swallowing lessened. The patient reported that she was able to swallow solids with less effort. Voice therapy then focused on optimizing speech by coordinating breath support with finger occlusion and adjusting lung air pressures for specific speaking situations. As she mastered TE speech, the patient became interested in an indwelling type of voice prosthesis. She had no previous trouble with yeast colonization on her voice prosthesis, and she was judged to be a good candidate for an indwelling prosthesis, which was tried with success. She then became interested in trying a tracheostoma valve for hands-free speech. Her speech rehabilitation resulted in good TE voice produced without the use of her hands, which allowed her to return to communication functioning that she judged to be very similar to her premorbid abilities.

✦ Conclusion

This chapter has focused on a variety of issues surrounding the head and neck cancer patient. Speech–language pathologists who work in a medical setting need a sound understanding of head and neck anatomy and physiology and a set of specialized skills for service provision to this group of patients. Speech and swallowing problems are common and varied. Head and neck cancer patients have optimal return of speech and swallowing function if they are provided with an intervention plan that is guided by knowledge of the changes in normal anatomy and physiology that can occur as a result of the disease and its treatment. Therapy that aims to address the impairment aspects of head and neck cancer and associated treatment but to also minimize the associated distress, disability and handicap aspects will ensure optimal patient satisfaction and communication success.

Study Questions

1. Why is it important to understand normal head and neck anatomy to best serve head and neck cancer patients?

2. What are the major internal compartments of the head and neck and the important structures for speech and swallowing found in each?

3. What are the symptoms of head and neck cancer?

4. What are the diagnostic procedures frequently used for head and neck cancer?

5. What is the TNM tumor classification system?

6. How does a multidisciplinary tumor board assist in patient care?

7. What are some of the considerations in pretreatment, immediate posttreatment, and extended posttreatment intervention periods?

8. What speech changes may be anticipated after surgery of the head and neck?

9. What rehabilitative measures are used to restore speech in head and neck cancer patients?

10. What swallowing changes may be anticipated after surgery of the head and neck?

11. What rehabilitative measures are used to restore swallowing in head and neck cancer patients?

References

Alessi, D.M., Hutcherson, R.W., & Mickel, R.A. (1989). Production of Lymphokine-Activated Lymphocytes: Lysis of Human Head and Neck Squamous Cell Carcinoma Cell Lines. *Archives of Otolaryngology Head and Neck Surgery, 115,* 725–730

American Cancer Society. (2002). *Cancer Facts and Figures.* Atlanta: American Cancer Society

Amrein, P. (1991). Current Chemotherapy of Head and Neck Cancer. *Journal of Oral Maxillofacial Surgery, 49,* 864–870

Andrews, J.C., Mickel, M.D., Monahan, G.P., Hanson, D.G., Ward, P.H. (1987). Major Complications Following Tracheoesophageal Puncture for Voice Rehabilitation. Laryngoscope, *97,* 562–567

Anthony, C.P., & Kolthoff, N.J. (1975). *Textbook of Anatomy and Physiology,* 9th ed. St. Louis: C.V. Mosby

Barnes, E.L. (1989). Pathology of the Head and Neck: General Considerations. In: E.M. Myers & J.Y. Suen (Eds.), *Cancer of the Head and Neck,* 2nd ed. (pp. 75–99). New York: Churchill Livingstone

Bastian, R.W., Collins, S.L., Kaniff, T., & Matz, G.J. (1989). Indirect Video Laryngoscopy Versus Direct Endoscopy for Larynx and Pharynx Cancer Staging: Toward Elimination of Preliminary Direct Laryngoscopy. *Annals of Otology, Rhinology, Laryngology, 98,* 693–698

Bauer, W.C. (1974). Concomitant Carcinoma in Situ and Invasive Carcinoma of the Larynx. *Canadian Journal of Otolaryngology, 3,* 533–542

Benninger, M.S. (1992a). Medical Liaisons for Continuity of Head and Neck Cancer Care. *Head and Neck, 14,* 28–32

Benninger, M.S. (1992b). Presentation and Evaluation of Patients with Epidermoid Head and Neck Cancers. *Henry Ford Hospital Medical Journal, 40,* 144–148

Benninger, M.S., Enrique, R.R., & Nichols, R.D. (1993). Symptom-Directed Selective Endoscopy for Evaluation of Head and Neck Cancer. *Head Neck, 15,* 532–536

Benninger, M., Gillen, J., Thieme, P., Jacobson, B., & Dragovich, J. (1994). Factors Associated with Recurrence and Voice Quality Following Radiation Therapy for T1 and T2 Glottic Carcinomas. *Laryngoscope, 104,* 294–298

Benninger, M.S., Shariff, A., & Blazoff, K. (2001). Symptom Directed Selective Endoscopy: Long Term Efficacy. *Archives of Otolaryngology Head and Neck Surgery, 127,* 770–773

Blom, E.D., Singer M., & Hamaker, R.C. (1982). Tracheostoma Valve for Postlaryngectomy Voice Rehabilitation. *Annals of Otology, Rhinology, and Laryngology, 91,* 576–578

Bush, S.E., & Bagshaw, M.A. (1982). Carcinoma of the Paranasal Sinuses. *Cancer, 50,* 154–158

Cachin, Y. (1989). Perspectives on Cancer of the Head and Neck. In: E.M. Myers & J.Y. Suen (Eds.), *Cancer of the Head and Neck,* 2nd ed. (pp. 1–16). New York: Churchill Livingstone

Casper, J.K., & Colton, R.H. (1993) *Clinical Manual for Laryngectomy and Head and Neck Cancer Rehabilitation.* San Diego: Singular

Citardi, M.J., Gracco, C.L., & Sasaki, C.T. (1995). The Anatomy of the Human Larynx. In: J.S. Rubin, R.T. Sataloff, G.S. Korovin, & W.J. Gould (Eds.), *Diagnosis and Treatment of Voice Disorders* (pp. 55–69). New York: - Igaku-Shoin

Cooper, J.S., Fu, K., Marks, J., & Silverman, S. (1995). Late Effects of Radiation Therapy in the Head and Neck Region. *International Journal of Radiation Oncology, Biology, and Physiology, 3,* 1141–1164

Decker, J., & Goldstein, J.C. (1982). Risk Factors in Head and Neck Cancer. *New England Journal of Medicine, 306,* 1151–1155

Delsupehe, K., Zink, I., Leiagere, M., & Delaere, P. (1998). Prospective Randomized Comparative Study of Tracheoesophageal Voice Prosthesis: Blom-Singer vs Provox. *Laryngoscope, 108,* 1561–1565

Department of Veterans Affairs Laryngeal Cancer Study Group. (1991). Induction Chemotherapy Plus Radiation Compared with Surgery, Radiation in Patients with Advanced Laryngeal Cancer. *New England Journal of Medicine, 324,* 1685–1691

Doyle, P.C. (1994). *Foundations of Voice and Speech Rehabilitation Following Laryngeal Cancer.* San Diego: Singular

Enderby, P. (1983). *Frenchay Dysarthria Assessment.* Austin, TX: Pro-Ed

Galati, L.T., & Johnson, J.T. (1999). Surgery of the Oral Cavity, Oropharynx and Hypopharynx. In: R.L. Carrau & T. Murry (Eds.), *Comprehensive Management of Swallowing Disorders* (pp. 141–146). San Diego: Singular

Groher, M.E. (1997). Mechanical Disorders of Swallowing. In: M.E. Groher (Ed.), *Dysphagia Diagnosis and Management,* 3rd ed. (pp. 73–106). Newton, MA: Butterworth-Heinemann

Hamlet, S.L., Patterson, R.L., & Fleming, S.M. (1992). A Longitudinal Study of Vowel Production in Partial Glossectomy Patients. *Journal of Phonetics, 20,* 209–224

Haughey, B.H., Fredrickson, J.M., Sessions, D.G., & Fuller D. (1995). Vibratory Segment Function After Free Flap Reconstruction of the Pharyngoesophagus. *Laryngoscope, 105,* 487–490

Hirano, M., Hirade, Y., & Kawasaki, H. (1985). Vocal Function Following Carbon Dioxide Laser Surgery for Glottic Carcinoma. *Annals of Otology, Rhinology, and Laryngology, 94,* 232–235

Johns, M.E.,& Papel, I.D. (1987). Carcinoma of the Oral Cavity and Pharynx. In: K.J. Lee (Ed.), *Essential Otolaryngology,* 4th ed. (pp. 475–492). New York: Medical Examination

Jones, K.R., & Weissler, M.C. (1990). Blood Transfusion and Other Risk Factors for Recurrence of Cancer of the Head and Neck. *Archives of Otolaryngology Head and Neck Surgery, 116,* 304–309

Keith, R.L., & Thomas, J.E. (1996). *A Handbook for the Laryngectomee,* 4th ed. Austin, TX: Pro-Ed

Koufman, J.A., & Burke, A.J. (1996). The Causes and Pathogenesis of Laryngeal Cancer. *Visible Voice, 5,* 26–46

Kronenberger, M.B., & Meyers, A.D. (1994). Dysphagia Following Head and Neck Cancer Surgery. *Dysphagia, 9,* 236–244

Lee, K.J. (Ed.). (1987). *Essential Otolaryngology.* New York: Medical Examination

Lehman, J.J., Bless, D.M., & Brandenburg, J.H. (1988). An Objective Assessment of Voice Production After Radiation Therapy for Stage I Squamous Cell Carcinoma of the Glottis. *Otolaryngology Head and Neck Surgery, 98,* 121–129

Llewellyn-Thomas, H.A., Sutherland, H.J., Hogg, S.A., Ciampi, A., Harwood, A.R., Keane, J.J., Till, J.E., & Boyd, N.F. (1984). Linear Analogue Self-Assessment of Voice Quality in Laryngeal Cancer. *Journal of Chronic Disease, 37,* 917–924

Logemann, J.A. (1983). Swallowing Disorders After Treatment for Laryngeal Cancer. In: J.A. Logemann (Ed.), *Evaluation and Treatment of Swallowing Disorders* (pp. 187–209). Austin, TX: Pro-Ed

Logemann, J.A. (1990). Effects of Aging on the Swallowing Mechanism. *Otolaryngology Clinics of North America, 23,* 1045–1056

McConnel, F.M., Pauloski, B.R., Logemann, L.A., Rademaker, A.W., Colangelo, L., Shedd, D., Carroll, W. Lewin, J., & Johnson, J. (1998). Functional Results of Primary Closure Versus Flaps in Oropharyngeal Reconstruction: A Prospective Study of Speech and Swallowing. *Archives of Otolaryngology Head and Neck Surgery, 124,* 625–630

McGuirt, W.F., Blalock, D., Koufman, J.A., & Feehs, R.S. (1992). Voice Analysis of Patients with Endoscopically Treated Early Laryngeal Carcinoma. *Annals of Otology, Rhinology, and Laryngology, 101,* 142–146

McKinstry, A. & Perry, A. (2003). Evaluation of Speech in People with Head and Neck Cancer: A Pilot Study. *International Journal of Language and Communication Disorders, 38,* 31–46

Morgan, D.A.L., Robinson, H.F., Marsh, L., & Bradley, P.J. (1988). Vocal Quality 10 Years After Radiotherapy for Early Glottic Cancer. *Clinical Radiology, 39,* 295–296

Nichols, R.D., & Mickelson, S.A. (1991). Partial Laryngectomy After Irradiation Failure. *Annals of Otology, Rhinology, and Laryngology, 100,* 176–180

Pearlstein, R.P., Benninger, M.S., Worsham, M., et al. (1997). 18Q Loss of Heterozygosity Is a Predictor of Poor Survival in Patients with Stage III Head and Neck Cancer. *Online International Journal of Otolaryngology, 2,* 1–8

Pellitteri, P.K., Kennedy, T.L., Vrobec, D.P., Beiler, D., & Hellstrom, M. (1991). Radiotherapy. The Main-Stay in the Treatment of Early Glottic Carcinomas. *Archives of Otolaryngology Head and Neck Surgery, 117,* 297–301

Pfister, D.G., Harrison, L.B., Strong, E.W., & Bosl, G.J. (1992). Current Status of Larynx Preservation with Multimodality Therapy. *Oncology, 6,* 33–38

Richard, J., Sancho-Garnier, H., & Micheau, C. (1987). Prognostic Factors in Cervical Lymph Node Metastasis in Upper Respiratory and Digestive Tract Carcinomas: Study of 1,713 Cases During a 15-Year Period. *Laryngoscope, 97,* 97–101

Robbins, J. (1984). Acoustic Differentiation of Laryngeal, Esophageal, and Tracheoesophageal Speech. *Journal of Speech and Hearing Research, 27,* 577–585

Robbins, J., Fisher, H.B., Blom, E.D., & Singer, M.L. (1984). A Comparative Acoustic Study of Normal, Esophageal, and Tracheoesophageal Speech Production. *Journal of Speech and Hearing Disorders, 49,* 202–210

Robins, K.T., (Ed.). (2001). *Pocket Guide to Neck Dissection Classification and TNM Staging of Head and Neck Cancer.* Washington, DC: American Academy of Otolaryngology-Head and Neck Surgery

Salmon, S.J. (1994). Artificial Larynxes: Types and Modifications. In: R.L. Keith & F.L. Darley (Eds.), *Laryngectomy Rehabilitation,* 3rd ed. (pp. 155–178). Austin, TX: Pro-Ed

Schaff, N.G. (1984) Maxillofacial Prosthetics and the Head and Neck Cancer Patient. *CA: A Cancer Journal for Clinicians, 54,* 2682–2690

Shu, C.H., Shiau, C.Y., Chi, K.H., Yen, S.H., & Li, W.Y. (1999). Salvage Surgery for Recurrent Nasopharyngeal Carcinoma in Anterior Marginal Mass After Radiotherapy. *Otolaryngology Head and Neck Surgery, 121,* 622–626

Silverberg, E., & Lubera, J.A. (1988). Cancer Statistics, 1988. *CA: A Cancer Journal for Clinicians, 38,* 5–22

Singer, M.I., & Blom, E.D. (1980). An Endoscopic Technique for Restoration of Voice After Laryngectomy. *Annals of Otology, Rhinology, and Laryngology, 89,* 529–533

Sisson, G.A., Toriumi, D.M., & Atiyah, R.A. (1989). Paranasal Sinus Malignancy: A Comprehensive Update. *Laryngoscope, 99,* 143–150

Spector, G. (1987). Cancer of the Larynx, Ear, and Paranasal Sinuses. In: K.J. (Ed.), *Essential Otolaryngology* (pp. 493–514). New York: Medical Examination

Stoicheff, M.L. (1975). Voice Following Radiotherapy. *Laryngoscope, 85,* 608–618

Stoicheff, M.L., Ciampi, A., Passi, J.E., & Fredrickson, J.M. (1983). The Irradiated Larynx and Voice: A Perceptual Study. *Journal of Speech and Hearing Research, 26,* 482–485

Tucker, H.M. (1993). Malignant Neoplasms. In: H.M. Tucker (Ed.), *The Larynx,* 2nd ed. (pp. 287–323). New York: Thieme

Weber, R.S., Ohlms, L., Bowman, J., Jacob, R., & Goepfert, H.. (1991). Functional Results After Total or Near Total Glossectomy with Laryngeal Preservation. *Archives of Otolaryngology Head and Neck Surgery, 117,* 512–515

World Health Organization. (2000). *The International Classification of Disease Processes.* Geneva: WHO

Zemlin, W.R. (1988). *Speech and Hearing Science,* 3rd ed. Englewood Cliffs, NJ: Prentice-Hall

Appendix 12–1 Competencies for Speech–Language Pathologists Working with Head and Neck Cancer Patients

1. Thorough knowledge of normal head and neck anatomy and physiology
2. Thorough knowledge of changes in head and neck anatomy and physiology as a result of cancer treatment
3. Ability to predict likely changes in speech and swallowing following head and neck cancer treatment
4. Provide parsimonious explanation of anatomic and physiologic alterations that result from head and neck cancer surgeries to patients.
5. Participate in a multidisciplinary tumor board meeting.
6. Counsel the patient with regard to changes in speech and swallowing.
7. Provide explanation and demonstration of alaryngeal voice restoration methods.
8. Assess patient for use of oral prosthesis.
9. Assess candidacy of patient for tracheoesophageal speech.
10. Perform esophageal insufflation and interpret results.
11. Fit a tracheoesophageal voice prosthesis.
12. Explain and demonstrate procedures for tracheoesophageal voice prosthesis care and use.
13. Explain and demonstrate procedures for use of tracheostoma valve.
14. Provide patients and medical personnel with updated information on speech, swallowing, and voice restoration products.
15. Assist patient in establishing most efficient communication method based on each patient's individual communication needs.
16. Apply appropriate swallowing strategies based on clinical and radiologic findings.

Appendix 12–2 Laryngectomy Counseling Checklist

Name

Address

Telephone

Sex

Date of Birth

Age

Medical Record Number

Contact Person

Surgeon Surgery Date

Surgical Procedure(s)

Type of Insurance

Discuss structural changes in respiration, speech, and swallowing.

Discuss the following:

Taste	Cough	Dentures	Water sports
Smell	Sneezing	Hygiene	Tissue versus handkerchief
Sniff	Throat clearing	Sex	Bathing
Sleeping	Smoking	Laughing	Crying
Showering	Lifting	Drinking	Shampooing
Blowing	Emergency help	Yelling	Shaving
Nose blowing	First aid	Radiation	Defecation
Humidity	Atomizer	Numbness	Cold air
Work	Body odors	Neck size	Jewelry
Whistle	Sun bathing	Vocal intensity	Musical instruments
Cooling food	Stoma covers	Swallowing	

Discuss stoma and oral hygiene.

Discuss laryngeal speech methods.

Discuss laryngectomy visitor and information resources.

Section 4

Topics in Clinical Collaboration and Service Delivery

13

Psychogenic Communication Disorders

Greg Mahr, Wendy Bertges Yost, and Barbara H. Jacobson

◆ **Terminology**

◆ **Classification**

◆ **Epidemiology**

◆ **Psychiatric Comorbidity**

◆ **Assessment**

◆ **Treatment**

After a violent assault, a young man suddenly develops dysfluent speech. His speech superficially resembles stuttering, but he blocks on every word, and has no struggle behaviors and no past history of speech disturbance. A woman newly diagnosed with leukemia suddenly stops talking, despite the absence of any neurologic pathology. In such cases, although the presenting symptom is a disturbance in communication, the underlying pathology involves emotional and psychological issues. These disorders are psychogenic; they superficially resemble physical illnesses but are in fact caused or exacerbated by emotional or mental factors.

Psychogenic communication disorders are very important in the practice of speech pathology in the medical setting. Psychogenic speech and voice disorders accounted for 4.5% of all acquired communication disorders evaluated at the Mayo Clinic between 1987 and 1990 (Duffy, 1995). As in most psychogenic disorders, an appropriate diagnosis of a psychogenic communication disorder is often established only after multiple costly medical evaluations. Patients with psychogenic problems tend to see many doctors and seek aggressive medical workups. Almost half of speech pathologists do not feel comfortable treating patients with psychogenic speech and voice disorders (Elias, Raven, Butcher, and Littlejohns, 1989). Effective and efficient diagnosis and treatment of these disorders requires a team approach and multidisciplinary collaboration. Speech–language pathology, mental health, and medical and surgical disciplines working as a team can minimize unnecessary and repetitive evaluations and provide effective coordinated care.

This chapter describes the various psychogenic speech and voice disorders, explores issues of psychiatric comorbidity, and discusses assessment and treatment.

◆ Terminology

Psychogenic symptoms have been called "functional," "histrionic" or "hysterical," "nonorganic," and "psychosomatic." None of these terms is satisfactory, including "psychogenic." The term *functional* implies a spurious dichotomy between structure and function. The terms *hysterical* and *histrionic* carry historical connotations that are sexist and pejorative. The term *hysteria* originally referred to the alleged wandering of the uterus in the female body. Historically, women's symptoms have been dismissed as "hysterical" by male physicians. The term *nonorganic* is clumsy and suggests a radical dichotomy between organic pathology and "other" pathology. The term *psychosomatic* refers specifically to illnesses like duodenal ulcer, ulcerative colitis, and asthma, in which some have suggested that chronic stress and autonomic overactivity leads to organic pathology.

Psychogenic is the least objectionable term available and the term that is used in this chapter. Although it still implies a dualistic view of mind and body, it is at least nonpejorative. This term also reminds the user that mental pathology is more than just the absence of organic pathology.

◆ Classification

Although psychogenic communication disorders in general have yet to be clearly described or categorized, several classification schemes have been devised for psychogenic voice disorders.

Aronson (1990) identified five groups of psychogenic voice disorders: (1) the musculoskeletal tension disorders involving excess muscle tension and vocal abuse, with resultant inflammation, nodules, and ulcers; (2) the conversion voice disorders, including conversion muteness, aphonia, dysphonia, and adductor spastic dysphonia; (3) mutational falsetto; (4) transsexualism; and (5) childlike speech in adults. Koufman and Blalock (1982) developed a similar classification scheme, but included a separate category for habitual hoarseness and postoperative dysphonia. Based on a retrospective review of 1000 patients, Morrison, Nichol, and Rammage (1986) described three types of psychogenic dysphonia: (1) muscle tension dysphonia, (2) functional or psychological dysphonia, and (3) spasmodic dysphonia. They detailed the anatomic and laryngoscopic findings in the various psychogenic voice disorders.

According to these schemes the muscle misuse or tension disorders are distinct from the conversion or psychological dysphonias. The misuse disorders are bad habits that may relate in a general way to personality style; the conversion voice disorders are specific symptoms of psychopathology and symbolically depict emotional conflicts. Morrison and Rammage (1993), in fact, argue that the term *psychogenic* should be restricted to the conversion voice disorders.

In practice, conversion and muscle misuse disorders are difficult to distinguish. In dysphonia, for instance, conversion symptoms necessarily involve changes in muscle tension. The diagnosis of conversion is based on theoretical constructs that must be inferred from observed data. Such inferences are often difficult to make. Distinctions between the two groups of disorders cannot be made on laryngoscopic or clinical grounds, but only on the basis of an interpretation of the nature and meaning of psychopathology. Such distinctions are inherently unreliable. Andersson and Schalen (1998) speculate that psychogenic voice disorders involve a disturbance of the reciprocal interactions among emotional awareness, laryngeal perception, and central motor control of phonation.

The three classification schemes described above are restricted to voice disorders and do not include closely related disorders of speech, like psychogenic stuttering. **Table 13–1** compares the classification schemes developed by Aronson, Koufman, and Morrison. **Table 13–2** lists our comprehensive classification scheme that encompasses the full range of the major psychogenic communication disorders.

Table 13–1   Classification Schemes for Psychogenic Speech and Voice Disorders

Aronson	Koufman	Morrison
Muscle tension	Voice abuse	Muscle tension
Conversion	Hysterical	Functional
Muteness	Aphonia	
Aphonia	Dysphonia	
Dysphonia		
Spastic dysphonia		Spasmodic
Mutational falsetto	Falsetto	
Transsexualism		
Child-like speech		
	Habitual hoarseness	
	Postoperative dysphonia	

Table 13–2   The Psychogenic Communication Disorders

Muscle tension disorders
Conversion communication disorders
Aphonia
Dysphonia
Psychogenic stuttering
Dysarthria
Aphasia
Mutational falsetto
Spasmodic dysphonia
Conversion type

Muscle Tension Disorders

Abnormal muscle tension is present in all the psychogenic communication disorders, but is particularly important in the muscle tension disorders. The laryngeal musculature responds to emotional stress with hypercontraction. As shown in **Fig. 13–1**, such tension can be observed and palpated by encircling the larynx with the thumb and middle finger in the region of the thyrohyoid space. In the relaxed state the larynx is mobile and the thyrohyoid space distinct and palpable; when the laryngeal musculature is tense, the larynx rises and the thyrohyoid space narrows (Case, 1996). Tension can also be palpated in the submandibular region.

Muscle tension or muscle misuse disorders develop when the laryngeal muscles are chronically and habitually misused or hypercontracted. Polyps, nodules, and scarring can develop as a result of chronic muscle misuse. Vocal nodules may account for 4% of an otolaryngology caseload, with at least two thirds of adult patients being female (Roy, Bless, and Heisey, 2000). Although patients with muscle tension disorders are sometimes anxious, they do not display the more specific forms of mental illness seen in conversion disorders. However, in individuals with vocal nodules, personality characteristics including a combination of sociable, dominant, and aggressive traits may lead to an increased risk for phonotraumatic patterns. In this group of patients, the excessive voice use coincides with an extraverted personality style (Roy et al, 2000). Patients with muscle tension voice disorders misuse their voices in one or more of the following ways: (1) overuse, (2) speaking with

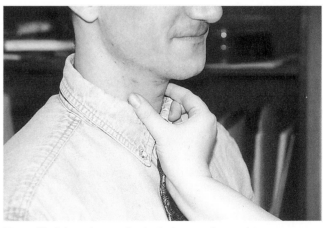

Figure 13–1 Assessing tension in the laryngeal musculature.

abnormal muscle tension in the larynx and neck muscles, and (3) using an abnormally low pitch (Koufman & Blalock, 1982).

Anatomic subtypes of muscle tension disorders have been described in detail by Morrison and Rammage (1993). Anatomic patterns seen in conversion and muscle misuse disorders may overlap, adding to the complexity of differential diagnosis.

The most common type is the laryngeal isometric, usually seen in untrained individuals who use their voice excessively, like cheerleaders or amateur singers. This pattern of misuse has also been called habitual hyperkinetic dysphonia and is one of the most common vocal complaints in adults. Sustained hypertonicity of the posterior cricoarytenoid muscle deflects the arytenoid cartilage and produces a posterior glottal chink. Phonation has a characteristic "whispery/breathy" quality, and secondary mucosal injury can occur.

Lateral contraction or hyperadduction, where the larynx is squeezed in a side-to-side direction, is also common. When this occurs at a glottic level it is usually as a result of poor vocal technique. Glottic contraction can be triggered by an upper respiratory infection, which causes hoarseness, and then is maintained by poor vocal technique after the viral irritation has resolved.

Supraglottic contraction is also known as ventricular dysphonia or plica ventricularis. This vocal pattern involves the abnormal participation of the false vocal cords in phonation. Supraglottic contraction commonly noted in the conversion dysphonias, but can occur in injury to the true vocal cords.

An anteroposterior contraction of the supraglottic larynx has also been described. Koufman labeled this disorder the "Bogart-Bacall" syndrome. Such patients display a tension dysphonia and effortful voice at the bottom of their vocal ranges but can talk freely at a higher pitch.

Hypokinetic dysphonia results from the inadequate movements of laryngeal muscles during phonation. Such patients have bowed vocal cords on indirect laryngoscopic exam and weak, husky breathy voices. Such patients typically suffer from conversion disorders, but hypokinetic dysphonia may result from habitual hoarseness following an upper respiratory tract infection.

Conversion Communication Disorders

The term *conversion disorder* describes a broad range of pseudoneurologic symptoms that develop as a result of emotional stress and conflict. In conversion psychic conflict is "converted" into a physical symptom. Conversion symptoms can be distinguished from true neurologic symptoms because conversion symptoms are *idiogenic.* They correspond not to the actual anatomy and physiology of a neurologic disorder, but rather to a person's idea of what such a disorder might be like. For instance, in a conversion paralysis of the arm a patient might be unable to move his arm from the elbow down. He does not understand the innervation of the arm, and does not realize that such a pattern of paralysis is implausible, but develops a symptom pattern that corresponds to his mental idea of a paralysis. Similarly, in conversion aphonia a patient might still be able to cough or sing, though he attests that he cannot phonate.

Conversion cannot be diagnosed by exclusion. Just because a symptom has no known anatomic or physiologic explanation does not mean that it is a conversion. To diagnose conversion a clear temporal relationship between a symptom and a psychological stressor must be present. In chronic conversion reactions such temporal relationships can be difficult to elucidate. The criteria for conversion disorder are listed in **Table 13–3**.

Table 13–3   Criteria for Conversion Disorder

Symptoms affecting voluntary motor or sensory function suggesting a neurologic condition
Psychological factors are temporally associated with the onset or exacerbation of the symptom
Symptom is not intentionally produced or feigned
Symptom cannot be explained by a medical condition

Initially a conversion reaction provides *primary gain.* The conversion symptom helps keep a painful emotional conflict out of conscious awareness. *Secondary gain* refers to those benefits that indirectly accrue from the conversion symptom, including time off work, disability benefits, extra nurturance from one's spouse, and relief from family responsibilities. Secondary gain helps maintain conversion symptoms and makes them more difficult to treat.

Conversion symptoms start early in life and are much more common in women than men. Cultural factors may explain the sex difference in the prevalence of conversion disorders. Sickness may empower a woman in a social context where she is otherwise without means of attaining power. There is some evidence that conversion disorders are more common in cultures where women are less empowered, such as in Mediterranean regions. Somatization disorders are also more common in daughters raised in alcoholic families, and in victims of sexual abuse.

A conversion disorder can be viewed as a kind of unconscious theatrical performance. Patients display or enact a symptom as a way of protecting themselves from emotional pain. They are not aware that they are performing; they are simultaneously actor and audience.

Malingering and factitious disorder can resemble conversion disorder. Unlike conversion, where patients are not aware that they are producing their symptoms, the malingering patient deliberately and consciously feigns symptoms for secondary gain. In factitious disorder, also known as Munchausen's syndrome, the patient deliberately and knowingly produces medical symptoms not for secondary gain, but for the purpose of assuming the sick role. In factitious disorder patients are aware that they are feigning symptoms, but not aware of their own motivations.

In practice, conversion disorder, factitious disorder, and malingering are difficult to distinguish. For instance, patients with a conversion symptom may consciously feign or magnify their illness when undergoing a disability evaluation. Jonas and Pope (1985) felt that these disorders were indistinguishable and should be called "dissembling disorders." In their view, all these patients dissembled or lied. Pure classical conversion patients lie to themselves and successfully fool even themselves. The relationship among conversion, factitious disorder, and malingering is depicted in **Table 13–4**.

Conversion speech symptoms are protean; their variety is limited only by the imagination of the sufferer. Conversion speech disorders are classified on the basis of the observed speech pattern. In conversion muteness the patient neither

Table 13–4   The Dissembling Disorders

Disorder	Symptom Production	Motivation
Conversion	Unconscious	Unconscious
Malingering	Conscious	Conscious
Factitious	Conscious	Unconscious

Table 13–5   Fluency Disorders

	Developmental Stuttering	Neurogenic Fluency Disorders	Psychogenic Stuttering
Age	Early childhood	Age of onset of neurologic illness	After trauma
Onset	Gradual	Same as neurologic illness	Sudden
Secondary mannerisms, struggle behaviors	Common	Rare	Rare
Improves with repetition, choral reading, delayed auditory feedback	Yes	No	No
Related psychogenic history	No	No	Other psychogenic illness or conversion symptoms

whispers nor articulates despite normal laryngeal and oral motor function. In conversion aphonia the patient whispers involuntarily despite normal vocal cord function on laryngoscopic exam and during nonspeech activities such as laughing or coughing. Conversion dysphonia is psychogenic hoarseness and can resemble laryngitis. The idiogenic nature of conversion symptoms is confirmed by the incongruities in the clinical presentation, like an inability to adduct the vocal cords during phonation in the presence of normal cough or laugh.

Psychogenic stuttering is also a form of conversion speech disorder. Like other conversion disorders, psychogenic stuttering shows idiogenic and atypical features. In contrast to typical developmental stuttering, psychogenic stutters show stereotyped repetitions, lack of improvement with choral reading, and the absence of islands of fluency, secondary symptoms or avoidance behaviors (Roth, Aronson, & Davis, 1989; Mahr & Leith, 1992). Developmental stuttering shows an insidious onset in early childhood, whereas psychogenic stuttering begins acutely and can occur at any age after an emotional trauma. Psychogenic stuttering must be carefully distinguished from fluency disturbances that can occur in brain diseases like Parkinson's or after traumatic brain injury. The differences among developmental stuttering, psychogenic stuttering, and neurogenic fluency disorders are summarized in **Table 13–5**.

Mutation falsetto or adolescent transitional dysphonia can be a habitual pattern or a form of conversion disorder. The adolescent male with mutational falsetto appears to resist the development of the normal lower pitch by adopting a falsetto voice. The larynx is raised and the glottis is tense and hyperadducted to maintain elevated pitch in the face of masculinized laryngeal anatomy. Mutational falsetto is relatively uncommon and represents only 2 or 3% of patients presenting for the treatment of voice disorders (Hammarberg, 1987). Most cases present in adolescence. Occasionally adults present because of pitch breaks, which actually are intervals of normal pitch in a mutational falsetto that has been habitually maintained for years or decades (Aronson, 1990).

✦ Epidemiology

Because psychogenic speech and voice disorders are not well defined and relatively uncommon, their incidence and prevalence in the general population are not known. As mentioned earlier, Duffy (1995) reported that psychogenic communication disorders accounted for 4.5% of all acquired communication disorders. Of these 215 cases, 80% had voice disorders. The most common psychogenic voice disorders

were aphonia and dysphonia, in that order. Functional dysphonia has been found to account for more than 10% of cases referred to multidisciplinary voice clinics (Schalen & Andersson, 1992). Disorders of fluency and prosody accounted for 20% of cases, most of those (11%) being psychogenic stuttering. In contrast, Bridger and Epstein's (1983) series of 109 patients with functional voice disorders showed a majority (87%) with dysphonia. Patients typically present for treatment of psychogenic speech and voice disorders in their early 40s (Butcher, Elias, & Raven, 1993; Koufman & Blalock, 1982). Psychogenic communication disorders are twice as common in women, probably because conversion disorders in general are much more common in women. Estimates of sex ratios in conversion disorder vary from 2:1 to 10:1 (American Psychiatric Association, 1994).

✦ Psychiatric Comorbidity

In past decades psychiatrists were quick to postulate psychological causative mechanisms for medical problems and symptoms. Many parents were inappropriately blamed for "causing" their child's asthma, schizophrenia, or autism. We now understand that many problems thought to be caused by emotional factors or childrearing are in fact medical illnesses in which emotional factors may be important, but not through simple causal mechanisms.

The relationship between emotional issues and psychogenic communication disorders is an example of this complex interplay between mind and body. Psychological issues may cause, maintain, or be a result of communication disorders. The older literature had focused exclusively on a search for the psychological *causes* of these illnesses.

Aronson (1990) has championed a stress model for the psychogenic voice disorders, suggesting that psychological issues cause psychogenic voice disorders through stress. He reported that those who suffer from muscle tension dysphonia are talkative, socially aggressive, and angry. In contrast, Aronson found patients with conversion dysphonias to be somatically preoccupied, immature, dependent, and superficial. According to Aronson, the laryngeal musculature is uniquely sensitive to stress, and that stress produces muscle hypercontraction. In susceptible individuals, hypercontraction of the laryngeal musculature produces the various psychogenic voice disorders.

Other research has not borne out Aronson's clear distinctions between the psychological traits of subgroups of psychogenic speech and voice disorders. Patients with psychogenic communication disorders, as a group, are anxious, somatically preoccupied, and complain of interpersonal stresses. It is not clear that muscle tension dysphonia patients are psychologically different from conversion patients.

The stress model has other weaknesses. It is not clear that psychogenic voice disorder patients have more stress, or that stress precedes the onset of their voice disorder. Furthermore, stress is ubiquitous. A stress model is not useful unless it offers specificity, or unless it suggests why some individuals are susceptible to specific pathology in response to stress.

Because we lack sufficient knowledge of the causes of the psychogenic speech and voice disorders, it is more useful to focus on comorbidity rather than cause. Comorbid disorders are associated with, but do not necessarily cause, an illness. Patients with psychogenic speech and voice patterns may also be anxious and depressed. Anxiety and depression may be a cause, a result, or simply a factor that exacerbates and maintains a voice disturbance. In any case, these comorbid disorders are highly treatable and must be identified and addressed in any comprehensive treatment program. To assess the psychological characteristics of patient's with functional dysphonias, Roy, McGrory, Tasko, Bless, Heisey, and Ford (1997) compared 25 individuals with functional dysphonia to 19 medical control patients. Compared with 90% of controls, 32% of those in the functional dysphonic group scored within the normal ranges on a personality measure, the Minnesota Multiphasic Personality Inventory (MMPI), and exhibited significantly more emotional problems and lower levels of adaptive functioning. Certain enduring psychological and personality dispositions likely contribute to the ongoing adjustment difficulties even after the remittance of voice symptoms.

Cognitive issues are also important comorbid factors in initiating and maintaining communication disorders. Cognitive models of mental disorders have become increasingly influential over the past decade. Aaron Beck (1976), a cognitive theorist, has proposed that ideas affect behavior and feelings. In cognitive models of depression, for instance, cognitive distortions and inappropriate generalizations like "I'm no good" lead to depressive feelings. Cognitive reeducation effectively treats mood related symptoms.

In somatoform disorders, pathologic beliefs and attitudes lead to somatic symptoms. Somatizing patients believe they are ill, so they become hypervigilant about their bodies. In their hypervigilance, they overinterpret normal somatic stimuli. A fleeting pain or sensation becomes a focus of attention and becomes magnified. In psychogenic dysphagia, for instance, a fleeting alteration in swallowing function becomes a chronic "globus hystericus."

Related to this somatizing hypervigilance is *spectatoring*. In spectatoring, a normally automatic function becomes distorted by the intrusion of conscious attention. Spectatoring is a common cause of male erectile dysfunction. After an episode of normal erectile failure, a male may become hypervigilant in his next sexual encounter about whether he can maintain an erection. This very hypervigilance precludes normal sexual arousal and causes the feared erectile failure.

Similar mechanisms may occur in dysphonia. Psychogenic dysphonia is often preceded by an upper respiratory infection with laryngitis. In vulnerable patients, concern about voice production leads to attempts at compensation, altered voice mechanisms, and chronic vocal strain.

Learned helplessness is a psychological construct proposed by Seligman (1975). He found that rats exposed to chronic but unpredictable punishment no longer attempted to avoid the aversive stimuli. The Seligman model has been applied to humans exposed to chronic illness. In response to chronic aversive consequences, patients come to feel that their actions have no bearing on the course or outcome of their illness. They become passive and develop an external locus of control. Patients with an internal locus of control and a strong sense of mastery tend to respond better to treatment and have more benign courses of illness. An external locus of control can be made more internal with cognitive therapy.

Cognitive models do not imply a causal relation between symptoms and emotions. In a cognitive model of dysphonia, spectatoring and anxieties about speaking at least perpetuate, maintain, or exacerbate a vocal problem. Effective interventions for psychogenic speech and voice disorders utilize cognitive as well as behavioral techniques.

In summary, potential comorbid factors associated with psychogenic communication disorders include depression, anxiety, and attitudinal factors like spectatoring and learned helplessness. Effective treatment must address such psychological comorbidity.

✦ Assessment

Assessment is the first step in treatment. The assessment should clarify and confirm the diagnosis, verify that a full and proper organic workup has been performed, and begin the process of exploring potential emotional factors in the speech or voice disorder. Exploration should be nonthreatening and nonjudgmental. Patients typically fear being ignored and abandoned because their problems are "in their head." Exploring organic issues first helps establish rapport and reassures the patient that their problems are being taken seriously. It may help to remind patients that their problems are indeed "organic" in the sense that the function of their laryngeal musculature and mucosa is central to their disorder.

Case (1996) offered the following model for initiating an exploration of emotional issues potentially related to a speech disorder: "It has been found that persons with voice patterns similar to yours are experiencing conflicts and stresses that might be affecting the voice. Is anything happening in your life that might be important for us to understand?" (p. 233).

Such phrasing normalizes the possibility that emotional factors may contribute to vocal pathology and does not diminish or trivialize symptoms. The main issues that are unique to each patient should be identified. Common stresses for individuals with psychogenic communication problems include problematic relationships, high level of family responsibilities, and inhibited emotional expression (Butcher & Cavalli, 1998). Initiating a dialogue about emotional issues begins the therapeutic process for patients with a psychogenic component to their communication problem.

Methods of assessment can include brief paper-and-pencil self-report measures such as the Beck Depression Inventory and Hospital Anxiety and Depression Scale, which can assist in identifying problematic comorbid issues (Beck, Ward, Mendelson, Mock, & Erbaugh, 1961; Zigmond & Snaith, 1983). Psychologists may use measures focused on understanding underlying personality characteristics, such as the MMPI, to assist in treatment planning (Hathaway & McKinley, 1972).

✦ Treatment

The process of speech therapy in patients with psychogenic communication disorders involves relaxation training, behavioral techniques, and cognitive techniques. There is a significant need for longitudinal and prospective studies regarding therapy effects.

Relaxation training is particularly important in the muscle tension dysphonias. Jacobson's progressive muscle relaxation is commonly used, but several techniques effectively produce sustained relaxation of voluntary musculature. Once generalized relaxation is obtained, specific techniques must be used to relax the laryngeal musculature. With experience and training patients learn how their muscle feels when they are relaxed and when they are tense. This feedback helps patients monitor their own tension states and reward themselves for successful relaxation.

Relaxed phonation can be digitally palpated as shown in **Fig. 13–2**. With one hand, the patient places a finger on the side of the nose, another on the face around the lips, and a third of the side of the larynx. In relaxed phonation vibration can be detected by all three fingers.

Behavioral techniques can help reestablish normal phonation in the conversion aphonias and dysphonias. The therapist begins a vocal retraining program by utilizing whatever phonation remains intact. When a patient can cough or grunt or hum, the therapist uses that phonatory response to rebuild normal speech. A cough or hum can be extended to form a vowel, then a monosyllabic word, then a phrase, and so forth until normal communication is restored (Case, 1996).

Such behavioral techniques involve indirect suggestion in contrast to direct suggestion. Direct suggestion means informing patients that whatever function was altered by their conversion is now restored, that is, simply telling patients that they can now talk or walk or move their arm. Direct suggestion is sometimes useful as a diagnostic tool. For instance, a diagnosis of a conversion paralysis can be confirmed by commanding a patient to move the affected limb under trance. When the paralyzed limb can move under trance, then the diagnosis of conversion reaction is confirmed. Direct suggestion is not useful as a therapeutic technique. Benefits are short-lived, and direct suggestion may humiliate or anger a patient and cause a psychogenic symptom to be even more deeply entrenched. If you simply tell patients to talk normally, they may cling more tightly to their symptom to show you that they cannot.

Indirect suggestion involves gradually showing patients that they can have normal vocal function. In this way the conversion symptom can be gradually abandoned, but the patient can save face. Specific behavior techniques are described in detail by Case (1996) and Aronson (1990).

Cognitive techniques are a natural and vital component of a therapy regimen for psychogenic voice disorders. Education about vocal functioning and proper vocal techniques helps patients gain a sense of mastery and control, and helps them be partners in their own care. Education helps negate the attitudes of passivity, helplessness, and self-blame that complicate the treatment of psychogenic speech and voice disorders.

A combination of cognitive and behavioral approaches to treatment may be used and is referred to as cognitive-behavioral therapy (CBT). Along with the standard voice therapy that provides the patient with skills better use of voice, CBT addresses the underlying psychological processes and offers alternative strategies to manage them. Even if patients come to acquire new skills to control their voice symptoms, they will likely need to alter cognitive-behavioral patterns. Otherwise, in times of stress they may revert to the maladaptive voice patterns that caused their symptoms.

Butcher et al (1993) provide specific guidelines on how CBT strategies can be used in speech therapy sessions. CBT techniques may focus on how to assess thinking processes, identify and modify dysfunctional thoughts, teach anxiety management strategies, train in assertiveness or communication, and teach general life management skills. **Table 13–6** presents examples of complementary aspects of voice therapy and CBT. CBT techniques can be an effective treatment tool for the speech therapist.

Several studies have confirmed the efficacy of voice therapy in the treatment of psychogenic dysphonia. MacKenzie, Millar, Wilson, Sellars, and Deary (2001) treated 70 patients with 6 weeks of voice therapy. Significant improvements in voice quality, as measured by self and observer ratings, occurred in the treatment group as compared with a group of 63 controls. In a long-term longitudinal study, Andersson and Schalen (1998) reported improvement in voice quality with minimal relapse 1.9 to 8.4 years after treatment. Bridger and Epstein (1983) found that about half of patients treated recover completely over 3 to 6 months, and another quarter are at

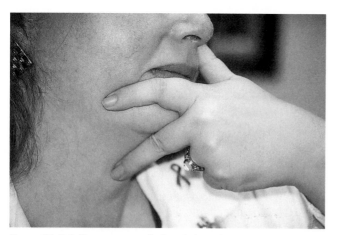

Figure 13–2 Self-assessment of relaxed phonation.

Table 13–6 Complementary Aspects of Voice Therapy and Cognitive-Behavioral Therapy (CBT)

Voice Therapy	CBT
1. Educate about voice production and sensitivity to muscle tension	1. Educate about role of dysfunctional thoughts/behaviors contributing to anxiety-related symptoms
2. Reduce tension in extrinsic and intrinsic laryngeal muscles using laryngeal manipulation techniques	2. Reduce muscle tension using systematic relaxation methods
3. Teach breathing techniques for voice to enable control of expiratory airflow for phonation	3. Teach diaphragmatic breathing for use as relaxation technique and for stress management
4. Monitor voice patterns and situations which trigger more severe symptoms	4. Utilize general stress management techniques with reduction of dysfunctional thoughts/behaviors

Flowchart for treatment

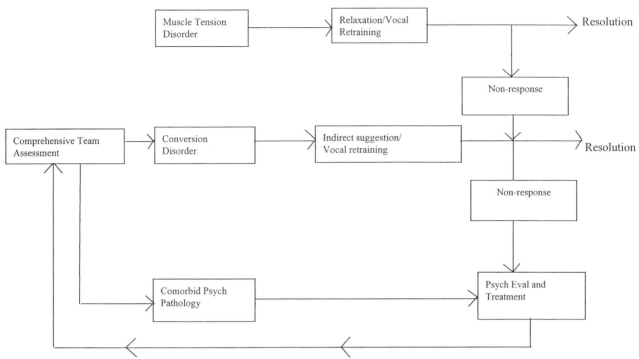

Figure 13–3 Flowchart for treatment.

least significantly improved by speech therapy. A significant minority of patients do not appear to do well. Butcher, Elias, Raven, Yeatman, and Littlejohns (1987) studied 19 nonresponders who were found to be anxious and to have significant problems with interpersonal relationships.

Referral to a mental health professional may be of benefit, especially in the treatment of nonresponders or those in whom emotional issues are clearly evident. Referral is also useful for the treatment of comorbid problems like anxiety, depression, and somatization. In Butcher et al's (1993) study of patients with psychogenic voice disorders who did not respond to standard speech therapy, nearly half improved in a conjoint therapy program with a psychologist and a speech pathologist.

Somatizing patients may reject mental health referrals. They may be very strongly investing in their problem being "medical," and a referral to a mental health provider may be seen as trivializing their voice problems. A referral to mental health treatment is best presented as an adjunct to speech therapy, not as a substitute for it.

A referral to a mental health professional might be worded as follows: "I have noticed that anxiety may be contributing to your voice problem. I work with Dr. X., who is an expert in anxiety problems and can help us with that aspect of your speech problem."

Unfortunately, the results of mental health referrals can be disappointing. Psychiatrists, psychologists and therapists often lack knowledge or experience in speech and voice problems. Few clinical settings allow for clinical interactions between speech–language pathologists and mental health professionals. In addition, most speech–language pathologists feel uncertain about when and to whom to refer patients. Treatment failures, patients less likely to benefit from any intervention, are usually the ones referred.

A multidisciplinary team approach can obviate some of these difficulties. A patient is more likely to accept a referral to a practitioner who is part of the team. Each team member brings unique expertise to the program and the team as a whole develops a comprehensive approach to patient care. Communication between disciplines is facilitated, allowing the patient's needs to be efficiently and effectively addressed.

✦ Conclusion

We have described the various psychogenic speech and voice disorders and presented methods for diagnosis and treatment. **Fig. 13–3** graphically depicts a model for the treatment of the psychogenic speech and voice disorders, including the role of psychiatric and psychological assessment.

Study Questions

1. What are the different types of psychogenic speech and voice disorders?

2. What is meant by comorbid pathology?

3. Why is it beneficial to differentiate comorbidity from cause?

4. How might treatment outcomes be improved for psychogenic speech and voice disorders?

5. What are some of the cognitive-behavioral techniques likely to be helpful in treatment of psychogenic dysphonia?

6. What are some of the common gender and cultural issues observed in conversion disorders?

References

American Psychiatric Association. (1994). *Diagnostic and Statistical Manual of Mental Disorders.* Washington, DC: APA Press

Andersson, K., & Schalen, L. (1998). Etiology and Treatment of Psychogenic Voice Disorder: Results of a Follow-Up Study of Thirty Patients. *Journal of Voice, 12,* 96–106

Aronson, A.E. (1990). *Clinical Voice Disorders.* New York: Thieme

Beck, A.T. (1976). *Cognitive Therapy and Emotional Disorders.* New York: International Universities Press

Beck, A.T., Ward, C.H., Mendelson, M., Mock, J., & Erbaugh, J. (1961). An Inventory for Measuring Depression. *Archives of General Psychiatry, 4,* 561–571

Bridger, M.W.M., & Epstein, R. (1983). Functional Voice Disorders: A Review of 109 Patients. *Journal of Laryngology and Otology, 97,* 1145–1148

Butcher, P., & Cavalli, L. (1998). Fran: Understanding and Treating Psychogenic Dysphonia from a Cognitive-Behavioral Perspective. In: D. Snyder (Ed.), *Wanting to Talk: Counseling Case Studies in Communication Disorders* (pp. 60–89). Hoboken, NJ: John Wiley

Butcher, P., Elias, A., & Raven, R. (1993). *Psychogenic Voice Disorders and Cognitive Behavioral Therapy.* San Diego: Singular

Butcher, P., Elias, A., Raven, R., Yeatman, J., & Littlejohns, D. (1987). Psychogenic Voice Disorder Unresponsive to Speech Therapy: Psychological Characteristics and Cognitive-Behavioral Therapy. *British Journal of Disorders of Communication, 22,* 81–92

Case, J.L. (1996). *Clinical Management of Voice Disorders.* Austin, TX: Pro-Ed

Duffy, J.R. (1995). *Motor Speech Disorders.* New York: Mosby

Elias, A., Raven, R., Butcher, P., Littlejohns, D.W. (1989). Speech Therapy for Psychogenic Voice Disorder: A Survey of Current Practice and Training. *British Journal of Disorders of Communication, 24,* 61–76

Hammarberg, B. (1987). Pitch and Quality Characteristics of Mutational Voice Disorders Before and After Therapy. *Folia Phoniatrica, 39,* 204–216

Hathaway, S.R., & McKinley, J.C. (1972). *The Minnesota Multiphasic Personality Inventory.* New York: Psychological Corporation

Jonas, J.M., & Pope, H.G. (1985). The Dissimulating Disorders: A Single Diagnostic Entity? *Comprehensive Psychiatry, 26,* 58–62

Koufman, J.A., & Blalock, P.D. (1982). Classification and Approach to Patients with Functional Voice Disorders. *Annals of Otology, Rhinology, and Laryngology, 91,* 372–377

MacKenzie, K., Millar, A., Wilson, J.A., Sellars, C., & Deary, I.J. (2001). Is Voice Therapy an Effective Treatment for Dysphonia? A Randomized Controlled Trial. *British Medical Journal, 323,* 658–661

Mahr, G., & Leith, W. (1992). Psychogenic Stuttering of Adult Onset. *Journal of Speech and Hearing Research, 35,* 283–286

Morrison, M.D., Nichol, H., & Rammage, L.A. (1986). Diagnostic Criteria in Functional Dysphonia. *Laryngoscope, 96,* 1–8

Morrison, M.D. & Rammage, L.A. (1993). Muscle Misuse Voice Disorders: Description and Classification. *Acta Otolaryngologica, 113,* 428–434

Roth, C.R., Aronson, A.E., & Davis, L.J. (1989). Clinical Studies in Psychogenic Stuttering of Adult Onset. *Journal of Speech and Hearing Disorders, 54,* 634–636

Roy, N., Bless, D.M., & Heisey, D. (2000). Personality and Voice Disorders: A Multitrait-Multidisorder Analysis. *Journal of Voice, 14,* 521–548

Roy, N., McGrory, J.J., Tasko, S.M., Bless, D.M., Heisey, D., & Ford, C.N. (1997). Psychological Correlates of Functional Dysphonia: An Investigation Using the Minnesota Multiphasic Personality Inventory. *Journal of Voice, 11,* 443–451

Schalen, L., & Andersson, K. (1992). Differential Diagnosis and Treatment of Psychogenic Voice Disorder. *Clinical Otolaryngology, 17,* 225–230

Seligman, M.E.P. (1975). *Helplessness.* San Francisco: Freeman

Zigmond, A.S., & Snaith, R.P. (1983). The Hospital Anxiety and Depression Scale. *Acta Psychiatrica Scandinavica, 67,* 361–370

14

Current Trends and Issues in Health Care Delivery: What Speech–Language Pathologists Need to Know

Janet E. Brown and Arlene A. Pietranton

◆ Background

◆ Current Picture of Speech–Language Pathology Practice in Health Care

◆ Knowledge and Skills Needed and Expected in the Health Care Workplace

◆ The Expanding Speech–Language Pathology Scope of Practice

◆ Evidence-Based Practice

◆ Culturally Competent Services

◆ Telepractice: The Wise Application of Technology to Clinical Service Delivery

◆ Reimbursement

◆ Health Insurance Portability and Accountability Act (HIPAA)

◆ Background

The last decade of the 20th century was one of unprecedented changes in access to and funding of clinical services. The preceding several decades were characterized by steady growth in the demand for and coverage of clinical services, including those of speech–language pathologists (SLPs). That growth was the result of a variety of factors, including (1) changing population demographics; (2) increased awareness of communication and related disorders and their impact; (3) scientific and technological advances; and (4) an expanding speech–language pathology scope of practice. It was also the result of a prevalent public policy theme, "funded mandates," and a dominant reimbursement methodology, "fee-for-service." Funded mandates (i.e., when a state or federal entity requires that certain services will be provided and allocates the funds necessary to pay for the required services) and fee-for-service reimbursement (i.e., when a provider's "reasonable and customary" charges are paid by the patient or an authorized third party/insurer) served health care recipients well, including individuals with communication and related disorders, as they helped to ensure that individuals had access to and coverage of services. However, that framework also contributed to the rapid escalation of health care costs in the later part of the 20th century. For example, in 1960 annual health care expenditures in the United States consumed 5.3% of the U.S. gross national product (GNP). By 1994 they had escalated to a point of consuming 16% of the GNP, with predictions that health care costs, if left unchecked, would extrapolate to consuming 100% of the GNP by the middle of the 21st century (Banja, 1994).

This startling financial reality unleashed a backlash of cost containment methodologies and a clear movement away from funded mandates and fee-for-service reimbursement as evidenced by congressional action and the phenomenal growth of managed care in the 1990s. A reality of health care in the United States is that the delivery of services is heavily influenced, some would even say driven, by the incentives and disincentives associated with reimbursement models. This chapter examines that complex relationship. It also addresses the critical reality of the rapidly increasing cultural and linguistic diversity in the United States and explores several important trends and issues [e.g., the expanding speech–language pathology scope of practice, telepractice, the Health Insurance Portability and Accountability Act (HIPAA)] related to the delivery of speech–language pathology services in the health care arena.

◆ Current Picture of Speech–Language Pathology Practice in Health Care

Health care changes in recent years have resulted in a new picture of the health care workplace for SLPs in terms of demographics, caseloads, opportunities, and challenges. According to the American Speech-Language-Hearing Association's (ASHA) 2004 membership count, approximately 35% of ASHA-certified SLPs work in a health care setting (ASHA, 2005c). The different settings—hospitals, rehabilitation hospitals, skilled nursing facilities (SNFs), home health agencies, outpatient clinics, private practice, and pediatric hospitals—each have unique characteristics that may appeal differently to SLPs who wish to practice in a health care environment.

One key variable is whether the employment arrangement is by salary, contract, or self-employment. Salaried employees most often work full time for their institution, and are likely to receive additional benefits, such as health insurance, paid vacation, and sick leave. According to ASHA's 2005 SLP Health Care Survey, 55% of respondents reported working as full-time or part-time salaried employees, and 19% described themselves as full- or part-time contract employees (ASHA, 2005e). SLPs who are self-employed may work in their own clinic or office, or they may contract with other health care settings. Those who are self-employed do not receive benefits from a contractor, but may negotiate a higher hourly rate to help offset the lack of a benefits package, typically valued as 20 to 25% of one's salary.

Health care clinicians may be held to a productivity target (i.e., the ratio of the number of hours spent in direct patient care to the total number of hours worked in a day or a week). On the 2005 ASHA survey of SLPs who work in health care settings, the largest percentage of respondents reported a productivity requirement in the range of 74 to 75%, which translates to about 6 hours of direct patient care a day in an 8-hour day. Home health settings were less likely to have productivity requirements because of the variable travel time required between patient visits. Forty-eight percent of respondents also indicated that SLP services are provided on weekends, most frequently in hospitals (particularly rehabilitation hospitals) and much less frequently in SNFs, home health, or outpatient clinics (ASHA, 2005e).

Adults in health care settings were most commonly treated for swallowing (45%), cognitive-communication disorders (20%), and aphasia (16%), although there is considerable variability depending on the type of setting (ASHA, 2005e). Although the majority of services are provided to children in pediatric hospitals, SLPs in home health reported that 48% of their services were delivered to infants and toddlers (ASHA, 2005e), most likely through early intervention programs. Across pediatric health care settings, swallowing and feeding (31%) and language (28%) were the most frequently treated disorders (ASHA, 2005e).

When the prospective payment system (PPS; discussed later in this chapter) was implemented in SNFs, there were predictions that changes in reimbursement and heightened demand for efficiencies would lead to a considerable rise in the volume of group treatment. Such has not been the case, with SLPs in rehabilitation hospitals reporting that 11% of their services are delivered via group treatment (Rosenfeld, 2002). Group treatment is reported to comprise less than 7% of SLP services in all other settings. Speculation about a sudden surge in the hiring of speech–language pathology assistants (SLPAs) in health care settings has also not been borne out, with only 2% of SLP reporting that their sites employ SLPAs (Rosenfeld, 2002).

Changes in reimbursement initiated by PPS and private health plans have affected other rehabilitation professionals as well. In our society where the workforce tends to be regulated by the principle of supply and demand, the staffing of health care institutions vacillates greatly by profession and by region. Although projected nursing shortages dominate concerns and discussion about the future of health care, the availability or shortage of various rehabilitation professionals may have a significant impact on how services are delivered in a specific facility.

For example, some SLPs work in settings that treat a large population of patients with tracheostomies or who are ventilator-dependent. These SLPs may find that they would like, or are expected, to become competent in performing suctioning. Principle II, rule B of ASHA's Code of Ethics states that members "shall engage only in those aspects of the professions that are within the scope of their competence, considering their level of education, training, and experience" (ASHA, 2003a). As SLPs obtain training beyond that which they receive during graduate education or clinical fellowship, they should ensure that their competency in these areas is documented. In addition to ASHA's Code of Ethics, accrediting organizations such as the Joint Commission on Accreditation of Healthcare Organizations (JCAHO) require that professional staff have competencies verified in writing, particularly for those skills that are either high volume (e.g., frequently occurring in that facility) or high risk (e.g., dysphagia, suctioning).

This dynamic environment and evolution of practice requires adaptation by SLPs both experienced and new to the profession. SLPs who meet the new Speech–Language Pathology Standards for Certification effective in 2005, including the requisite knowledge and skills in business practice, ethics, and dysphagia, should be well prepared for the challenges of health care settings. Similarly, experienced clinicians have the benefit of "on the job" learning about the value of their services and the limits of their competence. Challenges that SLPs sometimes face due to staff shortages or cost-containment efforts include pressure to provide treatment outside their personal scope of competence (e.g., to begin responding to referrals from the neonatal intensive care unit (NICU) without sufficient prior training, education, or experience), or to cross the boundaries into the scope of practice of another profession, or to provide training in areas of the SLP scope of practice to professionals in other disciplines. The clinician should respond by carefully reviewing the Code of Ethics and specific policies on multiskilled personnel and cross-training (ASHA, 1997, 2004h,i) to ensure that they are making an informed decision on behalf of the patient(s) rather than unquestioningly following an administrative policy.

◆ Knowledge and Skills Needed and Expected in the Health Care Workplace

Clinical practitioners who are determined to thrive and not merely survive in today's health care arena need to demonstrate clinical expertise related to the population(s) they serve, possess particular health care "business savvy," and exhibit a variety of key attributes to be viewed as highly valued contributors in the health care workplace. This reality of professional life is reflected in standard III-H of the Speech–Language Pathology Standards for Certification effective in 2005, which states, "The applicant must demonstrate knowledge of contemporary professional issues." Among the issues cited in the standard are "relevant legislation and regulations; . . . knowledge of policy and procedures at the federal, state, and local level; . . . business practices, and reimbursement issues" (American Speech-Language-Hearing Association Council on Professional Standards in Speech–Language Pathology and Audiology, 2000). ASHA's practice policy documents and publications on business practices (ASHA, 2003b, 2004a,c) specify requisite areas of health care business savvy such as:

+ Providing appropriate services that meet the business needs of the organization
+ Achieving compliance and professional practice
+ Achieving quality outcomes and performance improvement
+ Providing advocacy
+ Promoting and marketing professional services
+ Using technology
+ Obtaining payment for services

Research into workplace effectiveness has identified core skills that have been shown to correlate with success in any work environment. Several of those skills are essential for health care practitioners who wish to be effective in a leadership capacity in a highly challenging and increasingly competitive health care business environment (**Table 14–1**).

Table 14–1 Workplace Success Factors

Success Factors	Example of Application
Time management	Efficient use of clinical minutes to achieve goals and of nondirect time to fulfill responsibilities related to team meetings, insurance requirements, paperwork, etc.
Negotiation	Ensure that patients in need of speech–language pathology services receive referrals and sufficient minutes under skilled nursing facility prospective payment system
Conflict management	Discussions regarding the nature and amount of services needed with clinical colleagues, patients/family members, case managers
Priority setting/process management	Organize caseloads and provide effective clinical leadership across disciplines on a patient by patient basis
Interpersonal and organizational savvy	Effectively navigate the workplace and health care system on behalf of patients and profession
Entrepreneurialism	Ability to identify, seize, or create new approaches or opportunities to enhance the institution's or program's competitive edge

✦ The Expanding Speech–Language Pathology Scope of Practice

The domain of speech–language pathology includes human communication behaviors and disorders and swallowing or other upper aerodigestive functions and disorders. The most recent scope of practice in speech–language pathology includes prevention, diagnosis, habilitation, and rehabilitation of communication, swallowing, or other upper aerodigestive disorders; elective modification of communication behaviors; and enhancement of communication (ASHA, 2001). The overall objective of speech–language pathology services is to optimize patients' ability to communicate and/or swallow in natural environments, and thus improve their quality of life.

Speech–language pathology is a dynamic and continuously developing profession. Changes in service delivery systems, increasing numbers of people needing services, projected growth among cultural and linguistic minority populations in the United States, and technologic and scientific advances are a few of the factors that continue to expand the SLP scope of practice. Past decades witnessed dramatic expansions in the SLP scope of practice (e.g., language in the 1970s; dysphagia in the 1980s) and shifts in the focus of SLP caseloads. Current expansions are occurring in areas such as communication effectiveness and wellness, literacy, services to neonates in the NICU, upper aerodigestive functions, and telepractice (**Table 14–2**).

Table 14–2 Expansions to the Speech–Language Pathology Scope of Practice

Communication effectiveness and wellness: education and consultation to promote practices that develop and maintain optimal communication. A healthy lifestyle can promote good communication skills. Communication effectiveness, an aspect of communication wellness, concerns the development and maintenance of effective personal and professional communication in individuals without a communication disorder. For example, working with corporations to help employees become more effective communicators; or working with individuals on accent modification.

Literacy: Speech–language pathologists help children learn to read and write in several ways: building early speech and language skills to prevent later reading and writing problems; evaluating spoken language, reading, and writing skills and intervening as indicated; providing assistance to teachers and parents; and, conducting research.

Speech–language pathology services in the NICU: as communication, feeding, and swallowing specialists, SLPs may provide the earliest intervention in the NICU. Services include those provided to and for NICU staff, parents, and families of the infants and direct services to neonates in three primary areas: communication evaluation and intervention in the context of developmentally supportive and family focused care; feeding and swallowing evaluation and intervention; and parent/caregiver and staff education.

Upper aerodigestive functions: aeromechanical events related to communication, respiration, and swallowing (e.g., speaking valve selection, respiratory retraining for paradoxical vocal fold motion, stomal stenosis management, and insufflation testing after total laryngectomy).

Telepractice: the wise application of technology to increase patients' access to health care services, while saving costs and time of transportation for patients or clinicians.

◆ Evidence-Based Practice

Under the scrutiny of payers and sophisticated consumers, SLPs increasingly are being challenged to produce published research studies to justify their clinical decisions. "Evidence-based medicine" has evolved to "evidence-based practice" (EBP), and is having a dramatic impact on reimbursement and clinical practice (see Chapter 15 for a full discussion of levels of evidence and the development of practice guidelines). Given the limited number of studies at the highest level of evidence (e.g., randomized controlled trials) across the broad spectrum of disorders and populations in speech–language pathology, SLPs face the possibility of increasing denials of reimbursement for areas of practice where efficacy of treatment is not considered to be definitively established.

In response, ASHA developed policy documents on EBP (ASHA, 2004b, 2005a) and resources that integrate the concepts of EBP in graduate programs and clinical practice and that promote research using clinical trials. ASHA's National Center for Evidence-Based Practice (NCEP) has developed a registry for practice guidelines and is initiating a process for determining the research questions that have the highest priority in influencing policy and reimbursement in speech–language pathology.

◆ Culturally Competent Services

Every clinical interaction involves a cultural exchange between a patient/family and a clinician—an increasingly important reality as the ethnic, cultural, and linguistic makeup of the United States continues to become more and more diverse (**Table 14–3**). U.S. racial and ethnic projections for the years 2000 to 2015 indicate that the percentage of racial/ethnic minorities will increase to over 30% of the total U.S. population (U.S. Bureau of the Census, 2000) (**Table 14–4**).

Given the current and continually increasing cultural and linguistic diversity of the U.S. population, health care practitioners (including SLPs) already are providing and increasingly will provide services to individuals from diverse backgrounds. Recognizing that every clinician has a culture, just as every client/family has a culture, we must ensure that our services are provided in a culturally competent manner to be truly effective (ASHA, 2004d) (**Table 14–5**).

A related cultural reality in the U.S. is the rapidly growing numbers of older persons. According to the U.S. Bureau of the Census (2000), since 1900 the percentage of Americans 65

Table 14–3   Cultural and Linguistic Diversity in the United States

Nearly 1 of every 10 residents in the United States was born outside the U.S. and many speak languages other than a standard version of American English .
There are an estimated 32 million individuals over the age of 5 in the United States today who speak a language other than English at home.
It is anticipated that by 2010, children of immigrants will represent 22% of the school-age population.

From U.S. Bureau of the Census. (2000). *Statistical Abstract of the United States,* 119th ed. Washington, DC: U.S. Department of Commerce.

Table 14–4   U.S. Racial and Ethnic Projections

Racial/Ethnic Minority	Projected Percent of the 2015 U.S. Population	Percent Increase from 2000 to 2015
Hispanics	13.9	67.9
African Americans	13.4	11.9
Asian/Pacific Islanders	5.2	26.4
American Indians	0.9	13.1

From U.S. Bureau of the Census. (2000). *Statistical Abstract of the United States,* 119th ed. Washington, DC: U.S. Department of Commerce

years of age and older has more than tripled (4.1% in 1900 to 12.4% in 2000). The older population itself is getting older. Comparing 2000 to 1900 (U.S. Bureau of the Census, 2000):

◆ 65–74 age group was eight times larger
◆ 75–84 group was 16 times larger
◆ 85+ group was 34 times larger

The older population will continue to grow significantly in the future. By 2030, it is predicted that there will be 70 million older persons, more than twice the number in 2000. Minority populations are projected to represent 25.4% of the elderly population in 2030, up from 16.4% in 2000. Between 1999 and 2030, the white population aged 65+ is projected to increase by 81% compared with 219% for older minorities, including Hispanics (328%), African-Americans (131%), American Indians, Eskimos and Aleuts (147%), and Asians and Pacific Islanders (285%) (U.S. Bureau of the Census, 2000).

◆ Telepractice: The Wise Application of Technology to Clinical Service Delivery

Telepractice, also sometimes referred to as telemedicine, telehealth, or telerehabilitation, represents a growing trend for some health care disciplines, and an emerging trend for speech–language pathology. Potential benefits of telepractice

Table 14–5   Cultural Competence

Delivering Culturally Competent Speech–Language Pathology Services
Culturally competent speech–language pathologists must know:
How the persons in a patient's community communicate to be able to distinguish a communication disorder from a cultural or linguistic difference
About bilingualism, sociolinguistics, and second-language acquisition to make differential diagnoses and develop appropriate treatment plans
How to respectfully determine and provide for the patient/family's cultural beliefs and preferences (e.g., familial decision-making roles; attitudes about Western medicine, illness, disability, pharmacological interventions, technology, etc.
One's own cultural beliefs and biases

From American Speech-Language-Hearing Association. (2004d). *Knowledge and Skills Needed by Speech–Language Pathologists and Audiologists to Provide Culturally and Linguistically Appropriate Services.* http://www.asha.org/members/deskref-journals/deskref/default

include increasing patients' access to health care, including specialty care, while saving costs and time of transportation for patients or clinicians. Although telepractice will not replace face-to-face service delivery, it provides a means to help increase the efficiency and cost-effectiveness of patient care in an era of rising health care costs and staffing challenges.

In 2004, ASHA approved a position statement and technical report in which telepractice was defined as "the application of telecommunications technology to deliver professional services at a distance by linking clinician to client, or clinician to clinician for assessment, intervention, and/or consultation"(ASHA, 2004f,g). Although asserting that telepractice is an appropriate model of service delivery by SLPs, ASHA cautions that the quality of services must be consistent with those delivered in a face-to-face model.

The form of technology most likely to be used by SLPs is a synchronous visual and auditory connection such as videoconferencing. A telepractice session can be conducted over the Internet using a software application and one or more cameras and a microphone for the computer at each site. Stand-alone videoconferencing units offer an even simpler way of connecting patients and clinicians. An additional factor to consider is the bandwidth of the connection between the two sites. Narrower bandwidths such as telephone lines may provide slower and more limited transmissions, whereas digital connections such as DSL or ISDN offer faster and better image quality. The different connections must be evaluated in terms of cost and availability in different regions. Hospitals or schools that have already established networks may be able to deliver SLP services more readily because the technology and connectivity are being used by other disciplines as well. The privacy and security of the connection must also be protected.

Pioneering efforts by several SLPs have contributed to a growing body of knowledge about selecting appropriate patients for telepractice; training the patients, caregivers, or paraprofessionals to set up and utilize the technology; and types of interventions and disorders that best lend themselves to remote service delivery (ASHA, 2005d). Published studies describe current applications and research on telepractice by SLPs, including the area of voice (Mashima, Birkmire-Peters, Syms, Holtel, Burgess, & Peters, 2003), cognitive-communication for individuals with brain injuries (Brennan, Georgeadis, Baron & Barker, 2004; Georgeadis, Brennan, Baron & Barker, 2004), and instrumental swallowing studies (Perlman & Witthawaskul, 2002).

Significant expansion of telepractice in speech–language pathology depends on coverage by Medicare, Medicaid, and private insurers, as well as clarification of issues such as licensure, ethics, and training.

✦ Reimbursement

Speech–language pathologists and all other clinical practitioners in health care settings today need to be familiar with current models of health care reimbursement: Medicare, Medicaid, and private health plans. Medicare often serves as a model or foundation for the other reimbursement systems, so it is particularly important to be well versed in Medicare fundamentals.

Medicare

Medicare was created by the U.S. Congress in 1965 to provide acute care coverage for the nation's elderly (i.e., 62 years of age

and older). Over the years, it has grown into a complex program with variations in eligibility criteria and coverage policies depending on the type of health care setting (e.g., acute care, rehab unit or hospital, SNF, home health) in which the services are delivered. Medicare Part A, also known as Hospital Insurance Benefits for the Aged and Disabled, covers the first 90 days of an inpatient hospital stay, the first 100 days of a stay in an SNF, and the first 100 home health visits following a hospital or SNF stay. Social security beneficiaries receive Medicare Part A coverage at no additional cost. Medicare Part B, Supplemental Insurance Benefits, covers certain services or settings such as physician office visits, outpatient speech–language pathology, occupational therapy, physical therapy, and diagnostic audiology. Medicare Part B also covers inpatient services rendered after patients have exhausted their Part A days/visits and certain durable medical equipment (DME), such as augmentative and alternative communication devices (or, in Medicare terminology, "speech-generating devices") and wheelchairs. Under Medicare Part B coverage, a beneficiary is required to make a 20% co-pay to the provider of the services. Medicare Part B benefits are optional; to receive them, a Social Security beneficiary must pay a monthly premium (ASHA, 2004e).

Medicare is administered by the Centers for Medicare and Medicaid Services (CMS), an agency of the U.S. Department of Health and Human Services (DHHS). Medicare Part A claims are processed by fiscal intermediaries. Claims for Part B are processed either by carriers or fiscal intermediaries [i.e., regional entities contracted by Medicare that are being transitioned into regional Medicare administrative contractors (MACs)]. Coverage variations may exist among fiscal intermediaries and carriers from different regions. For example, some fiscal intermediaries (FIs) require that an instrumental swallowing assessment be performed when pharyngeal dysphagia is suspected; other FIs do not.

As payments to Medicare ballooned over the years, major cost-containment changes were put into place. In the 1980s diagnosis-related groups (DRGs) were implemented to control Medicare reimbursement for acute hospital stays. A single payment amount is allocated to each DRG based on the average cost associated with a hospital stay for that diagnosis. Factors that influence the cost include typical length of stay for the specific illness (e.g., pneumonia) or procedure (e.g., appendectomy), nature of services required, and cost of supplies. Hospitals break even or make money if they manage the patient's care efficiently and are able to discharge the patient by or before the anticipated length of stay associated with a particular DRG. When a patient experiences complications or inefficient coordination of care that leads to a longer or more costly stay, the hospital loses money. Diagnoses involving rehabilitation services were not included under DRGs, as there was insufficient data at the time to predict their cost accurately.

Further concern about growing Medicare expenditures led Congress to pass the Balanced Budget Act (BBA) of 1997 and the subsequent Balanced Budget Refinement Act (BBRA) and the Benefits Improvement and Protection Act (BIPA). The BBA introduced several cost-containment methodologies that affected rehabilitation services: prospective payment systems, the Medicare fee schedule, and therapy caps.

Medicare Prospective Payment Systems

The BBA mandated the expansion of the DRG cost-controlling concept for Medicare Part A services into other health care

Table 14–6   Medicare Prospective Payment Systems (PPS)

Health Care Setting	Name of PPS System	Payment Determined by	Time Frame Covered by Payment	Assessment Tool	Impact on Speech–Language Pathology Services
Hospitals	Diagnostic-related groups (DGRs)	Diagnosis category (rehab not included)	Length of stay	n/a	Shortened length of stay; heightened focus on assessment and acute intervention
Rehabilitation hospitals and rehabilitation units in hospitals	Inpatient Rehabilitation Facilities Prospective Payment System (IRF PPS)	Rehabilitation impairment categories (RICs) Case mix groups (CMGs)	Length of stay	IRF Payment Assessment Instrument (PAI)	Implemented in 2001; impact appears to be variable by facility
Skilled nursing facilities	Skilled Nursing Facilities Prospective Payment System (SNF PPS) (Part A = first 100 days of Medicare coverage)	Resource utilization groups (RUGS)	Daily rate	Minimum data set (MDS)	Need to negotiate with occupation therapy and physical therapy for allocation of minutes
	Part B = after first 100 days of Medicare coverage)	Medicare fee schedule (MFS)	Per procedure code	n/a	Establishes charge for each procedure; services may be limited by therapy cap or alternate cost containment methods
Home health care	Prospective payment system for home health agencies	Health resources groups (HRGs)	60-day episode of care	Outcome and Assessment Information Set (OASIS)	Home health agency receives increased reimbursement when rehab services are provided; efficient use of visits will be stressed
Outpatient	Outpatient Prospective Payment System (OPPS)	Ambulatory patient classifications (APCs) (not applicable to speech–language pathology services, which use the Medicare fee schedule)	Per procedure code	n/a	Not applicable to speech–language pathologists

From *Business Matters: A Guide for Speech–Language Pathologists*. ASHA, 2004. Copyright American Speech–Language-Hearing Association, with permission.

settings. The first setting the PPS system was implemented for was SNFs in 1998. Using a tool called the minimum data set (MDS) that gathers information about the level of care and services an individual needs, each patient fits in one of 53 categories called resource utilization groups (RUGs). Patients in need of intensive rehabilitation (i.e., more than 45 minutes per week) are assigned to one of 14 rehabilitation-specific RUG categories; in 2006 there will be nine additional categories for rehabilitation plus extensive services. Medicare pays the SNF a flat daily rate based on the patient's RUG, which covers all daily care and professional services, including speech–language pathology and other rehabilitation services. The maximum RUG category requires a minimum of 720 minutes of rehabilitation (i.e., speech–language pathology, occupational therapy, and/or physical therapy) per week. Instead of billing rehabilitation services as separate or additional services, SNFs now must provide Medicare Part A patients with all necessary care in exchange for the daily reimbursement rate established by the patient's RUG category. In the SNF PPS arena, rehabilitation professionals must negotiate to divide up the number of rehab minutes associated with the patient's RUG category in a manner that will best meet each patient's needs. The number of minutes of services provided each week must be carefully tracked to meet or exceed the number required by the patient's RUG category.

In the years following the implementation of PPS in SNFs, PPSs for Medicare Part A patients have also been implemented in home health care and inpatient rehabilitation facilities. Each is different, and each places unique constraints on the service delivery, documentation, and reimbursement in the particular setting (**Table 14–6**). Similarities exist among settings, such as using screening tools typically administered by nurses [e.g., Outcome and Assessment Information Set (OASIS) in home health; Inpatient Rehabilitation Facilities Payment Assessment Instrument (IRF PAI) in rehabilitation] to place patients into categories by medical complexity and need for services (e.g., home health resource groups in home health; rehabilitation impairment categories/case mix groups in rehabilitation). A key difference is that Medicare reimburses for Part A home care and rehabilitation services in a lump sum for an entire length of stay, similar to DRGs, whereas SNFs are reimbursed by a daily rate.

Regardless of the setting, PPS has heightened the emphasis on (1) shortened length of stay and the efficiency of services, and (2) achieving functional outcomes that facilitate discharge to the next (less costly) setting. In the PPS model, SLPs and other rehabilitation professionals no longer generate income for the facility by billing for their services on a fee-for-service basis, so they have to demonstrate the value their services contribute to the patient's functional improvement. This places a premium on reduced evaluation/assessment time and streamlined documentation that clearly demonstrates the medical necessity and functional benefit of the services provided.

Medicare Fee Schedule and Therapy Caps

The Medicare fee schedule (MFS) has been in existence and applied to physician services since the early 1990s. The Balanced Budget Act of 1997 made the MFS also apply to Medicare Part B rehabilitation services. In essence, the MFS establishes a set charge for a given rehab procedure, eliminating the longstanding previous Medicare Part B reimbursement model for rehab services that allowed for "usual and customary" rates. Under the MFS, charges are based on the Resource-Based Relative Value Scale (RBRVS), which assigns a total relative value unit (RVU) to each procedure performed. Each billable procedure is assigned a Common Procedural Terminology (CPT) code (described later in this chapter). Factors considered in establishing the RVU of a procedure include the amount of work (time, technical skill, physical effort, stress, and judgment); overhead costs; and professional liability costs. The RBRVS allows for geographic adjustments and is adjusted annually.

The Balanced Budget Act of 1997 also introduced a $1500 therapy cap as a means for controlling Part B costs for rehabilitation services in all settings except hospital outpatient departments. Under the provision of the BBA, each Medicare Part B beneficiary was eligible to receive Medicare coverage annually of up to a maximum of $1500 for (combined) speech–language pathology and physical therapy services, and a maximum of a separate $1500 for occupational therapy services. If beneficiaries exceeded the cap within a calendar year, they could transfer to a hospital outpatient site or choose to pay for the services out-of-pocket. The cap engendered strong resistance from beneficiary and therapy groups on the basis of the potential limitation of benefits to individuals in SNFs and to those with severe conditions whose rehabilitation needs could not be met with such limitations. Since the passage of the BBA, the caps have only been implemented for a short period of time, in 1999 and for several months in 2003. Alternatives to the cap are being proposed for 2006, when the cap will otherwise go back in effect. **Table 14–7** summarizes the impact of these strategies on clinical practice.

Table 14–7 Differential Impact of Balanced Budget Act Cost Containment Strategies

Medicare fee schedule: results in payment limitations on a per-session/ visit/procedure that are likely to result in:

  Decreased reimbursement to the provider for each visit/ session/ procedure

  Increased emphasis on clinical efficiency

  Increased emphasis on "billable" (versus "nonbillable") clinical time (i.e., productivity) to meet revenue requirements

Outpatient therapy cap: imposed coverage limitations on a per-patient basis that resulted in:

  Fewer sessions per patient

  Out-of-pocket costs to patients/family members to fund additional services needed beyond those that are covered

  Increased emphasis on clinical efficiency

  Increased competition among rehab disciplines for limited dollars/treatment time

Other Medicare Programs

The BBA also created Part C, or the Medicare Advantage program. The program provides Medicare beneficiaries new options to receive Part A and Part B coverage through a variety of plans such as health maintenance organizations, preferred provider organizations, etc. Part D is a new prescription benefit program that began in 2006.

Medicaid

Title XIX of the Social Security Act, Medicaid, was also created by Congress in 1965. It provides medical assistance for individuals and families with low incomes. Medicaid is jointly funded by the federal and state governments to assist states in the provision of adequate medical care to eligible needy persons. To receive federal matching funds, certain basic services must be offered to the categorically needy population in any state Medicaid program [e.g., inpatient hospital services; physician services; early and periodic screening, diagnosis, and treatment (EPSDT) services for individuals under age 21]. The federal government establishes broad national Medicaid guidelines. Each state in turn establishes its own eligibility standards; determines the type, amount, duration, and scope of services; sets the rate of payment for services; and administers its own program. As a result, Medicaid programs vary considerably from state to state in terms of coverage and payment policies. Federally, Medicaid is also administered by the Centers for Medicare and Medicaid Services. At the state level, it is typically administered through the state department of health.

Private Health Plans

In addition to the government-funded programs of Medicare and Medicaid, there are hundreds of private health plans. These are typically insurance companies to which a premium is paid by an individual or on behalf of the individual (e.g., by an employer) for a negotiated set of health benefits. A few of the larger private health plans include Aetna, Blue Cross/Blue Shield, CIGNA, Mutual of Omaha, and Travelers. Each of these companies in turn typically offers dozens of different plans, based on the nature and amount of the services offered, which in turn affects the amount of the premium to be paid. The two basic types of plans are either traditional indemnity fee-for-service plans, in which the health plan pays the provider a fee after the service was given, or managed care organizations, which have various forms (ASHA, 2005b).

Managed care organizations (MCOs) manage, or control, their health care costs by closely monitoring how providers treat their patients by evaluating the necessity, appropriateness, and efficiency of services (**Table 14–8** describes the types of MCOs). Managed care demonstrated a phenomenal rate of growth during the 1990s. With a focus on the "bottom line," MCOs may be more interested in "buying your outcomes" than "paying for your services." To survive in such an environment, clinical providers need to be able to prove the value of their services in measurable, meaningful, and preferably cost-savings terms. Although theoretically the patients are ultimately responsible for knowing what is and is not covered by their health plan, this is typically not something they think about until they need the services. Thus, it is in the facility's and health care provider's

Table 14–8 Managed Care

Types of Managed Care Organizations (MCO)
Health maintenance organization (HMO) The oldest type of MCO. HMOs offer comprehensive coverage for hospital and health care practitioner services for a prepaid, fixed fee. They employ or contract with participating health care practitioners (e.g., hospitals, physicians, and other practitioners). HMO members are either assigned to or may be able to choose among those providers for their health care needs. Visits to specialists usually require authorization by a primary care provider. The majority of HMOs are "federally qualified." Federally qualified HMOs are required to provide a minimum of 2 months or 60 visits (whichever is more) per condition for a combination of speech–language pathology, occupational therapy, and physical therapy services, if significant improvement can be expected within 2 months. Additional benefits are often offered by the HMO, depending on the plan purchased by the individual member or by the group through which the individual is covered.
Preferred provider organization (PPO): A health care benefit arrangement designed to supply services at an affordable cost to the employer by providing incentives to use designated health care providers who contract with the PPO at a discount. Financial incentives for enrollees to use preferred providers include lower co-payments or co-insurance and maximum limits on out-of-pocket costs for in-network use. Individuals who are enrolled in a PPO are also covered for services provided by practitioners who are outside of the PPO network, but at a higher out-of-pocket rate. Visits to specialists usually do not require authorization by a primary care provider. Most PPOs involve an arrangement between a panel or group of providers and the purchasers of care (e.g., employers or insurance companies). The group of providers agrees to a specified fee schedule in exchange for preferred status and is required to comply with certain utilization review guidelines.
Point of service (POS): These options combine HMO features and out-of-network coverage, with economic incentives for using network providers. Out-of-network coverage usually has a per-person cap or limit. The out-of-network providers are usually compensated on a fee-for-service basis, in which the health plan reimburses them for each procedure performed.

best interest to verify the eligibility and coverage requirements specific to their services (within their type of setting and geographic area) with each patient's health plan. Such requirements may include a variety of factors (**Table 14–9**).

Coding

Reimbursement relies on universally accepted coding systems that record the patient's diagnosis and the service that was provided. International Classification of Diseases (ICD) codes are developed by the World Health Organization and are used to identify the diseases or conditions that have caused a referral for treatment, including the patient's primary medical diagnosis (e.g., stroke, 437.1), other chronic conditions (e.g., hypertension, 401.0; diabetes, 250.0), and resulting conditions (e.g., aphasia, 784.3; dysphagia, 787.2; right hemiparesis, 438.21) (AMA, 2005a). If the ICD codes do not reflect a diagnosis associated with the treatment being provided, payment may be denied. For example, payers used to deny claims for swallowing evaluations for patients whose only diagnosis was postpolio syndrome, until published studies confirmed the increased incidence of swallowing problems in patients who had suffered polio many years earlier.

Current Procedural Terminology (CPT) codes are developed and owned by the American Medical Association with input from various professional groups (AMA, 2005b). The payer decides which codes it will reimburse and sets a payment rate for each code. The Medicare fee schedule often serves as a baseline for developing rates for other payers. Examples of CPT codes for speech–language pathology services include 92506 for speech–language evaluation and 92507 for speech–language treatment. There are also specific CPT codes for dysphagia, augmentative and alternative communication devices (called speech-generating devices) and services, for group (versus individual) treatment, and others.

✦ Health Insurance Portability and Accountability Act (HIPAA)

The Health Insurance Portability and Accountability Act (HIPAA) is a federal law that has large impact on health care facilities and providers. The Administration Simplification portion of HIPAA requires providers to comply with requirements for three different provisions: electronic data interchange (EDI), security, and privacy. The intent of these regulations is to protect patient confidentiality in exchanges that occur during electronic billing or sharing of patient information, and to increase awareness and security of conversations and information about the patient within and between facilities. SLPs in private practice are most directly affected by the EDI regulations; however, all SLPs and other health care providers who are covered entities need to be aware of and abide by the privacy regulations of HIPAA. Health care providers also need to be familiar with any related privacy requirements at the state level and make sure that they are complying with whichever of the two—federal or state law—is the most stringent.

HIPAA applies to covered entities (**Table 14–10**) that turn health data into electronic form or exchange information

Table 14–9 Examples of Private Health Plan Requirements

Referral: Although speech–language pathologists are autonomous practitioners and can legally make their own decisions regarding the need for, nature of, and amount of services, many payers require that a physician or other approved source such as a or case manager provide a referral.
Assessment: Payers often reimburse for only a single diagnostic or evaluation session. The results of the assessment must demonstrate the need for intervention and project the length, type, and functional benefit of those services.
Coverage exclusions: When there is a chronic or deteriorating condition such as multiple sclerosis or Alzheimer's disease, clinicians are often required to clearly indicate what change has occurred to warrant assessment and treatment; private health plans often exclude coverage of developmental disorders.
Coverage limitations: Many private payers have set limits for the number or duration of visits or services.

Table 14–10 Health Insurance Portability and Accountability Act (HIPAA) Covered Entities

Health Plans
Health care providers: transmit health information in electronic form
Health care clearinghouses: public or private entities that process health information received from another entity (e.g., billing companies, community health management information systems)

Table 14–11   HIPAA Protected Health Information (PHI)

Protected health information includes patient demographics and information that is:
Collected from an individual
Created by or received from a health care provider, health plan, employer or clearinghouse
Related to a past, present, or future physical or mental health or condition
Related to the provision or payment of health care
Identifies an individual or could be reasonably used to identify the individual
Transmitted or maintained in any form or medium (electronic, paper, or oral).

electronically. The HIPAA privacy provisions specify certain individually identifiable health information (**Table 14–11**) as protected health information (PHI). Permitted uses and disclosures of PHI include to the patient; to carry out treatment; for payment or health care operations (also referred to as T-P-O); pursuant to a valid authorization; by agreement of the patient; and as permitted or required by certain other laws (e.g., judicial proceedings, disease reporting requirements). Under HIPAA, except for certain limited circumstances, health care providers with a direct treatment relationship with patients are required to make a good faith effort to obtain a written acknowledgment from the patients that they received the provider's Notice of Privacy Practices.

The HIPAA security rule sets standards for limiting access to PHI only to those who should have access. These standards include administrative, physical, and technical safeguards (**Table 14–12**).

✦ Conclusion

Given the current and ever-emerging complexities of the health care workplace, it is imperative that SLPs be well versed in specific areas of clinical knowledge related to the population(s) served in health care settings as well as health care reimbursement and regulatory realities, and that they possess key workplace attributes that will enable them to thrive and to be highly effective and highly valued contributors in the health care workplace. (Further information about the issues covered in this chapter is available at the Web sites and sources listed in **Table 14–13.**) Providing speech–language pathology services in health care settings is challenging, stimulating, rewarding, and fulfilling. Thousands of individuals each day are able to communicate better, swallow more safely, and interact more successfully and independently with those around them as a result of the expertise and dedication of SLPs. Welcome to this exciting arena!

Table 14–12   HIPAA Security Rule

Administrative safeguards: assigning responsibility for security and training an individual within the facility
Physical safeguards: the mechanisms by which information is protected (e.g., passwords, off-site computer backups)
Technical safeguards: processes used to protect information, including encryption and verification of authority to access data

Table 14–13   Sources of Further Information

Web Sites	Topics
American Speech–Language-Hearing Association (ASHA) www.asha.org	SLP Practice Policy Documents
	Code of Ethics; Scope of Practice for SLP; Preferred Practice Patterns
	Knowledge and Skills in Business Practices Needed by SLPs in Health Care Settings
	Multiskilled Personnel
	Role of SLPs in Literacy, in the NICU
	SLPs Training and Supervising Other Professions in the Delivery of Services to Individuals with Swallowing and Feeding Disorders
	Telepractice
	HIPAA
	Multicultural Resources: culturally competent services, bilingual services, working with interpreters
	Reimbursement: Medicare, Medicaid, Private Health Plans
	Telepractice: report, survey, resources
Centers for Medicare and Medicaid (CMS) www.cms.hhs.gov	Medicare
	Medicaid
	HIPAA
American Telemedicine Association (ATA) www.american-telemed.org	Telehealth: conferences, publications, products, policy
Association of Telehealth Service Providers (ATSP) www.atsp.org	Telehealth: industry news, government news, business resources
Office for the Advancement of Telehealth (OAT) telehealth.hrsa.gov	Telehealth: services, publications, grants
U.S. Bureau of the Census www.census.gov	Demographic statistics and trends
Source	**Products**
American Speech–Language-Hearing Association 800–498–2071 – Action Center www.asha.org	Appealing Health Plan Denials
	Business Matters: A Guide for Speech–Language Pathologists
	Getting Your Services Covered: A Guide for Working with Insurance and Managed Care Plans
	Guidelines for Referral to Speech–Language Pathologists
	Guide to Speech–Language Pathology Assessment for Multicultural and Bilingual Populations
	Guide to Successful Private Practice in Speech–Language Pathology
	Guide to Verifying Competencies in Speech–Language Pathology
	Health Plan Coding and Claims Guide
	Let's Talk Health Care: Patient Education Illustrations and Handouts
	Medicare Handbook for Speech–Language Pathologists
	Mind Your Business Marketing Kits
	M-Power Box: The Power of One
	A Practical Guide to Applying Treatment Outcomes and Efficacy Resources
	Various Posters and Brochures

Study Questions

1. Select two core skills that would be important to develop to meet productivity requirements and describe your rationale.

2. Describe how the SLP's scope of practice has changed over the years and what have been the driving forces behind those changes.

3. Describe three ways in which the U.S. population is becoming more diverse; cite statistics to support your examples.

4. Describe a hypothetical patient (e.g., diagnosis, communication disorder(s), personal circumstances) and the services that could be delivered via telepractice that would benefit this patient.

5. What are the key differences among Medicare Part A, Medicare Part B, and Medicaid?

6. Describe two new reimbursement cost containment methodologies that were introduced by the Balanced Budget Act of 1997 and how they impact the delivery of speech–language pathology services.

7. Describe the difference between fee-for-service and the current reimbursement mechanism for one of the Medicare prospective payment systems and state how the change has affected SLPs.

8. What does CPT in "CPT Code" stand for and how are the CPTs' relative values determined?

References

American Medical Association. (2005a). *AMA Physician ICD-9-CM 2005.* Atlanta, GA: AMA Press

American Medical Association. (2005b). *CPT 2005 Standard Edition.* Atlanta, GA: AMA Press

American Speech-Language-Hearing Association. (1997, Spring). Position Statement and Technical Report: Multiskilled Personnel. http://www.asha.org/members/deskref-journals/deskref/default

American Speech-Language-Hearing Association. (2001). *Scope of Practice in Speech–Language Pathology.* Rockville, MD: ASHA

American Speech-Language-Hearing Association. (2003a). Code of Ethics (Revised). *ASHA Supplement, 23,* 13–15

American Speech-Language-Hearing Association. (2003b). Knowledge and Skills in Business Practices Needed by Speech–Language Pathologists in Health Care Settings. *ASHA Supplement, 23,* 87–92

American Speech-Language-Hearing Association. (2004a). *Business Matters: A Guide for Speech–Language Pathologists.* Rockville, MD: ASHA

American Speech-Language-Hearing Association. (2004b). *Evidence-Based Practice in Communication Disorders: An Introduction* [Technical report]. http://www.asha.org/members/deskref-journals/deskref/default

American Speech-Language-Hearing Association. (2004c). Knowledge and Skills in Business Practices for Speech–Language Pathologists Who Are Managers and Leaders in Health Care Organizations. *ASHA Supplement, 24,* 146–151

American Speech-Language-Hearing Association. (2004d). *Knowledge and Skills Needed by Speech–Language Pathologists and Audiologists to Provide Culturally and Linguistically Appropriate Services.* http://www.asha.org/members/deskref-journals/deskref/default

American Speech-Language-Hearing Association. (2004e). *Medicare Handbook for Speech–Language Pathologists.* Rockville, MD: ASHA

American Speech-Language-Hearing Association. (2004f). *Speech–Language Pathologists Providing Services Via Telepractice: Position Statement.* http://www.asha.org/members/deskref-journals/deskref/default

American Speech-Language-Hearing Association. (2004g). *Speech–Language Pathologists Providing Services Via Telepractice: Technical Report.* http://www.asha.org/members/deskref-journals/deskref/default

American Speech-Language-Hearing Association. (2004h). Speech–Language Pathologists Training and Supervising Other Professionals in the Delivery of Services to Individuals with Swallowing and Feeding Disorders: Position Statement. *ASHA Supplement, 24,* 62

American Speech-Language-Hearing Association. (2004i). Speech–Language Pathologists Training and Supervising Other Professionals in the Delivery of Services to Individuals with Swallowing and Feeding Disorders: Position Statement. *ASHA Supplement, 24,* 131–134

American Speech-Language-Hearing Association. (2005a). Evidence-Based Practice in Communication Disorders [Position statement]. http://www.asha.org/members/deskrefjournals/deskref/default

American Speech-Language-Hearing Association. (2005b). *Health Plan Coding and Claims Guide,* rev. ed. Rockville, MD: ASHA

American Speech-Language-Hearing Association. (2005c). *Highlights and Trends: ASHA Counts for 2004.* Accessed September 22, 2005. http://www.asha.org/about/membership-certification/member-data/member-counts.htm

American Speech-Language-Hearing Association. (2005d). *Knowledge and Skills Needed by Speech–Language Pathologists Providing Clinical Services Via Telepractice.* http://www.asha.org/members/deskref-journals/deskref/default

American Speech-Language-Hearing Association. (2005e). *SLP Health Care Survey 2005: Frequency Report.* Rockville, MD: ASHA

American Speech-Language-Hearing Association Council on Professional Standards in Speech–language Pathology and Audiology. (2000). *Standards and Implementation for the Certificate of Clinical Competence in Speech–Language Pathology.* Rockville, MD: ASHA

Banja, J.D. (1994). Ethics, Outcomes, and Reimbursement. *REHAB Management, 7(1),* 61–65, 136

Brennan, D.M., Georgeadis, A.C., Baron, C.R., & Barker, L.M. (2004). The Effect of Videoconference-Based Telerehab on Story Retelling Performance by Brain Injured Subjects and Its Implication for Remote Speech–Language Therapy. *Telemedicine and e-Health, 10(2),* 147–154

Georgeadis, A.C., Brennan, D.M., Barker, L.M., & Baron, C.R. (2004). Telerehabilitation and Its Effect on Story Retelling by Adults with Neurogenic Impairments. *Aphasiology, 18(5,6,7),* 639–652

Mashima, P., Birkmire-Peters, D., Syms, M., Holtel, M., Burgess, L., & Peters, L. (2003). Telehealth: Voice Therapy Using Telecommunications Technology. *American Journal of Speech–Language Pathology, 12,* 432–439

Perlman, A.L. & Witthawaskul, W. (2002). Real-Time Remote Telefluoroscopic Assessment of Patients with Dysphagia. *Dysphagia, 17,* 162–167

Rosenfeld, M. (2002). *Report on the ASHA Speech–Language Pathology Health Care Survey.* Rockville, MD: ASHA

U.S. Bureau of the Census. (2000). *Statistical Abstract of the United States,* 119th ed. Washington, DC: U.S. Department of Commerce

15

Evidence-Based Practice and Outcome Oriented Approaches in Speech–Language Pathology

Carol M. Frattali and Lee Ann Golper

- ✦ Current Requirements
- ✦ Evidence-Based Practice
- ✦ Outcomes Assessment: Definitions, Measures, and Methods
- ✦ Program Evaluation
- ✦ Using Outcomes Data for Decision Making

From an evidence-based perspective, it is fair to say that quality of care should be linked robustly to scientific evidence of its efficacy (in the laboratory sense) and effectiveness (in the clinic sense). Treatment efficacy studies provide evidence of cause and effect because stringent research controls must be in place to prevent any spurious intervening effects. Treatment effectiveness studies, however, although not providing evidence of cause and effect, nonetheless provide evidence related to outcome trends as well as associations of the treatment process with the outcome(s), and lend support to the findings of treatment efficacy studies. Thus, both laboratory and clinic work merge the ideal and real-world environments to amass sound collective evidence that what speech–language pathologists do makes a difference in the lives of persons with communication, swallowing, and related disorders.

From the introductory statement of this chapter, one can conjecture that only an evidence-based approach would result in optimal outcomes, and this is the approach taken here. This chapter begins with a discussion of the research-supported or evidence-based practices and clinical practice guidelines as the starting point for outcomes-oriented intervention. From there we explore the current accreditation and payer requirements that are driving the need for outcomes-oriented approaches, offer definitions and a conceptual model of patient outcomes and their measurement, and suggest ways in which outcomes data can be used for decision making.

✦ Current Requirements

The enterprise of health care today, given the choices of health plans and the active participation of consumers in making these choices, begs the question, "Whom do health care providers need to satisfy?" There would be little argument that, foremost, providers need to satisfy their patients by meeting their individual needs. Second, providers need to satisfy payers and regulators who have the tough job of managing limited resources. These parties, particularly in managed care environments, are largely responsible for the decisions surrounding provision of both effective and efficient care. In large measure, they determine what services will be provided to whom, by whom, in what setting, for how long, and at what cost. Their interest is in getting the best for the dollars spent. Thus, the primary measure of health care is in determining its value (good care at a low cost).

Particularly noteworthy, in terms consistent with a common mindset among payers, is a quotation from a payer who addressed an audience of rehabilitation professionals at a national meeting (Evidence-Based Medicine Working Group, 1992):

> If I (the buyer of care) give you (the provider of care) X dollars, I get one point on a functional status measure. If other providers can give me two points after the same treatment time, I'll buy from them. I'm a buyer. I want to get more for my money. I am paying you to maximize the level of independence.

What this buyer was seeking was, in his words, a "quantitative measure of a qualitative product" (i.e., rehabilitative services). Thus, functional status measures have become important among many payers because they speak in meaningful terms (e.g., levels of independence in daily life activities) and translate into dollars saved by suggesting the need of fewer health care resources as the patient's independence level increases. This cost perspective, which favors functional status as a desired or expected outcome of medical rehabilitation, is reflected in several important accreditation agency standards and payer guidelines (**Table 15–1**).

Table 15–1   Examples of Accreditation Agency and Payer Requirements

	Excerpts from Requirements/Guidelines
	Assessment of Patient Function (PE): "The goal of the patient assessment-function is to determine what kind of care is required to meet a patient's initial needs as well as his or her needs as they change in response to care" (p. 89).
	PE 1.3: Functional status is assessed when warranted by the patient's needs or condition. PE 1.3.1: All patients referred to rehabilitation services receive a functional assessment.
CARF, The Rehabilitation Accreditation Commission	Principle 4: Based on the informed choices of the persons served, the organization, using a team approach, provides coordinated, individualized, goal-oriented services leading to desired outcomes.
	Accreditation criterion 3: The organization meets the policy on outcomes.
	The organization should demonstrate that systems are in place to measure outcomes including effectiveness, efficiency, satisfaction of persons served, and status of the persons served after discharge (follow-up). These outcome measures should be in place for all programs for which the organization is seeking accreditation. The organization should demonstrate the utilization of outcome information throughout its planning activities. This information should be provided to the persons served, personnel, payers, and if requested, CARF.
American Speech–Language-Hearing Association's Professional Services Board	Standard 3.0 Performance Improvement and Program Evaluation
	Implementation:
	b. There is evidence that the program uses clinical outcomes that focus on meaningful changes in communication functions, such as measures of self-perceived hearing and balance functions and measures of function in speech, language, voice, and swallowing.
	c. The performance improvement process periodically addresses all areas of clinical practice, with particular attention to services that are high volume, that carry added risk, or that evidence problems.
	i. Patient/client evaluation or treatment outcomes are emphasized. These may include, but are not limited to, identification of disorder, acceptance of recommendations, functional change in status, and patient/client/family satisfaction.
Medicare: Intermediary Manual Part 3—Claims Process	Progress reports. Obtain:
	The initial functional communication level of the patient.
	The present functional level of the patient and progress. The medical reviewer may approve the claim if there is still a reasonable expectation that significant improvement in the patient's overall functional ability will occur. The speech–language pathologist may choose how to demonstrate progress. However, the method chosen and the measures used generally remain the same for the duration of treatment. The provider must interpret reports of test scores or comparable measures and their relationship to functional goals.
Medicare: Outpatient Rehabilitation Services Forms 700 (Plan of Care and Assessment) and 701 (Updated Plan of Care and Patient Progress)	Form 700 requires an initial assessment detailing the level of function at the start of care, and documentation of functional goals. Also requires documentation of the patient's functional level at the end of the billing.
	Form 701 requires an update of functional goals and a statement of functional level at the end of each billing period as compared with the previous month or initial assessment.

From Joint Commission on Accreditation of Healthcare Organizations.

Accreditation agencies and payers continue to emphasize the use of outcome measures, particularly for assessing functional status and patient satisfaction, to document the benefits of treatment. The requirements specify that these outcome measures should be used for comparative purposes (i.e., for comparing patient progress to baseline performance or one program's performance to another's). They do not, however, dictate which specific measures or methods should be used. These decisions are left to the practitioners who must identify, from the wide array of measures and methods available, the most appropriate for their particular patient populations and in their particular health care settings.

✦ Evidence-Based Practice

Referencing Empirical Evidence

The cornerstone of outcomes-oriented practice in medical speech–language pathology is empirical evidence. Empirical evidence allows us to determine if a given intervention is, in the first place, the right thing to do, and second, if the intervention is leading to the intended outcome. Making clinical decisions with reference to empirical evidence is called *evidence-based practice* (EBP), which is a generic term referring to the application of empirical evidence, along with clinical experience and expertise, to decision making in day-to-day clinical practice. In this section we discuss some of the basic principles of EBP. We look at the development of clinical practice guidelines (CPGs) as a natural outgrowth and consequence of EBP. We look at some of the points of departure between some proponents of EBP and the development of CPGs. Finally, we consider how various forms of empirical evidence, ranging from randomized control trials to our own clinical data, provide a reference upon which to base clinical decisions.

Origins

The roots of EBP come from a movement within medicine in the early 1990s, largely emanating from the Evidence-Based Medicine (EBM) Working Group led by Guyatt and his colleagues at

McMaster University in Canada, and then expanded further by Sackett, Rosenberg, Muir-Gray, Haynes, and Richardson (1996) through an affiliation and collaboration between McMaster University and Oxford University in the United Kingdom. It should be noted the stage had been set for a developmental base for EBM within the U.K., as the notions of EBM were aligned well with an established doctrine introduced in 1972 by British epidemiologist Archie Cochrane. Cochrane's (1972) landmark article on efficacy and effectiveness was well known in the medical community and the U.K.'s National Health Service. The use of epidemiologic data to guide decisions about the use of limited resources in health care was already a matter of public policy. Cochrane was one of the first to promote the use of randomized controlled trials (RCT), systematic reviews, and meta-analyses of medical research findings to evaluate existing and new treatment methods. He reasoned that resources would always lag behind the demand for health care services; consequently, research principles should be applied to inform decisions about treatment effects, side effects, risks and benefits, test selection in diagnosis, prognosis, and so forth. Over the course of little more than a decade, there has been an explosion of journal articles on the topics of EBM and EBP. There are now several journals solely devoted to the topic, and a networked clearinghouse for EBP has developed, the Cochran Collaboration, with centers in the U.K., North and South America, Africa, Asia, and Australia (Trinder & Reynolds, 2000).

Doing the Right Things Right

The basic notions of EBP come from clinical epidemiology. The field of clinical epidemiology seeks to apply data to achieve rational decision making in health care delivery. Epidemiologists examine and analyze data from populations (biostatistics) to determine how and where resources should be used for the best possible outcome, or "doing the right things right" (Muir-Gray, 1997). Doing the right things right is something we all seek, but it is especially important in a climate of heightened concern about excessive health care costs. This growing preoccupation with increasing cost and limited or decreasing resources, coupled with other factors such as widespread international access to electronic literature searches, good support for biomedical research in the United States, and consumer demand for consistent standards and reduced variations in the quality of care between providers, has caused many heath care disciplines to look to empirical evidence to find support for their interventions, and determine the most efficacious, effective, and efficient ways to deliver care. In addition to these political, economic and technological influences, Lohr, Eleazer, and Mauskoph (1998) suggest that a basic lack of training and sophistication in research methods among average clinicians in medicine and other disciplines has led them to look to experts for critiques and interpretation of research literature in their daily practices. Although the initial impetus behind EBM was aimed at an application of biostatistics and epidemiologic principles to physician practices, these same principles are now being applied in other health care as well as non–health care disciplines, and EBP is also of interest to policy makers, payers, and patients.

Research-Based Clinical Practice Guidelines

Clinical practice guidelines (CPGs) are formal conclusions and recommendations reached after expert reviews of the *available* best evidence (Lohr et al., 1998). Guidelines are developed and implemented with an eye toward changing practice patterns and eliminating untested/unproven assessment or treatment procedures, and standardizing the quality of care. The Institute of Medicine's *Guidelines for Clinical Practice* describes CPGs as "systematically developed statements to assist practitioner and patient decisions about appropriate health care for specific clinical circumstances" (p. 27) (Field & Lohr, 19xx). Guidelines are intended to bridge the research to clinic gap. They may or may not be restricted to one level or class of research evidence (e.g., RCTs). They should serve to point out where evidence is lacking or conflicting. They are intended to improve the quality of services, identify the most cost-effective intervention, prevent unfounded practices, and stimulate needed research (Johnston, Maney, & Wilkerson, 1988).

Proponents of EBP occasionally call into question the potential for bias within the evidence supporting the CPGs, basically asking: Can the evidence be trusted? (Trinder & Reynolds, 2000). Lohr et al. (1998) and Muir-Gray (1997) have pointed out that both EBP and CPGs are centered on scientific evidence and both are ultimately intended to improve patient outcomes and quality of life. One way to address that question is to provide tables listing all of the studies examined in the development of the guidelines, identifying the "classes" or "levels" of research represented. In addition, groups such as Miller, Rosenberg, Gelinas, et al. (1999) have clearly differentiated criteria for practice *standards, guidelines,* and *options* by distinguishing the levels of evidence required for each. In their development of practice parameters for amyotrophic lateral sclerosis, they took the position that a practice "standard" would require a stricter research support than a practice "guideline," and a guideline would reference stronger evidence than a practice "option" (**Table 15–2**).

The process of developing a CPG flows from gathering and systematically reviewing the biomedical research (efficacy findings) and health services research (effectiveness findings), analyzing the conclusions, and then disseminating the evidence tables and recommendations in the form of clinical decision-making algorithms and practice guidelines, standards, or options. Guidelines typically are the result of a consensus opinion drawn from a panel of experts (often multidisciplinary) who arrive at recommendations based on their assessment of the research evidence. That assessment introduces the risk of subjectivity, as there may be vested interests among the members of the panel. Guidelines are an interpretation and application of research findings. At best they are a filtered version of the available information about a given clinical question. In addition to being subject to the bias of the panel

Table 15–2 Differentiation of Standard, Guideline, and Option

Standard:	A recommendation for patient management that reflects a high degree of certainty based on class I or very strong class II evidence.
Guideline:	A recommendation for patient management reflecting moderate clinical certainty, usually based on class II, or a strong consensus from class III evidence.
Option:	A strategy for patient management for which the evidence is inconclusive or when there is some conflicting evidence or opinion.

From Miller, R.G., Rosenberg, J.A., Gelinas, D.F., et al. (1999). Practice Parameter: The Care of the Patient with Amyotrophic Lateral Sclerosis (An Evidence-Based Review). *Neurology, 52,* 1311–1325.

Table 15–3   Classifying or Ranking Research Evidence

Example 1: Centre for Evidence-Based Medicine (1999)

   Grade A: supported by one or more randomized controlled trials

   Grade B: supported by one or more retrospective, prospective, or outcome study(ies) with an internal control or comparison group

   Grade C: supported by case series of outcome studies without a control or comparison group

   Grade D: supported by expert opinion without explicit appraisal or by "bench research"

Example 2: Quality Standards Subcommittee of the American Academy Neurology (Miller et al., 1999)

   Class I: Evidence provided by one or more well-designed, randomized controlled clinical trials (RCTs)

   Class II: Evidence provided by one or more well-designed, observational clinical studies with concurrent controls (such as with single case control or cohort control studies)

   Class III: Evidence provided by expert opinion, case series, case reports, and studies with historical controls

of reviewers, guidelines also often take into account the perspective of patients or other consumers, potentially introducing more subjectivity in the application of the research findings (**Table 15–3**) (Miller et al., 1999).

What is Evidence?

As we discussed above, even though CPGs are a direct outgrowth of EBP, there is debate between evidence-based "purists" and those involved in practice guidelines development as to how one defines evidence, and the extent to which one includes or excludes certain types, or levels, of research evidence. Proponents of EBP, such as the Cochrane Collaboration, are criticized for tending to view randomized controlled trials (RTCs) and meta-analyses as the only valid forms of evidence to measure the benefit of a given procedure or to form a recommendation on a given intervention (Trinder & Reynolds, 2000). Some have suggested that criticism may reflect a misinterpretation of the writings and interests of groups tied to EBP principles, like the Cochrane Collaboration (Trinder & Reynolds, 2000). Geddes (2000) responds to the "RTC exclusivity" criticism of EBP by stating, "In fact, evidence-based health care makes no such claims for the universal pre-eminence of the randomised controlled trial for answering all types of clinical questions. Rather, the goal of evidence-based practice is to identify the study design best suited to providing the least biased answer to a question" (p. 83). A criticism sometimes leveled at both EBP and CPGs revolves around the potential risk for managed care groups and other third-party payers in enforcing a "cookbook" approach to care, without consideration of clinician autonomy, consumer demands, and real-life clinical practice decision-making, or for any payer source to require that only those services found to be efficacious (i.e., based on irrefutable, "gold standard" research evidence) would be covered for reimbursement (Centre for Evidence-Based Medicine, 1999; Craig & Smyth, 2002; Trinder & Reynolds, 2000). Proponents of EBP and CPGs respond by saying that "cookbook" care and referencing EBP as a cost-containment measure would go against the principles of EBP. Sackett et al. (1996) have clearly stated that the principles underlying EBP include the

practitioner's experience, clinical judgment and common sense. In their words:

> Evidence-based medicine is the conscientious, explicit, and judicious use of current best evidence in making decisions about the care of individual patients. The practice of evidence-based medicine means integrating individual clinical expertise with the best available external clinical evidence from systematic research. By individual clinical expertise we mean the proficiency and the judgment that individual clinicians acquire through clinical experience and clinical practice (p. 71).

Terminology and Conceptual Confusions

One of the problems contributing to misunderstandings about what EBP does or does not require is confusion in the use of terminology, especially when referring to *efficacy* research, *effectiveness* research, *efficiency* research, and studies of *outcome*. Wertz and Irwin (2001) defined an outcome broadly as a natural result, or a consequence, that is identified by a comparison of observations made at different points in time, such as pre- and posttreatment. Referring to well-established definitions of efficacy and effectiveness (Office of Technology Assessment, 1978), these authors reminded us that efficacy is the probability of benefit to individuals in a defined population from an intervention that is applied under *ideal* conditions, whereas effectiveness is the probability of benefit of a given intervention under *average* conditions and with average populations. Therefore, effectiveness, that is, whether or not doing something does more good than harm in the general population, cannot be tested, generally speaking, by RCTs. In RCTs, the conditions are "controlled" and the results may not apply to average conditions. To test for effectiveness with an RCT design requires having broadly represented cohorts of patients, of the sort found in multicenter clinical trials involving thousands of patients. Large numbers and randomly assigned clinical trials are one answer to the challenge of linking efficacy research to predict a general benefit, or effectiveness, in the less-than-ideal, or typical, situation. Wertz and Irwin (2001) also reminded us that the term *efficiency* refers to minimizing waste, expense, or unnecessary effort to achieve a high ratio of output to input, a concern that should be addressed after efficacy and effectiveness have been determined.

Wertz (2002) has suggested if all scientific inquiry were to proceed in perfect order, we would determine the efficacy of a given intervention before testing its effectiveness. Wertz proposes that Robey and Schultz's (1998) five-phase model be employed by scientific disciplines to answer specific questions in a systematic manner. In this model, exploring a question about the benefit or outcome of a given treatment would begin with an observation based on a hypothesis tested with a small *n*, or single-subject, experimental design to determine if the intervention is "active"—a Phase I study. Once promising findings are identified, an explanation of why the treatment might be efficacious or effective is refined by specifying the population, standardizing the protocol, establishing the validity and reliability of the measures, and so forth—a Phase II study. Following that, a RCT (or large multicenter RCT) with sufficient power (Cohen, 1988) and appropriate controls and under ideal conditions would be conducted to evaluate the efficacy of the intervention—a Phase III study. Once efficacy is established, then the effectiveness of the intervention under average conditions could be determined—a Phase IV study. Then the cost-benefit of the intervention could be addressed—a Phase V study. Unfortunately, with the exception of industry-supported, clinical trials of drug therapies and the like, clinical research has few multiphased clinical trials of the sort described by Robey and Schultz (1998). Suffice it to say, the general body of evidence is uneven and research on most of the interventions used in medical speech–language pathology, like every other health service, has not progressed in any kind of rational, systematic manner. There are good examples of RCTs to assess the efficacy of treatment in medical speech–language pathology (Wertz, Weiss, Aten, et al., 1986), and meta-analyses of clinical outcomes (Robey, 1998; Whurr, Lorch, Nye, 1992). But there are also a few poorly designed and poorly controlled RCTs that have been published, some lacking the basic expectations, such as random subject selection.

Randomized controlled trials and meta-analyses of two or more RTCs are unquestionably the "gold standard" for determining the *efficacy* of a procedure, but when these referenced studies are flawed, the findings are inconclusive. Wertz (2002) has pointed out that not all RCTs are created equal. We all need to be skeptical consumers of such research (Golper & Wertz, 2002), even with the conclusions reached through meta-analysis. The frequently cited criticisms of meta-analysis are that it is only as good as the studies included in the analysis, and it may generate misleading results by minimizing or ignoring meaningful heterogeneity among studies and entrenching biases through the process of pooling results (Naylor, 1997).

If we agree with the point of view proposed by Wertz and Irwin (2001) and Robey and Schultz (1998) that efficacy, by definition, can only be tested under highly controlled, ideal conditions, then we must question the use of RCT to test the *effectiveness* of a given intervention. In actual clinical application, a procedure that has been shown to be efficacious in ideal conditions ultimately may not be found to be effective with a given patient or in the hands of a given provider. Unfortunately, authors writing in the area of EBP have used often used the terms *effective* and *efficacious* as if they were synonymous. The descriptor statements for each of the levels of evidence proposed by the *British Medical Journal*'s clinical evidence Web site lists RCTs as the best indicator for the *effectiveness* of an intervention.

Appreciating that researchers may not have provided the answers to the questions they claim to have answered, that references to efficacy and effectiveness sometimes get confused, and that meta-analysis on RCT research is viewed as the "gold standard" by some and a meaningless pooling of data by others, we are left with the question, can we practice medical speech–language pathology in an evidence-based manner? For some clinical questions, empirical evidence may come from RTCs, meta-analyses, and other types of research, including treatment comparisons, case studies, and single-subject research designs. When the research literature is not conclusive, the best evidence source may be drawn from expert, consensus opinions, or from CPGs. Clinicians can look to the evidence tables and CPGs that are published with specific attention to medical speech–language pathology, such as those under development by the Academy of Neurologic Communication Disorders and Sciences (Academy of Neurological Communication Disorders and Sciences Web site). If research evidence and CPGs are not available, the best empirical basis for clinical decisions with a particular intervention will come from a clinician's own outcome measures, assuming that they are

objective. It is best if these outcome measures can be compared with some external standard (such at that provided by the National Outcomes Measurement Scales). The key requirement is objectivity.

In their discussion of what EBP (EBM) is and is not, Sackett et al. (1996) state that the practice of EBM is "a bottom up approach that integrates the best external evidence with individual clinical expertise and patient choice" (p. 71). To practice with an eye on the evidence requires us to look for and give credence to the *most unbiased* evidence available. If RCT evidence, for example, is not available to support a given procedure, Wertz (2002) suggested we "back up" (or step down) to the next level of evidence, appreciating that as we move away from carefully controlled research (treatment/no treatment comparisons), and down the evidence ladder (**Table 15–3**), there is an increasingly greater likelihood for bias within the data, and that a conclusive determination of the benefits or harms of a procedure has not been made.

Table 15–3 illustrates some of the schemas for ranking evidence. EBP asks us to consider if a given procedure or intervention approach is supported by any evidence and what the strength (ranking) of that evidence is. If there is no strong research to support an intervention, we should have heightened concern for what the benefit of this intervention is, and, more important, what the risk of harm is. Wertz (2002), for example, responded to the question, Is it ethical to withhold a given intervention for aphasia? by asking the question, Is it ethical to provide a given intervention for aphasia without knowing the potential for harm? What is the evidence that this intervention is efficacious? Are there any RCTs (for example, well-controlled, treatment-no-treatment comparisons) or meta-analyses available to support this intervention?

Before Treatment Begins

Before any clinical intervention is initiated, and certainly before applying a new procedure with a patient, clinicians should ask: What is the evidence that this intervention is efficacious? Is there any experimental evidence to indicate it would be effective with patients like this patient? Are there case reports or single-subject studies published to support this intervention? Is this patient similar to or different from those cases? Are there written clinical standards or guidelines of practice that support this intervention with patients like this patient? Is this intervention essentially an untested procedure? If so, what then are the outcomes that need to be monitored by the physician to find evidence that this procedure is of benefit to this patient? The subsequent sections of this chapter explore outcomes-oriented intervention in depth and discuss how outcomes assessments, outcomes-oriented treatment, and outcome comparisons can serve to augment formal research evidence or provide us with guidance in our decisions when formal research is lacking.

✦ Outcomes Assessment: Definitions, Measures, and Methods

Measuring outcomes is a complex activity because of the scope of their defining characteristics, the growing number of measures currently available with their varying purposes and psychometric properties, and the various methods of assessment. A simple comparison of the results yielded from pre- and posttreatment measures for individual patients can be considered outcomes assessment; so can statistical analysis of aggregate data generated from automated outcomes management systems that capture multiple outcomes of treatment while adjusting for various risks for large patient groups. Outcomes assessment can involve a case report or randomized controlled clinical trials. Outcome measures can be simple rating scales developed by group consensus, or highly standardized tests supported by rigorous psychometric research. Given the range of measures and methods that constitute "outcomes assessment," it is important to clarify what is meant by the term using currently accepted definitions and a conceptual model of patient outcomes.

Definitions of Terms

Simply defined, an outcome is the result of an intervention. In the context of health care, Donabedian (1980) describes the multifactorial nature of the term *outcome,* defining it as

> a change in a patient's current and future health status that can be attributed to antecedent health care. Change includes improvement of social and psychological function in addition to the more usual emphasis on the physical and physiological aspects of performance. By still another extension, [change includes] patient attitudes (including satisfaction), health-related knowledge acquired by the patient, and health-related behavioral change. All of these can be seen either as components of current health or as contributions to future health (pp. 82–83).

A clinical intervention, therefore, does not result in a single outcome; it results in several and reflects the varying perspectives of the patients and their agents, including families, physicians, payers, employers, and administrators. Thus, outcomes can be:

+ Clinically derived (e.g., ability to sustain phonation, accuracy in naming, type and frequency of disfluencies in a speech sample, integrity of the swallowing mechanism)
+ Functional (e.g., ability to communicate basic needs, use the telephone, read the newspaper)
+ Social (e.g., employability, ability to learn, community reintegration)
+ Patient-defined (e.g., satisfaction with treatment; quality of life)

Outcomes may also define programmatic characteristics and desired operational changes. Therefore, they can also be:

+ Administrative (e.g., patient referral patterns, average lengths of stay, rates of missed sessions, productivity levels in direct patient care)
+ Financial (e.g., cost-effective care, cost/benefit of care, rate of rehospitalization, levels of independence as an economic factor)

Outcomes as a Factor of Time

Outcomes can occur at any point during or after the course of clinical interventions, with their temporal order giving rise to the terms *intermediate, instrumental,* and *ultimate outcomes* (Rosen & Proctor, 1981). Intermediate outcomes determine,

from session to session, whether treatment is benefiting the patient. These outcomes allow investigation of the treatment process and, for example, can determine whether certain treatment methods (e.g., oral/facial exercises, head positioning) are necessary for adequate chewing and swallowing. Instrumental outcomes activate the learning process. These are outcomes that, when reached, trigger the ultimate outcome. Theoretically, once an instrumental outcome is reached, treatment is no longer necessary, for the patients will continue to improve on their own. It raises the "how long to treat" question, a question of particular interest to payers. Finally, ultimate outcomes are those that demonstrate the social or ecologic validity of interventions, such as functional communication, reemployability, and social integration. Ultimate outcomes are most meaningful to patients and their families: "How will this treatment make me a more effective communicator?" "How will it enhance my ability to learn in school or to get a job?"

Considering outcomes as a factor of time, both short- and long-term effects of interventions can be measured. Although most would agree that long-term outcomes are of greater significance as indicators of treatment benefit, they are the most difficult to measure for several reasons. First, patients can be lost to follow-up: patients die, develop secondary morbidities, relocate, or lose interest in participating in research activities. Second, it becomes more difficult to link treatment and outcome when other intervening variables outside the control of investigators fill the time gap. Finally, it requires considerable human and financial resources to conduct longitudinal studies, often an activity unsupported by payers of care who are focused on quick results and initial expenses of rehabilitation, rather than long-term savings to the health care system.

Measurable Aspects of Outcomes

In the field of speech–language pathology, a goal or desired outcome of treatment might be to improve the patient's functional communication. Thus, if a practitioner wants to capture functional communication, it must be measured in some manner. The focus on assessment, particularly if the clinician wants its features to be objective and measurable, requires operational definition. Thus, the practitioner must determine what exactly is meant by "functional." In the hospital setting, it may mean communicating basic needs to hospital staff. If focused at the outset of treatment on discharge, functional communication may be regarded as communication that allows the individual to function independently (e.g., telephone interactions, responding in an emergency, social communication, understanding TV/radio). As time passes, our focus on functional communication may involve the ability to become reemployed or return to school. Thus, functional communication becomes more individually defined and may involve higher level skills (e.g., writing business letters, completing forms, reading and comprehending books, following complex instructions, preparing and delivering oral presentations). The term *communication* must also be defined. For example, does it mean auditory comprehension and verbal expression only? Does it include nonverbal skills? With a partner? In a group? Does it include reading and writing skills? Does it include speech intelligibility or does it mean only that a message was conveyed regardless of articulatory precision? The questions lead to answers that form the content of operational definitions and, consequently, selection of appropriate instruments that are believed to accurately and sensitively capture the targeted behavior.

Deming (1982) devotes an entire chapter of his book *Out of the Crisis* to formulation of operational definitions as requisite to measurement:

> Adjectives like good, reliable, uniform, round, tired, safe, unsafe . . . have no communicable meaning until they are expressed in operational terms of sampling, test, and criterion. . . . We have seen in many places how important it is that buyer and seller understand each other. They must both use the same kind of centimetre. . . . This requirement has meaning only if instruments are in statistical control. Without operational definition, a specification is meaningless (p. 277).

Indeed, practitioners are best advised to measure "changes," whether clinically derived, functional, social, administrative, or financial, by means of instruments that stem from operational definitions. Further, these instruments must be reliable and valid if the derived data are to be meaningful. In addition, the perspectives of payers would add to the desired features of outcome measures in that they are quantitative (results expressed in scores or ratings) and comprehensible (written in language understandable or meaningful to the layperson).

A Conceptual Framework of Patient Outcomes

The range and interrelationships among patient outcomes, as well as their defining characteristics, have been expressed in several conceptual frameworks found in the professional literature. These models have been described and applied directly to the care of individuals in diagnosis and treatment, evaluation of treatment results, assessment for work and school, and facilitation of communication between various categories of health care workers and coordination between different levels of care. Although the international classification scheme of the World Health Organization (WHO) (2001) is perhaps the most widely known, other models have been proposed (e.g., Pope & Tarlov, 1991; Wilson & Cleary, 1995), with classifications distinguishing functional limitations and disabilities (instead of handicaps), and social science and biomedical paradigms becoming more accepted.

The World Health Organization's (2001) International Classification of Functioning, Disability, and Health (ICF), formerly the International Classification of Impairments, Disabilities and Handicaps (ICIDH), is a widely used model, particularly for identifying the consequential phenomena of disease or injury.

The ICF (WHO, 2001), based on a biopsychosocial approach, facilitates documentation of a range of human functioning from biologic, individual, and societal perspectives. The model links a chain of principal events that occur in the development of illnesses or injuries:

1. Something abnormal happens (a pathology occurs).
2. Someone becomes aware of such an occurrence.
3. The individual's performance or behavior may be altered and common activities may be restricted.
4. The individual is placed at a disadvantage relative to others, thus socializing the experience.

The WHO, then, defines the consequences of disease by means of two descriptive categories:

Body function and structure.   The body function component is the physiologic and psychological functions of body systems, whereas the structure component is the anatomic parts of the body such as organ, limbs, and their components.

Activities/participation.   These components are modified by four qualifiers: performance, capacity without assistance, capacity with assistance, and performance without assistance. Performance describes how patients function in their environment; capacity without assistance describes how patients function in a structured environment (e.g., a clinic room); capacity with assistance describes patients' functioning in a highly facilitative environment using both assistive devices and personal assistance; performance without assistance describes patients' functioning in their current environment without the benefit of assistive devices or personal assistance that would normally be present.

If the WHO framework is applied to the field of speech–language pathology, one can use the example of the patient with cerebral vascular disease who sustains a left-hemisphere stroke (body structure component). The resultant impairment at the body function component is aphasia (characterized by dysnomia, agrammatism, dysgraphia, and reduced auditory and visual comprehension). This, in turn, can lead to breakdowns within the activity/participation component, for example, a communication limitation manifested in the performance of daily life activities such as communicating with family members or friends, using the telephone, making grocery lists, and reading the newspaper. The activity limitation, in turn, can lead to participation restrictions of social isolation and loss of job.

For the purposes of discussion, it is useful to organize one's thinking by three levels of breakdown: impairment, activity limitation, and participation restriction. Each consequential phenomenon along the WHO continuum defines a class of patient outcomes, and thus a class of measures to capture these outcomes: (1) traditional diagnostic, instrumental, and behavioral measures to determine differential diagnosis and identify specific strengths and weaknesses; (2) functional communication measures to identify the effects of these deficits on communication in everyday life activities; and (3) quality-of-life or wellness measures that assess the social, environmental, and economic effects of impairments or disabilities from the perspectives of patients and their caregivers.

Although health-related consequences do not necessarily occur in a linear direction, the WHO model adequately portrays a problem-solving sequence in the context of clinical intervention. That is, intervention at the level of one element has the potential to modify or prevent succeeding elements. Batavia (1992) states, "With appropriate rehabilitative intervention, an impairment does not necessarily result in a disability. Similarly, with appropriate social and environmental interventions, a disability does not necessarily results in a handicap" (p. 3). The focus on problem solving, then, is largely considered to define the ultimate outcomes of medical rehabilitation, which are to optimize independence and quality of life.

Outcome Measures

Once the concept of outcomes assessment is described by way of definitions and accepted conceptual models, one can select appropriate measures from the array of available instruments. This, however, is not an easy task. Clinicians find it difficult to select the most appropriate or best measures: ones that are sufficiently sensitive, reliable, and valid; relatively quick and easy to administer; quantitative in their results; comprehensible and meaningful to key decision makers in patient care; and useful across the continuum of health care settings for defined patient populations.

At a minimum, practitioners must consider at least three classes of measurement to capture the impairments, activity limitations, and participation restrictions associated with disease, disorder, or injury. Also, practitioners need to select instruments with strong psychometric properties so that they can have confidence in the quality of derived test data.

Practitioners are advised to avoid the practice of *measurement generalization,* that is, the use of a measure beyond its intended purposes. For example, a functional communication measure will never yield the sensitive information necessary for differential diagnosis and thus appropriate treatment planning. Consider the patient with hoarseness who is found to have independent communication in daily activities as evidenced by scores on a functional status measure, but who has a malignant growth on the left vocal cord, only detectable by instrumental procedures such as laryngoscopy, that is causing the hoarseness. Consider also the patient with dementia who "looks good" on standardized tests of language processes but whose communication in everyday life situations, assessed by measures of functional communication, is markedly reduced. Such standardized tests typically are not designed to capture the integrative aspects or contextually based domains of functional communication.

Instrument sensitivity must also be addressed. One cannot, for example, expect to capture small increments of change using a measure designed as a minimum data set or screening tool, or using a general rather than condition-specific measure for particular patient populations.

Test Selection Considerations

Outcome measures should possess certain characteristics that can be used as a checklist against which to judge their appropriateness and ability to capture targeted behaviors. An outcome measure should be:

Valid: Measures what it claims to measure. A measure can be reliable but not valid. For example, the Functional Independence Measure (State University of New York at Buffalo Research Foundation, 1993) may be reliable but not valid as a measure of functional communication. The question of validity is raised by a school of thought in the discipline of communication sciences and disorders that upholds the concept of functional communication assessment as an integrated and contextually based (e.g., assessment domains of social communication, communication of basic needs) rather than modality-specific (e.g., assessment domains of verbal expression, auditory comprehension, reading and writing) construct.

Reliable: Consistent in results yielded across time and by different examiners. The chance of error can never completely be eliminated from a measure (e.g., due to the patient's anxiety level, quality and quantity of observations, time of day and fatigue factors), but to the extent that error is slight, scores derived from that measure are reliable.

Sensitive: Able to detect small but meaningful increments of change. An instrument is only sufficiently sensitive for its intended purposes. Thus, if it is a screening measure, it should be sensitive enough to identify problems versus no problems. If it is a diagnostic measure, it should be sufficiently sensitive to differentially diagnose among the patient populations for which it was validated. If it is a general measure it will seldom yield the depth of information sought by specialists for condition-specific populations. Therefore, tools should not be used beyond the limits of their intended purposes. If a measure is sensitive, it must be able to detect targeted change if change occurs.

Practical: Should be feasible for use by both examiners and examinees. The utility of an instrument typically is determined by the mode of administration required, the time it takes to administer, requirements in use of stimulus materials and other needed equipment, need for special training of examiners, burden to the respondent, and complexity of scoring.

Comprehensible: Should be understandable to end users of the information. Often, treatment decisions are made on the basis of test results. These decisions can include eligibility for services, payment for services, continuation of services, and judgments about the quality of services. Often, decision makers are not clinicians. The information yielded from tests, therefore, should be understandable to other professionals as well as the layperson.

These considerations should be incorporated into any evaluation of "best measures." Otherwise, measurement can become encumbered in conceptual, psychometric, and practical problems that can lead to misuse of time, effort, and resources.

Measures of Impairment

If the consequences of disease or injury are considered along a continuum, outcomes assessment usually begins with identification of modality-specific behaviors, and identification of changes in these behaviors over time. The WHO (2001) describes impairment as an exteriorization of a pathologic state. Thus, aphasia and dysphagia resulting from stroke, cognitive disturbances resulting from head injury or dementia, aphonia resulting from laryngectomy, and delayed speech and language resulting from mental retardation are examples of impairments.

The assessment of impairment historically has been the focus of the speech–language pathologist's evaluations. Included in this category are the instrumental and behavioral diagnostic procedures that assess specific anatomic structures, physiologic function, and behavioral processes of speech, language, voice, fluency, cognition, and swallowing.

Test Design Features Impairment-level measures are typically designed to test separate behavioral processes (e.g., speech, language, voice) that, considered collectively, constitute human communication. A range of behaviors within each modality (e.g., aspects of auditory comprehension and verbal expression for the modality of language) usually is measured by each instrument. Tests of acquired language dysfunction in adults, for example, could measure confrontation naming, word fluency, verbal repetition, grammatical structure, proverb interpretation, spontaneous speech, auditory comprehension of one-, two-, and three-step commands, auditory retention, and so on.

According to Sarno (1965), traditional clinical tests are designed to discover whatever residuals a patient may have in each modality. In this respect, these tests are more often a measure of communication potential than actual use. Examples include instrumental procedures, such as vocal tract visualization and imaging (e.g., flexible fiberoptic nasendoscopy, stroboscopy), instrumental diagnostic procedures for swallowing [e.g., fiberoptic endoscopic examination of swallowing (FEES), electromyography, ultrasonography], and evaluation for tracheoesophageal fistulization/puncture. Examples also include the standardized tests of acquired language disorders in adults, such as the Boston Diagnostic Aphasia Examination (Goodglass & Kaplan, 1972), Minnesota Test for Differential Diagnosis of Aphasia (Schuell, 1965), Porch Index of Communicative Ability (Porch, 1971), and Western Aphasia Battery (Kertesz, 1982).

Separate behaviors within a particular modality can also be assessed by a single test. Examples are found in the area of childhood language assessment, with tests designed to assess specific behaviors involving syntax, semantics, morphology, phonology, and pragmatics. They include the Peabody Picture Vocabulary Test (Dunn & Dunn, 1981), Expressive One-Word Picture Vocabulary Test—Revised (Gardner, 1990), mean length of utterance, Developmental Sentence Scoring (Lee, 1974), and Northwestern Syntax Screening Test (Lee, 1971).

Because of their clinical objectivity and psychometric strengths, standardized tests of impairment have been typically used for purposes of controlled clinical studies. Thus, the field of speech–language pathology currently knows more about the effects of interventions on impairment-level phenomena than on resultant functional abilities or quality of life.

Measures of Activities/Activity Limitations

Activity limitations, according to the WHO (2001), are the functional consequence of an impairment, manifested in the performance of daily life activities. In this context, specific speech, language, voice, fluency, and cognitive impairments can lead to communication breakdowns (e.g., problems in social communication, communication of basic needs, daily planning). Similarly, impairments in swallowing can lead to an eating problem that can interfere with adequate intake and nutrition.

Test Design Features Unlike impairment-level measures, functional communication measures typically are not designed to assess separate modalities. Rather, their designs coincide with the concept of communication as an integration of specific speech, language, and cognitive behaviors that allow the ability to perform everyday life activities. For example, the ability to use the telephone requires a range of specific skills (e.g., auditory comprehension, verbal expression, speech intelligibility, voice intensity and quality) that, considered together, allow the ability to perform the activity. Further, because disability often is measured by what patients do rather than can do (i.e., performance versus potential), many are designed to rate abilities on the basis of direct observations. A few examples of functional communication measures are the Functional Communication Profile (Sarno, 1969), Communication Activities of Daily Living, 2nd edition (Holland, Frattali, & Fromm, 1999), and the Functional Assessment of Communication Skills for Adults (Frattali, Thompson, Holland, Wohl, & Ferketic, 1995).

Measuring Participation/Participation Restriction

If participation restrictions pertain to the social, environmental, and economic effects of impairments or activity limitations, then outcomes assessment pertains largely to measuring health-related or communicative quality of life. By its very nature, quality of life is an inherently subjective concept, best judged not by clinicians but by the patients themselves. Thus, quality of life measurement reflects personal values, beliefs, and preferences. Environmental factors, such as societal attitudes and social/psychological supports also directly influence perceptions about quality of life.

Health-related quality of life (HQL) typically refers to the individual's ability to function in a variety of roles and derive satisfaction from them, despite the presence of an impairment or disability. These measures often assess multiple dimensions of life (the objective component) and attach values to each dimension (the subjective component). This area of outcomes measurement is perhaps the most important contribution made during the past 10 years, consistent with the growing consensus that the patient's point of view is central to measuring clinical outcomes. It is also an area in great need of research and development. Of particular interest in the field of speech–language pathology is the development of the American Speech–Language-Hearing Association Quality of Communicative Life Scale (Paul-Brown, Frattali, Holland, & Thompson, 2004), a self-administered visual analogue scale that measures dimensions of life quality from the perspective of an individual's communication. A unique feature of this scale is the use of universal icons, a vertically oriented scale presented in visual midfield, and simplified language that makes it possible for individuals with communication disorders to self-administer.

Test Design Features Assessment domains of HQL measures can be all encompassing and include performance of activities of daily living, social roles (e.g., return to work, school), social interaction, emotional state, intellectual functioning, and general satisfaction and perceived well-being. The concept, therefore, subsumes the narrower concepts of functional limitations or disabilities, but the dimensions of health-related quality of life are broader than those found in disability measures. Emotional well-being, overall life satisfaction, energy, and vitality are all legitimate components of quality of life.

The major distinguishing feature of HQL measures is that their dimensions are on the personal/social level; therefore, values are typically assigned by patients (or their family members) and reflect their personal values and beliefs. These measures often take the form of self-administered surveys, interviewer-administered questionnaires, and open-ended interviews.

Cost Measures

An outcome of primary interest to payers relates, not surprisingly, to cost. In the minds of payers, positive clinical outcomes must be viewed in terms of their relationship to total costs. This relationship often is expressed by dollars spent or length of stay. Two types of cost analyses can be conducted to determine how certain outcomes compare with their costs: cost-benefit and cost-effectiveness analyses. Both are conducted for comparative purposes in determining which provider can achieve the same or better outcomes at a lower cost. This type of analysis requires that cost and outcomes be linked.

A cost-benefit analysis determines the economic efficiency of a program expressed as the relationship between dollars spent to dollars saved. In contrast, a cost-effectiveness analysis explores the effectiveness of a program in achieving targeted intervention outcomes in relation to program costs (e.g., dollars spent or length of stay per points on a functional outcome measure).

The Uniform Data System for Medical Rehabilitation, which incorporates use of the Functional Independence Measure (FIM) (State University of New York at Buffalo Research Foundation, 1993), calculates what it calls a length of stay efficiency by dividing the FIM change by the length of stay to determine the mean change in FIM score per day. A higher length of stay efficiency denotes a more efficient program.

Satisfaction Measures

As health care becomes more patient centered, health care practitioners as well as administrators are turning their attention to patients' judgments about the quality of care. These measures, commonly designed as self-assessment questionnaires, solicit the judgments of patients about several dimensions of care and determine the extent to which a program fulfills patients' expectations. Dimensions of assessment address three basic areas:

1. Access to care (e.g., signs and directions to treatment facility, waiting room time, clinic hours)
2. Physical environment (e.g., cleanliness of reception area, noise level, condition of treatment space)
3. Care received (i.e., both interpersonal and technical aspects)

The adage "keep the customer happy" carries continued weight in the health care environment as managed care organizations compete for market share. Today's patients typically have a choice of provider, and they exercise this choice if dissatisfied.

Outcomes Assessment Methods

Any approach to outcomes assessment can be considered research if one attempts to systematically answer a question or test a hypothesis. A common question is, Does clinical intervention make a difference? Attempts to answer this inquiry lead to investigation. Although research usually carries a definition of scientific or scholarly investigation that implies explicit protocols and well-controlled conditions aimed at proving cause and effect, not all research proves causation. Thus, important differences have evolved between efficacy research and outcomes research.

Efficacy Research Versus Outcomes Research

Treatment efficacy is the ability of an applied treatment to produce a predicted result. It measures the results of treatment as it is applied under ideal circumstances. Conceptually, it is distinguished from outcomes research (which often is designed to investigate treatment effectiveness) that measures the results of treatment as it is applied to a typical circumstance. Outcomes studies seldom incorporate experimental research designs because their focus is on the influence of the applied treatment over numerous facets in the patient's life

that typically cannot be experimentally controlled. In general, efficacy research is designed to prove; outcomes research can only identify trends, describe, or make associations or estimates.

It is commonly held that efficacy research is reserved for the controlled conditions of a laboratory, and outcomes research for the variable conditions of the real-world including the health care setting. Interpretations of research findings, therefore, must be approached with caution. For example, statements of cause and effect (e.g., speech–language pathology treatment can shorten the length of stay for inpatients with dysphagia resulting from stroke) cannot be made when one has not adequately controlled for the possible intervening variables that could influence the outcome or outcomes under study (e.g., spontaneous recovery, severity of the clinical condition, age, type of clinical procedures, comorbidities, adherence to a treatment regimen).

Classifying Outcomes Assessment Methods

Outcomes assessment methodologies can be classified into three categories:

1. Experimental: Studies that involve random or fully specifiable assignment to intervention and control groups or phases. Examples include randomized controlled clinical trials and time series research using single subject designs.
2. Quasi-experimental: Studies that involve nonrandom and not fully specifiable assignment to intervention and control groups or phases. Examples include program evaluation studies and quality improvement studies. Epidemiologic studies also are often categorized as quasi-experimental.
3. Nonexperimental: Studies that involve no clear comparison groups or phases. Case reports and data registries are examples.

Two approaches of particular interest to individuals who work in health care settings are program evaluation and quality improvement processes. Over time, these two methods are losing their distinguishing features. Major components of both approaches are (1) measurement of patient outcomes, and (2) management of those outcomes to continually improve the quality of care.

✦ Program Evaluation

Program evaluation methods were designed primarily to determine whether a program is meeting its goals. Both clinical and administrative goals are monitored. The term *program evaluation* is defined by CARF, the Rehabilitation Accreditation Commission, as a system that enables the organization to identify the outcomes of its programs, the satisfaction of the persons served, and follow-up on outcomes achieved by the persons served. Patton (1982) describes program evaluation as the systematic collection of information about the characteristics (structure), activities (process), and outcomes of programs and services that help administrators reduce uncertainty in the decisions they make regarding those same program and services they administer. Program evaluation, therefore, is a planned process of gathering and analyzing data to help reduce the risk of decisions. Wilkerson (1998) refers to program evaluation as an enterprise that depends on aggregations of data collected about individuals receiving services. She details its key steps:

- Establish program goals, clarifying what outcomes are really important.
- Specify quantifiable objectives to meet those goals.
- Select measures that indicate progress toward objectives.
- Measure program performance on those measures.
- Compare performance to desired objective.
- Identify potential changes in the program likely to enhance performance toward desired objectives.
- Implement program changes.
- Measure program performance once again, comparing to the objective.
- Reenter the cycle.

Thus, both measurement and management components constitute the approach to program evaluation.

Quality Improvement

Both measurement and management are also the primary aspects of quality improvement methods. However, a greater emphasis is placed on measurement of work processes (which are directly attributable to desired or expected outcomes). Quality improvement methods were designed initially to determine whether actual care complies with preestablished gold standards (e.g., standards of practice, preferred practice patterns, practice guidelines, practice parameters, or critical/clinical paths). However, with recognition that methods can also be designed to acquire new knowledge, quality improvement activities can result in establishing or modifying gold standards.

Quality assessment and improvement are defined broadly by the Joint Commission on Accreditation of Healthcare Organizations (2003) as follows:

PI.3.1: The hospital collects data on important processes or outcomes related to patient care and organization functions.

PI.4.2: The hospital makes internal comparisons of its performance of processes and outcomes over time (pp. 134–135).

The methods typically involve a Plan-Do-Study-Act (PDSA) cycle:

Plan: A work process for study is selected and an improvement trial is developed. Baseline data are collected.

Do: The trial is performed, and data are collected.

Study: The data are studied and compared with previous knowledge (i.e., baseline data).

Act: Changes are made based on the new knowledge, or a new plan is developed and the cycle starts again.

The PDSA cycle, in fact, mirrors the clinical process. A clinician collects baseline data to document a patient's current condition and develops a plan of treatment to improve the condition (Plan). The clinician then carries out the plan (Do), observes and records the effects using objective outcome measures to determine if treatment results in improved abilities (Study). Finally, the clinician applies what is learned to continue, discontinue, or modify the plan of treatment (Act), thereby starting the cycle of learning and improvement over again.

✦ Using Outcomes Data for Decision Making

Once outcomes are measured, they must be managed if they are to have a purpose. This belief forms the basis of Ellwood's (1988) approach to outcomes management, which involves the use of outcomes data for decision making. Providers may find, for example, that the costs of certain clinical procedures do not justify the minimal progress made with certain patient populations, especially when less costly alternatives to treatment (e.g., family instruction or group treatment) have a similar result. Thus, a decision can be made to allocate more resources to underserved patient populations in which significant improvements can be documented.

The management of outcomes leads to the development of data-based standards of care and clinical management tools such as critical paths (i.e., treatment regimes, supported ideally by patient outcomes research, that include only those vital elements that have been proved to affect patient outcomes) to improve the effectiveness and efficiency of care.

The methods of program evaluation and quality improvement, described above, are examples of managing outcomes once they are measured. Both suggest a continuous cycle of investigation and change. Ellwood (1988) describes the field of outcomes management as:

A technology of patient experience designed to help patients, payers, providers make rational [health care]-related choices based on better insight into the impact of these choices on the patient's life. Outcomes Management consists of:

- Common patient-understood language of health outcomes;
- A national database containing clinical, financial and health outcome information and analysis that estimates as best we can the relationship between [health care] interventions and health outcomes, as well as the relationship between health outcomes and money;
- An opportunity for each decision-maker to have access to those analyses that are relevant to the choices they must make (p. 4).

Dissemination of outcomes data for the purposes of decision making not only by practitioners on a local level but by payers, legislators, and regulators on state, regional, and national levels becomes necessary. The ambitious work of the ASHA Task Force on Treatment Outcomes and Cost Effectiveness (ASHA, 1995) is a prime example of systematic collection and planned dissemination of outcomes data on a national level to improve access to and the quality of speech–language pathology services.

Good outcomes data can exist without the knowledge of professional groups. For outcomes to be managed, outcomes data must be translated into practice guidelines and protocols, which in turn should be distributed and applied widely in efforts to change ineffective or inefficient ways of rendering services.

✦ Conclusion

This chapter has addressed evidence-based practice and outcomes-oriented approaches to clinical intervention. It has included definitions of terms in current use and has also addressed some ways in which to proceed from measurement to management so that we may effectively improve care and, by extension, enhance patients' lives. Given the time demands of practitioners, the application of evidence-based practice and outcomes-oriented approaches is still largely perceived as a burden to busy clinical schedules. However, the demands for data should support and sustain these types of activities, if only to maintain patients' access to care and preserve its quality.

Established methodologies, the growing number of evidence-based practice guidelines and outcome measures in the field,

and advancing data management and analysis technologies allow their systematic and accurate application for answering some of the pressing questions being asked by both consumer representatives and payers. In this era of cost-constrained care, in which clinical outcomes form the basis of financial and clinical viability, the data are now necessary to most effectively provide health care to those in current and future need.

Study Questions

1. Explain the differences between efficacy, effectiveness, and efficiency studies.

2. Give an example of the type of study that would be ranked as a class I, or level I, study.

3. Discuss the factors that might cause a clinician to deviate from a clinical practice guideline.

4. Cite various payer and accreditation agency requirements for outcomes assessment.

5. Give three examples of outcomes that can be measured and identify the key stakeholders who would be most interested in each outcome.

6. Identify a measure of impairment, activities limitations, and participation restrictions in the profession of speech–

language pathology. How are they similar? How are they different?

7. Why is test reliability and validity important when measuring patient outcomes?

8. What is the difference between efficacy research and outcomes research?

9. What is the danger in looking at outcomes without regard for the antecedent process of care?

10. What might be your predictions for the future of evidence-based practice and outcome-oriented approaches in health care?

References

Academy of Neurologic Communication Disorders and Sciences Web site. *Practice Guidelines Project.* http://www.duq.edu./ancds

American Speech–Language-Hearing Association. (1995). *Task Force on Clinical Outcome and Cost Effectiveness.* Report Update. Rockville, MD: ASHA

Batavia, A.I. (1992). Assessing the Function of Functional Assessment: A Consumer Perspective. *Disability and Rehabilitation, 14,* 156–160

British Medical Journal Web site. *Categorisation of Treatment Effects in Clinical Evidence.* http://www.clinicalevidence.org/

CARF: The Rehabilitation Accreditation Commission. Accreditation Standards for Inpatient Rehabilitation Programs. Tucson, AZ: CARF

Centre for Evidence-Based Medicine. (1999). Levels of Evidence and Grades of Recommendations. Retrieved November 1999. http://cebm.jr2.ex.ac.uk/docs/

Cochrane, A.L. (1972). *Efficacy and Effectiveness.* Oxford, England: Nuffield Provincial Hospitals Trust

Cohen, H. (1988). *Statistical Power Analysis for the Behavioral Sciences,* 2nd ed. Hillsdale, NJ: Erlbaum

Craig, J.V., & Smyth, R.L. (2002). *The Evidence Based Practice Manual for Nurses.* Edinburgh: Churchill-Livingstone

Deming, W.E. (1982). *Out of the Crisis.* Cambridge, MA: Massachusetts Institute of Technology, Center for Advanced Engineering Study

Donabedian, A. (1980). *Explorations in Quality Assessment and Monitoring. Volume I: The Definition of Quality and Approaches to Its Assessment.* Ann Arbor, MI: Health Administration Press

Dunn, L.M., & Dunn, L.M. (1981). *Peabody Picture Vocabulary Test–Revised.* Circle Pines, MN: American Guidance Service

Ellwood P. (1988). Shattuck Lecture—Outcome Management: A Technology of Patient Experience. *New England Journal of Medicine, 318(23),* 1549–1556

Evidence-based Medicine Working Group. (1992). Evidence Based Medicine: A New Approach to Teaching the Practice of Medicine. *Journal of the American Medical Association, 268,* 2420–2425.

Field, M.J., & Lohr, K.N. (Eds.). (19xx). *Institute of Medicine's Guidelines for Clinical Practice: From Development to Use.* Washington, DC: National Academy Press

Frattali, C.M., Thompson, C.K., Holland, A.L., Wohl, C.B., & Ferketic, M.M. (1995). *Functional Assessment of Communication Skills for Adults.* Rockville, MD: ASHA

Gardner, M.F. (1990). *Expressive One-word Picture Vocabulary Test–Revised.* Novato, CH: Academic Therapy

Geddes, J. (2000). Evidence Based Practice in Mental Health. In: L. Trinder, & S. Reynolds (Eds.). *Evidence-Based Practice: A Critical Appraisal.* Oxford, England: Blackwell Science

Golper, L.A.C., & Wertz, R.T. (2002). Back to Basics: Reading Research. *Perspectives: Neurophysiology and Neurogenic Speech–Language Disorders, 12(2),* 27–31.

Goodglass, H., & Kaplan, E. (1972). *Assessment of Aphasia and Related Disorders,* 2nd ed. Philadelphia: Lea & Febiger

Holland, A.L., Frattali, C., & Fromm, D. (1999). *Communication Activities of Daily Living,* 2nd ed. Austin, TX: ProEd

Johnston, M.V., Maney, M., & Wilkerson, D.L. (1988). Systematically Assuring and Improving the Quality and Outcomes of Medical Rehabilitation Programs. In: J.A. DeLisa (Ed.), *Rehabilitation Medicine: Principles and Practices* (pp. 287–320). Philadelphia: Lippincott-Raven

Joint Commission on Accreditation of Healthcare Organizations. (2003). *Accreditation Manual for Hospitals.* Oakbrook Terrace, IL: JCAHO

Kertesz, A. (1982). *Western Aphasia Battery.* New York: Grune & Stratton

Lee, L.L. (1971). *Northwestern Syntax Screening Test.* Evanston, IL: Northwestern University Press

Lee, L.L. (1974). *Developmental Sentence Scoring.* Evanston, IL: Northwestern University Press

Lohr, K.N., Eleazer, K., & Mauskopf, J. (1998). Health Policy Issues and Applications for Evidence-Based Medicine and Clinical Practice Guidelines. *Health Policy, 46,* 1–19

Miller, R.G., Rosenberg, J.A., Gelinas, D.F., et al. (1999). Practice Parameter: The Care of the Patient with Amyotrophic Lateral Sclerosis (An Evidence-Based Review). *Neurology, 52,* 1311–1325

Muir-Gray, J.A. (1997). *How to Make Health Policy and Management Decisions.* New York: Churchill-Livingston

Naylor, C.D. (1997). Meta-Analysis and the Meta-Epidemiology of Clinical Research: Meta-Analysis Is an Important Contribution to Clinical Practice But It's Not a Panacea [Editorial]. *British Medical Journal, 315,* 617–619

Office of Technology Assessment. (1978). *Assessing the Efficacy and Safety of Medical Technologies.* Publication OTA-H-75. Washington, DC: U.S. Government Printing Office

Patton, M.Q. (1982). *Practical Evaluation.* Beverly Hills, CA: Sage

Paul-Brown, D., Frattali, C., Holland, A.L., & Thompson, C. (2004). *Quality of Communicative Life Scale.* Rockville, MD: ASHA

Pope, A.M., & Tarlov, A.L. (Eds.). (1991). *Disability in America: Toward a National Agenda for Prevention.* Washington, DC: National Academy Press

Porch, B.E. (1971). *Porch Index of Communicative Ability.* Palo Alto, CA: Consulting Psychologists Press

Robey, R.R. (1998). A Meta-Analysis of Clinical Outcomes in the Treatment of Aphasia. *Journal of Speech, Language, and Hearing Research, 41,* 172–187

Robey, R.R., & Schultz, M.C. (1998). A Model for Conducting Clinical Outcome Research: An Adaptation of the Standard Protocol for Use in Aphasiology. *Aphasiology, 12,* 787–810

Rosen, A., & Proctor, E.K. (1981). Distinctions Between Treatment Outcomes and Their Implications for Treatment Evaluation. *Journal of Consulting and Clinical Psychology, 49,* 418–425

Sackett, D.L., Rosenberg, W.M.C., Muir-Gray, J.A., Haynes, R.B., & Richardson, W.S. (1996). Evidence-Based Medicine: What It Is and What It Isn't. *British Medical Journal, 312,* 71–72.

Sarno, M.T. (1965). A Measurement of Functional Communication in aphasia. *Archives of Physical Medicine and Rehabilitation, 46,* 101–107.

Sarno, M.T. (1969). *Functional Communication Profile.* New York: Institute of Rehabilitation Medicine, New York University Medical Center

Schuell, H. (1965). *The Minnesota Test for Differential Diagnosis of Aphasia.* Minneapolis: University of Minnesota Press

State University of New York at Buffalo Research Foundation. (1993). *Guide for Use of the Uniform Data Set for Medical Rehabilitation: Functional Independence Measure.* Buffalo, NY: SUNY

Trinder, L., & Reynolds, S. (Eds.). (2000). *Evidence-Based Practice: a Critical Appraisal.* Oxford, England: Blackwell Science

Wertz, R.T. (2002). Evidence-Based Practice Guidelines: Not All Evidence Is Created Equal. *Journal of Medical Speech-language Pathology, 10,* xi–xv

Wertz, R.T., & Irwin, W.H. (2001). Darley and the Efficacy of Language Rehabilitation in Aphasia. *Aphasiology, 15,* 231–247

Wertz, R.T., Weiss, D.G., Aten, J.L., et al. (1986). Comparison of Clinic Home and Language Treatment for Aphasia: A Veterans Affairs Cooperative Study. *Archives of Neurology, 43,* 653–658

Whurr, R., Lorch, M.P., & Nye, C. (1992). A Meta-Analysis of Studies Carried Out Between 1946 and 1988 Concerned with the Efficacy of Speech and Language Treatment for Aphasic Patients. *European Journal of Disorders of Communication, 27,* 1–17

Wilkerson, D. (1998). Program Evaluation. In: C.W. Frattali (Ed.), *Measuring Outcomes in Speech–Language Pathology.* New York: Thieme

Wilson, I.B., & Cleary, P.D. (1995). Linking Clinical Variables with Health-Related Quality of Life: A Conceptual Model of Patient Outcomes. *Journal of the American Medical Association, 273(1),* 59–65

World Health Organization. (2001). *International Classification of Functioning, Disability and Health (ICF).* Geneva: WHO

16

Use of Data in Service Delivery

Nancy B. Swigert and Robert C. Mullen

✦ **Types of Data**
✦ **Uses for Data**
✦ **Examples of Data Use**

This chapter addresses ethical standards, research principles, and current professional and regulatory issues.

On an almost daily basis, speech–language pathologists (SLPs) practicing in medical settings are presented with difficult questions from a variety of sources. A physician may ask the likely locus of lesion based on the communication disorder. A nurse may want to know what the likelihood is that his patient will develop pneumonia if the family keeps giving the patient thin liquids. A patient may inquire how long she will have to come to therapy sessions before her speech is understandable to her friends. The facility administrator may demand proof that the services being provided are worth the cost before agreeing to approve a new staff position. A payer may request data to support the efficacy of the treatment approach selected before preauthorization will be given. A supervisor may ask if the SLP is meeting productivity standards. An accrediting agency may want to know why the SLP's aspiration pneumonia rate is higher than the national benchmark.

These and many other questions require that speech–language pathologists have access to, and understanding of, a variety of sources of data. Such data allow the clinician not only to answer these questions, but also to utilize an evidence base for all patient care and program management decisions. As noted in the previous chapter, evidence-based practice must be the standard and not the exception. The clinician must know how to collect, access, analyze, and use a variety of types of data. Each question posed may require a different type or types of data to provide a complete answer.

✦ Types of Data

Diagnostic Tests

One type of data used daily by clinicians, and with which clinicians are comfortable and experienced, is data obtained from administering a standardized or norm-referenced diagnostic test. Standardized tests apply psychometric principles

and are norm-referenced. The clinician obtains information in the form of standard scores, percentiles, or age equivalents. This allows the clinician to determine the severity of the disorder, which may help in determining prognosis. Such standardized tests are available to evaluate a variety of disorders in patients of all ages (**Table 16–1**).

Some tests are not standardized, and yet yield information useful in treatment planning. Such tests are often referred to as *criterion-referenced tests*. Salvia and Ysseldyke (1981) describe criterion-reference tests as measuring "a person's development or particular skills in terms of absolute levels of mastery .... Items on criterion-referenced tests are often linked directly to specific instructional objectives and therefore facilitate the writing of objectives" (p. 30) (**Table 16–2**).

Rating Scales

In addition to formal testing instruments, the speech–language pathologist may also utilize rating scales to assign a severity to some aspect of the impairment. These rating scales can be rescored during the course of treatment to document improvement, or decline, in function. An example of a rating scale that describes one component of swallowing is the eight-point, equal-interval scale developed by Rosenbek, Robbins, Roecker, Coyle, and Wood (1996) to describe penetration and aspiration during videofluoroscopic studies. These scores are determined primarily by the depth to which material enters the airway and whether or not it is expelled (**Table 16–3**).

Other rating scales are more comprehensive, allowing the clinician to rate the patient on more and broader areas. The ASHA Functional Assessment of Communication Skills for Adults (Frattali, Thompson, Holland, Wohl, & Ferketic, 1995) contains 43 items within four assessment domains: social communication; communication of basic needs; reading, writing, and number concepts; and daily planning. The patient is rated on a seven-point scale of independence and on five-point scales of qualitative dimensions of communication (e.g., adequacy, appropriateness, promptness and communication sharing).

Table 16–1   Examples of Standardized/Norm-Referenced Tests

Boston Diagnostic Aphasia Examination (Goodglass & Kaplan, 1972)

Minnesota Test for Differential Diagnosis of Aphasia (Schuell, 1965)

Western Aphasia Battery (Kertesz, 1982)

Peabody Picture Vocabulary Test (Dunn & Dunn, 1981)

Expressive One-Word Picture Vocabulary Test (Gardner, 1990)

Preschool Language Scale–3 (Zimmerman, Steiner & Pond, 1992)

Quality of Life Measures

Tools that measure patients' quality of life can also provide important data to the clinician. These measures may be in the form of a survey filled out by patients or their caregiver, or may be completed in an interview. Many of these are comprehensive in nature (that is, not specific to communication and swallowing disorders). They assess domains such as physical, mental, pain, mobility, psychosocial, self-esteem, and emotional. Others are more specific to the quality of life related to communication and swallowing. For example, the SWAL-QOL (McHorney, Bricker, Kramer, Rosenbek, Robbins, Chignell, Logemann, & Clarke, 2000a; McHorney, Bricker, Robbins, Kramer, Rosenbek, & Chignell, 2000b) is an outcomes tool to measure quality of life and quality of care for use by dysphagia researchers and clinicians.

Utilizing quality of life measures helps guide the clinician past a focus on the level of the impairment to a broader focus on the effect the impairment is having on the patient's daily life. These data can help the speech–language pathologist develop a treatment plan that is very functional.

Treatment Plans

After the evaluation is completed utilizing a variety of tools, the speech–language pathologist develops a treatment plan with short- and long-term goals and measurable objectives. The treatment plan, if developed in functional terms, can serve as a useful source for data to document the patient's progress.

Short-term goals are set with a specific target date in mind, and these may be accomplished within one level of care. For example, a clinician in an acute care setting may establish a short-term goal for the patient to "indicate basic needs through use of a picture communication board." In the next level of care, perhaps at an inpatient rehabilitation facility, the short-term goal for expressive language for the same patient might be for the patient to "use words and short phrases to indicate basic needs to staff and family." Short-term goals should be written in functional terms as well. This is accomplished by wording the goal to indicate the impact it will have

Table 16–2   Examples of Criterion-Referenced Tests

Rossetti Infant-Toddler Language Scale (Rossetti, 1990)

Bzoch-League Receptive-Expressive Emergent Language Scale for the Measurement of Language Skills in Infancy (Bzoch & League, 1991)

Apraxia Battery for Adults (Dabul, 1979)

Mini Inventory of Right Brain Injury (Pimental & Kingsbury, 1989)

Table 16–3   Eight-Point Penetration-Aspiration Scale

1. Material does not enter the airway.

2. Material enters the airway, remains above the vocal folds, and is ejected from the airway.

3. Material enters the airway, remains above the vocal folds, and is not ejected from the airway.

4. Material enters the airway, contacts the vocal folds, and is ejected from the airway.

5. Material enters the airway, contacts the vocal folds, and is not ejected from the airway.

6. Material enters the airway, passes below the vocal folds, and is ejected into the larynx or out of the airway.

7. Material enters the airway, passes below the vocal folds, and is not ejected from the trachea despite effort.

8. Material enters the airway, passes below the vocal folds, and no effort is made to eject.

From Rosenbek, J., Robbins, J., Roecker, E., Coyle, J., & Wood, J. (1996). A Penetration Aspiration Scale. *Dysphagia, 11,* 93–98. © 1996, Springer-Verlag New York, Inc., with permission.

on function, and perhaps by giving a specific example of the functional task on which improvement is sought (**Table 16–4**).

Long-term goals should predict what the patient will achieve by the end of the course of treatment, which may occur over several levels of care. Information obtained from quality of life measures can be particularly helpful in discussing with the patient and family what the patient hopes to accomplish and what issues are of priority. The patient's description of what the ultimate outcome of intervention should be is not necessarily the same as the clinician's. For example, the clinician might word a long-term goal as "Patient will exhibit optimal expressive language skills in activities of daily living." The patient might indicate that she wants to communicate well enough to rejoin her weekly bridge game. Clinicians should try to write long-term goals in functional terms understandable by patients, families, payers, and others.

Treatment objectives are small, measurable steps that help the patient achieve the short-term goals. Treatment objectives need not be written in functional terms, as they are usually deficit, or impairment, based. The clinician identifies the problem(s) or deficit(s) that are keeping the patient from accomplishing the short-term goal and writes one or more

Table 16–4   Nonfunctional and Functional Short-Term Goals

Goal Written in Nonfunctional Terms	Goal Rewritten in Functional Terms
Patient will increase intelligibility of speech.	Patient's speech will be understandable to familiar listeners on short phrases in structured conversations.
Patient will increase laryngeal closure during swallowing.	Patient will reduce the risk of food entering the airway by achieving better closure of the airway at the larynx.
Patient will improve short-term memory skills.	Patient will be able to remember basic events that have occurred on the same day.
Patient will improve receptive language skills.	Patient will be able to follow directions in activities of daily living.

Table 16–5 Functional Short-Term Goals and Treatment Objectives

Functional Short-Term Goal	Treatment Objectives
Patient's speech will be understandable to familiar listeners on short phrases in structured conversations.	Patient will imitate short phrases with adequate volume on 90% of trials.
	Patient will reduce rate of speech on repetition of phrases by utilizing a pacing board on 90% of trials.
	Patient will overarticulate words containing /s/ blends when reading words in phrases from a list on 90% of trials.
Patient will reduce the risk of food entering the airway by achieving better closure of the airway at the larynx.	Patient will use head rotation to the left with cues on 10 of 10 trials.
	Patient will perform correct use of supraglottic swallow with saliva on 90% of trials.
	Patient will perform tight breath-hold (Valsalva) maneuver on 90% of trials.
Patient will be able to remember basic events that have occurred on the same day.	Patient will listen to a three-sentence story and answer 80% of questions about facts in the story.
	Patient will repeat a sequence of four related words read to her after an imposed 5-second delay.
	Patient will use memory book to write down the names of any visitors to his room.
Patient will be able to follow directions in activities of daily living.	Patient will point to one of three objects named with 90% accuracy.
	Patient will point to one of three pictures of common objects when the function of the object is given on 8 of 10 trials.
	Patient will follow one-step directions with objects given maximum cues on 80% of trials.

treatment objectives to help the patient achieve the goal. These objectives parallel the activities that will occur in the treatment sessions, and on which data may be collected on the patient's performance (**Table 16–5**).

Periodic Summaries

The data contained in progress notes, then, reflects the patient's progress on the treatment objectives, and can be used to generate *periodic summaries*. The setting in which services are being rendered and the payer type determine how frequently these periodic summaries are to be written. For example, an outpatient receiving Medicare Part B services must have a recertification written every 30 days to be sent to the physician for signature to request more services. A similar report is written in home health every 60 days.

Facility-Specific Data

Facilities may collect data unrelated to the scope or quality of services provided to the patients. These facility-specific data may

instead focus on the type and quantity of service provided. These data are usually related to productivity of the clinician. A common format for these data are number of billable hours per day. The clinician may simply record the number of hours worked compared with the number of billable hours each day. The facility may utilize billing information tied to Current Procedural Terminology® (CPT) (AMA, 2002) codes to collect information on billable hours. The facility may also have any number of database programs that can analyze data such as cost per unit of service compared with a specific patient diagnosis. Facilities may also subscribe to a national database containing similar data, and that national data will be used as a benchmark. A benchmark is a standard against which other data are judged. The facility may set a goal for its staff related to the national benchmark. For example, a facility might strive to be at the 50th percentile for cost per unit of service (determined by dividing the cost of running that department by the number of billable units).

Outcomes Tools

Outcomes tools with national benchmarking data also exist and are widely used at different levels of care. These tools vary in the quality and quantity of information that is measured on communication and swallowing skills. The most widely used of these instruments is the Functional Independence Measure (FIM), developed by using the uniform data set for medical rehabilitation (UDSmr) (State University of New York, 1993). It is used mostly in inpatient rehabilitation facilities. The FIM has scales for measuring a variety of areas such as grooming, bathing, and bed and chair transfers. It has only two scales specifically for communication—comprehension and expression—and three scales related to communication—social interaction, problem solving, and memory. The scale for swallowing also contains measures of independent self-feeding. There is also a version of the FIM for use with the pediatric population in hospitals, known as the WeeFIM (State University of New York, 1991). Another instrument with a national database is the Level of Rehabilitation Scale–III (LORS-III) (Formations in Healthcare, 1991), which also contains some scales for communication and swallowing.

In 1994 the American Speech–Language-Hearing Association (ASHA) launched a project to collect and analyze data about the outcomes of services provided to patients with communication and swallowing disorders. Because analysis of the above-referenced national outcomes tools revealed a lack of detailed information on communication and swallowing, ASHA developed the ASHA National Outcomes Measurement System (NOMS). NOMS has three components, two of which can be used in health care settings: NOMS Adult and NOMS Pre-Kindergarten (ages 3 to 5). There is also a K-6 component for use in schools. Each of the components utilizes disorder-specific seven-point scales, called functional communication measures, to describe the communicative or swallow functioning. These scales balance clinical markers with functional terminology designed to make them understandable to relevant nonclinical audiences, such as payers, administrators, patients, and other health care professionals.

Data Collection Instruments

In recent years, Congress and the Centers for Medicare and Medicaid Services (CMMS) (formerly the Health Care Financing

Administration, HCFA) have mandated that data collection instruments be used in several health care settings. The Nursing Home Reform Act, part of the Omnibus Budget Reconciliation Act (OBRA) of 1987, mandated that patients in long-term care facilities be assessed with the Resident Assessment Instrument (RAI). The RAI consists of a tool called the Minimum Data Set (MDS) and Resident Assessment Protocols (RAPs). The stated purpose of the RAI is to provide for a comprehensive assessment when the resident is admitted, with any significant change in status, and then annually. The information is sent to a national database. The MDS contains several questions related to communication and swallowing.

In 1999, a similar tool, the Outcome and Assessment Information Set (OASIS), was mandated for use in home health care. Each of these tools fails to provide detailed information about the areas of communication and swallowing. For example, the OASIS contains one five- or six-point scale that addresses the following factors:

+ Hearing and ability to understand spoken language
+ Speech and oral (verbal) expression of language
+ Cognitive functioning

There is also a six-point feeding or eating scale that incorporates features of ability to self-feed along with ability to swallow safely. Caution should be used if data from such instruments are assumed to actually reflect the outcome of care in the areas of communication and swallowing. The tools may not accurately capture level of skill or capture changes in these skills.

Efficacy Data

One final type of data used by clinicians is efficacy data, which are found in studies reported in peer-reviewed journals. Efficacy research "provides evidence that treatment works by ruling out possible alternative explanations for client change. It also examines the various ways that treatment alters behavior" (Olswang, 1998, p. 135). Efficacy data are derived from carefully controlled studies and provide clinicians with information needed to determine if the approaches they are using with patients are evidence based.

✦ Uses for Data

Clinicians must assimilate data from many of the sources described above in a variety of ways on a daily basis. Some examples of common uses of data are described here.

Counseling Patients and Families

Parents of pediatric patients seek information about the nature and severity of their child's disorder. They are also interested in what might have caused the problem and how long it will take to remediate. Many parents are becoming more sophisticated consumers and also want information on how well this particular facility or practice will be able to provide the needed services compared with other facilities or settings. Adult patients and their families seek answers to similar questions about the nature and severity of their disorder and the prognosis for return to their premorbid status. They usually don't need data on possible etiologies, as the nature of acquired communication disorders is usually apparent.

Facility Case Planning

Multidisciplinary case management occurs at many types of facilities. This may be a formal weekly case conference, such as might occur in an inpatient rehabilitation facility, or an informal meeting of involved providers in the nursing station at an acute care facility. Regardless of the setting, these meetings are usually geared toward discharge planning. The exception is long-term care, which may be the patient's final stop on the continuum of care. Nevertheless, planning for discharge from rehabilitation services still occurs. Each discipline provides data about the patient's status, level of participation and progress, as well as prognosis for continued improvement and expected long-term goals. The team uses this information to work with the patient and family to plan for the patient's discharge.

Providing Information for Medical Diagnosis/Prognosis

Physicians have access to many streams of data to help determine a diagnosis and prognosis for the patient's medical condition. On occasion, they may request detailed input from the speech–language pathologist to help in making these decisions. In particular, information provided by the speech–language pathologist can help determine the site of lesion and whether or not the disorder is functional or organic in etiology.

Providing Information to Payers

Some payers, particularly managed care companies, ask for information before they will authorize the evaluation and treatment of a patient. Prior to the evaluation the insurance company usually requests information on the patient's diagnosis. Following the evaluation, it may request more detailed information about the severity and prognosis as well as the predicted length of treatment and even what specific types of treatment the clinician is going to render. Other payers, like Medicare, don't request information before the patient is treated. Instead, they may at any time decide to audit the patient's record according to some predetermined criterion (e.g., therapy has exceeded the typical number of visits for this disorder).

Patient-Specific Management Decisions

Clinicians utilize a variety of forms of data to help them determine questions about a patient's care. Data can be used to help the clinician determine if the patient is a candidate for treatment, how long the course of treatment might be, what treatment approaches would be appropriate, and what the prognosis is for return of function.

Facility/Practice Management Decisions

Data supplied by clinicians may also be used by the management of a facility or practice to make decisions about the most effective and efficient way to manage resources. Data may be collected to determine if there are an adequate number of staff members to serve the patients and to determine if the staff members are achieving desired levels of productivity. Such data can also be used to analyze the character of the caseload so that staff members with appropriate qualifications are hired when an opening occurs.

Performance Improvement/Quality Improvement

Most health care facilities have a program called Quality Improvement or Performance Improvement. These programs are designed to assess and improve the quality of care being provided to the patients of the facility. The activities may also be geared toward improving the cost effectiveness of such services. Accrediting agencies like the Joint Committee on Accreditation of Healthcare Organizations (JCAHO) and the Commission of Accreditation of Rehabilitation Facilities (CARF) carefully scrutinize the facility's performance improvement program and the outcomes of the program. In fact, JCAHO established a list of approved indicators and measures that can be utilized by facilities it accredits. This list is called ORYX. The Functional Communication Measures of the National Outcomes Measurement System (NOMS) are approved as ORYX indicators.

Forming Research Questions

One final way in which data should be used is not to answer questions but rather to form them. For example, if outcomes data revealed that children with receptive language disorders made progress more quickly when receiving services in clinical settings compared with home settings, this "answer" might actually pose additional questions. For example, what differences exist in those two settings that might account for the quicker progress at the clinic? Does the clinical setting provide a more stimulating environment? Are there more distractions in the home setting? Questions like these might lead to the design of a carefully controlled study to answer such questions.

✦ Examples of Data Use

This section gives examples of specific situations speech–language pathologists encounter daily in a medical environment that require the use of various forms of data. Suggested types of data and ways to interpret the data are given.

Pediatric Speech–Language Disorder: Determining Severity, Prognosis, Estimated Length of Treatment, and Best Service Delivery Model

You have evaluated a 4-year-old with limited expressive language that is very difficult to understand and who has some difficulty with receptive language. He has just begun treatment at your facility. Standardized diagnostic testing revealed that the child's receptive language skills are mildly delayed, with a standard score at just one standard deviation below the mean. The child's expressive skills, however, are more significantly impaired, with a standard score between one and two standard deviations below the mean. His articulation skills are 1 year below those expected of a child his age. With just this information at your disposal, you would be able to assess severity (though the assessment might be difficult for the parents to understand if they are unfamiliar with standardized testing). However, when answering their questions about prognosis, estimated length of treatment, and best service delivery model, you would only be able to draw on your experience. Because your facility participates in ASHA NOMS, you have also obtained additional information by scoring the child on three functional communication measures (FCMs): Spoken Language Comprehension (on which the child is at level 5), Spoken Language Production (level 3), and Articulation/Intelligibility (level 4). The parents accept that progress to full functionality (level 7) is unlikely to be a realistic near-term goal, and they ask you what would be needed for the child to progress to at least level 6 in all three areas. National NOMS data specific to this age group and level of functioning can help you determine the typical prognosis, length and amount of treatment, and optimal service delivery model.

The national data indicate that a child at level 4 on the comprehension FCM typically progresses to level 6 or above with 6 to 8 hours of treatment. The data on production are less encouraging. Even with extensive treatment, fewer than 10% of children nationally progress from level 3 to level 6 or 7 within a year's time. For both of these spoken language FCMs, the choice of service delivery model does not appear to have a significant impact upon outcomes.

National data on articulation, on the other hand, provide much more specific guidance. As seen in **Fig. 16–1**, children

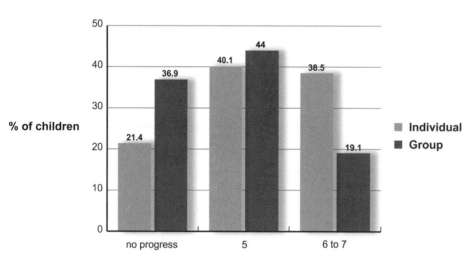

Figure 16–1 Progress on articulation functional communication measure (FCM) by service delivery model among children at FCM level 4 on admission.

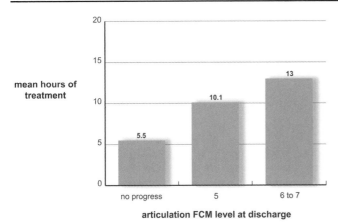

Figure 16–2 Progress on articulation FCM by hours of treatment among children at FCM level 4 on admission.

Table 16–6 Factors Affecting Children's Likelihood of Progressing from Level 4 to Level 6 or Higher on the Pre-Kindergarten Articulation FCM

	Articulation Level at Discharge		
	No Progress	5	6–7
Completed home program = yes At least 10 hours individual tx = yes	11.9%	23.9%	64.2%
Completed home program = yes At least 10 hours individual tx = no	31.6%	23.7%	44.7%
Completed home program = no At least 10 hours individual tx = yes	11.4%	42.9%	17.1%
Completed home program = no At least 10 hours individual tx = no	37.9%	49.5%	12.6%

who progress from articulation level 4 to level 6 or 7 are twice as likely to have received individual treatment as group treatment. Among children who did not progress at all, the relationship is almost exactly the reverse, with group treatment predominating. It is not only the model of treatment that affects outcomes; the amount of treatment does too. **Figure 16–2** indicates that children who make significant progress received markedly more treatment than those who did not.

You thus have valuable information to help you determine how much treatment will likely be needed to reach the child's goals, and how the treatment would best be delivered. The national data on articulation also provide another extremely valuable clue as to the factors affecting progress; successful completion of a structured home program is found to be a very important predictor of progress on articulation. From **Figure 16–3**, you see that over 50% of children who successfully complete a home program progress to at least FCM level 6, twice the rate at which other children achieve that level.

Putting all of these pieces together (**Table 16–6**) provides invaluable information to plan the treatment and help the parents set realistic expectations, using functional descriptions that they can understand more readily than clinical terminology.

Need for Instrumental Studies of Pharyngeal Dysphagia

One of the physicians on staff at your facility refuses to order any instrumental studies of dysphagia. He insists that you should be able to tell if the patient is aspirating based on observation at bedside, particularly using the 3-oz Water Swallow Test (DePippo, Holas, & Reding, 1992). You are preparing a presentation for the medical staff and want to provide evidence that documents the need for and benefits of instrumental studies. You research the literature and draw the following evidence-based facts that will serve as the basis for your presentation (**Table 16–7**).

Determining If Patient Is Ready for Discharge, or If More Treatment Is Indicated

A 56-year-old woman who suffered a closed head injury in a motor vehicle accident has been receiving outpatient services at your facility: hour-long sessions three times per week for the last 2 months. Her insurance company has requested a progress report and justification that more services are needed. Her treatment plan includes goals, with the amount

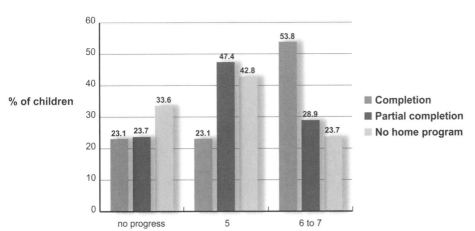

Figure 16–3 Progress on articulation FCM by completion of a structured home program among children at FCM level 4 on admission.

Table 16–7 Efficacy Studies Related to Instrumental Exams of Swallowing

Evidence of Importance of Instrumental Studies	Reference
The Water Swallow Test may miss many patients who aspirate, as up to 65% of patients who aspirate may do so without coughing.	Garon et al., 1995
Bedside evaluations are screening tools that can determine a risk ratio for aspirating. Some tools purport to predict the aspiration risk with 70–80% accuracy.	Logemann et al., 1999 Mann et al., 1999, 2000 Daniels et al., 1997
Predicting risk of aspiration is only a small part of the reason for dysphagia evaluation. A complete instrumental exam also allows you to determine appropriate diet and safe techniques for eating to eliminate the aspiration risk.	Splaingard et al., 1988 Logemann, 1998 Rasley et al., 1993 Langmore et al., 1988 Leder et al., 1998
One type of instrumental study, the modified barium swallow, has been shown to have multiple uses in addition to the above.	Martin-Harris et al., 2000

of progress reflected. She is clearly making progress on all treatment objectives (**Table 16–8**).

On admission to the facility you scored her at level 4 on the Adult NOMS Attention FCM, and at level 3 on the Memory FCM. She has now progressed one level on each scale. National NOMS data (**Fig. 16–4**) suggest that she would benefit from continued memory treatment.

Head-injured patients starting at level 3 on the Memory FCM are typically at level 4 after 2 months of outpatient treatment, which is precisely how your patient has progressed. After a third month of treatment, however, we see that most patients progress to level 5 or higher. You have accessed a national database of hundreds of similar cases to support your recommendation for continued treatment.

Requesting Precertification for Services

A 33-year-old woman, employed as an elementary school teacher, is referred by her otolaryngologist for treatment of hoarse vocal quality secondary to small bilateral vocal nodules. Her managed care company requests that you predict exactly how many sessions you will need before it will precertify the evaluation. You score her at level 4 on the Adult NOMS Voice FCM. National data from NOMS (**Fig. 16–5**) suggest that similar patients typically need 9 to 12 hours of treatment to reach at least level 6. At that level, her voice should sound normal most of the time and she should be able to use her voice in almost all situations.

Table 16–8 Sample Treatment Plan/Progress Report

Short-Term Goal/Treatment Objectives	Progress to Date
1. Patient will improve ability to remember sentence level material. a. Patient will repeat 8- to 10-word sentences read to her after an imposed 5-second delay. b. Patient will answer questions about an 8- to 10-word sentence read to her. c. Patient will follow two-step directions with objects after imposed 5-second delay.	1. a. Patient was initially able to complete this task on only 20% of attempts after a delay (she was 70% accurate without a delay). She can now complete this task 60% accurately after a delay. b. Patient has improved accuracy answering questions from 40% to 70%. c. Patient is now able to follow two-step directions 90% of the time in the absence of distractions, an improvement over initial performance of 55%.
2. Patient will use external memory aids to help her keep appointments and complete tasks. a. Patient will consistently write appointments in daily planner with cues. b. Patient will check the date off the calendar in her room each night without cues. c. Patient will follow daily schedule and check off each event as it occurs without cues.	2. a. Patient initially required maximum cues to use her planner, but now uses it with only occasional cues. b. Patient is doing this 100% without cues. c. Patient needs only small reminders to check off events as they occur during the day, but is not yet able to make changes in her schedule when they occur unless given lots of cues.
3. Patient will be able to pay attention to information in the presence of distractions (visual and auditory). a. Patient will be able to answer questions about a paragraph read to her when a radio is playing quietly in the background. b. Patient will be able to complete paper-and-pencil direction following activities while seated next to a window without redirection from the SLP.	3. a. Patient is able to answer 87% of questions asked with the radio on in the background. This is a significant improvement, as initially she could not complete this task at all with auditory distractions. b. Patient sometimes needs cues to ignore visual distractions, but then can complete these activities accurately.

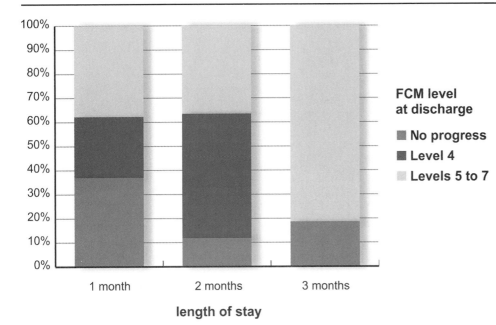

Figure 16–4 Progress on Adult National Outcomes Measurement System (NOMS) Memory FCM by length of time on outpatient SLP caseload among head-injured patients at level 3 on admission.

Requesting Approval for a New Full-Time Employee in the Department

You are the manager of the speech–language pathology department at an inpatient rehabilitation hospital with four full-time SLPs on staff. Each patient must receive at least 3 hours of combined physical therapy, occupational therapy, and speech–language therapy each day. Over the last 4 months, patients are averaging only ¾ hour of speech therapy a day, with the other therapies having to increase their length of treatment to reach the 3 hours. The productivity benchmark set by the hospital is for each SLP to have 6 hours billable time each day. The billable hours per day have averaged 6.75 hours over the last 3 months. (6.75 hours × 4 SLPs = 27 billable hours; 27 hours divided by ¾ hour indicates there are 36 patients on the caseload). If the current patients were to be given 1 hour of therapy daily, rather than ¾ hour, the extra ¼ hour a day for 36 patients would be another 9 billable hours a day. Staff

satisfaction is slipping. You present these data to administration to justify a request for another full-time employee (FTE) with a request that if the numbers remain steady, an additional one-half FTE would be indicated.

Performance Improvement

Example 1

The stroke team at your acute care facility has a goal to reduce cost while maintaining excellent service and outcomes. Each department that serves cerebrovascular accident (CVA) patients is challenged to meet this goal. Analysis of your NOMS data reveals that CVA patients scored on the Swallowing FCM at your facility were receiving an average number of 17.1 treatment units versus 12.7 nationally. Mean change in swallowing skills on the FCM was 1.2 compared with 1.0 nationally (considered similar).

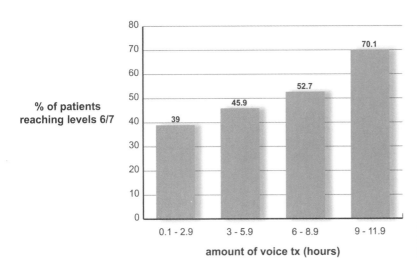

Figure 16–5 Likelihood of progressing from level 4 to level 6 or higher on the Adult Voice FCM by amount of treatment.

Table 16–9   Performance Improvement Data on Cerebrovascular Accident (CVA) Patients Scored on Swallowing FCM

	% Patients Recommended for Tx at Meals	Total No. of Treatment Units at Meals	Average No. of Treatment Units per Patient at Meals	Mean No. of Treatment Units by SLP Department (NOMS Data)	Mean No. of Treatment Units (National NOMS Data)	Mean Level of Change in Swallowing at Facility (NOMS Data)	Mean Level of Change in Swallowing (National NOMS data)
Baseline data	80%	35	2.3	17.1	12.7	1.2	1.0
After changes instituted	26%	15	3.0	10.8	11.9	1.1	1.2

The members of the department meet and discuss these findings and decide that one way to reduce the number of hours of intervention is to stop treating the patients at meal-times, and instead train nursing assistants on how to follow feeding precautions to keep patients safe. The department also decides to make more conservative recommendations at the time of the instrumental exam. For example, if it appears a patient is safe with thin liquids but only if she takes small sips and swallows twice (a recommendation that will require staff or family to be present during meals), but is safe with nectar-thick liquids in uncontrolled amounts, the recommendation will be for nectar-thick liquids at meals. Analysis of the data at the end of the quarter after instituting these changes revealed the department reduced the percent of patients for whom treatment at meals was recommended from 80% to 27%. The total number of treatment units at meals was reduced by more than 50%. For those patients still requiring treatment at meals, each patient was still getting the same (or more) units at meals. The total number of treatment units for stroke patients was less than the national average NOMS data, and yet the mean change in improvement in swallowing remained comparable to the national improvement. The department then used a cost per unit of service multiplied by the number of units not given to demonstrate cost savings to the hospital (**Table 16–9**).

Example 2

The Brain Injury Program at an inpatient rehabilitation hospital noted some worrisome findings in its performance improvement

data. The patients were not making as much progress on the Adult NOMS Memory FCM as the national benchmarks for brain-injured patients in that setting (**Fig. 16–6**).

The Program Improvement Committee first looked at the patient mix to see whether the national data were based on comparable populations. Although the committee knew that the treatment setting and diagnoses were comparable, it suspected that its patients might have been more severe. A comparison of the Memory FCM admission scores, however, showed that the patients reflected national norms. The committee next looked at the amount of memory treatment provided in its program (**Fig. 16–7**).

These data indicated that patients in the program received significantly less memory treatment than the national benchmarks. The committee knew from the national NOMS data (**Fig. 16–8**) that the amount of treatment is an important predictor of progress on this FCM.

The program increased the amount of time spent working on memory, and soon saw outcomes that equaled and surpassed the national benchmarks.

Forming Research Questions

One of the common misconceptions about outcomes data and research is that they are meant to replace, or somehow compete with, other types of research such as clinical trials. In fact, the various approaches should complement one another (see Chapter 15). Numerous questions arise from outcomes studies that can properly be addressed only through other research designs. Some examples:

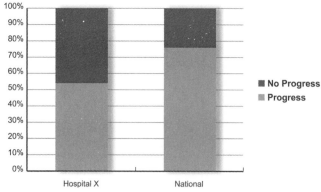

Figure 16–6 Progress on Adult Memory FCM by patients with brain injury in inpatient rehabilitation hospitals.

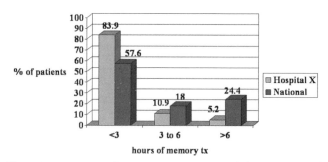

Figure 16–7 Amount of memory treatment provided to patients with brain injury in inpatient rehabilitation hospitals.

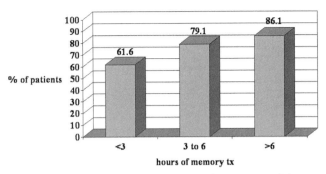

Figure 16–8 Progress on Adult Memory FCM by patients with brain injury in inpatient rehabilitation hospitals by amount of memory treatment provided (national data).

◆ What is the role of "spontaneous recovery" in the functional progress noted in stroke patients?

◆ How do the economic benefits associated with various outcomes compare with the costs of achieving them?

◆ Are there circumstances under which group treatment is more likely to be effective than individual treatment?

◆ Is the difference in function between one FCM level and the next, while clinically meaningful, also meaningful to the patient? If not, is that due to the need for more patient education or is it simply not meaningful?

◆ What is the spillover effect on an area such as spoken language comprehension resulting from treatment designed to affect a different but related area, such as spoken language production?

◆ Conclusion

Speech–language pathologists are continually confronted with questions that require data to answer accurately and completely. The data may be obtained from a variety of sources. Clinicians must understand the different sources of data and be able to critically evaluate the appropriateness of each type of data. The demands for data-based decisions will only grow in the future, requiring clinicians to continue to enhance their ability to understand and to utilize data.

Study Questions

1. Describe the distinctions between standardized tests, criterion-referenced tests, and rating scales.

2. What is the relationship among functional short-term goals, long-term goals, and treatment objectives?

3. Describe the difference in outcomes data and efficacy data.

4. Why has Congress mandated the use of data collection instruments in certain settings?

5. What is the ASHA National Outcomes Measurement System?

6. What kinds of decisions do speech–language pathologists make using outcomes data?

7. Describe daily situations in which some types of data are needed to adequately answer a question.

References

American Medical Association. (2002). *The Physicians' Current Procedural Terminology (CPT)*, 4th ed. Chicago: AMA

American Speech–Language and Hearing Association. (1994). *National Outcomes Measurement System*. Rockville, MD: ASHA

Bzoch, K.R., & League, R. (1991). *Receptive-Expressive Emergent Language Scale Second Edition*. Austin, TX: Pro-Ed

Dabul, B. (1979). *Apraxia Battery for Adults*. Austin, TX: Pro-Ed

Daniels, S.K., McAdam, C.P., Brailey, K., & Foundas, A.L. (1997). Clinical Assessment of Swallowing and Prediction of Dysphagia Severity. *American Journal of Speech–Language Pathology, 6*, 17–24

DePippo, K., Holas, M., & Reding, M. (1992). Validation of the 3-oz Water Swallow Test for Aspiration Following Stroke. *Archives of Neurology, 49*, 1259–1261

Dunn, L.M., & Dunn, L.M. (1981). *Peabody Picture Vocabulary Test–Revised*. Circle Pines, MN: American Guidance Service

Formations in Healthcare. (1991). *Level of Rehabilitation Scale–III*. Chicago: Formations in Healthcare

Frattali, C., Thompson, C., Holland, A., Wohl, C., & Ferketic, M. (1995). *Functional Assessment of Communication Skills for Adults*. Rockville, MD: American Speech–Language-Hearing Association

Gardner, M.F. (1990). *Expressive One-Word Picture Vocabulary Test–Revised*. Academic Therapy Publications

Garon, B.R., Engle, M., & Ormiston, C. (1995). Reliability of the 3-oz Water Swallow Test Utilizing Cough Reflex as Sole Indicator of Aspiration. *Journal of Neurologic Rehabilitation, 9*, 139–143

Goodglass, H., & Kaplan, E. (1972). *The Assessment of Aphasia and Related Disorders*, 2nd ed. Philadelphia: Lea & Febiger

Kertesz, A. (1982). *Western Aphasia Battery*. New York: Grune & Stratton

Langmore, S.E., Schatz, K., & Olsen, N. (1988). Fiberoptic Endoscopic Examination of Swallowing Safety: a New Procedure. *Dysphagia, 2*, 216–219

Leder, S.B., Sasaki, C.T., Burrell, M.L. (1998). Fiberoptic Endoscopic Evaluation of Dysphagia to Identify Silent Aspiration. *Dysphagia, 13*, 19–21

Logemann, J.A. (1998). *Evaluation and Treatment of Swallowing Disorders*. Austin, TX: Pro-Ed

Logemann, J., Veis, S., & Colangelo, L. (1999). A Screening Procedure for Oropharyngeal Dysphagia. *Dysphagia, 14*, 44–51

Mann, G., Hankey, G.J., & Cameron, D. (1999). Swallowing function after stroke—prognosis and prognostic factors at 6 months. *Stroke, 30*, 744–748

Mann, G., Hankey, G.J., & Cameron, D. (2000). Swallowing Disorders Following Acute Strokes: Prevalence and Diagnostic Accuracy. *Cerebrovascular Diseases, 10*, 380–386

Martin-Harris, B., Logemann, J.A., McMahon, S., Schleicher, M., & Sandidge, J. (2000). Clinical Utility of the Modified Barium Swallow. *Dysphagia, 15*, 136–141

McHorney, C.A., Bricker, D.E., Kramer, A.E., Rosenbek, J.C., Robbins, J., Chignell, K.A., Logemann, J.A., & Clarke, C. (2000a). The SWAL-QOL Outcomes Tool for Oropharyngeal Dysphagia in Adults. I. Conceptual Foundation and Item Development. *Dysphagia, 15*, 115–121

McHorney, C.A., Bricker, D.E., Robbins, J., Kramer, A.E., Rosenbek, J.C., & Chignell, K.A. (2000b). The SWAL-QOL Outcomes Tool for Oropharyngeal Dysphagia in Adults: II. Item Reduction and Preliminary Scaling. *Dysphagia, 15*, 122–133

Olswang, L.B. (1998). *Treatment Efficacy Research. Measuring Outcomes in Speech–Language Pathology*. New York: Thieme

Pimental, P.A., & Kingsbury, N.A. (1989). *Mini Inventory of Right Brain Injury*. Austin, TX: Pro-Ed

Rasley, A., Logemann, J.A., Kahrilas, P.J., Rademaker, A.W., Pauloski, B.R., & Dodds, W.J. (1993). Prevention of Barium Aspiration During Videofluoroscopic Swallowing Studies: Value of Change in Posture. *American Journal of Rehabilitation, 160,* 1005–1009

Rosenbek, J., Robbins, J., Roecker, E., Coyle, J., & Wood, J. (1996). A Penetration Aspiration Scale. *Dysphagia, 11,* 93–98

Rossetti, L. (1990). *The Rossetti–Infant-Toddler Language Scale.* Illinois: LinguiSystems

Salvia, J., & Ysseldyke, J. (1981). *Assessment in Special Remedial Education.* Boston: Houghton Mifflin

Schuell, H. (1965). *The Minnesota Test for Differential Diagnosis of Aphasia.* Minneapolis: University of Minnesota Press

Splaingard, M.L., Hutchins, B., Sulton, L.D., & Chaudhuri, G. (1988). Aspiration in Rehabilitation Patients: Videofluoroscopy Versus Bedside Clinical Assessment. *Archives of Physical Medicine and Rehabilitation, 69,* 637–640

State University of New York at Buffalo. (1991). *Functional Independence Measure for Children.* Version 1.5. Buffalo, NY: State University of NY at Buffalo

State University of New York at Buffalo. (1993). *Guide for Use of the Uniform Data Set for Medical Rehabilitation: Functional Independent Measure.* Buffalo, NY: Research Foundation

Zimmerman, I., Steinger, V., & Pond, R. (1992). *Preschool Language Scale-3 (PLS-3).* New York: Psychological Corporation

17

Clinical Documentation in Medical Speech–Language Pathology

Ann W. Kummer, Pete Johnson, and Katrina Zeit

✦ **Types of Documentation**
✦ **Purpose of Documentation**
✦ **Format of Documentation**

The word *document* usually refers to an official paper that provides information or proof of something (Merriam-Webster, 2001). In speech–language pathology, clinical documents serve to provide important *information* regarding the patient's history, current problem, and treatment. Clinical documents also provide *proof* that particular services have been provided and certain outcomes have been achieved.

Proper documentation is an important aspect of the practice of speech–language pathology, although it is usually not a high priority for the practicing clinician. In fact, the word *documentation* is similar to terms like *productivity* and *no-show* in evoking negative feelings from clinicians. Although documentation is required to obtain payment for services, insurance plans and governmental payers do not reimburse providers for the time spent in documentation. Furthermore, third-party payers often dictate the format and process of documentation (Marshall, 2000), increasing the workload and expenses in an era in which consumers are demanding a reduction in health care costs. Despite these concerns, proper documentation is critical for coordination of care, reimbursement, and even for accreditation. Therefore, as unpleasant as it may be for the clinician, the job is not complete without the necessary paperwork.

✦ Types of Documentation

If found in the medical chart, even a handwritten note on a scrap of paper can be considered part of the patient's clinical documentation. However, the most important speech–language pathology documents include the following:

✦ Diagnostic reports
✦ Treatment plans
✦ Progress/discharge reports
✦ Progress notes for each session

✦ Charge documents
✦ Letters regarding the patient

The exact format, style, and length of documentation reports varies widely across work settings, university programs, and even among clinicians working in the same setting (Shipley & McAfee, 1998). The lack of standards and wide variability can be frustrating to a speech–language pathology student or new clinician, and also to those who regularly receive the reports. Despite the lack of a standard documentation report model or format, it is important that each one of these documents contains basic identifying information and certain other key elements, depending on the type of document. For the "anatomy" of each document type, see **Tables 17–1** to **17–5**.

✦ Purpose of Documentation

The primary purpose of clinical documentation is to provide a means of communication between professionals regarding patient care. However, clinical documentation also serves as a means of recording and communicating for billing and reimbursement, providing proof of compliance and quality improvement, recording data for research purposes, and serving as a basis of legal evidence.

Documentation for Patient Care

In speech–language pathology, clinical documentation serves as the primary means for recording and communicating the patient's past medical history, current concerns, clinical evaluation findings, evaluator's impressions, assessment of potential causes or contributing factors, and recommendations for treatment. Documentation also serves to record and communicate the patient's plan of care, therapeutic interventions,

Table 17–1   Anatomy of a Diagnostic Report

Section	Usual Contents
Date	Evaluation date
	Billing period (30-day cycle for Medicare)
Identifying information	Name
	Birth date
	Medical record number
	May include address, phone number, social security number
	Caregiver or legal guardian (as appropriate)
Examiner	Examining SLP's name and degree initials (certification for Medicare)
Referral source	Usually a physician (Medicare requires Universal Physician Identification number)
Problem statement/ reason for referral	Statement of primary concern from patient/family
	Reason for referral as given by referral source
	Medical diagnosis(es): primary and secondary; some payers require date(s) of onset
	Speech–language pathology disorder/ diagnosis
Pertinent history	From sources such as:
	Parent/guardian or patient report
	Referral letter/form
	Medical record
	Medical history (pertinent to speech–language pathology diagnosis and treatment)
	Educational/occupational status
	Prior functional communication status (if disorder is acquired)
	Previous speech–language pathology or related evaluation results, treatment, and outcomes
	Length of previous treatment
Examination	Tests given
	Test scores or results
	Diagnostic observations
Impressions	Summary of professional judgment based on history and examination
	Current functional communication status
	Diagnosis and severity
	Prognosis
	Etiologic and contributing factors
Recommendations	Treatment type and amount
	Patient/family counseling or training
	Further evaluation
	Referral to other professional(s)

From Tjapkes, S. (1999). The What Works. *Health Management Technology, February.*

Table 17–2   Anatomy of a Treatment Plan

Section	Usual Contents
Date	Date of plan
Identifying information	Name
	Birth date
	Medical record number
	May include address, phone number, social security number
	Caregiver or legal guardian (as appropriate)
	Billing period (30-day cycle for Medicare)
Treating SLP	SLP's name and degree initials (certification for Medicare)
Treatment plan	Long-term goals, which should reflect the desired patient outcomes and expected level of communicative independence
	Short-term goals, which should be written in functional, measurable terms
	Treatment session length (e.g., 30-minute session), frequency (e.g., two times weekly) and expected duration (e.g., 6 months)
	Prognosis
	Statement of approval and involvement of patient/family
	Interdisciplinary conference dates, if applicable
	Statement of review schedule for treatment plan
Signature	Written or electronic signature
	Printed name with degree initials
	Professional title
Carbon copy section (if sent out)	Referring physician or source
	Primary care physician
	Patient/family
	Other treating professionals
	Third-party payers

(SLP) who provides the assessment or treatment is the responsible party for completing the patient's documentation. This information should be conveyed to the referral source, primary care physician, other treating professionals, and even to the patient and family.

Documentation for Billing and Reimbursement

Proper documentation, including the use of appropriate procedural and diagnostic codes, is also important for billing purposes. Reimbursement from third-party payers is usually based on the documentation and coding information. Several years ago, the American Medical Association (AMA), in concert with the Center for Medicare and Medicaid Services (CMS), formerly the Health Care Financing Administration (HCFA), drafted a manual describing the documentation guidelines for evaluation and treatment of patients. This manual continues to be updated regularly to ensure that the latest documentation guidelines are disseminated to practicing professionals.

and response to treatment. The American Speech–Language-Hearing Association (ASHA) reports that clinical documentation should justify the need for treatment, state the effectiveness of treatment, and be a legal record of events that occur in treatment (Paul-Brown, 1994). The speech–language pathologist

Table 17–3 Anatomy of a Progress/Discharge Report

Section	Usual Contents
Date	Date of report
	Billing period (30-day cycle for Medicare)
Identifying information	Name
	Birth date
	Medical record number
	May include address, phone number, social security number
	Caregiver or legal guardian (as appropriate)
SLP	Treating SLP's name and degree initials (and certification for Medicare)
Amount of therapy	Time period covered by report
	Date patient began treatment at present facility
	Number and length of sessions
Diagnostic summary	Taken from diagnostic report
Treatment plan summary	Short-term goals
	Long-term goals
	Prognosis
	Statement of approval and involvement of patient/family
Progress	Summary of response to treatment
	Treatment methods that work and those that don't work
	Status of goals (met, unmet, discontinued)
	Current status and concerns (include objective measures of performance in functional terms that relate to treatment goals such as pre- and posttesting results or comparable measures to those used in original assessment)
	Status on appropriate functional communication measures (FCMs) (pretreatment and current status)
	Any changes in prognosis and why
	Any changes in treatment plan
Recommendations	Further treatment (including type and amount) or discharge from treatment
	Parent/family counseling or training
	Further evaluation, if appropriate
	Referral to other professional(s)
Signature	Written or electronic signature
	Printed name with degree initials
	Professional title
Carbon copy section	Referring physician or source
	Primary care physician
	Patient/family
	Other treating professionals
	Third-party payers

Table 17–4 Anatomy of a SOAP (Subjective, Objective, Assessment, Plan) Note

Section	Usual Contents
Date	Date of note
Identifying information	Name
	Birth date
	Medical record number
Subjective	Patient's emotional, social, and physical status
	Patient's motivational level
Objective	Objective data as it relates to functional goals
	Progress reported in measurable terms (e.g., percentages)
	Document skilled interventions
	Document progress to previous documentation
Assessment	Patient response to therapy
	Functional progress
	Equipment utilized
	Deficits remaining
	Justify continued skilled need
	Staff/caregiver training
	Consultations
Plan	Plan for upcoming report period
	Goal or intervention changes
	Changes in frequency or duration
	Referrals needed
	Discharge plan
Signature	Written or electronic signature
	Printed name with degree initials
	Professional title
Carbon copy section (if sent out)	Referring physician or source
	Primary care physician
	Patient/family
	Other treating professionals
	Third-party payers

Billing Documentation Concepts

Several concepts are associated with proper and complete documentation for Medicare, fiscal intermediaries (insurance companies that are compensated by the government to administer the Medicare system), and many other third-party payers. These concepts include the following:

Medical Necessity The concept of medical necessity is important in clinical documentation because many health insurance plans base decisions of coverage or payment of services on determination of medical necessity. In fact, in 2001, the Department of Health and Human Services issued a report by the Office of the Inspector General that concluded that 14% of skilled nursing facility rehabilitation services were medically unnecessary, based solely on a sample review of medical record documentation (Swigert, 2002).

Definitions of medical necessity vary among insurance plans and often differ from a physician's use of the term (Ireys, Wehr, & Cooke, 1999). The Blue Cross–Blue Shield Association (2002, adapted from Clark, 1995) defines medically necessary services as

Table 17–5 Anatomy of a Charge Document

Section	Usual Contents
Date	Date of charge
SLP	Examining or treating SLP
Identifying information	Name
	Medical record number
	Account number
	Address
	Guarantor
	Insurance or third-party payer
Procedure	Appropriate CPT code
Diagnosis	Appropriate ICD-9 code
Units	Number of units, if time based
Charge	Total dollar amount

services or supplies as provided by a physician or other healthcare provider to identify and treat a member's illness or injury, which, as determined by the payor, are consistent with the symptoms, diagnosis, and treatment of the member's condition; in accordance with the standards of good medical practice; not solely for the convenience of the member, member's family, physician, or other healthcare provider; and furnished in the least intensive type of medical care setting required by the member's condition.

The SLP should be familiar with the patient's insurance plan and that plan's definition of medical necessity when requesting authorization or payment of services. Medicare guidelines recommend that the documentation indicate why the recommended treatment is appropriate for the patient's diagnosis and condition (ASHA, 2001a). Additionally, many insurance plans' definitions of medical necessity require that the patient improve significantly as a result of the treatment rather than allowing for treatment that will help maintain the patient's current level of functioning (Ireys et al., 1999). Therefore, the documentation of treatment goals should reflect that they are designed to improve the patient's condition rather than maintain the patient at current functional levels.

Change of Condition Medicare defines the concept of "change of condition" as a medical event that causes a need for skilled intervention. The information regarding the change of condition should be documented in the patient's history and the patient's plan of treatment. This change is usually viewed as permanent (Slominski, 1999). If the beginning of therapeutic services was delayed for a long period of time past the reported change of condition, Medicare expects a documented explanation for the time delay.

> If a patient suffered a stroke and was hospitalized with resulting aphasia on a particular date, then the change of condition would typically date from that hospitalization.

Previous Level of Functioning The patient's previous level of functioning (PLOF) prior to the change in condition becomes the ceiling for recovery. Therefore, the PLOF should be carefully documented and should include a description of the patient's prior abilities, previous attempts at remediation, and

the results of previous interventions. (Medicare and other insurers will question a plan of treatment that seeks to rehabilitate the patient beyond his or her level of function prior to the onset of the current change of condition.)

> A patient with a PLOF of normal speech intelligibility who suffers a stroke would likely have long-term goals that reflect normal speech intelligibility. Conversely, if the patient had suffered previous strokes, and, therefore, had reduced speech intelligibility prior to the most recent stroke, his long-term goals should reflect attaining the level of speech intelligibility present immediately before the last stroke (Slominski, 1997).

Reasonable and Necessary The amount, frequency, and duration of services must be considered appropriate (reasonable and necessary) for the diagnosis under accepted standards of practice (ASHA, 2001a). The frequency of the sessions should also reflect the patient's response to treatment. For example, the frequency of therapeutic sessions may decrease as the patient's progress improves and the patient is able to assume more independent function. With increased function, patients may be able to assume a greater role in their own remediation.

Specific Treatment must be targeted to preestablished and documented treatment goals (ASHA, 2001a). These goals must be stated clearly and in measurable terms.

Effective The treating SLP must have an expectation that the treatment will be effective and that the patient will improve "significantly" in a reasonable period of time (ASHA, 2001a). Therefore, the prognosis for improvement should be documented in the treatment plan and the progress toward achieving the goals should be documented in the progress report. Improving "significantly" means there is a "generally measurable and substantial increase in the patient's present level of communication, independence, and competence compared to their levels when treatment was initiated. Intermediaries must not interpret the term 'significant' so stringently that they may deny a claim because of a temporary setback in the patient's progress" (ASHA, 2001a, p. 10).

Skilled The treatment needs and the strategies to attain the goals must be so complex and sophisticated that it requires the knowledge, skills, and judgment of an SLP (ASHA, 2001a).

Functional Goals Medicare and most private insurers require that both short- and long-term treatment goals be stated in functional terms. Short-term goals reflect the steps to be taken to reach the long-term goals. Long-term goals reflect the communication or swallowing behaviors expected at the conclusion of treatment. Typically, short-term goals should be written for completion within the authorization/certification period. In the case of Medicare, the need for services must be documented at least every 30 days and at least every 60 days for home health agencies and certified outpatient rehabilitation facilities (CORFs) (Thompson, 2002).

Functional goals vary widely, depending on the patient's level of independence and competency. For instance, an appropriate functional communication goal may be to give a consistent yes/no response, or to use short phrases to communicate basic wants and needs, or to achieve conversational language skills (ASHA, 2001a). The goals become functional when they are related to the patient's activities of daily living. Examples of communication independence in activities of daily living are as follows:

+ Communicates basic physical needs and emotional status
+ Communicates personal self-care needs
+ Engages in social communicative interaction with immediate family or friends
+ Uses communicative means to interact in one's community (ASHA, 2001a)

The specific components of a functional goal should include an appropriate means of measurement and a time frame (Slominski, 1999). Functional goals should also include the patient and/or family's goals, preferably quoted verbatim, to reflect their involvement.

> A typical long-term goal for dysphagia: In order to tolerate the least restrictive diet without signs and symptoms of aspiration, the patient will utilize the following compensatory strategies (liquid assist, chin tuck) without cues with 90% accuracy over five consecutive sessions as reported by the SLP in 4 weeks' time. An example of a short-term goal to achieve this long-term goal: In 2 weeks, patient will demonstrate an appropriate chin tuck during liquid intake (nectar-thick) with minimal cues with 80% accuracy over three consecutive sessions as reported by the SLP.

Measurable Goals To authorize payment or continue coverage, third-party payers require documentation to show that the patient is making progress or has the potential for functional gains. Therefore, the goals must be designed to be measurable and to achieve appropriate outcomes. When documenting progress, one is in effect documenting outcomes that serve to justify the efficacy of the services. The SLP needs to choose the appropriate outcome measure that best shows the progress related to achievement of that goal (Marshall, 2000). Typically, measurable goals are written with an objective component that can be compared to previous levels, skills, or test scores, and that demonstrate progress toward a functional goal. If percentages are used for an objective measure, ASHA (2001a) recommends that they be based on real number counts.

Proper Coding For proper billing, the SLP needs to understand the relationship between the International Classification of Diseases, 9th Revision (ICD-9) and Current Procedural Terminology (CPT) codes. These codes are numeric and should be included in all billing documents. The use of these codes assists in reimbursement as well as in providing statistical information regarding mortality and morbidity.

The American Medical Association (AMA), in collaboration with CMS, developed both the ICD-9 codes and CPT codes. The ICD-9 codes are used to code etiologies, symptoms, diseases, and injuries that the health care provider is evaluating or treating. The CPT codes are used to describe the procedures, treatment, or service that health care providers use with patients. The nomenclature of CPT coding is divided between service and time-based codes. CPT codes are also divided between evaluation and therapeutic procedure codes. A list of speech–language pathology codes is available on the Internet at professional.asha.org/resources/reimbursement. Although

the CPT codes include the procedures SLPs use to evaluate and treat patients, the codes are not intended to be discipline specific. (Swigert & Fifer, 2002). Governmental and private insurance plans compare ICD-9 and CPT codes on billing documents to check for a reasonable relationship between the procedure and the disease (Slominski, 1997).

> If a patient with hypertension, laryngeal cancer, and a broken hip is being treated for voice therapy, the ICD-9 code for laryngeal cancer (the cause or reason for the voice therapy) should be used when billing for treatment.

It is always important that reports and progress notes support the codes and resulting charges. Techniques taught, exercises given, and concepts discussed with the patient or family need to be documented in a way that is consistent with the diagnosis and procedural coding used for billing. For Medicare, the SLP needs to document the exact start and stop times for each therapy session. The documentation of therapy time for the service-based codes should accurately reflect the length of time typically needed to provide the service. Service-based procedures are billed separately from time-based codes (Slominski, 1997).

It is important to note that not all CPT codes are recognized by every-third party payer or fiscal intermediary as appropriate for SLP services. Therefore, by checking with payers before billing for services, the SLP will greatly decrease the probability of a denial of payment for improper selection of codes. Often, hospitals and other health care employers ma0ke recommendations regarding the appropriate codes that SLPs can utilize for reimbursement of services.

Inappropriate use of CPT codes can lead to charges of fraud and abuse. For example, the use of too many CPT codes for one procedure can result in overpayment. In 1996, a congressional mandate called the Corrective Coding Initiative (CCI) was established to reduce such instances of fraud and abuse. As a result, CCI edits were implemented to reduce improper use of CPT codes.

In 1997, the Balanced Budget Act created a requirement that all claims for outpatient SLP services after April 1998 must be submitted utilizing a uniform coding system. The Health Care Financing Administration's Common Procedure Coding System (HCPCS) was the result. The CPT codes are included in the HCPCS system as level I HCPCS. Level II HCPCS are codes that are different in description or designation from the CPT codes and are specific to Medicaid and Medicare patients. The HCPCS coding system is required for Medicare Part B billing in hospitals, certified outpatient rehabilitation facilities (CORFs), skilled nursing facilities (SNFs), and home health agencies (Slominski, 1997).

Denials and Appeals Medicare, fiscal intermediaries, and private insurance plans employ reviewers who are trained to review documentation for justification of payment of those services. The reviewer may be a nurse, a doctor, or an SLP. (See **Table 17–6** for a partial list of reviewer guidelines.) Additionally, these payers establish an appeals process that may allow for multiple reviews. Therefore, this process can be lengthy. Because approval is based solely on the review of submitted documentation, careful and complete documentation from the start will increase the likelihood of payment and decrease the chance of denial.

Table 17–6 Medicare Documentation Reviewer Guidelines

Does the patient exhibit a pertinent medical history that is reflected in the plan of treatment? Avoid a "laundry list" of diagnoses. State precisely what happened and when a functional deficit occurred. If the diagnosis is chronic, state how it has caused the current functional deficit.

What did the patient do prior to therapy to attempt to correct the deficit? Were the attempts successful? Why does the patient need skilled intervention at this time?

Does the prognostic statement reflect rehabilitation potential to achieve the functional goal within a reasonable period of time?

What is the diagnosis and reason for referral?

Is the impairment related to a functional problem in activities of daily living?

What was the patient's prior level of functioning prior to onset of the deficit?

What specific measurements and tests substantiate the description of the functional deficit?

What is the patient's response to remediation?

What progress has the patient made toward meeting the functional and measurable short- and long-term goals?

Are progress notes present for each treatment date and do the notes specifically document all activities to support the charges?

Does the 30-day recertification documentation specifically address the justification for continuing skilled intervention?

Are all blanks in the documentation forms filled in or crossed through?

Does the patient understand what is expected, but is not motivated?

Does the certification or recertification (plan of care) include the physician and SLP signature and date?

Does the documentation merely reflect a temporary loss of function, a maintenance program involving repetitive activities, a program that is duplicative of other rehabilitation services, or a lack of progress owing to the inability (or refusal) of the patient to benefit from skilled intervention?

From Slominski, T.J. (1997). *Medicare Guidelines Explained for the Speech–Language Pathologist.* Gaylord, MI: Northern Speech Services.

For Medicare, the first level in the appeals process is a simple review of the current documentation. A second level consists of a review by another reviewer at the same level as the first reviewer. If the reviewer seeks more information, the SLP will receive a help letter requesting it. If the claim is denied, the family has the option to appeal the denial. In this case, the SLP sends documentation to "claims reconsideration." The SLP will be requested to substantiate why this claim should not be denied. When defending a denied claim, the SLP should refer to the Medicare guidelines described above (i.e., reasonable, necessary, specific, effective, skilled) and explain why the services provided fall within these guidelines (ASHA, 2001a). If the denial is upheld, the SLP can request a fair hearing with a hearing officer. If the hearing officer upholds the previous denial, the SLP has one final appeal to an administrative law judge. The decision of the administrative law judge is final (Slominski, 1997).

Documentation for Compliance and Performance Improvement

Accrediting agencies, such as the Joint Commission for Accreditation of Healthcare Organizations (JCAHO) and the Commission of Accreditation of Rehabilitation Facilities, Inc. (CARF),

have multiple standards for documentation of patient care. These standards require documentation of clinical information for adequate communication among providers. They also address the appropriate time frames for documentation and the need for confidentiality and security of patient records.

The Hospital Accreditation Standards Manual for JCAHO addresses documentation in several sections, but particularly under the patient-focused, organization-focused, and information management functions. According to the standards manual, the purpose of information management is to "obtain, manage, and use information to improve patient outcomes, and individual and hospital performance in patient care, governance, management and support processes" (JCAHO, 2002, p. 239).

Standards for Patient Care

The JCAHO Standards Manual (JCAHO, 2002) states that the patient's medical record should contain the following:

+ Sufficient information to identify the patient
+ Support the diagnosis; justify the treatment
+ Document the course and results; and facilitate continuity of care

Documentation of assessment results, treatment plans, interventions, progress towards goals, prognosis, and patient education are also important requirements for a complete patient record.

When the patient is referred, transferred, or discharged from treatment, there are basic standards for the continuum of care, as outlined by the standards manual. According to the standard (CC.5), the information that must be shared with other providers includes:

+ The reason for transfer, referral, discontinuation of services, or discharge
+ The patient's physical and psychosocial status
+ A summary of care provided and progress toward goals
+ Community resources or referrals provided to the patient (JCAHO, 2002)

The Standards Manual for CARF (CARF, 2002) also specifies what should be included in a patient's record. This includes:

+ Identification data
+ Pertinent history and relevant medical information
+ Information on impairments, activity limitations, and physical restrictions
+ Special communication needs
+ Assessment information
+ Predicted outcomes
+ Prescribed medications
+ Names and phone numbers of appropriate physicians or providers
+ Name of individual(s) coordinating the care
+ Various reports from other sources

As part of the treatment process, the record should include:

+ Assessment information
+ The plan of care with specific goals
+ Documentation of progress toward those goals
+ Critical incidents or interactions

Documentation must reflect active communication among the rehabilitation team members, and show the direct involvement of the patient and family in the rehabilitation process. As with JCAHO, CARF requires a written transfer or discharge summary at the appropriate time to show continuity of care.

Time Frames

Often, formal time frames for recording clinical documentation are established by accrediting bodies (national, state, and community), health care organizations, and the speech pathology departments. Typically, patient information (including evaluation, progress, and discharge reports) is expected to be sent to other professionals within 15 working days (Paul-Brown, 1994). ASHA recommends that clinical documentation be performed as soon as possible following the patient encounter, and JCAHO requires the transmission of information should be "timely" considering the data or information's intended use.

Confidentiality and Security

There are many specific standards for the confidentiality, storage, protection, and release of information in both the JCAHO and CARF standards manuals. In addition, the ASHA Code of Ethics (ASHA, 1994) contains several statements about the importance of confidentiality. Clinicians must not release or in any other way reveal any clinical information to unauthorized persons, unless required to do so by law or unless it is necessary to protect the welfare of the individual or other people. Electronic systems can help to protect confidentiality through the use of security IDs, passwords, and access codes. However, users need to be trained to avoid leaving confidential information on the screen unattended and to log out of the system when it is not in actual use.

Legislation has impacted patient confidentiality in documentation. The Health Insurance Portability and Accountability Act (HIPAA) of 1996 (ASHA, 1997–2002a) was originally designed to offer more insurance protection to working families. It was also intended to reduce the cases of families losing existing coverage due to preexisting conditions when they change jobs (Centers for Medicare & Medicaid Services, 2003). In addition to addressing access to insurance, the HIPAA privacy rule that was published by the Department of Health and Human Services (DHHS) is also pertinent to documentation.

The first finalized HIPAA rule specifies standard transaction formats and code sets for all health care professionals, including speech–language pathologists, who submit patient-related information electronically for a defined set of insurance transactions. In this context, faxing is not considered an electronic submission. Patient-related information includes claim submissions, eligibility inquiries, and coordination of benefits information.

HIPAA's second rule relates to privacy and requires written patient authorization for the release of medical information for purposes other than treatment, payment or operations (TPO). Under HIPAA, any identifying information is considered protected health information, including name, address, and Social Security number. Before disclosing any protected health information for reasons other than TPO, the treating health care professional must first obtain the authorization (consent) from the patient. The privacy regulations also require the provider to offer patients a notice of their privacy practices and request their acknowledgment of this notice. The notice must be presented to the patient with a summary statement of the providers' health information practices as well as a notification that patients have the right to request certain restrictions on how their information will be disclosed. An authorization is required for all nonroutine (other than TPO) uses of the information, such as distribution to employers or product marketers. Finally, HIPAA mandates that patients be able to view, copy, and request changes to their medical records.

The privacy rule is applicable not only to electronically stored patient information, but also to patient data in written form that is communicated through any means, including fax. For the field of speech–language pathology, HIPAA affects the practicing SLP in a variety of institutional settings, including hospitals, skilled nursing facilities, and home health agencies. HIPAA also has business associate provisions that apply to the speech–language pathologist who is a contracted provider for any entity that falls under HIPAA's jurisdiction. For more information on how HIPAA affects the practice of speech–language pathology, visit the Centers for Medicare and Medicaid Services Web site at http://www.cms.hhs.gov/hipaa.

Confidentiality and privacy must also be considered with storing patient documents. ASHA recommends that clinical documentation be stored in a secured place that can be accessed by authorized personnel only. Documentation should also be stored in a location that protects it from loss or destruction (JCAHO, 2002). For the treating SLP, current clinical records need to be accessible on a daily basis; however, historical documentation can be stored in a more remote location or be transferred to electronic means. Patient records should be disposed in a manner that also protects patient confidentiality (Paul-Brown, 1994).

Historical clinical records should be stored for as long as the state law mandates. In the absence of a state law, Medicare's record retention requirements should be followed. In most cases, health-care providers retain a patient's medical record for 5 to 7 years after the record or report is made. If the patient is a minor, the records may be retained longer.

Performance Improvement

Information from clinical documents is often used when designing and implementing a performance improvement program. Aggregate data taken from individual patient files can be collected, analyzed, and used to determine trends, problem areas, and outcomes. This information can then help to determine opportunities for improvement. For the data to be useful however, it must be collected in a consistent manner for all patients.

Documentation for Research

Accurate clinical documentation can provide data for research. However, for the documentation to be valuable for clinical research, it is important that the data are collected and documented in a consistent manner. The historical method of patient documentation included narrative descriptions of patient characteristics and test results. This form of documentation does not lend itself to research owing to the difficulty in finding the data and the inherent inconsistencies in the way that the data are reported. For data to be collected in a consistent manner, as required for research, checklists, standardized measures, and rating scales are recommended. These can be individualized for each patient and easily translated into outcomes measures for documentation purposes (Marshall, 2000). This type of format also allows the researcher to collect clean data that can be entered into a database for further analysis.

Outcomes research that shows that speech–language pathology services are efficacious and make a functional difference in the lives of patients is critical for the survival of the profession (Boston, 1994). If there is no research to support the efficacy of our services, third-party payers will further limit or even cease reimbursement. Efficacy research is also needed to determine "best practices" that are truly beneficial for the patient. Unfortunately, many common practices are based on clinical lore rather than solid evidence-based practice patterns. "The clinician, with the support of the academic community, must strive to justify his/her practices through rigorous investigations, or seeking of the truth rather than accepting the appearance of effectiveness" (Johnson & Huckabee, 2000, pp. 13–14). The only way to do this is to appropriately document the results of interventions and then collect and analyze the data.

To collect aggregate outcomes data on a national basis, ASHA developed the National Outcomes Measurement System (NOMS) for Speech–Language Pathology and Audiology in 1997. Through the use of the NOMS data, the value of speech–language pathology services can now be demonstrated to third-party payers, physicians, administrators, and consumers.

The data for NOMS are collected by using ASHA's Functional Communication Measures (FCMs). FCMs are a group of disorder-specific, seven-point rating scales that document the functional status of the patient at the time of the rating. FCMs are scored by a trained and certified SLP upon initiation of therapy and again at discharge. By comparing these ratings, clinicians document the amount of change in communication and/or swallowing function following intervention (see http://www.professional.asha.org/resources/noms/health.cfm).

Documentation for Legal Evidence

The medical record is a legal document that is admissible in a court of law and can be quoted verbatim. The document cannot be released to anyone other than treating professionals without a signed release from the patient, the parent, or the legal guardian. The medical record provides important proof for the patient in cases involving traumatic injury, medical or professional malpractice, corporate negligence, or disability determination. Because the professional may be called on to testify or provide evidence years after the patient was seen, it is particularly important to have complete and accurate information in the report. When there is a difference between the professional's verbal testimony and the written document, the court is more likely to give credence to a document that was completed close to the time that the patient was seen.

In addition to providing legal evidence for the patient, accurate and complete documentation can also provide legal evidence for the provider. This can help to show that appropriate procedures were followed in cases where the provider is accused of malpractice (Pannbacker, 2000).

Finally, billing documents must include the appropriate diagnostic and procedural codes for the patient. These documents must accurately reflect the patient's diagnosis or reason for services, the date the patient was seen, the amount of time that the patient was seen, and the services provided. Inaccurate or inappropriate billing documentation is very serious and can result in charges of fraud and abuse.

✦ Format of Documentation

Although there are standard types of documentation (e.g., diagnostic reports, treatment plans, progress reports, and discharge reports) that are generally completed for all patients, the format of these documents varies widely across settings and even among individual providers. These formats include completely handwritten reports, fill-in-the-blank-forms or checklists, dictated and typed reports, and computer-generated reports. Some SLPs generate very long, detailed reports, whereas others prefer to produce short, concise reports. The format used has a bearing on the ultimate quality of the professional communication, the cost of providing the documentation, and even the job satisfaction of the SLP.

Format that Meets the Customers' Needs

Because the primary purpose of clinical documentation is to communicate with other treating professionals, it is important to consider their needs. In general, the recipients of speech–language pathology reports are the physicians (referral and primary), other treating professionals, and parents or patients.

To determine what physicians need and want from our reports, the Speech Pathology Department at Cincinnati Children's Hospital Medical Center conducted a survey of referring physicians in October 2002 (**Table 17–7**); 108 physicians completed and returned the survey. The results revealed that most physicians read the "Summary and Impressions" and "Recommendations" sections of the report. However, only 27% stated that they read the "Examination" section. Of particular interest is the fact that the vast majority (88%) indicated that they prefer short, concise reports (about one page in length) rather than long, detailed reports (three or more pages). Most respondents (69%) preferred the testing results to be in a checklist format rather than in paragraph form. Finally, the majority of the surveyed physicians (71%) preferred the report to be easy to read with common terminology rather than technical language. Appendix 17–1 includes sample clinical reports.

The importance of making reports clear and concise for the readers has been stressed in the profession for many years. Although SLPs are expected to be experts in communication, we are often poor communicators when it comes to written documentation. As professionals, we tend to use terminology that only other SLPs understand. In addition, we often equate "comprehensive and thorough" with "long and wordy." The survey results noted above suggests that this practice does not meet the needs of those who receive the reports.

An additional concern is that long, technical reports may actually violate certain standards. For example, in the CARF standards manual it states that "all information, whether it is provided in writing or orally, should be provided in language and a format that can be understood by the person receiving

Table 17–7 Survey of Physician Documentation Preferences (*n* = 108 respondents)

What sections of a diagnostic report do you always read? (Check all that apply.)

41% (44)	Pertinent history
27% (29)	Examination (includes observations, tests given, and test results)
99% (107)	Summary and impressions
100% (108)	Recommendations

Which type of reports do you prefer?

12% (13)	Long and detailed (three or more pages)
88% (95)	Short and concise (one page)

Do you read the detail regarding the types of tests given, test scores, normative data, observations, etc?

25% (27)	Usually
60% (65)	Sometimes
15% (16)	Never

If information is included regarding formal tests, how would you prefer for it to be displayed?

31% (34)	Paragraph form within the report
69% (74)	Check list form as an attachment

What kind of language do you prefer in the reports?

30% (32)	Technical language
70% (76)	Common or simple language

How often do you want a progress report for a patient in therapy?

11% (12)	Monthly
72% (78)	Quarterly
1% (1)	Upon request only
16% (17)	Upon discharge from therapy

When do you typically read the report?

97% (105)	When the report is received
3% (3)	When the patient comes in for a visit

it" (Section 1. RP.-73, 3.a). Therefore, if the report is meant to meet standards and communicate with physicians and families, it is important that the report be fast and easy to read and contain terminology that is familiar to these readers.

Regardless of the form or length of the documentation, the SLP must have good writing skills (**Table 17–8**) and be able to communicate effectively in writing with other professionals and the patient and/or family. Because this is so important, the Council on Professional Standards of ASHA approved a requirement for "sufficient oral and written communication skills" (Standard III-A) in order to obtain a Certificate of Clinical Competence in Speech–Language Pathology, which took effect in 2005. The standard specifically states that the applicant must "be able to write and comprehend technical reports, diagnostic and treatment reports, treatment plans, and professional correspondence" (ASHA, 2001b).

Format and Effect on Cost

The documentation process can be very time-consuming, and thus very expensive. The more time spent on documentation, the less time the clinician will have for patient care and the generation of needed revenue. The challenges in obtaining reimbursement for services result in even more emphasis on productivity and the need to provide as much billable service as possible. Therefore, most settings cannot afford for the clinician to spend excessive time in documentation, especially because this activity is not directly billable.

The cost of documentation includes not only the clinician's time (and thus the salary expense), but also other related expenses such as transcription, copying, mailing, and storage. Of course, the more pages included in the report, the more professional time it takes to generate, and the more transcription expense if the report is typed by another person. If a secretary types 60 words per minute, it would take about a half-hour to type a three-page report. Assuming the secretary earns about $12 an hour plus benefits, the cost of typing that report would be about $7. Many organizations use transcription services that charge by line or character count. Charges per line vary, depending on the vendor, type of transcription, and the buyer's leverage abilities during the contracting phase. In the Midwest, transcription costs currently average 15 cents per line. With 42 lines on a standard page, this translates to approximately $6.30 per page. Therefore, a three-page report can result in almost $19 in transcription costs. Even

Table 17–8   Rules for Good Writing: A Tongue-in-Cheek Primer

Typos should never be toleratated so always spell chek.

Misspellings are never exceptable.

Lingering lame alliterations look lackadaisical.

Prepositions are not words to end sentences with.

It's not a good ideal to use words incorrectly in your righting. It's hard to reed.

One should always be orientated to the proper verb forms.

One word sentences. Eliminate.

No sentences without verbs.

Always end a sentence with a period

Its important to know when to use apostrophes.

Avoid cliches like the plague. (They're old hat.)

Don't be redundant and say the same things over and over again.

Don't use more words than absolutely, positively needed and really necessary.

Be more or less, but generally specific.

Analogies in writing are like feathers on a snake. You need 'em like a hole in the head.

Do you really need to use rhetorical questions?

Exaggeration is a billion times worse than understatement.

Foreign words and phrases are not apropos.

Y'all should be fixing to use standard grammar.

One should never generalize.

Parenthetical remarks (however relevant) are not necessary.

Never use ampersands & abbreviations, etc, etc.

Eliminate quotations. As Ralph Waldo Emerson once said, "I hate quotations."

He said to always reference pronouns before using them.

Table 17–9   Advantages of Computerized Documentation

Increases the quality and consistency of reports

Allows organizations to standardize their documentation through the use of templates

Reduces spelling errors, grammatical errors, and the use of unclear or unauthorized abbreviations

Increases accuracy of information and reduces errors with billing

Ensures that reports are legible

Decreases the redundancy of data entry

Reduces the time spent trying to think about appropriate wording when there are drop-down lists to select

Increases the ease of documentation

Increases the ability to generate reports quickly and provide timely documentation to physicians, third-party payers, patients, and families

Eliminates copying and mailing expenses if the reports can be e-mailed or faxed

Eliminates transcription costs

Increases access of information for providers at all locations and allows for seamless communication between locations

Increases access to policies/procedures, home programs, and other resources for all employees at all locations

Increases the security of protected patient information by blocking access to charts by unauthorized readers

Allows for supervision and management from a distance

Standardizes documentation templates, which can include the critical elements for hospital, JCAHO and CARF compliance

Provides the ability to collect, sort, calculate, and display information and generate management reports for use by supervisors, managers, hospital administrators, and other decision makers

Allows patient demographic information to be compiled for marketing purposes and program development

Reduces the need for storage of patient charts, handouts, and management documents, thereby saving costs in space

with computerized reports, there are costs associated with the clinician's time in generation of reports. Given these expenses, it is important for the documentation process to be efficient and the report to be concise.

On transcription costs: Approximately 6000 evaluations were performed by the Speech Pathology Department at Cincinnati Children's Hospital Medical Center in 2001. If our transcription service were used to generate the reports, the cost would have been about $151,200. Fortunately, patient documentation is computerized in the Speech Pathology Department, allowing staff to generate electronic reports themselves and therefore significantly reducing the costs associated with documentation.

Computerized Documentation

In response to the need for faster, more efficient, and streamlined documentation procedures, many organizations have turned to computer technology. The advantages of computerized documentation systems are numerous, as noted in **Table 17–9**. A computerized documentation system can increase the quality of services to the patient and family, improve service to referral sources and other health care providers, increase reimbursement from third-party payers, increase productivity and revenue, decrease expenses, increase available management information, and increase employee satisfaction and retention.

Although computerized documentation systems have significant benefits, there is an inherent danger to the use of standardized checklists. If providers become careless and complete the templates exactly the same for all of the patients they serve, this could have negative clinical and ethical implications. It could also affect reimbursement if the documentation is not individualized and fails to adequately justify the need for treatment (Marshall, 2000). If used appropriately, however, these templates can improve both the quality and consistency of the documentation, in addition to saving time and money.

The impact of computerization on a program can be dramatic and immediate. One study measuring the effects of computerization found a statistically significant decrease in total documentation time as a result of the computerization (Schumacher, Brodnik, Sachs, & Schiller, 1997). In the Speech Pathology Department at Cincinnati Children's Hospital Medical Center, all patient documentation and administrative functions have been computerized using the Chart Links software (Chart Links, Inc.) since 1996. (This product was originally developed by the Speech Pathology and Occupational/Physical Therapy Departments at Cincinnati Children's and these departments have remained active in suggesting enhancements to the product over time.) In 1996, an independent return-on-investment (ROI) study was done by International

Data Corporation (IDC) of the effects of computerization in these departments (International Data Corporation, 1998). This study showed a 264% ROI with development costs over a 3-year period, but a 668% ROI in 3 years when the initial development costs were deducted. The success of the computerization project in these two departments at Cincinnati Children's has been well documented (Medical Management Planning, 1997; Phillips, 1999; Tjapkes, 1999). Certainly, as hospitals and other health care facilities continue to compete for limited health care dollars, those facilities and programs that are fiscally solvent with the help of computer technology will be the ones to survive in the future. Therefore, the question should not be "Should we computerize?" but rather "How soon will we computerize?"

> The Chart Links system (Chart Links, Inc.), productivity ratios are calculated automatically for each SLP based on that person's billed charges and worked hours.

✦ Conclusion

Proper documentation of patient care is an important part of the practice of speech–language pathology. It should be the goal of each clinician to develop appropriate writing skills, and to document in a way that communicates effectively to the recipients, yet is done in an efficient and cost-effective manner. To achieve sufficient yet efficient documentation, the medical SLP must be knowledgeable of the documentation guidelines and criteria reviewed in this chapter. This is not an easy task, as a variety of organizations have established different guidelines and requirements, including governmental agencies, fiscal intermediaries, private third-party payers, and accrediting agencies. Furthermore, the guidelines and criteria continue to evolve, requiring medical SLPs to keep abreast of these changes on a yearly basis. Similar to clinical service delivery, documentation is an area of our practice that requires a *constant search for better ways to* meet the needs of the customers, demonstrate the value of our services, and be performed in a timely manner.

Study Questions

1. Describe the five primary purposes of documentation.
2. Why is the concept of medical necessity important in clinical documentation?
3. Identify and define six Medicare Documentation Guidelines.
4. Define a short-term goal and a long-term goal and provide an example of each. What criteria and/or components are needed to create a functional and measurable goal? Provide an example of a functional and measurable goal. Contrast this goal with a goal that is neither functional nor measurable.
5. What is the difference between CPT and ICD-9 codes? Why is it important that the SLP's documentation supports the codes used for each patient?
6. The accrediting agencies, JCAHO and CARF, have multiple standards for documentation of patient care. Identify the information that must be documented when a patient is referred, transferred, or discharged from treatment in order to meet JCAHO standards.
7. The Health Insurance Portability and Accountability Act (HIPAA) has impacted patient confidentiality in documentation. Under HIPAA's second rule, a patient's identifying information is considered protected health information. To comply with HIPAA standards, what must the treating health care professional obtain from the patient before disclosing any protected health information (for purposes other than treatment, payment or operations)? Additionally, HIPAA requires that providers offer patients a notice of their privacy practice. What must this notice include?
8. Research that supports the efficacy of our services is critical for the survival of the profession through continued reimbursement of services. What documentation formats are recommended for efficient and effective collection of research data?
9. Describe the three results of the survey on physician preferences for documentation (**Table 17–7**) related to length, format, and terminology. How will these results impact your documentation in the work setting?
10. Describe how a computerized documentation system can increase the quality of services to the patient and family while, at the same time, increase productivity and revenue. There are potential negative clinical and ethical implications from using computerized standardized checklists; describe how these implications can be avoided.

References

American Speech–Language Hearing Association. (1994). *Code of Ethics.* Rockville, MD: ASHA

American Speech–Language Hearing Association. (1997-2002a). *The Health Insurance Portability and Accountability Act of 1996 (HIPAA).* http://professional.asha.org/

American Speech–Language Hearing Association. (1997-2002b). *National Center for Treatment Effectiveness in Communication Disorders.* http://professional.asha.org/

American Speech–Language Hearing Association. (2001a). *Guidelines for Medicare Coverage of Speech-Language Pathology Services.* Rockville, MD: ASHA

American Speech–Language Hearing Association. (2001b). *Standards and Implementation for the Certificate of Clinical Competence in Speech–Language Pathology.* Rockville, MD: ASHA

Blue Cross-Blue Shield Association. (2002). *Glossary: Definition of Terms.* http://bluecrossblueshield.com/

Boston, B.O. (1994). Destiny Is in the Data: A Wake-Up Call for Outcome Measures. *ASHA November,* 35–38

Centers for Medicare & Medicaid Services (CMS). (2003). *Health Insurance Portability and Accountability Act of 1996 (HIPAA).* http://cms.hhs.gov/

Clark, B.W. (1995). Negotiating Successful Managed Care Contracts. *Healthcare Financial Management, 49,* 26–30

Commission on Accreditation of Rehabilitation Facilities, Inc (CARF). (2002). *Standards Manual: Medical Rehabilitation.* Tucson, AZ: CARF

International Data Corporation. (1998). *Children's Hospital Medical Center, Cincinnati, Ohio: Occupational Therapy, Physical Therapy and Speech Language Pathology Departments (Rehabilitation Professionals).* Cincinnati, OH: IDC

Ireys, H., Wehr, E., & Cooke, R. (1999). *Defining Medical Necessity: Strategies for Promoting Access to Quality Care for Persons with Developmental Disabilities, Mental Retardation, and Other Special Health Care Needs. The National Policy Center for Children with Special Health Care Needs, School of Hygiene and Public Health.* Baltimore: Johns Hopkins University Press

Johnson, P., & Huckabee, M.L. (2000). Research: The Pursuit of Truth. ASHA Special Interest Division 13. *Dysphagia Newsletter, 9,* 13–17

Joint Commission on Accreditation of Healthcare Organizations (JCAHO). (2002). *Hospital Accreditation Standards.* Oakbrook Terrace, IL: JCAHO

Marshall, R.C. (2000). Documentation in Medical Speech–language Pathology: Clinical-Friendly Suggestions to Keep the Tail from Wagging the Dog. *Journal of Medical Speech–language Pathology, 8,* 37–52

Medical Management Planning. (1997). Innovative Lotus Notes Program Streamlines Documentation in the Speech Pathology and OT/PT Departments CHCIN. *BENCH Press, 3,* 1–2

Merriam-Webster. (2001). *Collegiate Dictionary,* 10th ed. Springfield, MA: Merriam-Webster

Pannbacker, M. (2000). Whistleblowing in Speech–Language Pathology. *American Journal of Speech Language Pathology, 7,* 18–24

Pannbacker, M., Middleton, G., Vekovius, G.T., & Sanders, K.L. (2001). *Report Writing for Speech–language Pathologist and Audiologists,* 2nd ed. Austin: Pro-Ed

Paul-Brown, D. (1994). Clinical Record Keeping in Audiology and Speech–Language Pathology. *ASHA, 36,* 40–43

Phillips, S. (1999). Smothering in Paperwork, Healthcare Providers Seek a Cure in Groupware. *Group Computing, September/October*

Schumacher, K., Brodnik, M., Sachs, L., & Schiller, M.R. (1997). Therapists' Anxiety and Attitudes Toward Computerized Documentation in the Clinical Setting. *Journal of Allied Health, 26,* 151–158

Shipley, K.G., & McAfee, J.G. (1998). *Assessment in Speech–Language Pathology.* San Diego: Singular

Slominski, T.J. (1997). *Medicare Guidelines Explained for the Speech–Language Pathologist.* Gaylord, MI: Northern Speech Services

Slominski, T.J. (1999). *Medicare Documentation Requirements for Rehabilitation Services for Traditional Medicare and PPS Service Delivery.* Gaylord MI: Northern Speech Services

Swigert, N. (2002). Documenting What You Do Is as Important as Doing It. *The ASHA Leader, February,* 5

Swigert, N., & Fifer, R. (2002). Crafting Reimbursement Codes: CPT Coding Process Requires Time, Effort, & Expertise. *The ASHA Leader, October,* 8

Thompson, M. (2002). The Importance of Documenting What You Do. *The ASHA Leader, December,* 3

Tjapkes, S. (1999). The What Works. *Health Management Technology, February*

Appendix 17–1   Sample Clinical Reports

Anybody's Children's Hospital	Speech Pathology Evaluation
Patient Name: Ima Kidd	Date of Evaluation: 03/08/2001
Patient #: 0555555	Primary Physician: Dewey Hurt, M.D.
Date of Birth: 04/08/99	Referring Physician: Bill Jones, M.D.
Age: 1 year 11 months	SLP: John Q. Talker, M.A., CCC-SLP

Reason for Referral: Not talking.

Diagnosis: Intraventricular hemorrhage 431; Premature birth 765.1; Language disorder 784.5

PERTINENT HISTORY

Medical history includes prematurity (gestation of 24 weeks), low birth weight (2 lbs, 1 oz), and intraventricular hemorrhage (IVH) at birth requiring a 77-day stay in the NICU. Reflux has been diagnosed, but there are no other feeding or swallowing difficulties. Developmental milestones were accomplished with delay. Patient is not walking yet and she is currently using only a few words for communication.

EXAMINATION

Oral-Motor Function: Ima was able to imitate volitional oral movements. An assessment of oral-motor movement during feeding was performed and Ima was presented thin liquid (juice) via straw and crackers. The following observations were noted: good lip rounding and closure around the straw with no anterior loss of liquid; a strong internally stabilized and centered bite; tongue lateralization; diagonal chewing pattern; tongue tip elevation; adequate oral tone with no drooling.

Pragmatics: Age-appropriate skills were noted based on informal observation. Pragmatic skills demonstrated include maintaining eye contact; reciprocal smiling; turn-taking; joint attention.

Cognitive Play: Age-appropriate skills were noted based on informal observation and report. Skills are solid at the 21-month level with scatter skills to 30 months. Play routines observed included cause-effect play; vocal imitation; imitation of gestures and object manipulation; spatial problem solving (puzzles, shapes); functional and pretend play.

Receptive Language: Age-appropriate skills were noted based on informal observations and report. Skills are solid at the 21-month level with scatter skills up to 24 months. Receptive language skills observed included comprehension of: child's own name and names of family members; functional vocabulary/labels for common objects; labels for body parts; labels for pictures; labels for actions; one-step commands; simple yes/no questions; concepts and descriptors (emerging skills).

Expressive Language: Expressive language skills appear to be moderately to severely impaired based on informal observations and report and fall within the 6- to 9-month range with scatter skills up to 12 months. Ima's primary means of communication at this time is through gestures and some vocalizations. Expressive language skills observed included demonstration of: gestures, including pointing for showing an object (proto-declarative), reaching, giving, waving, and nodding for yes/no (appropriately); producing [Uh huh] in response to questions; vocalizations to call. Imitation skills observed include novel oral motor imitation; novel gestural imitation; limited and inconsistent verbal imitation.

Speech Production: Ima has developed the following sounds: /m, n, b, d, w, s, j, g/. Vowel repertoire includes /i, a, ae, o, ai, u/. Typical syllable shapes are CV and CVC; more advanced shapes such as CVCV are difficult to elicit. Mother reports that producing speech seems effortful for Ima; she notices oral groping patterns, especially when Ima is trying to vocalize. Ima produces a variety of clear sounds during babbling; sound variety decreases when she attempts to say words. The following words and sounds were elicited during the assessment using tactile cues: /o/ [open]; /bi/ and /ba/ [ball]; /guck/ [duck]; /mo/ [more]; /bo/ [blow]; /dis/ [this]; /dat/ [that]; /bu bu/ [bubbles]; /moo/ [cow]. Mother reports that Ima produced many word approximations for the first time during the assessment.

SUMMARY AND IMPRESSIONS

Ima Kidd, age 1 year 11 months, demonstrates a moderate to severe expressive language disorder, affecting her ability to communicate her functional wants and needs through verbalizations. Pragmatics, cognitive play, and receptive language skills appear to be age appropriate.

Appendix 17–1   *(Continued)*

Ima produces only a few words in simple consonant vowel (CV) structure. She exhibits difficulty in producing sounds in more advanced structures or sequences. Ima is very stimulable to speech and language therapy, as several new words were elicited during this assessment.

RECOMMENDATIONS

1. Speech and language therapy. Therapy goals should include eliciting word approximations through a hierarchical language stimulation approach; achieving more consonant sounds such as (p, t); achieving more complex syllable structures (i.e., CVCV, VCV, CVC2V, CVCV2, CVC2V2).

2. A formal audiology evaluation

3. A language stimulation home program: Handouts were provided describing language development activities to do in the home.

John Q. Talker, M.A., CCC-SLP

License number SP-XXXX

This document was electronically signed on 03/08/01.

cc: Health Information Management; Bill Jones, M.D.; Dewey Hurt, M.D.; Mr. and Mrs. Kidd

Anybody's Children's Hospital	**Videofluoroscopic Swallow Study**
Patient Name: Ima Kidd	Date of Evaluation: 06/11/2003
Patient #: 0555555	Primary Physician: Dewey Hurt, M.D.
Date of Birth: 05/03/99	Referring Physician: Bill Jones, M.D.
Age: 4 years 1 month	SLP: John Q. Talker, M.A., CCC-SLP

Reason for Referral: Swallowing concerns.

Diagnosis: Dysphagia 787.2

PERTINENT HISTORY

Ima is a 4-year-old boy with cerebral palsy/spastic quadriplegia. He presents at this time with clinical symptoms of coughing and choking during meals, primarily when eating too quickly. This video fluoroscopic swallowing study was requested to assess ability to maintain airway protection during intake of liquids and solids. This child's current status is as follows:

✦ Nutritional status: All nutritional intake is oral at this time. Ima reportedly accepts all textures. Higher textures are presented in a chopped form.

✦ Respiratory status: Respiratory status was unremarkable and there have been no episodes of pneumonia in the past 2 years by report.

CLINICAL OBSERVATIONS

Ima was positioned in the video fluoroscopy chair for lateral viewing without difficulty. Ima was cooperative throughout the entire examination.

DIAGNOSTIC IMPRESSIONS

The following study was done in conjunction with [Dr's. Name], radiologist, and was recorded on tape [number].

1. Oral motor skills were inefficient but functional for intake of liquid, purees, and easily managed solid food items.

2. Lip closure was adequate for intake of liquid via straw with sufficient sucking strength noted. Occasionally, shallow episodes of penetration were noted during intake of large boluses; however, airway protection was maintained.

3. Swallowing initiation was timely for intake of soft solids with satisfactory clearance through the hypopharynx. No episodes of penetration or aspiration were observed.

4. Per the radiologist, a screening view of esophageal function was within normal limits. Refer to [Dr's. Name] dictation under separate cover for more information.

RECOMMENDATIONS

The above findings were reviewed on the videotape with [Dr's. Name] and the following recommendations were jointly identified:

1. Continue with present speech pathology services.

2. Continue with spoon feeding of smooth and easily managed solid food consistencies.

3. Monitor size of bites and rate of feeding to maintain organization of swallowing and airway protection.

4. Monitor size of bolus and rate of swallowing when using a straw with intake of liquid for maintenance of airway protection.

John Q. Talker, M.S., CCC-SLP

License number SP-XXXX

This document was electronically signed on 06/12/03.

cc: Health Information Management; Bill Jones, M.D.; Dewey Hurt, M.D.; Mr. and Mrs. Kidd

18

Speech–Language Pathology in the Intensive Care Unit

Alice K. Silbergleit and Michael A. Basha

+ **Normal Respiration**
+ **Mechanical Ventilation**
+ **Medical Conditions that Require Treatment in an Intensive Care Unit Setting**
+ **Tracheotomy**
+ **Swallowing Issues**
+ **Case Vignettes**

Treating a patient in an intensive care unit (ICU) setting presents a series of unique and complicated issues. The feeling of loss of control that may occur when one is admitted to a hospital may be amplified for the ICU patient. The introduction of multiple tubes, the fear and anxiety associated with a serious medical illness, and the sudden loss of the ability to talk if a tracheotomy tube or mechanical ventilation is required may all contribute to a feeling of helplessness. The continued advances of medical technology have led to lifesaving techniques for individuals with stroke, traumatic brain injury (TBI), spinal cord injury (SCI), pulmonary disease, neurodegenerative disease, trauma, and cardiopulmonary conditions. The ICU patient may be of any age and have any one of a myriad of disorders that affects his or her communication or swallowing abilities.

The involvement of speech–language pathologists (SLPs) in the care of ICU patients has increased over the past several years. For this reason it is imperative that clinicians have a working knowledge of the breathing and speaking changes that occur in individuals who require tracheotomy tubes or ventilatory assistance. In the earliest stages of admission to an ICU, medical stability is the primary concern; speech–language pathologists may be asked to assist at this early stage by identifying a mode of communication or establishing a safe method of nutritional intake for a patient. The current trend of limiting hospital stays to decrease medical costs may be one of the reasons for early consultation among a variety of health care specialists who would previously have delayed consultation until a patient was transferred to a regular medical unit.

This chapter familiarizes the practicing SLP with some of the more common terminology and issues specific to the ICU environment. Our discussion includes an explanation of the basic processes of normal respiration and mechanical ventilation as well as common illnesses seen in an ICU setting. Because the role of SLPs working with tracheostomized patients is becoming more popular, we present a review of various methods of voicing with tracheostomy tubes and speaking valves. In addition, we discuss decision-making issues regarding a patient's candidacy for oral feeding and various methods of testing for and treating dysphagia, including some ethical considerations related to feeding severely ill patients. The importance of a team approach to diagnosing and treating ICU patients is emphasized throughout. This information will help the practicing SLP to understand the complexities of working with an ICU patient and thus facilitate effective communication and swallowing care for individuals in an ICU setting.

+ Normal Respiration

In most cases admission to a medical ICU indicates a problem in respiration. To fully understand such disorders, it is essential for us to have sound knowledge of the normal respiratory process.

The respiratory system is relatively easy to comprehend when one understands the function of its two major components: the lungs and the respiratory, or ventilatory, pump. The lungs are primarily involved in gas exchange; they are responsible for moving oxygen from the atmosphere into the alveoli and then into the pulmonary capillary blood and for moving carbon dioxide from the pulmonary capillary blood to the alveoli where it can be exhaled into the atmosphere. Hence, the lungs ensure a constant supply of oxygen to the blood, which is then distributed to the cells, tissues, and organs of the body, providing the necessary maintenance of normal biochemical and metabolic function (Weinberger, Schwartzstein, & Weiss, 1989). Likewise, the ability of the lungs to excrete carbon dioxide, the major waste product of metabolism, prevents accumulation of this potentially deadly gas in the body. Diseases that primarily affect the working tissue of the lung (lung parenchyma) (e.g., pneumonia, congestive heart failure, pulmonary hemorrhage) interfere with the gas exchange process and lead to low blood oxygen, called hypoxemia, or occasionally to elevated blood carbon dioxide, or hypercapnia (West, 1971).

Ventilation is the process of eliminating carbon dioxide from the body through the lungs. The function of the respiratory, or ventilatory, pump of the respiratory system is more complex than that of the lungs and involves those elements that are included in the bellows function of the system. The respiratory cycle begins in the brainstem in the respiratory centers of the pons and medulla, with the generation of a nerve impulse and the transmission of that stimulus to the respiratory muscles, primarily the diaphragm (**Fig. 18–1**). The contraction and flattening of the diaphragm result in the shortening of its muscle fibers as it descends in the thorax. When this occurs, intrapleural pressure becomes more negative as intrathoracic volume increases. This increase in negative intrapleural pressure is transmitted to the alveoli and allows intraalveolar pressure to be lower than atmospheric pressure. The gradient between the atmosphere and alveoli causes air to move into the lungs until alveolar and atmospheric pressures are equal (Murray, 1986). At end-inspiration, when atmospheric pressure equals intraalveolar pressure, airflow into the lungs ceases and expiration begins.

Usually expiration is a passive process dependent on the elastic recoil of the lungs, the presence or absence of airway resistance, and the use of the abdominal and intercostal expiratory muscles. At end-expiration, intrapleural pressure has increased back to –2.0 cm H_2O and the whole process is repeated (Roussos & Macklem, 1982). The negative intrapleural pressure at end-expiration is created by the opposing forces of the lungs, which want to collapse, and the chest wall, which wants to spring outward. These opposing forces keep the lungs expanded and prevent them from collapsing, create negative intrapleural pressure at end-expiration, and allow a volume of air in the lungs prior to the next inspiration, termed functional residual capacity.

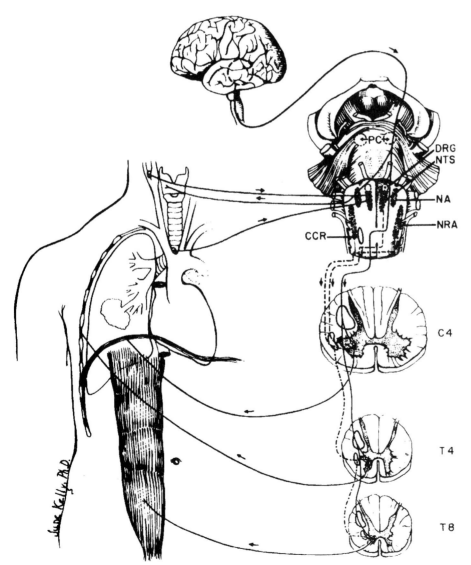

Figure 18–1 Summary of the route of respiration. [From American College of Chest Physicians. (1991). The Diagnosis and Management of Neuromuscular Diseases Causing Respiratory Failure. *Chest, 99*, 1485–1494, with permission.]

Functional residual capacity is the beginning point for a new respiratory cycle. Therefore, the normal respiratory cycle in a spontaneously breathing person depends on opposite pressure and volume changes that allow air to move in and out of the lungs. Tidal volume is the volume of air moving into the lungs depending on their compliance. If the lung is stiff (as in idiopathic pulmonary fibrosis), less volume moves into the lung. Conversely, if its compliance is great (e.g., obstructive lung disease), a greater amount of air constitutes the patient's tidal volume.

✦ Mechanical Ventilation

Patients in an ICU setting are frequently assisted in their respiration by mechanical ventilation. Respiratory failure, whether secondary to hypoxemia, hypercapnia, or both, is the primary reason why critically ill patients eventually require ICU care and mechanical ventilation (Pingleton, 1988). The majority of patients seen in an ICU have a fulminant course with a dramatic presentation, and the institution of mechanical ventilation can be lifesaving once the primary insult is treated or reversed. However, in some cases patients with neuromuscular disease or chest wall abnormalities experience slowly progressive, chronic respiratory failure and are unable to be weaned from the ventilator.

Most adult patients requiring mechanical ventilation in an ICU will be ventilated via positive-pressure, volume-cycled ventilators. This means that gas that is above atmospheric pressure is delivered into the lungs, raising intraalveolar pressure during inspiration. During inspiration from a ventilator, a preset tidal volume is delivered to the patient, and both intrathoracic volume and pressure increase. Therefore, intrathoracic pressure and volume move in the same direction, unlike that of a spontaneously breathing individual. The amount of delivered tidal volume is constant and the pressure is variable, depending on lung compliance and airway resistance (Tobin, 1994). Airway pressure will be high if lung compliance is low (e.g., idiopathic pulmonary fibrosis) or airway resistance is high (e.g., tumor, foreign-body aspiration, increased pulmonary secretions), or both. At end-inspiration, an exhalation port valve is opened and exhalation is essentially passive, dependent on lung elastic recoil, airway resistance, and the use of expiratory muscles as in a spontaneously breathing patient.

The next breath is either triggered by the patient or automatically given to the patient by the ventilator. If the patient is alert or able to initiate a breath, the patient sets the rate of breathing. This mode of mechanical ventilation is referred to as the assist-control (AC) mode and is the preferred mode of early ventilation in patients who develop respiratory failure from a variety of causes. If the patient is unable to set the respiratory rate, the physician can determine the number of minimum breaths per minute. The product of delivered tidal volume and respiratory rate is termed minute volume or minute ventilation; this value varies from patient to patient depending on the underlying disease process. All ventilator settings are adjusted by a physician, usually a pulmonologist, or respiratory therapist or nurse who follows the orders of a physician. Some patients are uncomfortable with artificial ventilation, which causes them to be anxious and agitated. In those instances, sedation, and in extreme cases, drug-induced paralysis, may be necessary to ensure good patient-ventilator synchrony.

There are other types of noninvasive modes of respiration that may be implemented in less ill patients who may not require conventional ventilation or to forestall more conventional ventilation in patients whose primary disease process can be reversed or controlled. These alternative modes of ventilation deliver positive pressure to the airway via a tight fitting nasal or full facial mask, which are meant to augment the oxygenation and ventilatory processes and reduce the patient's work of breathing (Meduri, Cook, Turner, et al., 1996). Noninvasive ventilation may also serve as a bridge to more normal spontaneous ventilation as a patient's medical status improves and he or she is ready to be weaned from full mechanical ventilation. Noninvasive airway ventilatory management that is typically seen in an ICU setting may include continuous positive airway pressure (CPAP), pressure support ventilation (PSV), and inspiratory/expiratory positive airway pressure (BiPAP).

Continuous Positive Airway Pressure

Continuous positive airway pressure (CPAP) is the application of positive pressure to the airways throughout the respiratory cycle (i.e., during both inspiration and expiration). This mode of ventilation can be used only for a spontaneously breathing person. The amount of airway pressure applied is determined by a physician and is usually between 5 and 10 cm H_2O. CPAP may be applied through the ventilator in an intubated patient or via a tight fitting nasal or full face mask in a nonintubated patient. It can be used to assist in weaning a patient from mechanical ventilation or for breath support in patients with frank or impending respiratory failure. CPAP works by splinting open atelectatic alveoli, increasing end-expiratory lung volume, and assisting the inspiratory muscles in reducing the work of breathing (Katz & Marks, 1985).

Pressure Support Ventilation

This method of ventilation, which is patient initiated, has been relatively recently described and used. It is a physician-determined mode that is pressure cycled and flow limited in a spontaneously breathing patient with an intact respiratory center. That is, pressure is applied to the airway only during the inspiratory phase of the respiratory cycle (pressure cycled), and the pressure applied (determined by the physician) ceases once the inspiratory flow drops below a certain level, [e.g., 5 L/min (flow-limited)]. Exhalation is then passive and no pressure is applied during this part of the respiratory cycle. PSV can be used to entirely support the patient or assist in the weaning of the patient from mechanical ventilation. The more pressure used, the more the patient is assisted and the less the work of breathing for the patient.

Like CPAP, PSV can be used via a mask or through an endotracheal tube in an intubated patient. PSV reduces the work of breathing by unloading the inspiratory muscles. It may be of special value in patients who have increased inspiratory resistance (e.g., central airway mass/tumor, etc.) (MacIntyre, 1986).

Inspiratory/Expiratory Positive Airway Pressure

BiPAP is a technique of noninvasive ventilation in which pressure applied to the airway can be adjusted for both the inspiratory and expiratory phases of the respiratory cycle. Hence, the differential pressures may be used to assist in the ventilation of patients with different disease processes. This modality is used in a spontaneously breathing patient by a tight-fitting nasal or full face mask. The pressure applied during inspiration is inspiratory positive airway pressure (IPAP) and during expiration is expiratory positive airway pressure (EPAP). IPAP is very similar to PSV and EPAP is similar to positive end-expiratory pressure (PEEP). BiPAP helps to unload the respiratory muscles, reduce the work of breathing, splint open collapsed alveoli, and raise end-expiratory volume. BiPAP is often used in patients who require partial ventilatory support or in those who have impending respiratory failure who might be spared endotracheal intubation if the primary disorder can be quickly reversed (Brochard, Isabey, Piquet, et al., 1990).

Mechanical Ventilation Weaning

Although the literature is replete with articles suggesting the best approaches or proper timing for weaning a patient from mechanical ventilation, this process is as much an art as a science (Tobin & Yang, 1990). Numerous weaning parameters have been established to aid physicians in the decision-making process, but these parameters do not always predict a successful outcome (Sahn & Lakshminarayan, 1973). As a general rule, the less time a patient is mechanically ventilated and the more quickly reversible the primary insult is, the more accurate these weaning guidelines are for predicting successful weaning. In addition, younger patients and surgical patients tend to wean more quickly from mechanical ventilation than older patients, patients with multiple or complex medical problems, or those with multiple organ dysfunction.

A rapid shallow breathing index, which provides a ratio of respiratory frequency divided by tidal volume in liters, seems to predict successful weaning in several patients if this ratio is less than 105 (Yang & Tobin, 1991). Ultimately, many experienced critical care physicians base the decision to wean on general impressions of patient status. However, as a general principle, weaning usually occurs when patients assume a greater part of the work of breathing as their clinical condition improves and when gas exchange, as assessed by arterial blood gases, shows stable oxygenation and ventilation.

✦ Medical Conditions that Require Treatment in an Intensive Care Unit Setting

This section reviews the most common pulmonary and neurologic illnesses that are typically seen in an ICU setting.

Pulmonary Disease

Chronic Obstructive Pulmonary Disease

Chronic obstructive pulmonary disease (COPD) encompasses a group of lung diseases characterized by slow progression and long continuance as well as the presence of expiratory airflow limitation or obstruction. Emphysema and chronic bronchitis are two of the more important diseases that fall under this large category, but chronic bronchial asthma, cystic fibrosis, bronchiectasis, small airway disease, and bronchiolitis all fulfill the broad definition of COPD. About 15 million people in the United States have emphysema and chronic bronchitis, and another 15 million suffer from asthma (total 30 million, or 11 to 12.5% of the U.S. population) (Feinleib, Rosenberg, Collins, et al., 1989). The differences in these diseases are based on histologic, physiologic, radiologic, clinical, and other criteria.

Emphysema

Emphysema is characterized by the permanent destruction and enlargement of the distal air spaces, most commonly caused by cigarette smoking (active or passive) (Snider, Kleinerman, Thurlbeck, et al., 1985). Patients tend to be limited mostly by dyspnea and have significant air trapping and hyperinflation. Because they work so hard to maintain normal or near-normal blood gases, they are often referred to as "pink puffers." They are usually thin and cachectic and rely on pursed lip breathing.

Acute Respiratory Distress Syndrome

Acute respiratory distress syndrome (ARDS, formerly adult respiratory distress syndrome) is a catastrophic disease characterized by significant and acute lung injury leading to respiratory failure usually within 48 hours of the insult. The majority of these patients have profound impairment in gas exchange, are severely hypoxemic, and spend variable amounts of time on a mechanical ventilator. ARDS is most commonly caused by pneumonia, aspiration, polytrauma, multiple transfusions, gram-negative sepsis, and pancreatitis. Other organ system involvement and failure occur and the mortality is high (40%) (Ashbaugh, Bigelow, Petty, et al., 1967).

Cardiopulmonary Illness

Congestive Heart Failure

Congestive heart failure (CHF) is caused by several diseases in which impairments in cardiac output allow blood to pool in the pulmonary veins, capillaries, and pulmonary arteries. This pooling of blood leads to lung congestion and gas exchange impairments. Etiologies that can cause CHF include myocardial infarction, valvular heart disease, hypertensive heart disease, cardiomyopathy, and pericardial diseases. The condition can be acute or chronic and almost all patients suffer with dyspnea, fatigue, exercise intolerance, and lower extremity edema.

Cardiac Failure

Cardiac failure is a nonspecific condition of cardiac or heart dysfunction caused by a variety of diseases, including hypertensive and ischemic heart disease, pericardial disease, and valvular disease. During cardiac failure, cardiac output is impaired and end-organ perfusion suffers. Patients with cardiac failure may develop stroke, kidney disease, liver failure, and other organ dysfunction. A majority of these patients also have CHF.

Pulmonary Edema

Pulmonary edema is a condition of excess lung fluid that often leads to respiratory failure because the fluid-filled alveoli are unable to participate in normal gas exchange. CHF and ARDS are causes of pulmonary edema. Important in the evolution of this disease is the type of accumulated lung fluid. Protein-poor edema fluid (as in CHF) is more responsive to diuretic therapy than is protein-rich edema fluid (as in ARDS). Pulmonary edema usually causes dyspnea, fatigue, weakness, exercise intolerance, and peripheral edema.

Neurologic Disease

Amyotrophic Lateral Sclerosis

Amyotrophic lateral sclerosis (ALS) is a degenerative neuromuscular disease that involves the upper motor neurons in the cortex and lower motor neurons in the brainstem and spinal cord (Mulder, 1957). To date, the etiology of ALS is unknown. Viral, toxic, and genetic causes have been speculated (Mulder, 1957). In the United States the ratio of men to women who acquire the nonfamilial form of the illness is 2:1, and the cause of death is usually respiratory failure or pneumonia (Mulder, 1957). Although muscle cramping is commonly the initial symptom of the disease, nearly one quarter of patients present with dysarthria as their initial symptom (Mulder, 1984; Rosen, 1978). This illness eventually involves the musculature of speech, swallowing, and respiration. Patients who have made the decision to undergo a tracheotomy and/or mechanical ventilation to assist or prolong their respiratory status may be seen in the ICU. If a patient is anarthric, speech via a tracheostomy tube will not be functional and alternative methods of communication are necessary.

Guillain-Barré Syndrome

Adams and Victor (1985) describe this illness as a rapidly progressing ascending inflammatory disease that affects people of all ages and both sexes. The usual clinical presentation is muscle weakness, which can result in total muscle paralysis and death due to respiratory failure within a few days of onset. Facial diplegia occurs in approximately half of the cases and arises along with other cranial nerve signs after the arms are affected. The use of plasmapheresis within 2 weeks of onset has been known to expedite recovery, including the length of time patients require mechanical ventilation. The focus of medical treatment is respiratory assistance and careful nursing care as the disease resolves naturally. Recovery is complete in the majority of cases. A flaccid form of dysarthria is seen with this disorder, and careful speech assessment and short-term treatment may be necessary as the patient recovers.

Stroke

Many forms of stroke require ICU placement for a patient. Stroke may result from an intracranial hemorrhage or a thrombotic or embolic event. Patients who develop brainstem strokes are likely to spend their acute phase of hospitalization in an ICU because respiration may be compromised. As the course of the illness progresses, the patient should be followed closely from a communication and swallowing standpoint.

Traumatic Brain Injury

A patient with an acute TBI sometimes has an evaluation for basic cognitive stimulation in the ICU by an SLP. Because intubation and eventual tracheotomy are common occurrences in such situations, thorough diagnostic therapy from a communication and swallowing standpoint is imperative. TBI patients may exhibit rapid changes in neurologic status in a short period of time, and thus constant contact with nursing and medical staff are necessary for anticipating the patient's ability to try new methods of communication and feeding, particularly as this relates to voicing and swallowing with a tracheostomy tube.

Spinal Cord Injury

Patients with acute SCI above the level of C3 likely have breathing problems and require mechanical ventilation (Rowland, 1985). As the patient stabilizes, communication and swallowing issues arise. Communication may progress from simple eye blinks for yes/no responses to voicing with a tracheostomy tube as the patient's condition improves. Ongoing monitoring and diagnostic therapy are necessary to provide the most effective and efficient methods of communication for the patient.

Laryngeal Injury

According to Tucker (1993), the larynx is relatively protected within the neck by the sternocleidomastoid muscles laterally, the cervical vertebrae and other muscles of the neck posteriorly, and the mandible from above. Laryngeal injuries occur from several causes ranging from blunt trauma to the larynx, as seen in seat belt or steering wheel injuries in car accidents, to penetrating trauma-bullet or knife wounds. Blunt injury to an older, more calcified larynx may result in arytenoid dislocation or laryngeal fracture of the cartilaginous structures of the larynx, whereas the same blow may produce little damage to a young, flexible larynx.

The ICU patient with a laryngeal injury commonly has a tracheostomy tube. It is important to discuss the full extent of the patient's laryngeal injuries and the surgical repair procedures with the physician to anticipate short- and long-term voicing conditions. Counseling regarding voice use in the early stages of hospitalization is recommended with close monitoring, and voice therapy, with or without the presence of a tracheostomy tube, may be necessary.

✦ Tracheotomy

During their initial days in the ICU patients may be ventilated via nasal or oral intubation with an endotracheal tube. However, many of these patients require a tracheotomy to facilitate respiration. Decisions about the proper timing and indications for changing the airway access to a tracheostomy tube seem to be less controversial than in the past, but a variety of opinions still exist. The trend in recent years has been toward earlier insertion of tracheostomy tubes after initial nasal or oral intubation in critically ill patients. For spontaneously breathing patients a tracheostomy tube is placed to improve ventilation. It provides direct access to the lower respiratory tract. The patient inhales and exhales directly via the tracheostomy tube, which is usually inserted at or below the second or third tracheal ring, thus bypassing the nose and mouth. A tracheotomy is usually performed in cases when upper respiratory obstruction occurs owing to illness, injury, or surgery (Nash, 1988).

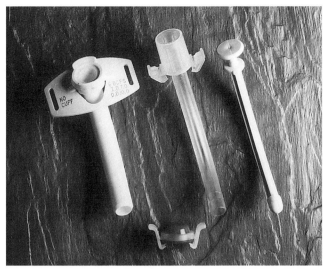

Figure 18–2 Shiley outer cannula, inner cannula, and obturator (left to right). (Courtesy of Mallinckrodt Medical, Inc.)

Figure 18–3 Shiley cuffed tracheostomy tube. (From left to right: outer cannula, inner cannula, obturation). (Courtesy of Mallinckrodt Medical, Inc.)

Components of a Tracheostomy Tube

There are three basic parts to a tracheostomy tube: the obturator, the outer cannula, and the inner cannula (**Fig. 18–2**) (Nash, 1988). The obturator is used for insertion of the outer cannula of the tracheostomy tube and is replaced by the inner cannula once the outer cannula is securely in place. The inner cannula remains in place to collect secretions that could potentially obstruct the airway. At times these secretions may be viscous or may collect and dry within the inner cannula. If the inner cannula is not in place and secretions become encrusted within the outer cannula, the potential for airway obstruction exists, which, in extreme cases, may require a total tracheostomy tube change. For this reason it is highly recommended that the inner cannula remain in place and undergo cleaning on a regular basis. Disposable inner cannulas are available that may be replaced without cleaning, and single cannula tracheostomy tubes are also available that are made of a silicone plastic and do not require the use of an inner cannula. The silicone material is intended to reduce the risk of encrustation of secretions (Dikeman & Kazandjian, 1995b).

Types of Tracheostomy Tubes

Tracheostomy tubes may be cuffed (**Fig. 18–3**) or uncuffed (**Fig. 18–4**). The cuff is inflated and deflated via a syringe that inserts into the pilot balloon. When the cuff is inflated, the route of air travel is directly via the trachea to the lower airway, thus bypassing the nose and mouth as shown in **Fig. 18–5**. In most cases, as a patient's medical status improves, the cuff may be deflated or a cuffless tracheostomy tube inserted. In either of these scenarios, air is then able to pass through the upper airway and vocal folds, enabling the patient to voice with a tracheostomy tube as shown in **Fig. 18–6**.

Many manufacturers offer tracheostomy tubes of varying sizes, yet, as noted in **Table 18–1**, tube sizes are usually not comparable among the different manufacturers. For example, a standard No. 6 Shiley tracheostomy tube (Mallinckrodt Medical, Inc., Irvine, CA), does not have the same dimensions as a No. 6 tracheostomy tube made by Portex (Smiths Medical, Hythe,

Kent, UK). For this reason, it is important to know the inner and outer cannula dimensions, and not just the given size of the tube, when substituting tubes from one manufacturer to another.

Advantages to Tracheostomy Tube Placement

As with any procedure there are advantages and potential complications to the placement of a tracheostomy tube. In addition to the primary advantage of providing airway access, advantages to the placement of a tracheostomy tube include (Dikeman & Kazandjian, 1995b; Nash, 1988):

1. Ease of access to the lower respiratory tract for suctioning
2. A decrease in the risk of laryngeal granuloma and subglottic stenosis owing to the elimination of constant pressure of an orotracheal tube at the level of the vocal folds and subglottis

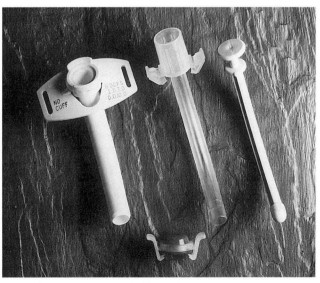

Figure 18–4 Shiley uncuffed tracheostomy tube (left). (Courtesy of Mallinckrodt Medical, Inc.)

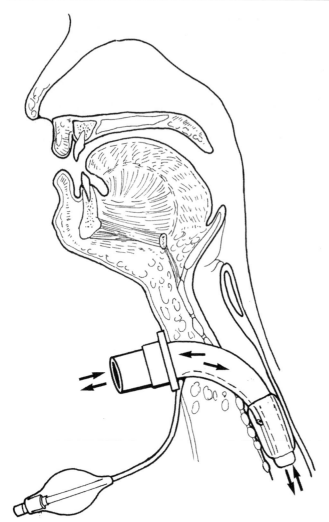

Figure 18–5 Route of airflow to and from the lower airway (arrows) with an inflated tracheostomy tube cuff.

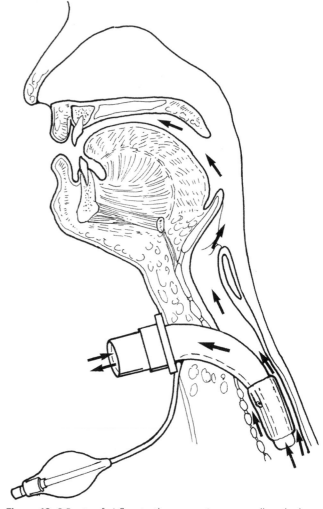

Figure 18–6 Route of airflow to the upper airway as well as the lower airway (arrows) when a tracheostomy tube cuff is deflated.

3. Improved weaning from mechanical ventilation because (a) the design and placement of a tracheostomy tube lessens the resistance to airflow that is seen in endotracheal tubes; and (b) air volume is delivered directly to the lungs, thereby reducing the amount of dead space in the airway (areas within the airway that do not participate in gas exchange) and allowing for greater volumes of inspired air available for oxygen exchange

4. An increase in patient comfort compared with nasal or orotracheal intubation

5. Improved options for oral communication and swallowing compared with nasal or orotracheal intubation

6. Improved oral hygiene owing to improved access to the oral cavity without the presence of an endotracheal tube

Complications of Tracheostomy Tube Placement

The following are some complications of tracheostomy tube placement (Dikeman & Kazandjian, 1995b; Heffner, Miller, & Sahn, 1986; Logemann, 1983; Mason, 1993a; Nash, 1988):

1. Loss of taste and smell owing to an absence of airflow through the nose and mouth

2. An increase in secretions secondary to the presence of the tracheostomy tube as the body reacts to the presence of a foreign object

3. Tracheal granuloma secondary to abrasion at the stoma site

4. Tracheomalacia, a softening or degeneration of the elastic and connective tissues of the trachea, which may occur when there is any trauma to the tracheal walls that exposes the cartilage and leads to tissue breakdown

5. Tracheal stenosis occurs when the trachea narrows as part of the healing process after trauma. Stenosis may occur at the stoma site or near the cuff of the tracheostomy tube. Tracheal stenosis at the stoma site may result from frequent infections, tube changes, a stoma that is too large and begins to close as part of the healing process, or continuous tugging on the tracheostomy tube from ventilator tubing. Constant pressure on the tracheal mucosa or abrasive movements of the cuff as the tube moves up and down during breathing, swallowing, or changes in body position may contribute to tracheal stenosis at the cuff site.

6. Limitation of laryngeal elevation with a cuffed tracheostomy tube during swallowing, which may lead to aspiration

7. Tracheoesophageal fistula, a connection between the trachea and the esophagus, may occur from pressure on the

Table 18–1   Cross-Reference Chart of Tracheostomy Tube Sizes

Adult Tracheostomy Tube Cross Reference

BIVONA CODE NO.	ID mm	OD mm	APPX French	APPX Jackson	Length mm	SHILEY CODE NO.	ID mm	OD mm	APPX French	APPX Jackson	Length mm	PORTEX CODE NO.	ID mm	OD mm	APPX French	APPX Jackson	Length mm
850150	5.0	7.3	22	3	60												
850160	6.0	8.7	26	4	70	4DCT	5.0	8.5	26	4	67	503060	5.0	8.5	26	4	67
850170	7.0	10.0	30	6	80	6DCT	7.0	10.0	30	6	78	503070	6.0	9.9	30	6	73
850180	8.0	11.0	33	7	88							503080	7.0	11.3	34	7	78
850190	9.0	12.3	37	8	98	8DCT	8.5	12.0	36	8	84	503090	8.0	12.6	38	8	84
850195	9.5	13.3	40	10	98	10DCT	9.0	13.0	39	10	84	503100	9.0	14.0	42	10	84
850150	5.0	7.3	22	3	60	5SCT	5.0	7.0	21	3	58						
850160	6.0	8.7	26	4	70	6SCT	6.0	8.3	24.9	4	67	530060	6.0	8.3	24	4	55
850170	7.0	10.0	30	6	80	7SCT	7.0	9.6	28.8	6	80	530070	7.0	9.7	30	6	75
850180	8.0	11.0	33	7	88	8SCT	8.0	10.9	32.7	7	89	530080	8.0	11.0	33	7	82
850190	9.0	12.3	37	8	98	9SCT	9.0	12.1	36.3	8	99	530090	9.0	12.4	36	8	87
850195	9.5	13.3	40	10	98	10SCT	10.0	13.3	39.9	10	105	530100	10.0	13.8	40	10	98
670150	5.0	7.3	22	3	60												
670160	6.0	8.7	26	4	70	4FEN	5.0	8.5	26	4	67	513060	5.0	8.5	26	4	67
670170	7.0	10.0	30	6	80	6FEN	7.0	10.0	30	6	78	513070	6.0	9.9	30	6	73
670180	8.0	11.0	33	7	88							513080	7.0	11.3	34	7	78
670190	9.0	12.3	37	8	98	8FEN	8.5	12.0	36	8	84	513090	8.0	12.6	38	8	84
670195	9.5	13.3	40	10	98	10FEN	9.0	13.0	39	10	84	513100	9.0	14.0	42	10	84

(Continued)

Table 18–1 *(Continued)*

Uncuffed Tracheostomy Tube Cross Reference

BIVONA CODE NO.	ID mm	OD mm	APPX French	APPX Jackson	Length mm	SHILEY CODE NO.	ID mm	OD mm	APPX French	APPX Jackson	Length mm	PORTEX CODE NO.	ID mm	OD mm	APPX French	APPX Jackson	Length mm
60N025	2.5	4.0	12	000	30												
60N030	3.0	4.7	14	00	32	00NT	3.1	4.5	14	00	30	553025	2.5	4.5	13	00	30
						0NT	3.4	5.0	15	0	32	553030	3.0	5.2	15	0	32
60N035	3.5	5.3	16	0/1	34	INT	3.7	5.5	17	1	34	553035	3.5	5.8	16	1	34
60N040	4.0	6.0	18	2	36						36						
60P025	2.5	4.0	12	000	38							555025	2.5	4.5	13	00	30
60P030	3.0	4.7	14	00	39	00PT	3.1	4.5	14	00	39	555030	3.0	5.2	15	00	36
60P035	3.5	5.3	16	0/1	40	0PT	3.4	5.0	15	0	40	555035	3.5	5.8	16	01	40
60P040	4.0	6.0	18	2	41	1PT	3.7	5.5	17	1	41	555040	4.0	6.5	18	02	44
60P045	4.5	6.7	20	3−	42	2PT	4.1	6.0	18	2	42	555045	4.5	7.1	19	03	48
60P050	5.0	7.3	22	3+	44	3PT	4.8	7.0	21	3	44	555050	5.0	7.7	21	4−	50
60P055	5.5	8.0	24	4	46	4PT	5.5	8.0	24	4	46	555055	5.5	8.3	23	4+	52
60A150	5.0	7.3	22	3	60												
60A160	6.0	8.7	26	4	70	4CFS	5.0	8.5	26	4	67	550060	6.0	8.3	24	4	55
60A170	7.0	10.0	30	6	80	6CFS	7.0	10.0	30	6	78	550070	7.0	9.7	30	6	75
60A180	8.0	11.0	33	7	88							550080	8.0	11.0	33	7	82
60A190	9.0	12.3	37	8	98	8CFS	8.5	12.0	36	8	84	550090	9.0	12.4	36	8	87
60A195	9.5	13.3	40	10	98	10CFS	9.0	13.0	39	10	84	550100	10.0	13.8	40	10	98

Source: Courtesy of Bivona Medical Technologies.

anterior esophageal wall from an overinflated tracheostomy tube cuff in conjunction with the presence of a large nasogastric feeding tube. Necrosis of the tracheal and esophageal walls then takes place. Infection and poor nutrition may contribute to this problem.

8. Tracheoinnominate fistula occurs when a tracheostomy tube is inserted too low within the trachea, usually below the third cartilaginous ring. The tube may impinge on the innominate artery, causing eventual erosion, the creation of a fistula, and potentially life-threatening hemorrhage. This is a dangerous but rare complication of tracheostomy.

9. Respiratory infection owing to changes in bacterial colonization within the airway following tracheotomy. Tracheal wound infections, a severely ill patient, and a reduction in tracheal mucociliary clearance after tracheotomy all contribute to the risk of pneumonia in tracheostomized patients.

Communication with a Tracheostomy Tube

Patient Assessment

Before recommending voicing with a tracheostomy tube, patients should be assessed to determine whether they are viable candidates for use of this mode of communication. Evaluation includes a review of the patient's medical condition, vocal fold status, oral-motor status, and general communicative/cognitive condition.

Medical History

A thorough review of the patient's medical history facilitates anticipating any problems with verbal communication from a linguistic/cognitive, speech, and voice standpoint. In particular, the patient's respiratory and neurologic status should be discussed thoroughly with the patient's physician.

Otolaryngologic Examination

A laryngeal evaluation is important so that any problems with voicing arising from vocal fold paralysis or granulation tissue in the posterior commissure of the glottis may be anticipated. These findings do not preclude the use of a tracheostomy tube for voicing but will prepare the patient for changes in expected vocal quality.

Oral-Motor Status

This evaluation is necessary for determining if a patient is a candidate for verbal communication. Severely restricted lingual, labial, and buccal movements secondary to neurologic impairment or head and neck surgery may limit the effectiveness of voicing with a tracheostomy tube, making alternative modes of communication necessary. In many cases patients with mild to moderate dysarthria are able to effectively communicate verbally via their tracheostomy tubes.

Voicing Options for Patients with Deflated or Cuffless Tracheostomy Tubes

Several different options are possible for voicing with a tracheostomy tube. In almost all cases the cuff must be deflated

or a cuffless tube must be in place. Medical clearance is always necessary when manipulating a tracheostomy tube. When a tracheostomy tube is in place and the cuff is inflated, air is being inhaled and exhaled directly to and from the trachea. Therefore, to redirect the air through the vocal folds, the cuff must be deflated so that air can then travel around the distal end of the tracheostomy tube and up through the vocal folds. The proximal opening of the tube should be occluded during voicing so airflow will not escape through the tracheotomy tube to the atmosphere outside, but will be completely redirected through the vocal folds and out the patient's mouth and nose. There are several ways of doing this:

1. Keep the inner cannula in place while using digital occlusion over the proximal opening of the tracheostomy tube. The patient inhales, the inner cannula is digitally occluded, and the patient voices on exhalation.

2. If the tube is fenestrated, use a fenestrated inner cannula or remove a nonfenestrated inner cannula in order for air to flow both around the distal end of the outer cannula and up through the fenestration, thus allowing for greater airflow and a stronger voice while the proximal end of the outer cannula is digitally occluded or capped. Because air will flow through the path of least resistance, it is important to occlude the outer cannula for more efficient use of breath support and a louder voice, otherwise air will flow both out of the tracheostomy tube and the patient's mouth and nose, and a weak, breathy voice will occur.

3. Remove the inner cannula in a cuffless or cuff-deflated nonfenestrated tube and use digital occlusion or capping of the outer cannula for voicing.

4. Use a one-way speaking valve with the inner cannula in place.

If a fenestrated tube is in place and cuff deflation is not an option from a medical standpoint, the inner cannula may be removed for short periods and voicing may occur through the fenestration alone when the outer cannula is digitally occluded. However, if the cuff cannot be deflated, this is probably the result of an excess of oropharyngeal and tracheal secretions. Therefore, thorough suctioning prior to removal of the inner cannula should be done to limit the risk of a patient aspirating secretions that may fall through the fenestration. This method usually produces a weaker sounding or strained voice because airflow is limited to travel through the small fenestration and is recommended for vocalization of only a few phrases, for a short time.

One-Way Speaking Valves   Although digital occlusion of a tracheostomy tube is usually effective for voicing under the proper conditions, patients are at risk for infection if they or the person occluding the tracheostomy tube are not wearing gloves. Also, digital occlusion may not be an option if the patient or caregiver is unable to occlude the tube because of extremity weakness. A speaking valve eliminates the need for digital occlusion of a tracheostomy tube for voicing or swallowing. Speaking valves continue to allow inhalation via the tracheostomy tube, but exhalation occurs via the nose and mouth as the valve closes and air is then redirected to the upper airway. Many long-term tracheostomized patients become accustomed to airflow through the tracheostomy tube, which bypasses the nose and mouth. When the patient is ready to begin weaning from a tracheostomy tube, a speaking valve may be less anxiety provoking than sudden capping (and

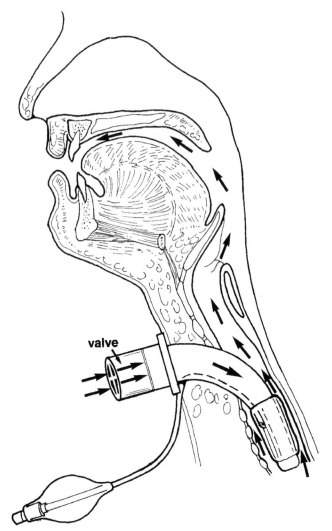

Figure 18–7 Route of inhalation through a speaking valve and exhalation via the upper airway (arrows) with a speaking valve in place and the tracheostomy tube cuff fully deflated.

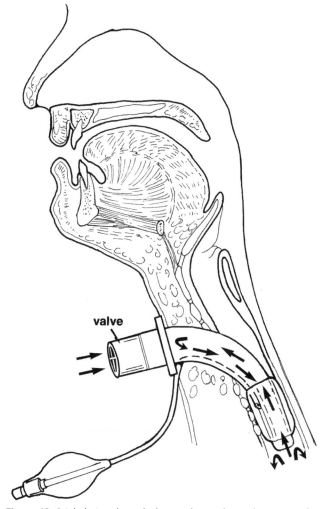

Figure 18–8 Inhalation through the speaking valve and trapping of air within the trachea (arrows) during attempts to exhale when a speaking valve is in place and the tracheostomy tube cuff is inflated.

redirecting of inhalation and exhalation through the upper airway) of the tracheostomy tube. The valve thus may act as an intermediate step between full breathing from a tracheostomy tube and capping of the tube.

All speaking valves must be used with a completely deflated cuff or cuffless tracheostomy tube. In addition, the use of a speaking valve is not recommended with foam-cuffed tracheostomy tubes because a foam cuff usually does not completely deflate and spontaneously reinflate. If a cuff is inflated while a speaking valve is in place, the patient is not able to exhale. Air becomes trapped beneath the level of the cuff, unable to travel to the upper airway owing to the inflated cuff and unable to travel through the outer opening of the tracheostomy tube because of the seal of the valve, which occurs during exhalation. **Figs. 18–7** and **18–8** demonstrate the route of airflow when a speaking valve is attached to a tracheostomy tube when the cuff is deflated and when it is inflated. The amount of pressure required to open a speaking valve varies between valves (Fornataro-Clerici & Zajac, 1993). The following are common valves currently on the market.

Passy-Muir Tracheostomy and Ventilator Swallowing and Speaking Valve (Passy-Muir Ventilator, PMV) (Fig. 18–9)   This valve attaches

to the standard 15-mm hub of all inner cannulas. An adapter for metal tracheostomy tubes is available. It is unique from other speaking valves in that it is biased toward the closed position. The valve is continuously closed, and it opens only when the patient inhales. The valve then begins to close prior to the completion of the inspiratory cycle (Mason & Watkins, 1992).

The advantage of having the valve resume a closed position prior to the completion of inhalation is that a column of air then becomes trapped within the valve and tracheostomy tube. This column of air acts as a buffer and helps prevent occlusion of the valve by tracheal secretions. An additional advantage to the biased closed position is that it requires less effort for a patient to close than valves that have an open bias (Mason & Watkins, 1992). It has been reported that the use of the PMV improves oxygen saturation and assists in patient tolerance of the ventilatory weaning process (Frey & Wood, 1991). Frey and Wood reported that the use of the PMV led to independent breathing in 33% of a group of long-term mechanically ventilated patients.

The PMV is available in several different models as seen in **Fig. 18–9**. The aqua valve is designed specifically for in-line use with ventilators to accommodate the ventilator tubing; it

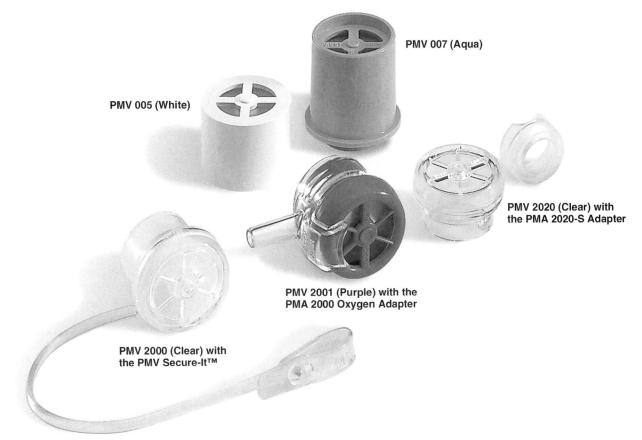

PMV 007 (Aqua)

PMV 005 (White)

PMV 2020 (Clear) with
the PMA 2020-S Adapter

PMV 2001 (Purple) with the
PMA 2000 Oxygen Adapter

PMV 2000 (Clear) with
the PMV Secure-It™

Figure 18–9 Passy-Muir tracheostomy and ventilator swallowing and speaking valves. (Courtesy of Passy-Muir, Inc., Irvine, CA.)

can also be used with nonmechanically ventilated patients with tracheostomy tubes. The clear and purple valves are low profile and are available with an optional oxygen attachment and an attachment to secure the valve to the tracheostomy tube collar so that the valve remains near the patient should it become dislodged (e.g., during a cough).

*Hood Speaking Valve (**Fig. 18–10**)*   This is a one-way valve designed to adapt to all 15-mm connectors for tracheostomy tubes (Hood Laboratories, Pembroke, MA). The valve is also available in a model designed to attach to two sizes of the Hood stoma stent, thus eliminating finger occlusion for voicing for patients wearing the stent.

*Montgomery Tracheostomy Speaking Valve (**Fig. 18–11**)*   This valve fits onto the standard 15-mm hub of an inner cannula. It has a unique cough release feature that helps prevent the valve from popping off of the tracheostomy tube during a cough. When coughing occurs, the silicone diaphragm partially dislodges. It is easily tucked back into its housing following the cough (Boston Medical Products, Westborough, MA,1996). This valve is also available in a model specifically designed for in line use with a ventilator, called the VENTRACH speaking valve (**Fig. 18–11**).

*Shiley Phonate Speaking Valve (**Fig. 18–12**)*   This valve attaches to the standard 15-mm hub of an inner cannula. It is available with or without an oxygen port to allow for supplemental oxygen and/or humidification. It has a flexible diaphragm that can be easily pushed back into the housing should it become displaced after a cough or sneeze (Mallinckrodt Medical, Inc., Irvine, CA, 1994).

Suggested Protocol for Placement of a Speaking Valve

Preplacement Issues   In some instances the SLP may be consulted at the first signs of alertness from a patient. This is particularly true if a patient has had a long hospital course and the medical staff and family members are anxious to communicate

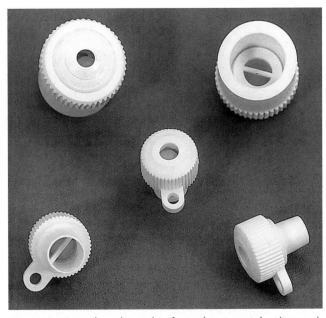

Figure 18–10 Hood speaking valves for tracheostomy tubes (top row). Hood speaking valves that attach to the Hood stoma stents (middle and bottom rows). (Courtesy of Hood Laboratories, Pembroke, MA.)

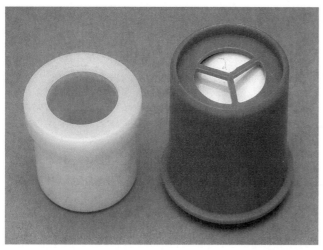

Figure 18–11 Montgomery speaking valve (left) and Montgomery VENTRACH speaking valve (right). (Courtesy of Boston Medical Products.)

with the patient. Once consideration for a speaking valve is made, several preplacement issues should be addressed. Many of the following suggestions are also applicable when voicing with a cuffless tracheostomy tube without the use of a speaking valve, as mentioned earlier.

1. Normal, or near normal, oral motor examination: Although a dysarthric patient may be a candidate for a speaking valve, a patient who is anarthric or has had extensive oral or head and neck surgery and has limited lingual or mandibular movement may not be an effective speaker with a valve. In such instances, the patient may be a more effective communicator via nonverbal methods.

2. Patients attempting to communicate: Patients may have a normal oral-motor and speech and voice examination, but if they are not motivated to verbalize, have diminished cognition, or are too fatigued or ill to speak, they may not be appropriate candidates for a valve. Placement may then have to be postponed until medical status, cognitive status, or motivation improves.

3. Alertness for most of the day for at least 2 consecutive days: A speaking valve may be used for short periods for communication of needs or questions to health care

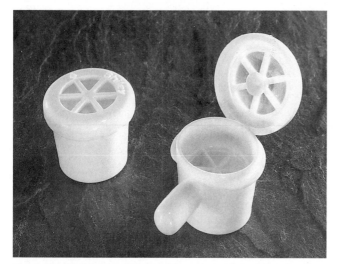

Figure 18–12 Shiley phonate speaking valve with (right) and without (left) oxygen port. (Courtesy of Mallinckrodt Medical, Inc.)

providers or brief conversation with family members. However, in general, ongoing communication is best facilitated in a patient who is alert for most of the day and interested in communicating with people within the environment. Speaking valves may also be used in patients with low levels of cognitive awareness as a means of coma stimulation. Stimulation of airflow to the upper airway may provide tactile feedback to that area, and auditory feedback from vegetative vocalizations may encourage further attempts to vocalize.

4. Tracheostomy tube in place 24 hours: Allowing a day of healing from the tracheotomy procedure is frequently recommended prior to valve placement. However, some facilities introduce speaking valves the day of tracheostomy tube placement.

5. Normal laryngeal examination by an otolaryngologist, or at least identification of laryngeal pathology that may compromise vocal quality: Knowledge of vocal fold pathology enables the clinician to prepare a patient for changes in voice. The ear, nose, and throat (ENT) examination is also necessary to rule out vocal fold pathology, which may preclude speaking valve use such as bilateral adductor paralysis of the vocal folds.

6. Cuff deflation is allowed or cuffless tracheostomy tube is in place: For a patient to use a speaking valve, the cuff of a tracheostomy tube must be fully deflated or a cuffless tube must be in place as previously described.

7. Assessment of viscosity of secretions: If tracheal or oropharyngeal secretions are too thick and thus have the potential to obstruct the airway or interfere with communication, the patient may not be a candidate for a speaking valve until the secretions lessen or become thinner. However, the use of a speaking valve may improve a patient's ability to swallow and thus more effectively clear oropharyngeal secretions. As reported by Eibling and Gross (1996), the use of the PMV assisted in significantly reducing or eliminating aspiration in a group of patients known to have aspiration without the PMV in place.

8. Assessment of upper airway: Note any upper airway obstruction that may exist such as tracheal or glottal stenosis or granulation tissue. This information is usually obtained through the case history or the physician's reports after viewing the nasal, oral, tracheal, and bronchial structures, usually via endoscopy. Mason (1993a) points out that assessment of the upper airway may also be made by the clinician's digitally occluding the tracheostomy tube and listening or observing exhaled airflow through the nose and mouth. Any sights or sounds of difficulty breathing, such as an excessively gurgly voice or strained or loud breathing, may indicate problems with upper airway airflow, in which case trials of a valve should be postponed until the problem is investigated further by the patient's physician.

9. If the valve is being used with a ventilator dependent patient, a physician must approve deflation of the cuff and modification of ventilator volumes: To ensure that adequate airflow is reaching the lungs during cuff deflation, an increase in tidal volume is sometimes necessary when a speaking valve is being used with a ventilator dependent patient. Increasing the tidal volume accommodates the new air leakage around a deflated cuff. With the cuff deflated, air flows up and around the tracheostomy tube as well as into the lungs, and therefore close monitoring of

tidal volumes is important. Readjustment of the rate of breathing from the ventilator may also be necessary at times when a speaking valve is in place.

10. Arrange for a respiratory therapist and physician or nurse to be in attendance during initial placement trials with ventilator dependent patients: The SLP is usually not formally trained to monitor respiratory function. For this reason it is important that a health care expert in the area of ventilators and pulmonology, usually a registered respiratory therapist (RRT) or pulmonologist, be present during the initial placement trials of a speaking valve. A respiratory therapist and SLP may perform subsequent treatment trials as a team. Utilization of a team approach between respiratory therapy, speech–language pathology, and the nursing

and medical staff is imperative for achieving success when using the PMV and to maximize patient safety and comfort when using the valve.

Constant education is required for new staff in all areas of the ICU. At Henry Ford Hospital, Detroit, Michigan, the Division of Speech–Language Sciences and Disorders, Department of Neurology, has a policy and procedure (P&P) for care and use of the PMV encompassing all of the areas reviewed in this section. To provide a unified approach to placement of the PMV, Speech–Language Pathology and Respiratory Therapy (RT) at Henry Ford Hospital worked together to develop the P&P for the Respiratory Therapy Department. A summary of the P&P is outlined below and may serve as a guideline for other health care facilities (**Tables 18–2** and **18–3**).

Table 18–2 Passy-Muir Tracheostomy and Ventilator Swallowing and Speaking Valve (PMV)

Purpose	To provide a consistent method of placement, care, removal, and cleaning of the PMV for tracheostomized, ventilated, and nonventilated patients.
Articles needed	PMV (provided by speech–language pathologist)
	15 × 22 mm adapter (provided by speech–language pathologist for attachment to ventilator circuit)
	Tracheostomy tube (unfenestrated or fenestrated with fenestrated inner cannula)
	Syringe
	Suction catheter
	Suction apparatus
	Pulse oximeter
	Pure soap (Ivory)

Procedure	Key Points
1. Check physician's written order.	1. To verify request. Initial order should request speech–language pathology (SLP) referral for PMV evaluation. If PMV placement is deemed appropriate by SLP, subsequent physician orders should specify frequency and duration of PMV placement as recommended by SLP.
2. Review chart to ensure appropriateness of therapy.	2. Refer to selection criteria and contraindications as noted above.
3. Notify patient's nurse of intended procedure.	3. To ensure cooperation and promote team collaboration
4. Wash hands.	4. To prevent the spread of pathogens
5. Wear appropriate protective garments.	5. According to Infection Control Standard Precaution guidelines
6. Identify patient by name and Medical Record Number (MRN).	6. To ensure procedure is performed on proper patient
7. Explain procedure to patient; initial explanation performed by SLP.	7. To alleviate patient concerns or anxiety
8. Position patient upright.	8. Promotes a patent airway and facilitates proper diaphragmatic movement
9. Suction patient mouth and tracheostomy.	9. Prevents secretion aspiration and/or facilitates airway clearance
10. If tracheostomy tube is uncuffed, proceed to step 11. Insert syringe into pilot balloon of trach and slowly aspirate air from cuff. Repeat suction, if necessary. Observe patient toleration of cuff deflation.	10. IMPORTANT: TRACH TUBE CUFF MUST BE *COMPLETELY DEFLATED* BEFORE PLACING THE PMV. PATIENT WILL BE UNABLE TO BREATHE IF CUFF IS NOT DEFLATED. Slow cuff deflation facilitates patient adjustment to airflow through upper airway.
11. If patient is not vented, SLP may occlude trach and observe patient ability to voice.	11. If patient is unable to phonate, consult among SLP/MD/RRT for trach downsize/troubleshooting.
12. Place appropriate speaking valve on patient.	12.
a. *If trach shield is in use*, place connector side of purple PMV 2001 directly to trach. Stabilize trach tube neck plate with one hand and attach the PMV to the 15-mm hub of trach with the other hand using an approximate ¼-clockwise twist. Continue to deliver humidified oxygen at prescribed FiO₂ using the trach collar.	a. Valve is designed with a friction fit to prevent patient pop off. Do not place forcefully on trach as that may make it difficult to remove the PMV. Note: The PMV must be removed prior to tracheal suction when patient is on trach shield.

(Continued)

Table 18–2 *(Continued)*

Procedure	Key Points

b. *If patient is on the ventilator*, with closed suction system:

✦ Place 22 mm end of 22 × 15 mm adapter to end of suction catheter T that connects to patient Y.

✦ Attach open end of PMV to 15 mm end of adapter.

✦ Attach a short piece of standard 23-mm disposable corrugated ventilator tubing to the other end of the PMV, then attach to patient Y (www.passy-muir.com).

13. Assess leak associated with PMV application. Modifications to the ventilator may be necessary owing to leak through upper airway. Discuss and obtain order for all ventilator changes with MD. Document changes and MD name on PMV flow sheet.

   a. *Volume ventilation patient:* Note post-PMV PiP and exhaled ventilator tidal volume (Vt). Increase tidal volume in 50-cc increments for a total of 300 cc above set Vt to achieve previous PiP. DO NOT EXCEED PRE-CUFF DEFLATION PiP.

   b. Peak inspiratory pressure *(PEEP):* Assess PEEP level.

   c. *CPAP/PSV:* Assess degree of leak. Consider change in PSV level, ventilator mode or trach-shield application.

13. Modifications include: Additional flow added to expiratory side of ventilator PB 7200, decrease in flow rate, change in mode of ventilator, and/or increase in FiO_2.

   a. When PMV is in use, PiP is a more accurate monitor of patient ventilation because exhaled tidal volume escapes through upper airway and will not be measured by ventilator.

   b. PEEP may be lowered due to increase in physiologic PEEP with PMV.

14. Assess patient humidification needs if heat and moisture exchanger (HME) is in use. HME should be placed between PMV and the patient.

14. *IMPORTANT:* HME performance is reduced owing to patient exhalation through upper airway. Change to heater wire circuit may be warranted.

15. Evaluate all ventilator alarms for appropriate adjustment. NO VENTILATOR ALARM WILL BE DISABLED. Assess alarm settings before, during, and after PMV use to avoid compromise of patient safety.

   Note: If ventilator alarms cannot be alleviated with adjustment, terminate PMV trial and reassess valve use the following day.

15. Volume alarms may be adjusted to reflect volume loss through upper airway. High- and low-pressure alarms should be set to notify personnel of airway obstruction and/or patient disconnect.

   Document ventilator alarm setting on PMV assessment sheet.

16. Observe patient to ensure valve of PMV opens during inspiration and remains closed on expiration. Exhaled tidal volume from patient upper airway may be measured with Wright's spirometer.

16. Assess proper function and position of PMV on airway. Assess exhaled tidal volume.

17. Closely monitor patient tolerance of valve placement and record vital signs on PMV assessment sheet.

   a. Record vital signs with initial trials (trials 1–3) every 5, 15, and 30 minutes.

   b. Once speech pathologist approves RT to place valve without SLP present, RT will initiate trials in collaboration with the RN and record vital signs every 2 hours.

   If ordered, obtain arterial blood gas (ABG) 30 minutes after valve placement. If significant negative changes are observed, remove PMV and adapter (if ventilated) immediately as outlined in step 20 and support patient ventilation and oxygenation as appropriate. Notify physician. Document patient assessment and actions taken on critical care record.

17. Close observation of the patient by all team members for objective and subjective signs of respiratory distress is mandatory during PMV trial.

   Refer to Table 18–3, Patient Assessment/Monitoring and Troubleshooting/Indications for PMV Removal.

18. After PMV placement, encourage the patient to say "ahh," count to 10, or clear throat to help acclimate to voice/speech production.

18. Speech production should occur during *exhalation* only to maintain adequate ventilation.

19. Assure placement of manufacturer caution labels on pilot balloon and at patient bedside after initial patient trial.

19. Labels alert personnel of cuff deflation with PMV use.

20. To terminate PMV trial:

   a. Remove PMV and adapter from trach tube or vent circuit.

   b. Reinflate trach cuff, if applicable.

   c. Return alarm and vent parameters to original settings.

   d. Document patient vital signs and tolerance of trial on PMV assessment sheet.

20. Length of patient trial and wear schedule is dependent on patient tolerance of valve and doctor's order. Patient progress may vary from day to day depending on patient's medical condition.

21. Clean PMV valve *daily*:

   a. Place warm water in basin. Lather soap in gloved hands. Place lathered hands in basin.

   b. Place valve and 15 × 22 mm adapter in emesis basin.

   c. Swish valve and adapter around in soapy water.

   d. Rinse thoroughly in warm water.

   e. Set valve and adapter on sterile 4 × 4 gauze inside of open PMV container. Allow to air dry.

   f. When dry, remove 4 × 4 from container and discard. Place dry PMV and adapter in plastic container and cover. Be sure patient name/MRN appears on container.

21. *PMV important points:*

   ✦ PMV is single-patient use.

   ✦ Recommended duration of valve is 2 months.

   ✦ To avoid damage to valve: Do not use hot water, peroxide, bleach, vinegar, or alcohol. Do not use brushes or other instruments on valve (Passy-Muir, 2000).

Table 18–3 Indications for PMV Removal/Troubleshooting
(Passy-Muir, 2000)

A. Inability to exhale through upper airway/PMV repeatedly pops off or is difficult to place on trach (increased airway resistance)—stridor may be present; if patient is mechanically ventilated, increase in peak inspiratory pressure or high-pressure alarm may result.

  1. Ensure cuff deflation

  2. Consult with SLP and physician to downsize trach or change to cuffless tube.

  3. Physician assesses for airway obstruction/patency.

  4. Position patient to optimize ventilation.

  5. Suction airway.

B. Continuous rush of air through mouth and nose—low exhaled tidal volume/minute ventilation alarm or low-pressure alarm may result.

  1. Adjust ventilator settings: flow rate, tidal volume, or ventilator mode.

  2. If PSV (pressure support ventilation) mode is in use, consider decrease in PSV or change ventilator mode until glottic function returns. When a leak occurs in PSV mode, vent continues to deliver flow until either preset pressure level or allotted time limit is reached.

  3. Coordination of voicing and breathing retraining by SLP

C. Increased or excessive coughing—usually caused by airflow through upper airway moving secretions upward

  1. Suction patient.

  2. Assess patient for air trapping.

D. Patient anxiety

  1. Educate patient on valve use and ensure patient of close monitoring by staff.

  2. Distraction techniques

E. Patient unable to voice

  1. Reassess laryngeal status.

  2. Reassess upper airway patency.

F. PMV valve is noisy or vibrates

  1. Reassess placement on trach or in ventilator circuit.

  2. Assess cleaning techniques—refer to PMSV manual.

  3. Replace valve (recommended usage is 2 months).

Contraindications to Using a Speaking Valve

As described by Dikeman and Kazandjian (1995a), the following situations are contraindications to using a speaking valve:

1. Evidence of airway obstruction: For the patient to fully expel air, a patent airway is necessary.

2. Laryngectomy: A speaking valve is not to be confused with a voice prosthesis such as those used in laryngectomy patients with tracheoesophageal punctures. Laryngectomees are not candidates for use of a valve because their only means of air exchange is directly through the lower airway, thus completely bypassing the upper airway.

3. Cuff inflation or foam-cuffed tracheostomy tubes: As previously mentioned, the tracheostomy tube cuff must be completely deflated to use a speaking valve. Foam cuffs do not deflate completely and spontaneously reinflate. Therefore, foam cuffs are a contraindication to speaking valve use.

4. End-stage pulmonary disease: Patients with end-stage pulmonary disease tend to retain air in their lungs and may therefore have difficulty tolerating a speaking valve, as a valve may increase their work of breathing.

Three Voicing Options for Patients with a Tracheostomy and Ventilator Dependency

It has been reported that the inability to talk is the primary cause of feelings of fear and anxiety or panic in tracheostomized or ventilator dependent patients (Bergbom-Engberg & Haljamae, 1989). In addition to the importance of daily communication, voicing while on mechanical ventilation may be a very important goal to achieve in terminally ill patients who wish to make their medical, financial, or personal needs and desires known to their caregivers, family, and friends. Three basic options are available for voicing in patients who have tracheostomy tubes and are ventilator dependent. We have reviewed the use of the PMV in facilitating communication and swallowing in tracheostomized and ventilator-dependent patients. There are two other options for voicing: voicing with a deflated cuff by timing phonation with the inhalation cycle of the ventilator, and using a "talking" tracheostomy tube with an inflated cuff.

Speaking on the Inhalation Phase of the Ventilator Cycle

When a patient is on a ventilator and the cuff of the tracheostomy tube is deflated, the patient may be able to time voicing as the inspiratory cycle begins and a breath is given by the ventilator. During inhalation, air is forced into the lungs, but if a deflated cuff is in place, some of that air escapes around the cuff and travels up through the vocal folds, enabling the patient to phonate. During exhalation, recoil of the respiratory system takes place and air is expelled through the ventilator tubing, thus preventing voicing from occurring on exhalation. Hoit, Shea, and Banzett (1994) studied the timing of voicing of four men and three women who were mechanically ventilated for at least 3 years. They reported that their subjects initiated speech 0.3 to 0.7 seconds after the onset of inspiratory flow and terminated their utterances 0.7 to 1.1 seconds after the offset of inspiratory flow (or 0.1 to 0.5 seconds after the opening of the expiratory valve). Extemporaneous speaking and reading resulted in earlier speech initiation, later speech termination, and longer speech duration than repetition of sentences and sustained phonation of /a/. The authors also discovered that in conjunction with voicing during inspiratory flow, their subjects continued to speak during end-inspiratory pause and early expiration.

Because the process of initiating phonation on inhalation is completely contrary to voicing prior to mechanical ventilation, it may be difficult for a patient to adjust to this type of communication. However, most patients are glad to use their own voices for communication and are able to learn how to time speaking with the respiratory cycles provided by the ventilator. Hoit et al (1994) suggest some minor ventilator adjustments and training strategies for optimizing speaking in this manner:

1. Lengthen the time of the end-inspiratory pause that patients appear to speak through.

2. Use PEEP to prolong inspiration.

3. Encourage the patient to continue speaking as far into the expiratory portion of the cycle as possible until voicing fades. This likely results in linguistically inappropriate silences within an utterance, but the pauses mid-utterance may also serve as a cue to the listener that the patient intends to continue talking.

Talking Tracheostomy Tubes

A talking tracheostomy tube is specially designed for patients on mechanical ventilation who are unable to tolerate cuff deflation for voicing. A talking tracheostomy tube has exterior tubing that connects from an outside source of compressed air, such as a wall-mounted oxygen flow unit usually seen at a patient's bedside, to the outer cannula. There is an open port on the connector tube that, when occluded, directs air from the outside oxygen air source through a fenestration that sits above the cuff in the outer cannula of the tracheostomy tube, up through the vocal folds for phonation to take place. When a talking tracheostomy tube is in place, the patient is breathing and phonating from two separate channels.

Ventilation takes place as usual, but because the cuff is inflated, there is no connection between the lower and upper respiratory airways. Phonation occurs when the outside source of compressed air travels through the extended exterior tubing of the tracheostomy tube, through the fenestration(s) on the outer cannula of the tracheostomy tube, and then up through the vocal folds. The Portex talk tube (**Fig. 18–13**) is an example of a talking tracheostomy tube. The same criteria for candidacy for speaking valves apply to talking tracheostomy tubes except, of course, for the ability to tolerate cuff deflation.

Advantages: The advantages of talking tracheostomy tubes include the following:

1. They provide voicing for patients who are unable to have the cuff of their tracheostomy tubes deflated;
2. Ventilator cycles are not adjusted when talking tracheostomy tubes are in place because breathing and speaking occur from two separate mechanisms;

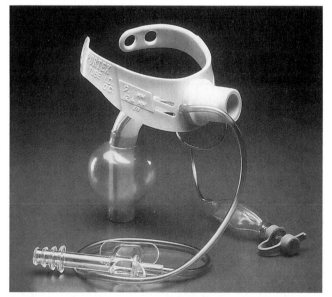

Figure 18–13 Portex "trach-talk" tube. (Courtesy of Sims Medical Systems.)

3. The patient is able to continually phonate without having to time speaking with the breathing cycle of the ventilator.

However, this continuous flow of air leads to complaints of dryness by some patients. It can be alleviated by humidifying the air source, occluding the port on the extended tubing only when speaking occurs, physically turning the exterior air source on and off for speech, or using an environmental control unit (ECU) for patients who are unable to digitally occlude the port.

An ECU allows a patient with upper extremity weakness to activate the air source only during speaking times while the port is permanently occluded, such as when tape is wrapped around the port. The on-off switch to the compressed air source may be activated by, for example, a sip and puff or head activation switch; this is usually best determined by a rehabilitation engineer. Activating the compressed air only when speaking eliminates the constant flow of air through the pharynx that causes dryness. Another strategy for reducing dryness is to reduce the amount of airflow per minute through the external airflow line.

One method of determining optimal airflow is to ask the patient to phonate /a/ for an extended period of time while adjusting the airflow rate of the compressed air source until optimal comfort and speaking volume are obtained. Kluin, Maynard, and Bogdasarian (1984) reported that 5 L/minute produces an audible whisper with the Portex talking tracheostomy tube, whereas 8 to 10 L/minute provides normal speaking intensity. As with any new device, training and counseling are necessary when introducing a talking tracheostomy tube to a patient. It has been reported that an average of 5.6 days may elapse before adequate voicing occurs with some talking tracheostomy tubes, likely owing to prolonged intubation (Leder & Traquina, 1989).

Disadvantages: There are certain disadvantages to talking tracheostomy tubes that clinicians should be aware of when instructing patients and caregivers in their use:

1. The exterior speaking tube or the fenestrations in the tube may become occluded with secretions, and frequent suctioning of the speaking tube and oropharynx may be necessary.
2. The exterior air source must be turned off when the patient is eating. The constant rush of air up through the pharynx competes with the oral and pharyngeal phases of swallowing as the patient is trying to propel food posteriorly through the oral cavity and inferiorly through the pharynx.
3. The exterior air source must be turned off when the patient is not involved in a conversation or when the patient is sleeping. If the patient's mouth is closed for an extended period of time, the potential exists for the patient to swallow air, and subsequent abdominal distention and discomfort may occur.

Suctioning

The authors recommend suctioning a patient orally, pharyngeally, and transtracheally prior to deflating the cuff of a tracheostomy tube for voicing or swallowing purposes. Resuctioning the trachea should take place after the cuff is deflated to remove any secretions that may have collected above the cuff while it was inflated. After secretions are suctioned, the voice is usually clearer, breathing is easier, and the risk of aspiration of secretions that have collected above the inflated cuff is lessened. Suctioning should be performed only by a trained individual. This usually includes a respiratory therapist, nurse, or family member. In some cases the speech pathologist is also trained in suctioning technique.

Nonverbal Methods of Communication in an Intensive Care Unit Setting

Nonverbal methods of communication, in general, may range from a simple letter or picture board to speech generating devices. An ICU patient's initial need for communication may be to request pain medication or suctioning, or to convey requests concerning medical decisions. For these reasons it is important that the SLP establishes a reliable method of communication for the patient. This may include, for example, the use of eye blinks, foot movement, or any other consistently and accurately established muscle movement to indicate a yes/no response. A slightly more advanced method of communication via eye movements is the Frenchay E-Tran Frame (Speechmark Publishing, Ltd., Bicester, Oxfordshire, UK) board. This clear acrylic board has strategically placed clusters of letters on its four corners that the patient looks at while the communication partner decodes the message, seated across from the patient, asking for confirmation that he or she has identified the correct letter of the word the patient is spelling. The patient responds and the next letter is chosen.

In most cases, at least initially, nonverbal methods of communication for ICU patients will likely focus on quick and simple strategies that relate to getting basic needs met. The complexity of the system may increase as the patient's skills and medical status improve.

In summary, key ingredients to successful communication for an ICU patient include a thorough knowledge of the patient's condition, a strong background of voicing options with tracheostomy tubes and speaking valves, patience, counseling, and a team approach.

✦ Swallowing Issues

Aspiration of oropharyngeal secretions is known to occur in healthy adults as well as critically ill patients. In a study by Huxley, Viroslav, Gray, et al (1978), 20 healthy adults and 10 individuals in a coma or stuporous state were studied for aspiration. The results revealed that 45% of the healthy adults aspirated during deep sleep and 70% of the adults with depressed consciousness aspirated. Aspiration was more extensive and occurred more frequently in the latter group. Healthy subjects who did not aspirate awakened frequently during the night or slept poorly, whereas the subjects who did aspirate slept soundly throughout the night. It is suspected that pulmonary infections owing to oropharyngeal aspiration are likely related to the frequency, volume, and character of the aspirated material and usually are avoided in healthy individuals because of their ability to more efficiently clear bacteria by pulmonary defense mechanisms (Huxley, et al., 1978; Bartlett & Gorbach, 1975). Healthy elderly patients may also be at an increased risk for aspiration that may be compounded by the introduction of an illness. Pontoppidan and Beecher (1960) found that individuals in their 70s and 80s have reduced laryngeal sensitivity. This finding may contribute to silent aspiration and eventually lead to pneumonia in the elderly.

Aspiration Pneumonia

Treating patients with oropharyngeal aspiration is common practice for SLPs working in an ICU setting, particularly because most of the patients likely have several of the risk factors for aspiration pneumonia. These risk factors include acute stroke (Gordon, Hewer, & Wade, 1987; Horner, Massey, Riski et al., 1988), seizure, alcoholism, tracheostomy tubes, older age, a reduction in mental status, a previous history of pneumonia (Cogen & Weinryb, 1989), and, in general, any state of depressed consciousness (Bartlett & Gorbach, 1975). Russin and Adler (1989) described three distinct syndromes of aspiration that can lead to pneumonia. These include aspiration of oropharyngeal secretions, inert fluids (e.g., saline or barium solutions), and aspiration of acidic gastric contents. The latter syndrome is considered the most severe because of its rapid progression, which causes irreversible lung damage, and its high mortality rate. Hypoxia is the most characteristic physiologic feature of aspiration of gastric contents (Bartlett & Gorbach, 1975) and may occur within 2 hours after aspiration (Russin & Adler, 1989). Sitzmann (1990) found that any form of upper enteric feeding such as nasogastric or gastrostomy tubes significantly increased a patient's risk of developing aspiration pneumonia owing to a reduction in tone of the lower esophageal sphincter, which may lead to reflux of gastric contents.

Predicting Risk of Aspiration

Many patients in the ICU are at high risk of aspiration. The ICU patient may be in a stuporous state, have a feeding tube, and be elderly with multiple medical problems. All these factors should be considered prior to initiating the evaluation and should play a role in the planning stages of swallowing treatment. Predicting a patient's likelihood of aspiration during oral feeding may be the first step to take in the intervention process. Several studies have attempted to predict aspiration based on clinical presentation (Horner, Massey, Riski et al., 1988; Linden & Siebens, 1983; Martin, Corlew, Wood et al., 1994). Horner et al (1988) reported that aspiration occurred equally in left and right hemisphere stroke patients, but more frequently in patients with bilateral stroke. The incidence of aspiration in stroke was further broken down by location of the lesion as studied on computed tomography. The highest percentage of aspiration occurred in patients with combined bilateral cerebral and brainstem strokes (six of six, 100%), followed by unilateral cerebral and brainstem stroke (six of seven, 85.7%), brainstem strokes alone (four of six, 66.7%), and cerebral strokes (14 of 33, 42.4%).

The most prominent clinical feature of aspirating patients was dysphonia. This included a dry or wet sounding hoarse voice. A diminished or absent gag reflex was equally present in aspirating and nonaspirating patients and therefore was not a prognostically valuable sign for predicting aspiration. The most prominent videofluoroscopic feature of aspirating patients was a delayed swallow response in conjunction with reduced pharyngeal peristalsis. Poor oral motility did not correlate well with aspiration. Interestingly, a single chest x-ray was not predictive of aspirating versus nonaspirating patients. However, the authors concluded that this may have resulted from the NPO status of most of the patients, the degree of aspiration, the acute stage of the patients' illnesses, or the protective nature of the cough reflex.

Linden and Siebens (1983) studied clinical signs in 15 patients with pharyngeal dysphagia in an attempt to predict laryngeal penetration on videofluorography. They reported a wet-hoarse voice and impaired pharyngeal gag among 11 patients with laryngeal penetration. Their findings also revealed that laryngeal penetration occurred more frequently with liquids as opposed to semisolids and that a cough was an unpredictable clinical indicator of laryngeal penetration.

Martin et al (1994) reported significantly slower oral transit time during videofluoroscopic swallowing studies in nine patients with aspiration pneumonia compared with seven patients with nonaspiration pneumonia. However, most of the patients in the aspiration pneumonia group were neurologically impaired and one had undergone head and neck surgery.

A retrospective review of poststroke patients with and without aspiration during videofluorography was analyzed by Schmidt, Holas, Halvorson, et al (1994). Their results revealed that the odds of patients developing pneumonia were 7.6 times greater if they aspirated during the videofluoroscopic examination. In addition, patients who aspirated thick or solid consistencies were 5.6 times at greater risk of developing pneumonia than those who did not aspirate or aspirated thin liquids.

In summary, although predicting aspiration based on clinical findings depends on the nature of the illness and the mental and neurologic status of the patient, a voice evaluation should be standard practice and the presence of dysphonia should be an indication to the clinician that the patient is at risk to aspirate. In addition, it is important to remember that the presence of a gag reflex does not reliably indicate that the patient will not aspirate (Bleach, 1993). During videofluorographic examinations for swallowing, treatment strategies should be attempted whenever possible to assess the effectiveness of therapy or the patient's potential to learn a compensatory swallowing technique and avoid aspiration.

Tracheostomy Tubes in Patients with Swallowing Disorders

Adding to the complexities involved in treating an ICU patient for dysphagia is the presence of a tracheostomy tube. The introduction of a tracheostomy tube in any patient presents a series of unique swallowing problems. According to Logemann (1983), an inflated tracheostomy tube cuff creates the possibility of tracheal irritation and the restriction of laryngeal elevation during swallowing. Nash (1988) further reports that pressure on the distal esophagus from an inflated cuff may occur when swallowing. Cameron, Reynolds, and Zuidema (1973) reported an increased incidence of aspiration of oropharyngeal secretions in hospitalized patients with tracheostomy tubes versus orally intubated patients.

As in speech, a patient's swallowing skills are improved when cuff deflation is allowed. Cuff deflation provides improved laryngeal excursion during the swallow (Logemann, 1983) and releases the pressure placed on the distal esophagus from a potentially overinflated cuff. In addition, placing a one-way valve, capping, or digitally occluding the outer opening of the tracheostomy tube will assist in restoring subglottic pressure and the ability to cough and clear the airway should laryngeal penetration or aspiration occur (Siebens, Tippett, Kirby, et al., 1993).

Suiter, McCullough, and Powell (2003) studied the effects of the PMV on 18 individuals with dysphagia and tracheostomy tubes. Each participant swallowed liquid and puree barium under three different conditions: tracheostomy tube cuff inflated, cuff deflated, and cuff deflated with a one-way valve (the PMV) in place. Their results revealed that aspiration of liquids was significantly reduced when the subjects swallowed with the PMV in place. The authors speculated that the restoration of subglottic air pressure likely improved the swallowing function in their subjects. Their results also revealed that there was an increased incidence of laryngeal penetration along with a reduction of tracheal aspiration. Improved laryngeal sensation may have assisted the patients in their ability to sense and expel material with a cough from the laryngeal vestibule. The authors further reported an increase in oral and pharyngeal residue in patients who wore the one-way valve during swallowing. This finding warrants further investigation to prevent postswallow aspiration.

Assessing the Intensive Care Unit Patient with Dysphagia

As in all patients with dysphagia, a careful review of the ICU patient's medical condition is mandatory prior to evaluation and treatment. In this population, the SLP must ascertain the following: (1) the patient's level of consciousness, (2) length of time the patient was intubated, (3) if and when patient underwent a tracheotomy, (4) type and size of the tracheostomy tube, (5) presence of cuffed or cuffless tracheostomy tube, (6) anticipated weaning schedule from the ventilator, and (7) cranial nerve status. Because many ICU patients are not able to travel to a videofluorographic swallowing study because of positioning problems in the presence of multiple tubing and equipment, other forms of assessment may need to be initially explored. The following sections review swallowing assessment techniques that may be performed in the ICU setting.

Blue Dye Testing

In 1973 Cameron et al described a method of testing for aspiration of oropharyngeal secretions in 61 patients with a tracheostomy tube and 25 patients with oral endotracheal tubes. A 1% solution of Evans blue dye was placed on the patients' tongues every 4 hours for up to 48 hours as routine suctioning took place. The results of the study revealed that 69% of the patients with tracheostomy tubes had evidence of the blue dye marker on suctioning and none of the patients with oral endotracheal tubes exhibited aspiration of oropharyngeal secretions. Since that time, blue dye testing has become a common method of assessing dysphagia in the ICU setting.

This method usually takes place when a patient is unable to travel for a videofluorographic swallowing study and the physician is interested in upgrading the patient's nutritional status to oral intake after prolonged tube feeding. Typically this method involves the insertion of a small amount of blue food dye into a small amount of barium, food, or liquid (usually beginning with 1 cc) and having the patient swallow. Blue is used to differentiate the swallowed material from secretions or gastric contents that may be aspirated. This procedure is applied to patients with tracheostomy tubes who are either on or off of a ventilator. The patient is usually suctioned immediately after a swallow and periodically during the hour after swallowing. Dikeman and Kazandjian (1995a) advise suctioning every 15 minutes for 1 hour after swallowing.

The obvious limitation to blue dye testing is that if a patient aspirates during swallowing, it is impossible to know where along the oropharyngeal tract the difficulty occurred to cause the aspiration. In addition, the absence of blue dye in tracheal secretions during suctioning does not indicate without a doubt that the patient did not aspirate. It is possible that aspiration prior to or between suctioning occurred and the secretions may have traveled too low in the bronchial tree to be completely suctioned. In addition, residual material in the pharynx may remain for an extended period of time, placing the patient at risk to aspirate from pharyngeal residue entering the airway after suctioning has ceased. Although these limitations exist, if a patient's blue dye test is positive, it does provide the clinician with the knowledge that the patient is aspirating and likely is not ready to eat until further testing can be performed such as videoendoscopy or videofluoroscopic evaluations of dysphagia.

If a patient appears to tolerate a small amount of blue dyed liquid, careful monitoring of pulmonary status is strongly suggested as bolus size and texture of consistencies are upgraded. Any signs of difficulty breathing, fever, increase in tracheal secretions, or change in mental status may indicate aspiration and feeding trials should be terminated until further investigation takes place.

Blue dye may also be injected into a feeding tube by a physician or nurse to assess the presence of aspiration of gastric contents. It should be noted that the Food and Drug Administration recently issued a warning about the use of FD&C Blue No. 1 in enteral feedings as there have been reports of patient deaths and organ discoloration with this product (ASHA, 2003). Even though the amount of blue coloring used for oropharyngeal dysphagia assessment is minimal, practicing SLPs should be familiar with their health care facility's policy regarding the use of blue dye.

Fiberoptic Endoscopic Evaluation of Swallowing (FEES)

As previously mentioned, many ICU patients are unable to undergo a videofluoroscopic swallowing evaluation because of positioning difficulties or the presence of multiple tubes and equipment. In such cases, evaluating a patient's potential to swallow may be assisted by the use of a nasopharyngeal endoscope as discussed by Langmore, Schatz, and Olson (1988). This technique requires the insertion of a flexible fiberoptic endoscope into the patient's nasopharynx. Viewing the anatomy and physiology while patients swallow may lead to information regarding aspiration and patients' ability to clear their pharynx.

Unfortunately, this type of assessment does not allow full analysis of the oral phase of swallowing, and the view of the larynx is obliterated as the patient swallows, precluding analysis of timing of the swallow response and the ability to assess whether aspiration occurred during or after the swallow response. Both factors provide necessary information for planning the appropriate treatment strategies. However, despite these limitations, this technique offers information regarding premature spillage of material, the occurrence of aspiration before a swallow response and insight into the status of pharyngeal peristalsis as noted by any residual material unilaterally or bilaterally in the pharynx after the swallow. These findings, coupled with clinical signs, may be useful in recommending the initiation of swallowing trials with careful clinical monitoring or may provide enough information to recommend withholding swallowing until the patient's medical status improves and

a videofluorographic swallowing study can be performed. As with all swallowing evaluation and treatment techniques, formal training is necessary prior to performing FEES.

Auscultation

Cervical auscultation may be useful to determine if a patient is aspirating during swallowing by detecting bubbling sounds during or immediately after swallowing (Takahashi, Groher, & Michi, 1994). Typically a stethoscope is placed along various areas of the neck while the patient swallows. The subjective nature of this technique has been made more objective via acoustic analysis of the swallow sounds as reported by Takahashi et al. (1994). However, it may be an impractical assessment technique because many facilities may not have the equipment necessary to objectify the data collected. The study may provide general information but should not be a substitute for other methods of swallowing assessment such as videofluorography.

The Use of Videofluorography to Assess Swallowing in Mechanically Ventilated Patients with Tracheostomy Tubes

If a ventilator-dependent patient meets the same criteria for candidacy for a videofluorographic swallowing study as would be expected in any patient, that patient should be allowed to travel to the radiology suite and undergo the examination. These criteria include medical stability, secretion control, adequate oral motor and laryngeal status, and intact cognition so that the patient may follow the instructions provided during the examination and later during swallowing therapy. Ideally, cuff deflation is recommended, coupled with the placement of a one-way speaking valve to facilitate an efficient swallow (Siebens et al., 1993).

Siebens et al (1993) described a technique of using the inspiratory phase of the ventilator to clear the larynx and pharynx from aspirated or residual pharyngeal material in mechanically ventilated patients with cuffless or cuff-deflated tracheostomy tubes. During videofluoroscopy, aspiration and pharyngeal residue were noted after the patient swallowed. The force of air that was introduced during the inspiratory phase of the ventilator essentially pushed the food up from the trachea and pharynx to then be swallowed by the patient. In their study, this method proved the only way for one of the patients to safely swallow until her respiratory illness improved.

Ethical Issues

Besides the physical aspect of tolerating oral feedings, there is usually a complex, psychological advantage given to patients and their families when a patient is able to obtain nutrition orally after prolonged tube feeding. It should be noted that tube feeding does not necessarily preclude a patient's ability to orally eat. In many cases, eating for pleasure occurs in combination with tube feeding for nutritional maintenance. One of the more difficult situations that may arise when treating a patient in an ICU setting is the decision to allow a patient to eat even when obvious signs of aspiration are present. These decisions are not easy to make and depend on the individual case. For example, a patient with a terminal illness and documented tracheal aspiration may decide to eat by mouth. In such instances the SLP must consider the quality-of-life issues involved in the patient's case. Teaching patients compensatory swallowing strategies to minimize their risk of aspiration while eating may be the best route of treatment in some cases. Of course, these decisions are complex and vary depending on the background training of the SLPs, their personal philosophical beliefs regarding quality of life issues, the policy of the health care facility, and the decisions expressed by the patient and agreed to by the medical staff. According to Groher (1994), the final decision to feed a patient with known tracheal aspiration ultimately may be more anecdotal than empirical.

✦ Case Vignettes

Case One

M.H. is a 29-year-old woman who was involved in an auto accident and has been in the ICU for 3 weeks. Her course of recovery was complicated by pneumonia, cardiac arrest, and coma for 10 days. She has now been awake and alert for short periods of time several times throughout the day. She underwent emergent oral endotracheal intubation at the time of hospital admission and a tracheotomy 10 days later. She is on a ventilator. The patient's family is interested in giving the patient ice chips and fluids as she complains of a dry mouth. The medical and nursing staff is hesitant to allow the family to give anything by mouth to the patient as their attempts to do so resulted in immediate coughing by the patient and they are concerned that she is aspirating. The speech pathology service was consulted for cognitive/communicative and swallowing assessment and treatment.

Initial language and cognitive testing with written responses and mouthing words by the patient revealed intact orientation, intact auditory comprehension for simple commands and questions, mild semantic paraphasia in her writing samples, and mild-moderate short-term memory impairment. A right facial droop and mild right lingual weakness were also noted. Prior to evaluating the patient's swallowing skills, the speech pathologist requested an otolaryngologic evaluation to obtain information regarding her vocal fold status. The patient was found to have small bilateral granulomatous tissue formation on the vocal processes and a mild right vocal fold paresis resulting in a mild glottal chink. Her pulmonologist approved cuff deflation trials with a speaking valve to further assess speech, voice, communication/cognition, and swallowing.

The patient's overall medical status improved daily and she tolerated cuff deflation trials well for voicing with a speaking valve in line with the ventilator. During this trial period of voicing and adjusting to the speaking valve, the patient was instructed to practice dry swallows using a modified supraglottic swallow strategy, with the focus on voluntary breath-holding during the swallow. The goal was to begin preparing the patient for swallowing in a modified manner given the knowledge of her vocal fold paresis and incomplete glottal closure. Anticipation for a swallowing evaluation via bedside assessment of blue-dye testing or endoscopic assessment prior to the patient's ability to travel to radiology for a videofluorographic swallowing study was initially planned. However, M.H. was rapidly improving from a medical standpoint and was fully weaned from the ventilator 5 days after speech pathology's initial consultation. She remained tracheostomized with a No. 6 cuffed tracheostomy tube. She was able to travel to the radiology suites for a videofluorographic swallow study

with her tracheostomy tube cuff deflated and a Passy-Muir speaking and swallowing tracheostomy and ventilator speaking valve (PMV) in place. Initial liquid trials resulted in penetration of barium into the laryngeal vestibule as a result of impaired timing and coordination of the oropharyngeal swallow. However, with the PMV in place, the patient was able to effectively cough and clear the supraglottic area and thus, prevent tracheal aspiration. When M.H. consistently used a modified supraglottic swallow strategy, laryngeal vestibule penetration was avoided on all liquid and solid consistencies. It was recommended that M.H. swallow all consistencies using a modified supraglottic swallow strategy and that the PMV remain on the tracheostomy tube during all eating times to improve subglottic pressure during swallowing and promote an effective cough should tracheal aspiration occur.

Case Two

J.M. is a 33-year-old man hospitalized in the ICU for the past 2 weeks with a medical diagnosis of Guillain-Barré syndrome. The speech pathology service was consulted on day 7 of his hospitalization. At that time he was orally intubated and mechanically ventilated. He was almost completely paretic; however, he was observed to have ocular movements. After a short training period of 2 days he was able to consistently move his eyes up and down for a yes and no response. Because J.M. appeared accurate in his yes/no responses, communication via an E-Tran board was attempted. This method of communication was successful, but it was slow, and the patient's family members were frustrated by their inability to quickly and accurately understand his needs and thoughts. The patient underwent a tracheotomy after 2 weeks of oral endotracheal intubation. Assessment of the patient's oral-motor movements revealed slow and imprecise lip and tongue motion during isolated tasks; however, J.M. continually tried to communicate by mouthing words. Therefore, a cervical electrolarynx was attempted as a mode of communication, and although he was severely dysarthric, the patient was able to approximate simple single words with enough accuracy and guesswork on the part of the listener to make simple needs known. As the patient's medical status improved over the next 2 weeks, cuff deflation and PMV trials were approved by the patient's physician. Although J.M. had a weak, breathy voice with an overall moderate-severe flaccid dysarthria, the patient and his family preferred verbal communication over nonverbal methods. Cuff deflation and PMV trials occurred twice a day for only 10 minutes at a time because of fatigue by the patient. Gradually the patient's medical condition improved as did his dysarthria. He was able to tolerate longer periods of cuff deflation and voicing with or without the PMV. When his cuff was inflated, an electrolarynx was used for quick verbal communication needs. J.M. continued to use a speaking valve after he was weaned from the ventilator. He was discharged from the hospital using the PMV with a cuffless tracheostomy tube with the goal of decannulation in the near future.

✦ Conclusion

The need for speech–language pathology services is great in the ICU. This chapter has described many voicing, communication, and swallowing options for the tracheostomized and/or ventilator-dependent patient. The ICU setting is a challenging, ever-changing environment. Like most patients in a medical setting, the ICU patient's condition may change on a daily basis and SLPs must be flexible and ready to alter assessment or treatment strategies on a moment's notice.

Key ingredients to successful management of communication and swallowing include a thorough knowledge of the patient's condition, a strong background in voicing options with tracheostomy tubes and speaking valves, the ability to provide appropriate counseling and support, and good team skills. Frequently, SLPs find themselves working with physicians, nurses, respiratory therapists, psychiatrists, psychologists, and the patient's family along with the patient. When possible, we recommend that SLPs accompany the medical staff on rounds. This opens doors to improved understanding of the patient's medical condition and enables SLPs to address communication and swallowing needs and to answer questions from other team members in an efficient manner. Clinical experience has shown that this approach allows the SLP to intervene, consult, and educate in an effective and efficient manner and truly act as part of the patient care team. Appendix 18–1 lists the competencies that the clinician should have.

Acknowledgment

The authors wish to acknowledge Kathy Raniszeski, RRT, Henry Ford Hospital for her role in developing the P&P guidelines for PMV use.

Study Questions

1. You have a 25-year-old TBI patient on your caseload who recently underwent a tracheotomy after 2 weeks of oral endotracheal intubation. He is still on a ventilator, but is expected to be fully weaned from mechanical ventilation within the next 2 to 3 weeks. He has been attempting communication on a regular basis via eye and head movements and facial expressions. His physician has approved cuff deflation trials. Which modes of verbal communication will you attempt with this patient?

2. There is a patient in the ICU who has a tracheostomy tube and is mechanically ventilated. She is intermittently awake for short periods each day. The medical and nursing staff would like you to provide her with a means of verbal communication as soon as possible because it is difficult for them to know what the patient's needs are. Would this patient be a candidate for a speaking valve? Why or why not? If a speaking valve is not an appropriate method of communication at this time, what other types of communication would you recommend?

3. One of your patients is very anxious when his speaking valve is in place and reports difficulty breathing while using the valve. Pre- and postplacement assessment of vital signs and airway clearance have all turned out to be normal. What are some strategies for improving acceptance of the valve that you could apply with this patient?

4. A 32-year-old alert, tracheostomized, and ventilator-dependent patient appears to be aspirating during the initial clinical trials of fluid intake by mouth. What assessment techniques would you pursue? You may assume that cuff deflation during eating has been medically approved.

5. You have a new patient on your caseload who recently had a stroke. He is 89 years old and was orally intubated for 10 days while in a semiconscious state. Following extubation the nursing staff began giving the patient sips of water and noted that he coughs and chokes every time he drinks. What are some of this patient's risk factors for aspiration? What specific clinical signs will you look for that may predict the patient's likelihood of aspiration prior to assessing his swallowing abilities with videofluorography?

References

Adams, R.D., & Victor, M. (1985). Diseases of Peripheral Nerve and Muscle. In: R.D. Adams, & M. Victor (Eds.), *Principles of Neurology*, 3rd ed. (p. 968). New York: McGraw-Hill

ASHA. (2003). FDA Issues Public Health Advisory on Blue Dye. *ASHA Leader Newsmagazine, November*, 22

Ashbaugh, D.G., Bigelow, D.B., Petty, T.L., et al. (1967). Acute Respiratory Distress in Adults. *Lancet, 12*, 319–323

Bartlett, J.G., & Gorbach, S. (1975). The Triple Threat of Aspiration Pneumonia. *Chest, 68*, 560–565

Bergbom-Engberg, I., & Haljamae, H. (1989). Assessment of Patient's Experience of Discomforts During Respiratory Therapy. *Critical Care Medicine, 17*, 1068–1072

Bleach, N.R. (1993). The Gag Reflex and Aspiration: A Retrospective Analysis of 120 Patients Assessed by Videofluoroscopy. *Clinical Otolaryngology, 18*, 303–307

Boston Medical Products. (1996). *The Montgomery Speaking Valve* (p. 18). Boston: Boston Medical Products Product Catalog

Brochard, L., Isabey, D., Piquet, J., et al. (1990). Reversal of Acute Exacerbations of Chronic Obstructive Lung Disease by Inspiratory Assistance with a Face Mask. *New England Journal of Medicine, 323*, 1523–1530

Cameron, J.L., Reynolds, J., & Zuidema, G.D. (1973). Aspiration in Patients with Tracheostomies. *Surgical Gynecology and Obstetrics, 136*, 68–70

Cogen, R., & Weinryb, J. (1989). Aspiration Pneumonia in Nursing Home Patients Fed Via Gastrostomy Tubes. *American Journal of Gastroenterology, 84*, 1509–1512

Dikeman, K.J., & Kazandjian, M.S. (1995a). Airway management techniques. In: K.J. Dikeman, & M.S. Kazandjian (Eds.), *Communication and Swallowing Management of Tracheostomized and Ventilator-Dependent Adults* (pp. 35–60). San Diego: Singular

Dikeman, K.J., & Kazandjian, M.S. (1995b). Endotracheal tubes and tracheostomy tubes. In: K.J. Dikeman, & M.S. Kazandjian (Eds.), *Communication and Swallowing Management of Tracheostomized and Ventilator-Dependent Adults* (pp. 61–96). San Diego: Singular

Dikeman, K.J., & Kazandjian, M.S. (1995c). Oral communication options. In: K.J. Dikeman, & M.S. Kazandjian (Eds.), *Communication and Swallowing Management of Tracheostomized and Ventilator-Dependent Adults* (pp. 141–195). San Diego: Singular

Dikeman, K.J., & Kazandjian, M.S. (1995d). Program development. In: K.J. Dikeman, & M.S. Kazandjian (Eds.), *Communication and Swallowing Management of Tracheostomized and Ventilator-Dependent Adults* (pp. 311–334). San Diego: Singular

Eibling, D.E., & Gross, R.D. (1996). Subglottic Air Pressure: A Key Component of Swallowing Efficiency. *Annual of Otology, Rhinology, and Laryngology, 105*, 253–258

Feinleib, M., Rosenberg, H.M., Collins, J.G., et al. (1989). Trends in COPD Morbidity and Mortality in the United States. *American Review of Respiratory Disease, 140*, S9–S18

Fornataro-Clerici, L., & Zajac, D.J. (1993). Aerodynamic Characteristics of Tracheostomy Speaking Valves. *Journal of Speech and Hearing Research, 36*, 529–532

Frey, J.A., & Wood, S. (1991). *Weaning from mechanical ventilation augmented by the Passy-Muir speaking and swallowing valve.* Presented at the International Conference of the American Lung Association and the American Thoracic Society, Anaheim

Gordon, C., Hewer, R.L., & Wade, D. (1987). Dysphagia in Acute Stroke. *British Medical Journal, 295,* 411–414

Groher, M.E. (1994). Determination of the Risks and Benefits of Oral Feeding. *Dysphagia, 9,* 233–235

Heffner, J.E., Miller, K.S., & Sahn, S.A. (1986). Tracheostomy in the Intensive Care Unit, Part 2: Complications. *Chest, 90,* 430–436

Hoit, J.D., Shea, S.A., & Banzett, R.B. (1994). Speech production during mechanical ventilation in tracheostomized individuals. *Journal of Speech and Hearing Research, 37,* 53–63

Hood Laboratories. *Hood Speaking Valve Product Information.* Pembroke, MA: Hood Laboratories

Horner, J., Massey, E.W., Riski, J.E., et al. (1988). Aspiration Following Stroke: Clinical Correlates and Outcome. *Neurology, 38,* 1359–1362

Huxley, E.J., Viroslav, J., Gray, W.R., et al. (1978). Pharyngeal Aspiration in Normal Adults and Patients with Depressed Consciousness. *American Journal of Medicine, 64,* 564–568

Katz, J.A., & Marks, J.D. (1985). Inspiratory Work with and Without Continuous Positive Airway Pressure in Patients with Acute Respiratory Failure. *Anesthesiology, 63,* 598–607

Kluin, K.J., Maynard, F., Bogdasarian, R.S. (1984). The Patient Requiring Mechanical Ventilatory Support: Use of the Cuffed Tracheostomy "Talk" Tube to Establish Phonation. *Otolaryngology Head and Neck Surgery, 92,* 625–627

Langmore, S.E., Schatz, K., & Olson, N. (1988). Fiberoptic Endoscopic Evaluation of Swallowing Safety: A New Procedure. *Dysphagia, 2,* 216–219

Leder, S.B., & Traquina, D.N. (1989). Voice Intensity of Patients Using a Communi-Trach I Cuffed Speaking Tracheostomy Tube. *Laryngoscope, 99,* 744–747

Linden, P., & Siebens, A.A. (1983). Dysphagia: Predicting Laryngeal Penetration. *Archives of Physical Medicine and Rehabilitation, 64,* 281–284

Logemann, J. (1983). Evaluation of Swallowing Disorders. In: J. Logemann (Ed.), *Evaluation and Treatment of Swallowing Disorders* (pp. 87–125). Boston: Little-Brown

MacIntyre, N.R. (1986). Respiratory Function During Pressure Support Ventilation. *Chest, 89,* 677–683

Mallinckrodt Medical. (1994). *Shiley Phonate Speaking Valve: Product Information Pamphlet.* Irvine, CA: Mallinckrodt Medical

Martin, B.J., Corlew, M.M., Wood, H., et al. (1994). The Association of Swallowing Dysfunction and Aspiration Pneumonia. *Dysphagia, 9,* 1–6

Mason, M.F. (1993a). Airway Issues. In: M.F. Mason (Ed.), *Speech Pathology for Tracheostomized and Ventilator Dependent Patients* (pp. 106–125). Newport Beach, CA: Voicing

Mason, M.F. (1993b). Vocal Treatment Strategies. In: M.F. Mason (Ed.), *Speech Pathology for Tracheostomized and Ventilator Dependent Patients* (pp. 336–381). Newport Beach, CA: Voicing

Mason, M., & Watkins, C. (1992). Protocol for Use of the Passy-Muir Tracheostomy Speaking Valves. *European Respiratory Journal, 5(suppl),* 148s–153s

Meduri, G.U., Cook, T.R., & Turner, R.E., et al. (1996). Noninvasive Positive Pressure Ventilation in Status Asthmaticus. *Chest, 110,* 767–774

Mulder, D.W. (1957). The Clinical Syndrome of Amyotrophic Lateral Sclerosis. *Mayo Clinic Proceedings, 32,* 427–436

Mulder, D.W. (1984). Motor Neuron Disease. In: P.J. Dyck, P.K. Thomas, E.H. Lambert, & R. Bunge (Eds.), *Peripheral Neuropathy,* vol. 2 (p. 1526). Philadelphia: WB

Murray, J.F. (1986). The Normal Lung, 2nd ed. Philadelphia: WB Sanders

Nash, M. (1988). Swallowing Problems in the Tracheostomized Patient. *Otolaryngologic Clinics of North America, 21,* 701–709

Passy-Muir. (2000). *Passy-Muir Tracheostomy and Ventilator Speaking Valve Instructional Booklet and Videotape.* Irvine, CA: Passy-Muir. www.passy-muir.com

Pingleton, S.K. (1988). Complications of Acute Respiratory Failure. *American Review of Respiratory Disease, 137,* 1463–1493

Pontoppidan, H., & Beecher, H.K. (1960). Progressive Loss of Protective Reflexes in the Airway with the Advancement of Age. *Journal of the American Medical Association, 174,* 2209–2213

Rosen, A.D. (1978). Amyotrophic lateral sclerosis. *Archives of Neurology, 35,* 638–642

Roussos, C., & Macklem, P.T. (1982). The Respiratory Muscles. *New England Journal of Medicine, 307,* 786–797

Rowland, L.P. (1985). Clinical Syndromes of the Spinal Cord. In: E.R. Kandel, & J.H. Schwartz (Eds.), *Principles of Neural Science,* 2nd ed. (pp. 469–477). New York: Elsevier

Russin, S.J., & Adler, A.G. (1989). Pulmonary Aspiration—The Three Syndromes. *Postgraduate Medicine, 85,* 155–161

Sahn, S.A., & Lakshminarayan, S. (1973). Bedside Criteria for Discontinuation of Mechanical Ventilation. *Chest, 63,* 1002–1005

Schmidt, J., Holas, M., Halvorson, K., et al. (1994). Videofluoroscopic Evidence of Aspiration Predicts Pneumonia and Death but Not Dehydration Following Stroke. *Dysphagia, 9,* 7–11

Siebens, A.A., Tippett, D.C., Kirby, N., et al. (1993). Dysphagia and Expiratory Air Flow. *Dysphagia, 8,* 266–269

Sitzmann, J.V. (1990). Nutritional Support of the Dysphagic Patient: Methods, Risks, and Complications of Therapy. *Journal of Parenteral and Enteral Nutrition, 14,* 60–64

Snider, G.L., Kleinerman, J., Thurlbeck, W.M., et al. (1985). The Definition of Emphysema: Report of a National Heart, Lung and Blood Institute, Division of Lung Diseases workshop. *American Review of Respiratory Disease, 132,* 182–185

Suiter, D.M., McCullough, G.H., & Powell, P.W. (2003). Effects of Cuff Deflation and One-Way Tracheostomy Speaking Valve Placement on Swallowing Physiology. *Dysphagia, 18,* 284–292

Takahashi, K., Groher, M.E., & Michi, K. (1994). Methodology for Detecting Swallowing Sounds. *Dysphagia, 9,* 54–62

Tobin, M.J. (1994). Mechanical Ventilation. *New England Journal of Medicine, 330,* 1056–1061

Tobin, M.J., & Yang, K. (1990). Weaning from Mechanical Ventilation. *Critical Care Clinics, 6,* 725–747

Tucker, H.M. (1993). Laryngeal Trauma. In: H.M. Tucker (Ed.), *The Larynx,* 2nd ed. (pp. 199–215). New York: Thieme

Weinberger, S.E., Schwartzstein, R.M., & Weiss, J.W. (1989). Hypercapnia. *New England Journal of Medicine, 321,* 1223–1231

West, J.B. (1971). Causes of Carbon Dioxide Retention in Lung Disease. *New England Journal of Medicine, 284,* 1232–1236

Yang, K.L., & Tobin, M.J. (1991). A Prospective Study of Indexes Predicting the Outcome of Trials of Weaning from Mechanical Ventilation. *New England Journal of Medicine, 324,* 1445–1450

Appendix 18–1   Competencies

Tracheostomy and Mechanical Ventilation

The clinician should be able to perform the following tasks:

1. Discuss a patient's respiratory status with team members and subsequently plan appropriate methods of communication for the patient.

2. Anticipate short- and long-term communication needs of an ICU patient, particularly if progression from oral intubation to tracheostomy tube is expected.

3. Identify situations that preclude the use of a speaking valve.

4. Recommend the appropriate type of speaking valve.

5. Explain to a patient, the family, and the medical staff why a speaking valve must be used with a fully deflated cuff or cuffless tracheostomy tube.

6. Educate a patient regarding the use of a speaking valve and identify signs of patient anxiety related to initial use of a speaking valve.

7. Perform cursory tests of upper airway patency when a speaking valve is in place.

8. Identify signs of breath stacking in a patient using a speaking valve.

Appendix 18–1 *(Continued)*

9. Identify signs of patient intolerance to a speaking valve.

10. Suggest methods to improve timing of speaking patterns for patients with tracheostomy tubes and cuff deflation who are phonating on the inhalation phase of the ventilatory cycle.

11. Troubleshoot when a patient is unable to voice with a "talking" tracheostomy tube in place.

Swallowing

The clinician should be able to perform the following tasks:

1. Identify clinical features of a speech and voice assessment that may predict aspiration during a videofluorographic swallowing study.

2. Present the rationale for recommending cuff deflation for swallowing purposes to a patient's physician.

3. Present the rationale for recommending use of a speaking valve, digital occlusion or capping of a deflated tracheostomy tube during swallowing.

4. Discuss the advantages and limitations to alternate methods of assessing dysphagia in an ICU patient who is unable to undergo a videofluorographic swallowing study.

5. Discuss common swallowing problems associated with the presence of a tracheostomy tube.

6. Discuss the importance of suctioning a patient who is undergoing blue-dye testing for dysphagia.

7. Discuss ethical issues regarding swallowing treatment in a patient with known tracheal aspiration with the patient and team members.

8. Plan in-service meetings on communication and swallowing issues for members of the ICU team.

19

Speech–Language Pathology Practice in the Acute Care Setting: A Consultative Approach

Alex F. Johnson, Anne Marie Valachovic, and K. Paige George

◆ Consultative Approach to Service Delivery in Acute Care
◆ Description of the Acute Care Setting
◆ Key Issues in Speech–Language Pathology Acute Care Practice
◆ The Process of Consultation
◆ Education in the Acute Care Setting

The acute care environment represents a part of the health care "culture" that provides an exciting and creative opportunity for the speech–language pathologist (SLP). Most SLPs have been prepared extensively for work in various rehabilitation settings, whereas few SLPs have been specifically educated for practice in the acute care environment. Miller and Groher (1990) describe acute care as "a stage in an individual's medical care where symptoms are severe and the duration of the immediate illness is short." It is important for the practicing clinician to appreciate the important differences between this point in the health care continuum and other points of care. In addition, we believe that the role of the SLP in acute care is unique and contributes to positive outcomes for the patient.

◆ Consultative Approach to Service Delivery in Acute Care

A general framework for consideration of key issues in acute care practice is presented in this chapter. Consultation in acute care involves three key professional activities: evaluation/diagnosis of the communication/swallowing disorder, intensive monitoring of clinical symptoms and intervention, and education/counseling. These services are referred to as consultative because ideally they are delivered to the patient with consideration of the information needs of the patient, family, and referral source. During the acute hospital stay the patient is rarely able to tolerate long periods of treatment that are more typical of rehabilitative care. This emphasis on consultative practice (as opposed to a traditional rehabilitative approach) is called for because of the short length of stay in acute care, the period of rapid change exhibited by most acute

patients, and, most important, the need to produce the best outcome in a short time frame. **Figure 19–1** presents a schema for considering these factors and their relationship to achieving the best patient outcome.

Implementation of the consultative model for acute care requires a rethinking of the traditional speech–language pathology service delivery system that is currently taught in most graduate programs. Key elements of current training-differential diagnosis, report writing, patient education, clinical supervision, treatment planning, and follow-up are components of service delivery in acute care. However, the unique arrangement of this environment demands a slightly different emphasis and packaging of patient care. The short-term nature of the patient contact; the demands for quick, accurate, and advanced levels of information and communication; the day-to-day interaction with many different types of professionals; and the observation and treatment of patients during critical points in illness and recovery dictate adjustments in the standard practice of our discipline.

The role of the acute care SLP is to assist patients and their health providers and caregivers to *prepare* for the rehabilitation activities that will follow discharge (**Table 19–1**). The activities of preparation for long-term rehabilitation or recovery include:

◆ Differential diagnosis of the communication and swallowing disturbance

◆ Assessment of the severity of the problem as the patient progresses (or worsens)

◆ Aggressive communication with the referring physician, primary care doctor, and other specialists

◆ Manipulation of the environment to facilitate immediate communication and swallowing

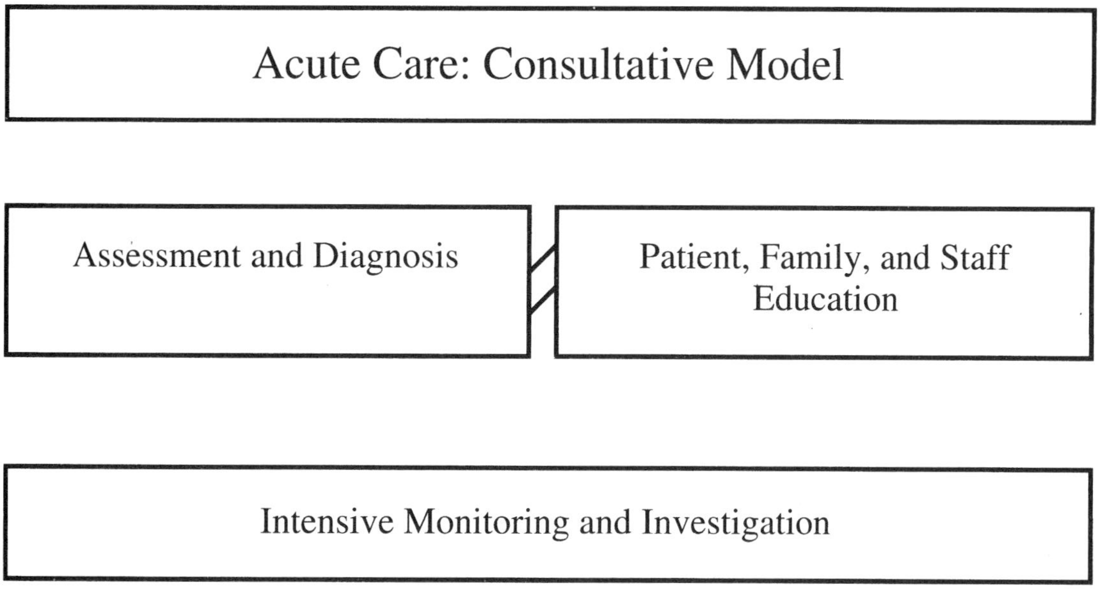

```
┌─────────────────────────────────────────────────────────────┐
│                                                             │
│            Acute Care: Consultative Model                   │
│                                                             │
└─────────────────────────────────────────────────────────────┘
```

```
┌──────────────────────────────┐  ┌──────────────────────────────┐
│                              │  │                              │
│   Assessment and Diagnosis   │  │   Patient, Family, and Staff │
│                              │  │          Education           │
│                              │  │                              │
└──────────────────────────────┘  └──────────────────────────────┘
```

```
┌─────────────────────────────────────────────────────────────┐
│                                                             │
│        Intensive Monitoring and Investigation               │
│                                                             │
└─────────────────────────────────────────────────────────────┘
```

Figure 19–1 The acute care consultative model.

◆ Education of the family and the patient about the communication disorder

◆ Intensive monitoring of changes in communication and swallowing function

◆ Development of a discharge plan and plan for follow-up

◆ Provision of short-term treatment

◆ Description of the Acute Care Setting

Acute care hospitals can be organized in a variety of ways. Acute care services are provided in small community hospitals, large medical centers, or university hospitals. Most acute care facilities include an emergency department through which many patients are admitted, a variety of surgical and medical departments by which physician services are organized, operating rooms, intensive care units, and a range of other services designed to support the primary medical and surgical functions. Some institutions are designed to function in managing the

Table 19–1   Main Reasons for Consultation in Acute Care and Examples of How the Speech–Language Pathologist May Fulfill the Purpose of Each Type of Consultation

Reasons for Consultation	Role of Speech–Language Pathologist (Examples)
Advice on diagnosis	Aphasia classification
	Lesion localization
Advice on management	Feeding status
	Feeding tube placement
Performance of a test	Videofluoroscopic assessment of swallowing

most acutely ill patients. These hospitals tend to be large, technologically advanced, and specialized in the way in which services are delivered. For a basic review of the major functions of the full range of various medical and surgical specialties, see the texts prepared by Miller and Groher (1990), or Golper (1992).

Common Referral Sources

A few specialties tend to be major referral sources, and the SLP in the hospital setting should have a keen appreciation for the scope of interest of each of these key specialists as well as an understanding of typical referral concerns and questions. In the acute setting, SLPs receive a significant number of referrals from neurologists, neurosurgeons, otolaryngologists, psychiatrists, and pulmonary specialists. Because of the rapidly expanding scope of practice of SLPs, new referral and collaboration relationships are constantly being formed, and so in some institutions the "high-volume" list may include many other specialties.

Neurologists and Neurosurgeons

These physicians provide medical diagnosis and care for patients with diseases of the nervous system. In larger centers, neurologic services tend to be subspecialized, with providers concentrating in one area of practice. Major subspecialties of neurology that interact frequently with speech–language pathology include cerebrovascular disease (stroke), epileptology, neuromuscular disease, movement disorders, behavioral neurology, neuro-oncology, and pediatric neurology.

The neurologist has much to offer the SLP in the acute care setting. The detailed neurologic examination, when observed by the astute SLP, can reveal important information that may serve to complement the working diagnosis and the ongoing treatment of the communication disorder.

Neurosurgeons provide surgical and postoperative care to patients with tumors, malformations, or neurotrauma. Some of the more common groups of patients referred by neurosurgeons include patients with traumatic brain injury, spinal cord injury, or those with cranial nerve tumors.

In some centers, SLPs are involved in presurgical evaluation for patients at risk for postsurgical changes in speech, language, or swallowing.

Otolaryngologists

These specialists provide surgical and medical care to patients with diseases of the head and neck. Otolaryngologists are frequently involved in surgical placement of tracheostomy tubes to assist patients with breathing difficulty. They are typically the referral source to SLPs for patients with vocal fold paralysis as well as those with malignancies involving the jaw, tongue, or larynx.

Psychiatry

In the acute care setting, SLPs come into contact with patients exhibiting a variety of psychiatric disorders. The SLP's interaction with psychiatrists and other mental health professionals (psychologists, clinical social workers) usually occurs when both groups are asked to consult on patients exhibiting some behavioral difficulty. Patients with speech, language, or swallowing disorders may also exhibit serious psychological problems that need to be addressed with drugs or other therapies. Likewise, some patients with primary psychological disturbances may exhibit disturbances of communication or swallowing.

Pulmonary Medicine

These subspecialists of general internal medicine evaluate and treat patients with diseases of the respiratory system. Pulmonary specialists frequently refer patients from the intensive care setting for communication and swallowing evaluation. Typically, referred patients are seriously compromised at the time of referral and may be dependent on artificial ventilation for oxygen exchange. In addition to these predictable referrals from the intensive care unit, pulmonary physicians may refer patients who are admitted for workup of suspected functional breathing disorders such as paradoxical vocal fold movement. Jacobson and Silbergleit (1994) have presented such a patient who was admitted to the hospital in acute distress.

✦ Key Issues in Acute Care Speech–Language Pathology Practice

Appreciation and comprehension of the circumstances that guide the distinctive practice of acute care SLPs are critical to effective service delivery. Understanding of these issues adds clarity and provides direction for the SLP and benefits patients. Themes central to the practice of acute care speech–language pathology include:

✦ Understanding the distinctive characteristics of the consultative model of practice

✦ Provision of expert level diagnostic services

✦ Delivery of skilled provision of patient performance monitoring information over time

✦ Provision of multifaceted educational services

Given these important themes, as guideposts, the following specific points are offered as factors that are more specific to the practice of acute care speech–language pathology:

1. *Appreciation of the importance of timely (rapid) access to information by all members of the health care team.* Patients change rapidly in the acute care setting. Acute disease processes tend to be highly variable over time, and patients are observed to improve or worsen frequently during their stay. Additionally, patient stays continue to decrease in length. These changes are due to improved ability to provide advanced outpatient and home-based care, as well as the high cost of inpatient services. Thus, timely response and provision of information is critical to good patient care. The decrease in length of stay increases the complexity of scheduling inpatient tests and procedures, managing communication, and discharge planning. SLPs need to develop communication styles (oral and written) that are conducive to effective relay of information in the medical setting. **Table 19–2** provides an example of communication guidelines developed in one major hospital program.

2. *Knowledge of appropriate observation and treatment methods for patients seen during periods of rapid change.* The approaches to patient care used by the SLP in the acute care setting should be different from those provided in rehabilitation or long-term-care programs. The most effective approach, regardless of the type of disorder, is typically one that integrates consultative activities with differential diagnosis and careful patient monitoring.

3. *Communication with a broad audience of other professionals.* The issue of time pressure around professional communication in acute care has been cited as a key characteristic of this practice setting. Another issue of communication relates to the diverse audience of professionals with whom the SLP must converse. This factor interacts with the important variable of time to complicate the communication arrangement.

   Why is the nature of the audience important or of concern to the SLP? Given that one of the major goals of care in the acute setting is to participate in the medical and rehabilitative care of the patient, it is very important that the interaction among care providers be clear, concise, and directed toward

Table 19–2   Sample Acute Care Professional Communication Issues and Guidelines

1. Complete all documentation immediately following the patient encounter. This includes chart notes, patient instructions, and counseling with staff or families.

2. For initial consultations, complete the consultation form and place it at the front of the chart and then page the referring physician and review your findings and recommendations.

3. For patients with dysphagia, attempt to communicate on a daily basis with referring physician.

4. Always complete all documentation and place it in the patient's chart by the end of the working day.

5. Document every encounter with your signature, degree, CCC-speech–language pathologist, and your pager number.

6. Return all pages immediately when on the inpatient service.

From Henry Ford Hospital, Division of Speech–Language Sciences and Disorders.

patient care. The SLP in acute care can affect little change with the patient without the cooperation of other providers. Careful observation, appropriate and accurate diagnosis, and good interaction with the patient, while essential, will not ensure that the patient is positioned properly for eating, has the appropriate level of communication interaction, is using his/her communication device appropriately, has the necessary dietary accommodations, or is receiving appropriate therapies. All these activities and decisions, which might be recommended by a SLP, need to be performed by someone else in the patient's array of care providers. Thus, it is essential that the SLP in acute care settings has communication skills that allow for very specific explanations that provide a clear (and brief) rationale for any recommendation or request; anticipation of the varying information needs of different providers (physician, nurse, occupational therapist, psychologist); and the ability to provide background information (justification) for any unusual or unexpected recommendations. It is important to remember also that the SLP is as much a receiver as a sender of information. Therefore, good listening skills and the ability to respond critically without confrontation become important. In general, a communication style that is respectful and diplomatic, balanced with directness, and targeted toward a specific professional's interest or concern is desirable.

4. *Dealing with patients and families during times of crisis.* Admission to an acute care situation is never trivial for a patient or the patient's family. In many cases, admissions are nonelective, and both the patient and the family are under considerable stress. It is important for clinicians to remember that they are rarely seeing the "best" communication ability when they evaluate the patient for the first time. Regardless of the etiology of the patient's condition, the psychological state of the patient at the time of evaluation is always an issue. The SLP's role is to demonstrate appropriate concern and empathy for the patient and the family, advocate for the patient (especially around issues of communication and swallowing), and assist the family in finding resources that might be helpful to the patient. Under very stressful critical care situations, families can exhibit anger, extreme emotionality, withdrawal, and defensiveness. SLPs should obtain appropriate information about desirable communication skills in these situations and seek the help of other professionals (social workers, psychologists, pastoral care professionals) when they are not sure how to deal with a difficult patient or family.

5. *Providing information that has immediate effect on patient care.* SLPs in acute care need to appreciate the pace with which information transfer occurs. Once information is entered into a paper or electronic record, it becomes available for use by anyone with access to the record. This places pressure on the clinician to provide accurate, clear, and essential recommendations. The rapid growth of feeding and swallowing practice in our discipline has highlighted the need for clear communication of results of dysphagia evaluation. Frequently nurses are waiting for these results so that they can feed the patient with the correct food consistency, or physicians are waiting to determine if a feeding tube is necessary for the patient. Because of the implications of these types of recommendations on cost of care, length of stay, and patient outcome, it is essential that information be transmitted as soon as possible. It is equally important that the SLP appreciates others' need for information and also

understands that once information is provided, follow-up actions will ensue in a timely manner.

6. *Potential for significant clinical errors in judgment or practice.* The SLP in acute care practice has a responsibility that affects patient care, satisfaction with treatment, and patient outcome. More than in most other settings, the fast-paced acute care environment affords the opportunity for clinical errors. Some of these errors may cause inconvenience to the patient or caregivers; others can cause serious complications to an illness; and still other bad decisions can be life threatening. A keen knowledge of common clinical pitfalls can serve to prevent clinical errors. A sampling of common errors can be found in **Table 19–3**.

Speech–language pathologists should *always* be knowledgeable about any potential negative effects that could occur as the result of recommendations or actions on their part. The SLP has the responsibility of informing families, physicians, nurses, and other professionals of any potential adverse effects associated with any recommended or completed procedures.

In the unfortunate situation that an adverse effect occurs as the result of a speech–language pathology recommendation or procedure, the first issue to be addressed (following

Table 19–3 Potential Significant Errors in Speech–Language Pathology Practice

1. Failure to communicate results of high-risk or invasive procedures accurately or in a timely manner

2. Failure to document detailed recommendations in the chart (especially diet changes or aspiration precautions)

3. Failure to respond to referrals or requests for information from families or physicians in a timely manner, especially when this delay causes interruption of other care or delays discharge from the acute care setting

4. Performing any procedure without having demonstrated competency

5. Failure to supervise noncertified personnel when they are completing procedures

6. Failure to communicate results from language, speech, or swallowing testing that have diagnostic significance and could change the medical plan of care

7. Failure to observe or report significant changes in patient behavior that may signal an alteration in the medical or psychological status

8. Performing procedures outside the scope of practice

9. Performing procedures that are experimental or of questionable benefit without appropriate informed consent

10. Making diagnostic statements or drawing conclusions that are not substantiated by observation or test data

11. Failure to make appropriate referrals when indicated

12. Failure to follow up on recommendations previously made

13. Failure to explain and document important information to the patient and/or the family

14. Failure to ensure patient confidentiality

15. Providing services that would be viewed as incomplete or faulty by a group of your peers

16. Failure to limit opinions and decisions to topics directly related to speech, language, swallowing, cognition disorders, and their sequelae

17. Failure to follow basic procedures for infection control, universal precautions, and safety

appropriate and careful attention to the needs of the patient) should be the reduction of the possibility for the same adverse effect to reoccur. The second issue should involve the careful study of the problem that was presented so that one can learn all that is possible from the situation toward the goal of improved patient care.

7. *Observing immediate effects of illness, drugs, and surgical management on patient performance, function, and outcome.* One of the most unique learning opportunities for learning afforded to the SLP in the acute care setting is the study of the effects that various medical interventions have on the speech, language, cognitive, motor, or swallowing systems. Because these effects can be immediate, sustained, or short or long term, it is essential that the clinician come to appreciate the significance of the most common interventions. Many clinicians find it helpful to obtain some of the common manuals used by physicians that present these effects in outline or tabular forms for quick reference. A few of these sources are listed in **Table 19–4**.

8. *Dealing with issues related to patient advocacy and ethics.* Another recent development in health care that has affected patient decision making and also involves high-level problem solving and communication among practitioners is the study and practice of ethics. Many institutions have established interdisciplinary teams that include clinicians who have developed expertise in the study of ethical problem solving, members of the clergy, and professionals from behavioral medicine. The recent technologic advances that have extended the viability of the patient combined with media attention on these issues have emphasized the role of the patient and the family in decision making about life and death issues as well as quality of life. SLPs tend to be involved in these discussions from a variety of perspectives: Can a patient comprehend a situation and make an informed decision? Will the patient ever be independent in communication or cognitive functioning? What are the implications for a given patient when the decision is made to continue oral feedings when chronic aspiration is documented?

Many SLPs have not had, as part of their formal training, coursework in medical ethics, death and dying, grief

counseling with families, or other topics related to end-of-life issues. Participation in discussions with ethics teams can be a valuable learning experience for the clinician interested in learning more about this type of decision making. Most important, however, is the need for SLPs who are working in tertiary care settings to become familiar with ethical principles and with issues related to death, dying, chronic disability, and interprofessional and family consultation around these topics. When these issues arise in the course of patient care, it is important for the SLP to inform the patient's primary physician of patient-family concerns, and seek advice from those experienced in management of these issues. These issues are rarely addressed by the SLP alone.

9. *Understanding the role of the SLP in ensuring the best outcomes—both rehabilitative and medical.* A final point regarding the role of the SLP in acute care is that in addition to providing immediate consultation, diagnosis, and treatment for the patient and the referring physician, the SLP has the responsibility to ensure that the more long-term needs of the patient begin to be addressed. Frequently these issues relate to the postdischarge placement of the patient for rehabilitation or nursing care. It is not uncommon for discharge planners or physicians unfamiliar with the complexities of managing communication issues to overlook these needs in planning postacute care services. SLPs have the responsibility of pointing out these needs and recommending suitable referrals or community resources. Every patient should leave the hospital with an appropriate plan for communication treatment (when indicated), and discussion with professionals who will be providing follow-up is an important ingredient to quality care. SLPs also have an important role in family education about the patient's communication or swallowing disorder. This can frequently be accomplished in bedside discussions with the patient and the family. For more complex problems, it may be necessary to provide written materials, videos, or other resources designed for patient education. Ideally, patients and families should be given a written plan for follow-up, including scheduling of necessary return appointments, to ensure that patients are likely to receive those services that will best meet their communicative needs.

Table 19–4 Examples of Common Sources that Summarize Effects of Drugs and Procedures on Cognitive, Communicative, and Motor Systems

The Little Black Book of Neurology: A Manual for House Officers, 2nd ed. J. S. Bonner and J. J. Bonner, Mosby (1991).

Handbook of Symptom Oriented Neurology, 2nd ed. W.H. Olson, R.A. Brumback, V. Iyer, G. Gascon, Mosby (1994).

Pocket Guide to Assessment in Speech–Language Pathology, M.N. Hegde, Singular (1996).

Otolaryngology, 3rd ed. M.M. Paparella, D.A. Shumrick, J.L. Gluckman, W.L. Meyerhoff (eds.), W.B. Saunders (1991).

Interpretation of Diagnostic Tests, 6th ed. Wallach, J., Little, Brown (1996).

Current Medical Diagnosis and Therapy, 36th ed. L.M. Tierney, S.J. McPhee, M.A. Papadakis (Eds.), Appleton and Lange (1997).

Harrison's Principles of Internal Medicine, 13th ed. K.J. Isselbacher, E. Braunwald, J.D. Wilson, J.B. Marin, A.S. Fauci, D.L. Kasper (Eds.), McGraw-Hill (1994).

The Merck Manual, 16th ed. R. Berkow (ed.), Merck Research Laboratories (1992).

✦ The Process of Consultation

Consultation is an essential component of acute medical care. For the SLP, the consultative model is one that can be contrasted with the rehabilitative SLP model. Although all assessments in SLP include both a diagnostic and rehabilitative focus, it is probably safe to say that in the consultative model, the information provided is "tipped" in the direction of diagnosis and explanation of the communication disorder, with the opposite emphasis occurring in rehabilitative settings. It is a highly complex process that is most effective when a model is used to guide the consultation from referral to discharge. The following process is presented as a successful model for guiding consultative activities. A condensed version is provided in checklist format in **Appendix 19–1**. It may be used as a resource for training fellows or new medical SLPs to be effective consultants. Consultation is a skill that should be taught formally and perfected through experience, rather than learned in a trial-and-error manner.

Anatomy of an Effective Consultation

Referral Process

The referral of a patient for a speech–language pathology consultation is usually made by a staff or resident physician from the patient's primary service. Typically, referrals are generated directly by the patient's physician, although they may be prompted by a nurse, patient, or family member who reports a concern to the physician. Finally, referrals may be prompted by other consulting services via recommendations.

Once the referral is received, there is a general rule that a response from the consultant is expected within 24 hours. Horwitz, Henes, and Horwitz (1983) found that internist's consultations performed within 24 hours of referral had a significantly increased impact on diagnosis or management than those performed more than 24 hours from initial referral. Note that the study cited above was completed many years prior to the onset of the current system of shortened stays. It is likely that the expectations for "fast response" have increased significantly in the current environment.

Preparation for the Consultation

Once a patient has been referred for consultation, the SLP begins with a comprehensive review of the patient's medical chart. The medical chart contains a wealth of information that provides the astute SLP with the background of the case and a strong starting point. The following list of medical chart components should be carefully examined and understood by the SLP:

✦ The history and physical form provides the reason for admission, findings of the initial examination, and past medical history.
✦ Chart notes, or progress notes, are important in understanding the patient's treatment regimen and clinical course since admission.
✦ Review of findings from all tests or procedures
✦ Review of the reports from other consultants

During the chart review, the SLP must be aware of signs that indicate significant clinical information. This requires the medical SLP to have a working knowledge of pertinent information from related areas of medicine and other disciplines. For example, if the chart indicates that a patient has been intubated for 3 weeks, a voice or swallowing impairment may be suspected; similarly, it is of clinical significance that the patient had progressive mental status changes 6 months prior to admission rather than an acute onset of changes. A history of stroke, pneumonia, or cancer may lead to hypotheses regarding current communication or swallowing disorders. Therefore, the consultation process involves application of traditional speech–language pathology skills, as well as the acquisition and practical use of new knowledge from multiple disciplines.

Referral Question   The key to a successful consultation is to accurately identify the referral questions. According to Lee, Pappius, and Goldman (1983), "consultants must identify the reasons for which their expertise has been sought." Only when a question has been identified can it be answered. At times, the referring physician may specify the reason for the consultation in verbal communication or in writing on the consultation re-

port. However, in many consultations, no question has been specified. This then becomes a problem-solving endeavor. A thorough medical chart review is critical for identifying the referral question, and if the question does not become clear through chart review alone, a call to the referring physician to clarify the reason for the consultation is indicated.

Physicians most commonly request consultations for the following:

1. Advice regarding diagnosis
2. Advice regarding management
3. Assistance in scheduling or performing a test or procedure

The SLP may be consulted for any of these purposes. Typical referral questions encountered by the medical SLP include:

✦ Is it safe to the patient to eat?
✦ What type of aphasia does the patient have?
✦ Is the patient a good rehabilitation candidate?
✦ Is the presenting behavior consistent with a diagnosis of X disease?

Once the medical chart has been reviewed and the referral question clearly identified, the SLP must formulate a plan for the examination.

Plan for the Examination   Based on information from the medical chart review, the SLP is able to formulate hypotheses about which communication disorders to expect on examination. A list of differential diagnoses may then be compiled in order of likelihood. This facilitates the plan for diagnostic testing because each of the diagnoses must systematically be confirmed or ruled out during the examination.

Formal and informal test measures are selected based on the communication parameters that need to be assessed. In acute care, the main areas to be tested usually include language, cognitive communication, speech, and swallowing, with perhaps an emphasis in one area based on the referral question. Even if the referral question involves one area, such as swallowing, all parameters are assessed or at least screened. Owing to the limited time for testing in the acute setting, brief formal tests are often preferred over more lengthy formal tests that may be better suited for the outpatient clinical setting. Formal tests may be given in part if they cannot be administered in whole. Informal testing is heavily relied on in acute care owing to poor patient tolerance, lack of ability to comply with formal testing, or poor testing conditions.

The organization and sequence of the testing session also must be determined. In general, it is best to first perform the testing needed to answer the referral question. In this manner, the SLP has at least obtained the information necessary for addressing the reason for the consultation. Examinations can be limited because of patient fatigue or interruptions for routine medical care or medical tests that temporarily take patients away from their hospital room. Thus, it is important to address the most important issues early in the testing session.

Examination and Diagnostic Testing   In the acute care setting, patients are seen and examined in their hospital room or in the intensive care unit. Examination of the patient involves the administration of formal tests and informal measures according to the plan of action that was developed based on the medical chart review. Even the most experienced and organized SLP may not be able to examine the patient according to the original plan because of the unique challenges of the acute care environment. Invariably, modifications in the original plan are necessary as a result of the condition or performance of the patient. A patient may be lethargic owing to a neurologic condition or the effects of medication, resulting in a limited assessment and a reliance on behavioral measures; or a patient with severe aphasia may be struggling with formal aphasia tests, requiring the use of informal language measures. These modifications represent an on-line decision-making process that is done throughout the evaluation. It requires skill and experience to determine when such modifications in testing are necessary.

The primary goal of the examination is to obtain sufficient data to answer the referral question; the assessment is not considered complete until this has been accomplished. It is also important to systematically rule out or confirm the presence of each item on the list of differential diagnoses. Finally, the information from the initial assessment provides an important baseline for measuring change.

Documentation: Generation of the Written Consultation Report

The written consultation report is the means by which the consultant's expertise is translated into usable information. Typically, the consultant's report is limited to less than one page. This necessitates that it be brief, specific, informative, and to the point. Although at times it is difficult to record the necessary information in such a limited fashion, effective consultants are able to relay their findings in a concise manner, with as much content and impact as in a much longer report. The standard information contained in the written consultation report is presented in three sections: the body of the report, impressions, and recommendations. (See **Appendix 19–2** for an example of written consultation reports.)

Body of the Consultation Report

The first statement of the consultation report usually includes information regarding the patient's age, sex, date of admission, and reason for hospitalization. This is followed by a statement listing the patient's past medical history. In the next section, the SLP consultant provides objective clinical data and key observations obtained during the patient examination. People reading the report benefit from organization by subheadings representing the main areas tested. For example, the subheadings commonly used in reports for patients with neurogenic communication disorders include:

✦ Cognitive-communication language
✦ Physical examination of the speech structures and functions
✦ Speech
✦ Swallowing

Impressions   Following the documentation of objective data, the consultant records diagnoses in the impressions section of the report. Diagnoses are usually given in a list, and it is not uncommon for acutely ill patients to have a list of three to five diagnosed communication or swallowing disorders. All are listed, whether or not they are related to the referral question. Each diagnosis should be qualified by a severity level (i.e., mild, moderate, severe). It is also beneficial and often appreciated if the suspected etiology of the communication disorder is in-

cluded in the report to the referring physician. For example, a phonatory disturbance may occur as a result of prolonged intubation or may have a neurologic etiology. If the patient is found to have aphasia or dysarthria, classification according to the traditional profiles should be attempted and stated whenever possible. It is not sufficient to report impressions as "aphasia" or even "receptive aphasia." Referral sources are typically good observers of behavior and know the superficial categories of impairment exhibited by the patient. *They seek the expertise of the SLP for diagnosing the type of communication or swallowing disorder and interpreting the presenting problem in the context of the patient's physiologic or anatomic disturbance.* Many neurologists and neurosurgeons are familiar with the Aphasia Classification System proposed by Goodglass and Kaplan (2000), or the Mayo Clinic Dysarthria Classification (1995). Using these types of systems may improve communication with physicians and be helpful as they attempt to use the information to localize the lesion or clarify the medical diagnosis.

Recommendations   The last section of the consultation report is the recommendations section. Based on clinical impressions, the SLP provides recommendations to the referring physician regarding patient management. Recommendations should be presented in a concise list and address pertinent issues, including:

✦ Feeding status: NPO (nothing by mouth) or diet order (e.g., pureed, soft, regular) if it is judged that the patient may safely eat
✦ Treatment/management issues: for example, recommendation for modified barium swallowing study; ongoing assessment and treatment of communication/language, swallowing, speech, or voice; or augmentative/alternative communication
✦ Discharge status: recommendation for continued speech-language follow-up, if indicated, and in what setting (i.e., outpatient clinic, rehabilitation center, home health care, nursing home). In the majority of cases it is not too soon to address this at the time of the initial evaluation.
✦ Referrals to other services if indicated: the examination may reveal issues that warrant attention from a discipline not already involved in the case. For example, a patient with prolonged dysphonia after extubation may benefit from an examination by otolaryngology. In this case, the recommendation may be written as follows: "Recommend otolaryngology consultation to rule out laryngeal pathology."

In all cases, the referring service may be more compliant with recommendations when they are made aware of the reason for the recommendation. All recommendations must be supported by objective information presented in the Consultant's Remarks section of the report. The SLP must be prepared to provide the rationale for each recommendation to increase compliance. It is best to recommend tests and treatments that are likely to make a difference in management.

Communicative and Swallowing Monitoring and Intervention

The acute care SLP needs to provide information to the patient, family, and referral sources about the evolution of speech, language, cognitive, and swallowing abilities of the patient. Through serial testing and precise behavioral monitoring over time changes in these abilities can be demonstrated. Selected tests that provide quantitative measures of performance can be useful indices of change. This section reviews the process of monitoring patient change. Because the most complex type of patient monitoring, in our experience, focuses on documenting change in patients with neurologic problems, we have chosen to present examples from the neurocommunication point of view. Note, however, that patients with swallowing and speech problems owing to damage of respiratory, laryngeal, or motor systems also require systematic observation and monitoring.

Neurocommunication Monitoring Measurement Tools

Depending on the findings from the initial consultation, one or more neurocommunication monitoring tools may be used in combination to monitor the communication processes of interest (**Table 19–5**). For example, a patient with aphasia might be tested daily with the Aphasia Diagnostic Profile (ADP) (Helm-Estabrooks, 1992) to track the evolution of language behavior. A patient with a traumatic brain injury might be evaluated daily with the Ranchos Los Amigos Scale (Hagen and Malkmus, 1979) and the Galveston Orientation and Amnesia Test (GOAT) (1979). The choice of test is important because it may be used to predict

Table 19–5 Neurocommunication Monitoring Tools for the Acute Setting

Behavioral scales

Glasgow Coma Scale (Teasdale & Jennett, 1974)

Ranchos Los Amigos Scale (Hagen, 1979)

Cognitive measurement tools

Mini-Mental State Examination (MMSE) (Folstein, Folstein, & McHugh, 1975)

Galveston Orientation and Attention Test (GOAT) (Levin et al., 1979)

Brief Test of Head Injury (BTHI) (Helm-Estabrooks & Hotz, 1991)

Ross Information Processing Assessment (Ross, 1986)

Clock Drawing (Freedman et al., 1994)

Rehabilitation Institute of Chicago Evaluation of Communication (Burns, Halper, & Mogil, 1985)

Mini-Inventory of Right Brain Injury (MIRBI) (Pimental & Kingsbury, 1989)

Language monitoring tools

Frenchay Aphasia Screening Test (FAST) (Enderby, Wood, & Wade, 1983)

Aphasia Diagnostic Profiles (ADP)

Bedside Evaluation Screening Test (BEST) (Fitch-West & Sands, 1987)

Boston Assessment of Severe Aphasia (BASA) (Helm-Estabrooks et al., 1989)

Multilingual Aphasia Examination (MAE) (Benton, Hamsher, & Sivan, 1994)

Boston Naming Test (BNT) (Kaplan, Goodglass, & Weintraub, 1983)

Functional communication measures

ASHA Functional Communication Measures (FCMS) (ASHA, 1983)

ASHA Functional Assessment of Communication Skills for Adults (FACS) (Frattali et al., 1995)

Table 19–6 Ranchos Los Amigos Scale of Cognitive Levels and Expected Behavior

Level I	Response: unresponsive to all stimuli
Level II	Generalized inconsistent, nonpurposeful, nonspecific reactions to stimuli; responds to pain, but response may be delayed
Level III	Localized response; inconsistent reaction directly related to type of stimulus presented; responds to some commands; may respond to discomfort
Level IV	Confused, agitated, disoriented and unaware of present events; response with frequent bizarre and inappropriate behavior; attention span is short, and ability to process information impaired
Level V	Confused, nonpurposeful random or fragmented inappropriate responses when task complexity exceed nonagitated abilities; patient appears alert and responds to simple commands; performs previously learned tasks but is unable to learn new ones
Level VI	Confused, behavior is goal-directed; responses are appropriate to the situation with incorrect response because of memory difficulties
Level VII	Automatic, correct routine responses that are robot-like; appropriate, appears oriented to setting, but insight, response judgment, and problem solving are poor
Level VIII	Purposeful, correct responding carryover of new appropriate learning; no required supervision, poor response tolerance for stress, and some abstract reasoning difficulties

From Hagen, C., Malkmus, D. (1979). *Intervention Strategies for Language Disorders Secondary to Head Trauma.* Atlanta: American Speech–Language-Hearing Association.

future recovery levels. Levin, O'Donnell, and Grossman (1979) found that the period of posttraumatic amnesia as documented serially with the GOAT corresponded to eventual outcome levels. Assessment of outcome was completed on 32 patient 6 months after injury. Subjects with posttraumatic amnesia less than 2 weeks in duration had a "good outcome" as measured on the Glasgow Outcome Scale (**Table 19–6**). In addition, monitoring tools must detect subtle change in communication skills while being relatively quick to administer and score. Johnson, George, and Valachovic (1996) found the ADP sensitive to subtle change in language performance in the acute setting.

When selecting tools for a particular diagnosis, be aware of several key features that make for a good neurocommunication monitoring instrument. Neurocommunication monitoring tools should be:

✦ Brief: The tool needs to be easy to administer and score, ideally taking 30 minutes or less. There is a time pressure to have results available quickly, and patient's testing tolerance may be limited.

✦ Sensitive: The tool needs to detect subtle change in communication and cognitive skills. The sensitivity of the instrument depends on the degree of disorder severity. Screening tools may detect the presence of a problem, but not be effective for detecting subtle change in performance.

✦ Quantifiable: The tool should allow for accurate measurement of the communication behavior under consideration. Quantification provides one important index for measuring change and progression of symptoms.

Table 19–7   Features of Selected Neurocommunication Monitoring Tools

Instrument	Brief	Sensitive	Quantifiable	Standardized
Glasgow Coma Scale	+		+	+
Ranchos Los Amigos Scale	+		+	+
Mini–Mental State Examination	+		+	+
Galveston Orientation and Attention Test	+	+	+	+
Brief Test of Head Injury	+/$\tilde{+}$		+	+
Clock Drawing	+		+	+
RIC Evaluation of Right Hemisphere Dysfunction	+/$\tilde{-}$		+	+
Mini Inventory of Right Brain Injury	+/$\tilde{-}$		+	+
Frenchay Aphasia Screening Test	+		+	+
Aphasia Diagnostic Profiles	+/$\tilde{-}$	+	+	+
Bedside Evaluation Screening Test	+		+	+
Boston Assessment of Severe Aphasia	+		+	+
Multi-Lingual Aphasia Test	?		+	+
ASHA FACS	.$\tilde{}$/		+	+
ASHA FCMS	+		+	+

FACS, Functional Assessment of Communication Skill; FCMS, Functional Communication Measurement System; RIC, Rehabilitation Institute of Chicago.

✦ Standardized: Measures that meet the criteria for differentiating levels of impairment, identifying normal and atypical individuals, and reliably identifying changes over time are useful in the acute setting.

These features are guidelines for choosing a "good" monitoring tool. Several widely used scales, tests, and functional assessments meet all or some of these criteria (**Table 19–7**). In addition to these measures, clinicians may have developed their own language and cognitive assessment tools to meet their needs.

Clinical Observations   Clinicians make many observations that provide insight into a patient's medical, neurologic, and communication status that extends beyond performance on standard tests. Changes in these initial observations over time help clinicians to formulate tentative hypotheses about the communication impairment and are later used to signal improvement or decline in function. For the more severely impaired patient, formal testing may be impossible and precise behavioral description may be the only measure of ability. In addition, clinical observations provide information about preserved communication skills not formally tested, the influence of the environment and communication partner on communication abilities, the patient and family's emotional and psychological adjustment, and the patient's rehabilitation potential. The following areas should be considered as the SLP interacts with the patient over time.

Mental Status   The degree of alertness, attention, and orientation must be observed and documented daily. Patients who have decreased alertness or an inability to focus, maintain, and shift their attention will not provide valid and reliable responses on tests of language and cognition. Poor performance, may result from decreased arousal and attention, and not a deficit in higher cognitive or language processing. Formal testing should not continue if a patient cannot maintain an alert state.

General Appearance and Behavior   It is important to note the patient's physical appearance and overall behavior. How does the patient look and behave during the session? What are the patient's mood and affect? Does the patient tend to his/her hygiene and grooming? Is behavior appropriate to the context? Behavioral changes can either be increased or decreased. Both are significant. For example, the abulic patient will show a flat affect, indifferent attitude, and a decreased responsiveness. In contrast the manic patient may be euphoric and impulsive with increased activity.

Medical Status   It is important to appreciate the patient's medical status. Many acutely ill patients are medically unstable, which can result in fluctuations in language and cognitive function. A review of the medical chart, nursing notes, and daily laboratory values combined with clinical observation can help clinicians determine the patient's medical status. It is beneficial to note the patient's vital signs including temperature, pulse, respiration, and blood pressure. Fluctuations and irregularity may signal medical instability. There are a wide array of factors that may adversely affect language and cognition. Some of these include cardiovascular dysfunction (e.g., reduced cardiac output, causing a reduction in blood flow to the brain), infection or fever, drug intoxication, metabolic and nutritional imbalance (e.g., hyperthyroidism, dehydration, electrolyte disturbance), neurologic disorders of traumatic, vascular, or infectious origin, and disorders associated with hospitalization (e.g., confusion following anesthesia) (Albert, 1988).

Medical Interventions/Medication   Different tests, medical procedures, and therapies may influence patient performance. Patients may fatigue more readily following a day of tests, or they may have received certain medications that cause drowsiness or confusion. It is important to be aware of the patient's activities and schedule of medications. See Vogel and Carter (1995, 1999) and Chapter 23 in this text for a review of medications that influence communication.

Medical Devices   It is common for patients in the acute setting to be managed with certain medical devices such as catheters, feeding tubes, intravenous tubes, and oxygen. These devices help clinicians to identify other variables that could influence overall medical and communication functioning.

Motor Function   Observation of posture and motor function has important diagnostic and prognostic indications. Often patients present with a new physical impairment such as complete or partial paralysis of one side of the body. The functional impact of these limitations should be observed and the compensations a patient implements should be noted.

Prosthetics   Many patients wear glasses, hearing aids, dentures, or another prosthetic device. The clinician should note if the patient wears any prosthetic devices and ensure that they are readily available to the patient. Patients might be misdiagnosed if they are tested without the aid of their glasses or hearing aid.

Insight and Awareness   Insight and awareness into one's deficits are important prognostic indicators. In the acute setting it is not uncommon for patients to have a lack of awareness about their medical condition and associated deficits. This lack of awareness may be the result of the neurologic insult as in the case of right hemisphere patients or it may be due to a global cognitive decline as seen with demented patients. Patients and family members may show a lack of awareness because the behavioral consequences of an acute illness are so new and foreign. There may also be a degree of denial that serves as a coping mechanism.

Testing and Treatment Tolerance   Another sign of change is testing or treatment tolerance. Patients who fatigue easily may not be candidates for full inpatient rehabilitation and may need a less intensive treatment program following discharge.

Distractibility   Patients with brain injuries commonly suffer from attentional impairments and are easily distracted by competing stimuli. Distractions may be internal such as worries or intrusive thoughts or may be caused by background stimuli, such as bright lights, noises, or other conversations. What is the patient's response to distractions? Can he or she stay on task? What happens when the clinician reduces the distractions by modifying the environment (i.e., turning the television down, drawing the curtain)? The influence of distractions is important to note and may signal improvement when they have less of an impact.

Testing the Limits   At times, strict adherence to standardized testing procedures may not elucidate the underlying cause of failure on a given test item. Clinicians should do what Lezak (1980) calls "testing the limits" of the patient. Testing the limits refers to the practice of going beyond the standard test procedures to exploit an individual's full capacities. For example, if a patient is unable to mentally perform arithmetic on an orally administered math test, the cause of the failure is unknown. Does the patient not understand the problem? Does the patient's level of attention and concentration interfere? Is the patient unable to hold the numbers in short-term memory long enough to perform the calculation? If the reason for failure is unclear, the examiner can extend the test by giving the patient a pencil and paper and repeating the failed test items; if the patient completes the calculations, then attention, concentration, or short-term memory problems may be at the root of the deficit. Testing the limits is done after standard test procedures have been completed, and may yield additional insight about the underlying cause of the deficit.

Response to Cues   Toglia (1991) emphasized the importance of investigating a patient's response to cues during an assessment. What effect do cues and the type of cues have on a patient's performance? It is often beneficial to start with the cue of least strength and progress to stronger cues. Toglia describes three levels: (1) error detection and awareness, (2) focusing attention, and (3) strategy use. At the lowest level, feedback cues are given, such as, "How do you think you did?" The examiner is interested in determining the patient's awareness of errors, and whether or not this question may prompt the recognition of an error. At the next level, attention is focused on the error. For example, for a right-hemisphere stroke patient with neglect, this level of cue would be, "Did you find all the information on the left?" Finally, at the highest level of cuing, a strategy is provided and the response observed. Patients who are aware of their errors and more responsive to cues typically show greater rehabilitation potential.

Patient and Family Strategy Use   Often the patient and family members develop compensatory communication strategies without any direct intervention. It is important to observe these strategies and develop related strategies. In addition, note maladaptive strategies or behaviors that impede communication and modify them. For example, talking louder may not necessarily aid comprehension, but shortening instructions will.

Practice   Neurocommunication monitoring also allows for observations of changed performance with practice. Does the patient recognize items that were difficult on the previous day's testing? Are previously demonstrated strategies spontaneously used by the patient to maximize performance?

Modalities   Which modalities does the patient respond to most/least accurately? Does the patient exhibit greater comprehension in the written or auditory modality? Does the patient write the names of common objects better than he says the names?

Through observation and interaction with the patient, an experienced clinician can often make a tentative diagnosis of the communication disorder before administering a formal test. Behavioral observations are invaluable as they can be used to demonstrate evolution of communication abilities as well. These observations may capture change in communication more effectively than test data. Objective results from test data combined with behavioral descriptions provide great insight into a patient's speech–language diagnosis, communication strengths and weaknesses, rehabilitation potential, counseling and education needs, and expected level of recovery.

Utilizing Results to Influence Patient Care   As mentioned previously, the information gained through neurocommunication monitoring is used to influence management of the patient acutely and following discharge. The SLP can have a primary impact in several specific ways.

Documenting Improvement or Decline of Function   Neurocommunication monitoring data provide an objective measure for demonstrating the evolution of speech, language, cognition, and communication. Data are reported comparatively across sessions both quantitatively and through precise behavioral description.

Determining Functional Communication Abilities   The SLP interprets test performance and behavioral observations in functional terms. This is very important as typical test scores alone do not reflect the impact of the impairment on communication function.

Establishing Short-Term Goals   The results from neurocommunication monitoring are used in setting goals. These might include (1) more in depth assessment, (2) patient/family education, (3) provision of communication strategies, (4) establishment of an augmentative communication system, and (5) reduction of communication frustration through communication repair strategies.

Determining Prognosis   Tracking the rate and pattern of communication change in the acute phase allows for more accurate judgments of prognosis. If there is no other neurologic event, most patients go through some degree of spontaneous recovery. Several studies have examined prognosis in aphasic patients (Basso, 1992; Pedersen, Jorgenssen, Nakayama, et al., 1995). Initial severity level, persistence of deficits, and a host of medical factors are predictive of outcome, and SLPs should be familiar with this information in all its complexity. In general, the more severe the initial aphasia, the poorer the outcome. Lengthier hospital stays and hemiplegia at discharge have also been shown to be predictive of poorer recovery of language function in persons with aphasia, as well as those with right-hemisphere communication deficits poststroke (Kertesz & McCabe, 1977). Finally, for patients with head injury, a different set of predictors has been suggested (Teasdale & Jennett, 1974).

Communicating and Charting Significant Changes   As mentioned earlier, communication is of key importance in the acute setting. Findings from test performance and behavioral observation are documented in the chart and discussed directly with physicians, nurses, and other care providers. Chart notes should include the findings from repeated assessment and the change noted since the previous visit. Any education and counseling activities involving the patient and family should be charted as well. Notes should be clear and concise and convey significant findings. Progress notes can be written either narratively or following a SOAP (Subjective, Objective, Assessment, Plan) format. In this format, specific topics are consistently addressed under each of the major categories. Subjective information includes how patients report how they feel and any complaints, and a description of their mood mental status. Objective information includes data from communication assessment tools, specific behavioral observations, and the results of any behavioral or environmental interventions. Assessment includes evaluation (interpretation) of the data and any significant conclusions that can be drawn and where feasible, an estimate of the prognosis based on data and observations. Plan includes identification of needed follow-up including referrals, strategies that might enhance communication in the hospital environment, short-term goals or interventions that might be helpful, and discharge plans.

✦ Education in the Acute Care Setting

In this chapter a case has been made for emphasizing education in the context of acute care service delivery. To some readers this may come as a surprise, because educational activities are rarely discussed as part of service delivery discussions. However, there are several compelling reasons for including specific educational activities as part of an integrated clinical program. Educational activities in acute care can be considered in three broad categories: (1) patient and family education, (2) interdisciplinary education about communication and swallowing disorders, and (3) clinical education and competency development for SLPs at various professional levels.

Patient and Family Education Programming

Patient and family education is essential in the acute care setting and serves several important functions: providing basic information about the patient's communication or swallowing disorder, assisting the patient/family in developing an understanding of the expected course of treatment, serving as a focus for discussion of patient questions or concerns, and assisting with identification of information gaps.

Provides Basic Information

As soon as the SLP has a relatively clear picture of the problem, he or she should begin to provide an explanation for the patient, including a basic description of the speech and language diagnosis and a label for the problem. At first, it is best to provide basic and limited information, based on the patient's current and premorbid abilities. A brief, clear, direct explanation of clinical characteristics followed by an opportunity for patient/family questions will go far to allay concern and build trust.

Following this first conversation, the nature of the educational activity becomes more specific. Fortunately, there is a wide variety of resources to assist with educational goals. Some patients can benefit from pamphlets or booklets or other commercially developed written or video materials. In general, patients with communication disorders need some direction and guidance to benefit from such resources.

Assist the Patient/Family to Develop an Understanding of the Course of Treatment

Patients should not leave the hospital without having learned about their problem, including the necessary follow-up, the expected outcomes, community resources for assistance, and contact information for an SLP for follow-up. To the degree possible, patients should be given written instructions, which should be supplemented with clear verbal explanation and opportunity for questions and conversation.

Serve as a Focus for Discussion of Patient Questions or Concerns

Interruption in the independent use of swallowing, communicating, speaking, understanding, or reading and writing is tragic, representing a serious loss for most patients. The SLP in the acute setting, regularly confronted with these ideas, must resist the inclination to become desensitized to their profound impact. The clinician needs to listen to the concerns, expectation, fears, and confusion of the patient and family. The SLP can then respond to these specific concerns, gauging the response to the linguistic or cognitive abilities of the patient. Drawings or visual aids can be useful to help assist with comprehension. If the patient is showing signs of depression or very difficult adjustment to the problem, then appropriate referrals should be implemented.

Assist with Identification of "Information Gaps"

A final component of patient education addresses the area of information gaps that may be obstacles to progress in treatment. These gaps in knowledge about communication, swallowing, or health service delivery are common. For example, a common confusion exhibited by families (and some health professionals) relates to misunderstanding of the significance of not being able to speak. Those communicating with the patient may not appreciate the level of preserved comprehension and will speak to the patient in a childish or demeaning way. The solution for such a problem is a brief but clear explanation to the family member, perhaps followed by a demonstration of the patient's comprehension level. Some other common information gaps are listed in **Table 19–8**.

Preprofessional Education

The acute care environment affords a significant learning environment for students in graduate education program in speech–language pathology. Students are usually able to see

Table 19–8 Common "Information Gaps" for Patients, Families, and Staff in the Acute Care Environment

Information gap: Overestimation of patient's ability
Common statement: "I know he understands what I'm saying."
Results: Information overload to patient, frustration from family when patient does not respond
Solution: *Highlight strengths and weaknesses;* teach family to focus on strengths with patient; focus on compensatory strategies to assist with comprehension; teach strategies in context of every contact with the family
Information gap: Lack of differentiation between language and cognitive disturbances
Common statement: "He seems so confused when he's talking."
Results in: Misinterpretation of patient's behavior, frustration
Solutions: Clarify differences for family; provide opportunities for family to see patient's strengths and weaknesses, highlighting areas of strength; involve family in daily sessions
Information gap: Poor understanding of the cause of a comprehension deficit
Common statement: "You need to talk louder so he can HEAR you."
Results: Patient annoyance or misinterpretation of loud speech as angry speech
Solutions: Patient/family education concerning specific strengths and weaknesses; provide family with observation tools to observe progress with patient; model appropriate communication style; provide basic reading material for family
Information gap: Failure to understand NPO status of patient
Common statement: "They keep refusing to feed my husband. He's going to starve."
Results in: Anger and frustration
Solution: Explain risks related to oral feeding; explain the alternative method of feeding that is being used; include family/patient in discussions of results of ongoing swallowing monitoring and evaluation

patients in conjunction with an experienced SLP. Because of the nature of the inpatient environment in most hospitals, students can be afforded a variety of educational opportunities and challenges. The most unique learning opportunities are related education about the specific nature of diseases and their effects on human communication and swallowing and the opportunity to learn from other disciplines. In most cases, competence for independent functioning as an SLP cannot be obtained during a graduate internship lasting only a few months. It is reasonable, however, to expect students to advance their knowledge about their discipline, to become skilled at bedside communication and swallowing examination, and to develop basic skills in documentation, communication, and intervention in the acute care setting.

Because most programs are not equipped to provide clinical opportunities that prepare a student for entry into acute care, it is important for practicum sites to commit to a broad-based educational approach. Ideally, this approach should include such activities as observation of a variety of clinical activities, interaction with physicians and nurses, experience in basic assessment, participation in specialty clinics, participation in grand rounds, attendance at staff meetings, or presentation of cases to more experienced clinical staff.

Clinical Fellowship

The Certificate of Clinical Competence in Speech–Language Pathology, as well as most licensing boards, require the completion of a clinical fellowship. This 9- to 12-month experience can provide a capstone to the clinical preparation of SLPs that was initiated in their graduate education.

Johnson (1993) described a medical SLP fellowship program that was used at Henry Ford Hospital in Detroit, Michigan, over a 10-year period. This program included rotations in neuroscience, otolaryngology, critical care, psychiatry, and pediatrics as well as participation in several multidisciplinary clinics. Achievement of specific competencies in several areas was also achieved and served as the "outcomes" for demonstrating successful completion of the fellowship program. The areas in which competency was demonstrated included inpatient consultation, dysphagia, speech production laboratory, tracheostomy/ventilator communication and swallowing, and adult neurogenic disorders. This model places serious time and skill demands on the SLPs involved in supervision and clinical teaching. Despite this limitation, the investment ensures the development of a qualified supply of individuals for practice in medical settings. Although time constraints are often offered as a rationale for denying access to positions to entry level SLPs, there is no other obvious approach to ensuring the development of quality providers.

✦ Conclusion

This chapter discussed the science and the art involved in delivering speech–language and swallowing services to patients in the acute care environment. It discussed the role of the clinician in providing effective consultation through skilled diagnoses, effective educational programming, and intensive patient monitoring.

Study Questions

1. Discuss the differences between consultative and rehabilitative SLP practice.

2. What tools and tests are most useful for the SLP in acute care settings?

3. What are the techniques that are most useful for patient instruction and education?

4. How could you apply "intensive communication and swallowing monitoring" in your setting?

5. Consider the cases example at the end of this chapter and answer the following questions.

A. Who was the referral source and what was the referral question?

B. How did the findings presented address the referral question?

C. What would be the expected outcomes if the recommendations were followed? What if they were not followed?

6. Evaluate your own information needs regarding practice in the acute setting. What steps will you need to take to improve your own effectiveness?

References

Albert, M. (1988). Acute Confusional States. In: M. Albert, & M.B. Moss (Eds.), *Geriatric Neuropsychology.* New York: Guilford Press

American Speech–Language-Hearing Association. (1983). *Functional Communication Measures.* Rockville, MD: ASHA

Basso, A. (1992). Prognostic Factors in Aphasia. *Aphasiology, 6,* 337–348

Benton, A.L., Hamsher, K., & Sivan AB. (1994). *Multilingual Aphasia Examination.* Iowa City, IA: AJA Associates

Burns, M., Halper, A.S., & Mogil, S.I. (1985). *Clinical Management of Right Hemisphere Dysfunction.* Rockville, MD: Aspen

Enderby, P.M., Wood, V.A., & Wade, D.T. (1983). The Frenchay Aphasia Screening Test: A Short Simple Test for Aphasia Appropriate for Non Specialists. *International Journal of Rehabilitation Medicine,* 166–170

Fitch-West, J., & Sands, E. (1987). *Bedside Evaluation and Screening Test of Aphasia.* Rockville, MD: Aspen

Folstein, M.F., Folstein, S.E., & McHugh, P.R. (1975). Mini Mental State: A Practical Method for Grading the Cognitive State of Patients for the Clinician. *Journal of Psychiatric Research, 12,* 189–198

Frattali, C.M., Thompson, C.K., Holland, A.L., Wohl, C.B., & Ferketic, M.M. (1995). *ASHA Functional Assessment of Communication for Adults.* Rockville, MD: ASHA

Freedman, M.L., Leach, L., Kaplan, E., et al. (1994). *Clock Drawing: A Neuropsychological Analysis.* New York: Oxford University Press

Golper, L. (1992). *Sourcebook for Medical Speech–Language Pathology.* San Diego: Singular

Goodglass, H., & Kaplan, E. (1983). *The Assessment of Aphasia and Related Disorders.* Philadelphia: Lea & Febiger

Hagen, C., & Malkmus, D. (1979). *Intervention Strategies for Language Disorders Secondary to Head Trauma.* American Speech–Language-Hearing Association annual meeting, Atlanta, GA

Helm-Estabrooks, N. (1992). *Aphasia Diagnostic Profiles.* Chicago: Riverside

Helm-Estabrooks, N., & Hotz, G. (1991). *Brief Test of Head Injury.* Chicago: Riverside

Helm-Estabrooks, N., Ramsberger, G., Moran, A., & Nicholas, M. (1989). *Boston Assessment of Severe Aphasia.* Chicago: Riverside

Horwitz, R.I., Henes, C.G., & Horwitz, S.M. (1983). Developing Strategies for Improving the Diagnostic and Management Efficacy of Medical Consultations. *Journal of Chronic Disease, 36,* 213–218

Jacobson, B.H., & Silbergleit, A.K. (1994). *Improvement of Functional Cough.* Philadelphia: The Voice Foundation

Johnson, A. (1993). *Two Year Fellowship in Medical Speech–Language Pathology.* American Speech–Language-Hearing Association annual meeting, Anaheim, CA

Johnson, A.F., George, K.P., & Valachovic, A.M. (1996). *Acute Aphasia: Predicting Outcome One and Three Months Post Stroke.* American Speech–Language-Hearing Association annual meeting, Seattle

Kaplan, E., Goodglass, H., & Weintraub, S. (1983). *Boston Naming Test.* Philadelphia: Lea & Febiger

Kertesz, A., & McCabe, P. (1977). Recovery Patterns and Prognosis in Aphasia. *Brain, 100,* 1–18

Lee, T., Pappius, E., & Goldman, L. (1983). Impact of Interphysician Communication on the Effectiveness of Medical Consultations. *American Journal of Medicine, 74,* 106–112

Levin, H.S., O'Donnell, V.M., & Grossman, R.G. (1979). The Galveston Orientation and Amnesia Test. *Journal of Nervous and Mental Disease, 167,* 675–684

Lezak, M. (1980). *Neuropsychological Assessment.* New York: Oxford University Press

Miller, R.M., & Groher, M.E. (1990). *Medical Speech–Language Pathology.* Rockville, MD: Aspen

Pedersen, P.M., Jorgenssen, H.S., Nakayama, H., et al. (1995). Aphasia in Acute Stroke: Incidence, Determinants, and Recovery. *Annals of Neurology, 38,* 659–666

Pimental, P., & Kingsbury, N. (1989). *Mini-Inventory of Right Brain Injury.* Austin, TX: Pro-Ed

Ross, D. (1986). *Ross Information Processing Assessment.* Austin, TX: Pro-Ed

Teasdale, G., & Jennett, B. (1974). Assessment of Coma and Impaired Consciousness: A Practical Scale. *Lancet, 2,* 81–84

Toglia, J. (1991). Generalization to Treatment: A Multicontext Approach to Cognitive Perceptual Impairment in Adults with Brain Injury. *American Journal of Occupational Therapy, 45,* 505–516

Vogel, D., & Carter, J.E. (1995, 1999). *The Effects of Drugs on Communication.* San Diego: Singular

Appendix 19–1   Inpatient Consultation Competency Checklist

Preparation for the consultation

__Medical chart review

__Working knowledge of pertinent medical information and case history information

__Identification of referral question

Appendix 19–1   *(Continued)*

Plan for the examination

___List of differential diagnoses in rank order from most to least likely

___Selection formal and informal measures

___Organization/sequence of test administration

Examination/diagnostic testing

___Administration of tests and informal assessments

___Appropriate modification in initial plan throughout examination

___Sufficient data to answer the question

Documentation: Generation of written consultation report

___Organization of report with subheadings representing the main areas tested

___Accurate diagnostic statement, including severity levels

___Suspected etiology of diagnostic impressions

___Classification of aphasia or dysarthria types

___Suspected lesion localization of the neurologic communication disorder

___Recommendations appropriate to findings/impressions

___Recommendations for referral to other professionals

___Clear answer to the referral questions

Follow-up/management issues

___Contact referring physician to report impressions/recommendations

___Arrange diagnostic/therapeutic examinations as indicated

___Repeated testing to monitor changes in communication disorders over time

___Ongoing patient/family counseling

___Treatment of communication disorders

___Discharge planning

Appendix 19–2   Example of a Consultation Report

Referring Service: Neurosurgery

Location: Intensive Care Unit

Reason for Consultation: 36-year-old man status post–multiple gunshot wounds to the head with left frontoparietal hemorrhage and right frontal contusion. Please evaluate.

SLP Remarks:

Significant History: Pt. was admitted on Jan. 17 with multiple gunshot wounds to the head. He is now status post–left frontotemporal craniotomy for evacuation of hematoma. He was intubated secondary to respiratory failure and was extubated on Jan. 31.

Clinical Examination: Pt. lying in bed, fully alert, oriented to person only based on yes/no responses with head nod. Shows good eye contact with examiner.

Comprehension: Patient follows axial command only, unable to follow commands involving extremities. Executed commands with left upper extremity to imitation only. Reliable yes/no response with head nod to simple questions, unreliable for complex questions. Patient often gestured with left upper extremity to indicate that he did not understand question/commands.

Expression: Patient is mute; no verbal output and no vocalizations, and no phonation. Patient attempted to vocalize to command and to imitation but was unable to phonate.

Oral Examination: Right facial weakness, tongue deviated to right on protrusion. Decreased left palatal elevation and absent gag response.

Speech Production: No speech production, no phonation

Swallowing: Excess secretions in oropharynx; patient unable to manage oral secretions. Spontaneous coughing on secretion ×2. Assessment of swallowing with food was deferred to reduce risk of aspiration.

IMPRESSION:

1. Global aphasia with mutism

2. Severe oropharyngeal dysphagia

3. Oral verbal apraxia (severe)

4. Probable dysarthria

(Continued)

Appendix 19–2   *(Continued)*

Recommendations:

1. NPO: Continue tube feedings

2. Follow for ongoing assessment and treatment of communication and swallowing

3. Recommend inpatient rehabilitation after discharge

Speech–language pathology follow up activities during subsequent patient contacts:

1. Patient/family education and provision of communication strategies

2. Implementation of methods to increase vocalization and verbal output and to maximize auditory comprehension

3. Trials with augmentative communication systems

4. Ongoing monitoring of neurocommunication status with reclassification of aphasia from global aphasia to Broca's aphasia

5. Diagnostic classification of dysarthria (spastic) established after pt. began to verbalize

6. Modified barium swallow study completed 1 week post–initial assessment

Section 5

Medical Perspectives

20

Issues in Geriatric Medicine

Thomas R. Palmer and Murray B. Hunter

◆ **Issues in Treating the Elderly**
◆ **Nutritional Needs of the Elderly**
◆ **Nonoral Feeding**
◆ **Pneumonia in the Elderly**
◆ **Delirium and Dementias**
◆ **Ethical Issues in Geriatric Practice**
◆ **Case Vignettes**

Elderly adults are the most rapidly growing age group among Americans. As of the 2000 United States Census, 12.4% of the population was older than 64, whereas 1.5% was 85 or older (U.S. Census Bureau, 2000). By 2050, 20.4% of the population is projected to be older than 64, with 4.8% age 85 or older (U.S. Census Bureau, 2000) (**Fig. 20–1**). Thus, the "old old" group, 85 and older, is the most rapidly growing segment of senior adults. This is the group with the most functional and cognitive impairments. The need for professionals to help them will continue to increase.

Geriatrics is the area of medicine that deals with the elderly. Elderly people cannot be treated as if they were young adults who happen to be chronologically older. Because of physiologic differences, a higher frequency of functional and cognitive impairments, a lack of physiologic reserve, a higher frequency of multiple chronic illnesses, a greater number of sensory impairments, and an increased chance of being on multiple potentially interacting medications, the elderly must be approached in a specific age-appropriate manner. Although these factors make adverse consequences of ill-advised treatments more likely, they also increase the beneficial impact of a well-chosen intervention. For functionally impaired bedridden older adults, for example, the simple act of becoming able to transfer from their bed to a wheelchair makes a tremendous difference in their enjoyment of life.

This chapter discusses issues that are specific to the management of illness in elderly persons, especially during hospitalization. These include nutritional status, nonoral feeding, pneumonia, dementia and delirium, and ethical considerations. Although this is not meant to be an exhaustive coverage of geriatric medicine, we have highlighted the most frequently occurring conditions and concerns for this group of patients.

◆ Issues in Treating the Elderly

The frail elderly are the group most in need of an age-specific, multidisciplinary approach. The frail elderly can be defined as those with a diminished ability to carry out the important practical and social activities of daily living (Brown, Renwick, & Raphael, 1995). Many factors can contribute to frailty (Winograd, Gerety, Chung, et al., 1991), and the more factors present, the more dependent a person is likely to be (**Table 20–1**). Certain problems are more common in the elderly. These include polypharmacy, dementia and delirium, fecal and urinary incontinence, arthritis, visual and hearing deficits, pressure ulcers, malnutrition, osteoporosis, and falls. Because the multiple, complex issues involved in their care are more than an individual professional can deal with alone, these patients benefit from a multidisciplinary team approach to their care.

Functional Status

The most important objective in the care of the elderly is to maximize functional status. For example, there is no value in giving older patients a medication to help normalize an abnormal laboratory value if in the process they become stiff and unable to walk to the bathroom or if a mild degree of confusion becomes more severe as a result. Assessing functional status is more important than documenting physical findings such as arthritis of the knees or a heart murmur. Functional status is the end result of multiple interacting factors including illnesses, cognitive problems, medications, nutrition, and social interaction that combine to affect the person's overall wellness.

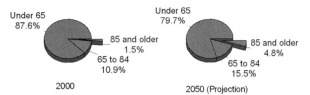

Figure 20–1 Percent distribution of elderly in the United States. (From U.S. Census Bureau: Census 2000 and Population Projections Program.)

Functional status is commonly defined by a person's ability to perform the activities of daily living (ADLs) and the instrumental activities of daily living (IADLs). In the commonly used Katz scale of ADLs, transfers (such as from bed to a wheelchair), dressing, bathing, toileting, continence, and feeding are all evaluated to see whether individuals can do the activity independently, need help, or are totally dependent (Katz, Ford, & Moskowitz, et al., 1963). To be able to safely live alone without help, a person must be independent in ADLs. Likewise, an improvement in the ability to perform ADLs adds to independence and quality of life. The IADLs are using the telephone, traveling, shopping, preparing meals, doing housework, taking medication, and handling money (Lawton & Brody, 1969). Assessment of ADLs is also useful in determining how much help a person might need and in monitoring decline or improvement in function over time.

Polypharmacy

Polypharmacy refers to the tendency of many older people to be on numerous medications. Every medication has potential side effects. For example, nonsteroidal antiinflammatory drugs such as ibuprofen can cause gastric ulceration (sometimes with bleeding), kidney impairment, edema, liver enzyme elevation, drowsiness, and dizziness, among other side effects. Medications can also have potential side effects as a result of interactions with other drugs. Ibuprofen can decrease the effect of the diuretic furosemide owing to a specific drug interaction. When

Table 20–1   Criteria for Frailty

Cerebrovascular accident
Chronic and disabling illness
Confusion
Dependence in ADLs
Depression
Falls
Impaired mobility
Incontinence
Malnutrition
Polypharmacy
Pressure sore
Prolonged bedrest
Restraints
Sensory impairment
Socioeconomic/family problems

From Winograd, C.H., Gerety, M.B., Chung, M., et al. (1991). Screening for Frailty: Criteria and Predictors of Outcomes. *Journal of the American Geriatrics Society, 39*, 778–784.

ibuprofen is taken with the anticoagulant warfarin, the chances of gastrointestinal bleeding are greatly increased over what might be expected from each drug independently. Thus, each additional medication that a person takes can cause side effects not only by itself but also from drug–drug interactions. The more medications a person is taking, the greater the risk of having a single adverse drug reaction. The risk of adverse drug interactions increases exponentially as the number of medications increases (Colley & Lucas, 1993).

Another complication of polypharmacy is the increased risk of noncompliance with taking prescribed medications. Medication costs may consume a larger proportion of a senior's income, which may be limited. Older persons faced with taking a handful of pills several times a day may more easily decide that they need not take them.

For these reasons, medications should only be given to older people if they are clearly needed and clearly benefiting the recipient. Over-the-counter medications must also be considered when reviewing an elderly person's medications. A helpful strategy is to ask the patient or family to place all the medications being used in a bag and to bring them to appointments or to the hospital. Often, a medication will emerge that was not previously mentioned. Removing unneeded medications can result in an improvement in daily functioning or in cognition.

✦ Nutritional Needs of the Elderly

Dietary Requirements

In general, the nutritional needs of healthy elderly people do not differ much from those of younger healthy adults. The major physiologic changes that occur with aging are a decrease in total body protein, an increase in the proportion of total body fat with a redistribution of fat stores, a reduction in total body water, and a decrease in bone density (Chernoff, 1995). Despite the decreased body protein, dietary protein requirements are greater in the elderly than in younger adults (Kerstetter, Holthausen, & Fitz, 1993). Total energy expenditure is slightly reduced in older women compared with younger women but approximately 20% less in older men compared with younger men. The elderly also have a lower resting metabolic rate (Morely, 1993), which results in less caloric intake being required in the elderly on average. An average calorie requirement for a bed-bound senior to maintain weight is 25 kcal per kilogram of body weight. If malnourished, a goal for nutrient intake is 35 kcal per kilogram (Lipschitz, 1995). At least 10% of the calories in the elderly should consist of fat to ensure adequate fat-soluble vitamins and essential fatty acids. Usually, this is not a problem because the average American diet consists of 40% fat (Chernoff, 1995). Carbohydrates should be of the complex variety, which are less easily digested and add bulk to the stool, and constitute 55 to 60% of calories (Chernoff, 1995). Fiber is most easily added in the form of fresh fruits and vegetables, but may also be given as bran supplements, cereals, or psyllium.

Hydration

Drinking fluids is a natural part of life and young adults have no difficulty responding to their thirst sensation by drinking more fluids. The elderly, however, have more problems with dehydration owing to various physiologic as well as situational causes. Thirst sensation is not as reliable as in younger people and the kidneys do not concentrate urine as well. Often because of problems with incontinence or edema, the elderly purposely may not drink as much as they should. Conditions such as dementia or immobility may prevent adequate fluid intake. Diuretic medicines may contribute to the problem. Hot weather, exercise, or febrile illness may more easily combine with all the above conditions to cause dehydration. Dehydration can often be prevented by educating the elderly person and encouraging fluid intake.

Vitamins

Vitamin deficiency is a cause of concern in the elderly, especially of vitamins B_{12}, C, D, and folate. Vitamin B_{12} deficiency can occur from dietary deficiency, medication interactions, atrophic gastritis, or pernicious anemia, and can result in anemia, peripheral neuropathy, unsteadiness in walking, and dementia. It is one of the reversible causes of dementia and a part of the laboratory screen for evaluating dementia. Replacement can be given with an intramuscular injection, if poor absorption is the cause, or orally. Vitamin C is a water-soluble vitamin often found to be deficient in the elderly. Deficiency can cause capillary fragility and poor wound healing. Vitamin D is most important in calcium metabolism, and exposure of the skin to sunlight helps convert it to its active form. Deficiency is most common in immobile elderly people in nursing homes or at home with little exposure to sunlight. Replacement is important to optimize calcium absorption, and the typical multivitamin contains 400 IU of Vitamin D, which is enough to ensure adequate amounts. Folate deficiency also can cause anemia. Absorption of folic acid is decreased by ulcer medicines that lower gastric acidity such as antacids (Silver, 1991).

Malnutrition

Malnutrition is more common in the elderly, especially the frail elderly. It should be suspected in any thin or frail-appearing senior. In its more severe form, it may present as the cachexia seen in end-stage cancer, heart disease, and other illnesses. In cachexia there is severe muscle wasting and atrophy, with prominent bones and a concave abdomen. The goal, however, is to identify malnutrition at an early stage, when intervention may be of most benefit.

Risk Factors

There are many risk factors for malnutrition (**Table 20–2**). Alcoholism occurs in the elderly, and appropriate screening questions should be asked in any malnourished person. Persons with even a mild dementia may forget whether they have eaten and may not prepare an adequate meal. Those with more advanced dementias are usually thin and often have aphasia, agnosia (the failure to recognize sensory stimuli), and apraxia (difficulty with automatic movements), all of which have a major effect on eating (Cohen, 1994). A lack of appetite is one of the symptoms used in the diagnosis of major depression, and as the depression improves, the appetite typically improves. Other mental illness (such as psychosis) commonly affects one's ability to function, thus impairing the ability to prepare or eat food.

Table 20–2 Malnutrition Risk Factors

Alcoholism
Dementia
Depression
Psychosis
Illness causing decreased appetite
Impaired taste, smell, or vision
Limited finances
Living alone and social isolation
Polypharmacy
Poor dentition or edentulous
Poor functional status
Poor nutritional knowledge

From Rauscher, C. (1993). Malnutrition Among the Elderly. *Canadian Family Physician, 39*, 1395–1403.

Many medical illnesses, both acute and chronic, affect the appetite adversely. In addition, some conditions cause increased nutritional needs, such as wound healing and hyperthyroidism. Impaired sensory input is common in the elderly, and impaired taste, smell, or vision can make it more of a chore to eat than an enjoyment. When teeth are in poor condition or absent and dentures are ill fitting, it may be easier to eat less than to find foods of a texture and nutritional value that can be chewed and ingested well.

As functional status decreases, the risk of malnutrition increases. An inability to shop or prepare meals (IADLs) may result in less food with less variety on the table at mealtime. Difficulty transferring to the table and feeding (ADLs) will also impair nutrition.

Medications can either independently or via drug–drug interactions adversely affect appetite. Many medications, including some common antidepressants such as amitriptyline, have anticholinergic side effects that result in dryness of the mouth. Antiinflammatory medications for arthritis might cause anorexia from irritation of the stomach or small intestine. Most antibiotics can cause gastric upset. This risk is another reason for older persons to be taking only essential medications.

Knowledge of good nutrition is important for all older people, including the importance of eating foods from the basic food groups. This knowledge may be less available to those from minority groups, especially if they need to follow a special diet for a medical condition incorporating their preferred ethnic foods (Dwyer, 1994). Special diets (renal, low salt, low fat, or diabetic) are often tasteless. The need for a certain diet for a medical condition must be balanced against the need for adequate nutrition, especially in the frail elderly. Poor elderly may not have enough money remaining after other expenses to afford an adequate diet. The less human contact a person has, the easier it is for harmful nutritional patterns to continue. Social isolation and living alone are risk factors for malnutrition. Elderly persons may have several risk factors for malnutrition at the same time, and the more factors present, the greater the risk.

Measurement of Nutritional Status

Malnutrition can be suspected by clinical appearance, as mentioned earlier. Certain measurements give more objec-

Table 20–3 Important Indicators of Malnutrition

Body mass index (BMI) = Wt (kg)/(Ht (m))^2

    <22 = probable malnourished

    22 to 27 = desirable

    >27 = obese

Serum albumin

    Normal 4.0 to 6.5, <3.5 suggestive of protein calorie malnutrition

Total lymphocyte count

    Total white cell count 3% lymphocytes in differential

    <1500 is significant

Significant weight loss over time

    >5.0% of body weight in 1 month

    >7.5% of body weight in 3 months

    >10.0% of body weight in 6 months

    >10 pounds of involuntary weight loss in 6 months

From Barrocas, A., Belcher, D., Champagne, C., & Jastram, C. (1995). Nutrition Assessment: Practical Approaches. *Clinics in Geriatric Medicine, 11*, 675–713.

tivity to the evaluation and can be followed serially in an individual to show improvement or deterioration over time. Body weight is the most basic measurement. A significant weight loss over time is an important indicator of malnutrition (**Table 20–3**). Malnutrition can also be suspected in anyone over 65 with a body mass index (BMI) less than 22. BMI is defined as the weight in kilograms divided by the height in meters squared. A desirable BMI is 22 to 27; a BMI over 27 suggests obesity (Dwyer, 1994). Triceps skinfold (TSF) measurement is a measure of subcutaneous fat using calipers, but is less reliable in older people because of physical changes with aging such as a redistribution of fat. Mid-arm muscle circumference can be calculated using standardized tables from the mid-arm circumference measurement. A mid-arm muscle circumference falling below the 10th percentile indicates poor nutritional status (Barrocas, Belcher, Champagne, & Jastram, 1995).

Albumin is a simple protein found in blood that is a good indicator of nutritional status. Like all indicators of malnutrition, it is not perfect and has some limitations. Because of its relatively long half-life it is a reasonable measure of nutritional status during the previous month or so, but not over the previous few days. Conditions such as dehydration may cause it to appear to be higher than it really is. Normal levels are 4.0 to 6.0 g/dL, and levels less than 3.5 g/dL are suggestive of protein calorie malnutrition. Serum albumin levels less than 2.5 g/dL have been shown to be helpful prognostic indicators for a limited life expectancy (Stuart et al., 1996).

Serum albumin levels are also important in certain drug actions. For example, the anticonvulsant phenytoin is a seizure medication that partly binds to albumin in the blood. However, the active portion of phenytoin is the unbound portion. When elderly malnourished patients are given phenytoin, they need a smaller dose because of the lower amount of albumin available to bind the drug, leaving a larger unbound active portion.

Other useful laboratory measures suggesting malnutrition include the total lymphocyte count and hemoglobin. Lymphocytes are a type of white blood cell. Total lymphocyte counts less than 1500 can be caused by malnutrition. Hemoglobin

measures the red blood cell concentration. It normally ranges from 12.0 to 16.0 g/dL in women and from 14.0 to 18.0 g/dL in men. In malnutrition, the body is not able to make enough red blood cells, and a mild anemia with normal sized red blood cells is common. Specific nutritional deficiencies of B_{12} and folate also may cause anemias, but the red cells are usually larger than normal in these cases.

Treatment of Malnutrition

Once a senior is found to be malnourished, or at nutritional risk, solutions vary as much as causes. A simple generic multivitamin taken daily is an inexpensive way to help specific deficiencies such as lack of vitamin D. Finding ways to help increase food intake with a diet that is tasty but also nutritious is important. Community programs such as Meals on Wheels and congregate nutrition programs are nutritionally helpful; they also provide regular social contact to elders who might otherwise be more isolated. Commercial nutrition supplements can be used for those unable to eat a regular diet, and feeding tubes can be considered for those unable to take adequate food and liquids orally.

✦ Nonoral Feeding

William Beaumont, a physician assigned to Mackinac Island, Michigan, in 1822, treated a French trapper who had suffered a shotgun wound to his abdomen. It healed, leaving a direct opening to his stomach. Beaumont did experiments putting various substances, such as meat, into the stomach and observing what happened (Bald, 1954). In a similar way percutaneous endoscopic gastrostomy (PEG) tubes deliver nutrition through a hole in the abdominal wall into the stomach. Their placement has become so technically easy that the current protocol might be described as "the patient can't swallow safely or is malnourished; therefore, place a feeding tube." This attitude among health professionals should be discarded and replaced. A more appropriate process should include a thorough discussion of both the risks and benefits of feeding tubes with patients or their decision makers, so they can make an informed decision.

Nutrition not taken by mouth can be divided into two main groups: parenteral and enteral. Parenteral nutrition is given intravenously into either a peripheral vein, or more commonly into a large central vein such as the jugular or subclavian. A central vein allows hypertonic (more concentrated) solutions to be infused. It bypasses the gastrointestinal system. Enteral nutrition refers to nutrition given directly into the gastrointestinal system, allowing more natural absorption of nutrients to occur. It can be given through nasogastric (NG) tubes manually placed, PEG, or percutaneous endoscopic jejunostomy (PEJ) tubes placed endoscopically, and gastrostomy or jejunostomy tubes placed surgically or percutaneously with radiologic guidance (**Fig. 20–2**).

Parenteral Nutrition

Parenteral nutrition is indicated in elderly patients needing nutritional supplementation with contraindications to enteral nutrition. The only absolute contraindication to enteral nutrition is mechanical obstruction of the small or large intestine. Relative contraindications include massive small bowel resection and acute pancreatitis (Rolandelli & Ullrich, 1994). Par-

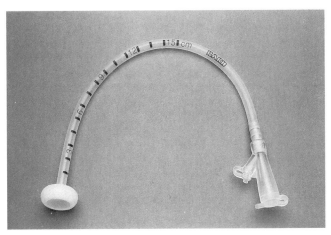

Figure 20–2 Percutaneous endoscopic gastrostomy (PEG) tube. The opening on the left is inserted inside the stomach. The opening on the right is outside the abdomen. (Courtesy of Bard International Products, Billerica, MA.)

Table 20–4 Common Potential Problems with Gastrostomy Tubes

Large residual volume
Wound infection
Aspiration
Bleeding
Diarrhea
Tube obstruction
Tube leakage
Accidental tube removal
Peritube leakage
Hyponatremia or hypernatremia
Restraint use to prevent removal:
　Resulting in immobility
　Leading to pressure sores
　Causing agitation

From O'Keefe, K.P. (1994). Complication of Percutaneous Feeding Tubes. *Emergency Medical Clinics of North America, 12,* 815–826.

enteral nutrition is often used after attempts at enteral nutrition have failed or had complications, or after major abdominal surgery. Ideally, it is employed for a short time and discontinued once enteral nutrition can be resumed. Complications include pneumothorax or bleeding during placement of the central line, infection, and venous thrombosis. Confused elderly patients may require restraints or sedation to keep them from pulling out the intravenous line.

Enteral Nutrition

Nasogastric Tubes

Nasogastric tubes are commonly used in hospital and nursing home settings. The standard rigid polyvinyl tube is uncomfortable and can be irritating to the nasal, esophageal, and gastric tissues. Smaller, more flexible tubes made of silicone or polyurethane are more comfortable and thought to be less irritating to the oropharynx, esophagus, and esophageal sphincter (Drickamer & Cooney, 1993).

In addition to discomfort, NG tubes can cause various complications. The tube can be placed inadvertently into the respiratory tract, a potentially lethal problem if nutritional supplements are infused through it. This can be checked by chest x-ray, physical exam, or aspiration of gastric contents to determine pH. Tracheobronchial secretions tend to be alkaline with a pH over 7, whereas gastric aspirates usually have an acidic pH less than 5.19. Aspiration can occur in patients with NG tubes, and gastrointestinal bleeding can result from tube irritation. As with all feeding devices, restraints may be required to keep patients from pulling them out. When restraints are used, there is increased risk for pressure sores, loss of mobility, incontinence, and delirium.

Gastrostomy/Jejunostomy Tubes

Gastrostomy or jejunostomy tubes are preferred for long-term enteral nutrition. With their use, patients no longer have to deal with the nasopharyngeal irritation associated with NG tubes. With intermittent bolus feeding, clothing can cover the tube when the patient is not receiving feedings, allowing fuller freedom to participate in activities without being obvi-

ous to others that there is a tube present. In those with a tendency to pull tubes out, an abdominal binder can be used to lessen this possibility.

Complications　Gastrostomy tubes have numerous potential complications associated with their use (**Table 20–4**). Aspiration can still occur despite precautions such as elevating the head of the bed 30 to 45 degrees (Metheny, 1993). Studies have found rates of aspiration pneumonia to be 23 to 58% in patients with PEG or PEJ tubes (Drickamer & Cooney, 1993). Wound infection or bleeding can occur immediately postoperatively or long after the tube has been inserted. Bleeding might be related to irritation of the gastric or intestinal lining, resulting in ulceration either adjacent to the tube or where the tube tip hits the mucosa. Diarrhea can occur from hyperosmolar formula, rapid bolus feedings, and lactose intolerance. Strategies for alleviating diarrhea include using a more dilute formula, switching to continuous pump feedings, and using a lactose-free formula (Galindo-Ciocon, 1993). Most commercial formulas are lactose free. Blocked feeding tubes are a recurrent problem. The blockage may occur from precipitation of medicines given through the tube or from formula solidifying. This is most common with continuous feedings. Periodic flushing as often as every 4 hours with water is the best preventative (Galindo-Ciocon, 1993). Once blockage occurs, irrigation of the tube with cola sometimes unplugs it, but often the only solution is replacing the feeding tube, which may involve another surgical intervention depending on which type of device is present.

Confused patients may pull the tube out, or it may otherwise come out. Once this occurs, the opening quickly closes within hours, again requiring a hospital visit to replace it. Large residual volumes in the stomach are commonly due to gastric atony (a lack of peristaltic waves in the stomach) or other problems. If gastric atony has been identified as the cause, medications are available that can help. Peritube leakage is more likely to occur with large gastric volumes, but most often results from a chronic infection at the abdominal opening leading to a gradual increase in the size of that opening. Finally, because of the loss of volitional control over intake, fluid imbalance with hyponatremia, hypernatremia, overhydration, and dehydration can occur.

Issues in Decision Making   When a feeding tube is being considered for a patient with a chronic illness, it is important to discuss all available information with the patient and family. If the patient's decision-making capacity is not intact, a surrogate decision maker needs to be involved. The insertion of a feeding tube is such a major decision that, ideally, a meeting should be scheduled so all interested family members can be present. The topic of the meeting should be given to family and caregivers beforehand, so that they can be prepared with questions and concerns. It is also wise to have present as many members of the care team as possible to give the perspective of different disciplines and provide the various implications of tube placement.

Several questions must be answered by the care team and family members to help arrive at the best decision regarding tube placement (**Table 20–5**). It is important to know the underlying condition that resulted in feeding tube placement. In addition, the prognosis based on the illness needs to be known. For example, a benign stricture of the esophagus in a functionally active person would have a very different prognosis than dysphagia in a bedridden, aphasic patient with end-stage Alzheimer's disease. If the need for a tube is expected to be short term—for an otherwise healthy senior to recover from pneumonia, for example—that need would be much clearer than in a patient with a progressive terminal illness.

If patients' decision-making capacity is intact, they can decide for themselves, after being given all the information. If they are grossly confused, then family or a guardian will need to make the decision. Advance directives or living wills are very helpful in establishing a cognitively impaired patient's wishes. These documents might be at home or in a safe deposit box and often are not present at the hospital. If they are not available, then the family should be asked about whether the patient ever expressed any opinions about feeding tubes in the past when he or she was cognitively intact.

The benefits as well as the risks of feeding tubes should be discussed by the care team. Sometimes a temporary trial of tube feeding is warranted. Ethically, there is no difference between not starting a feeding tube and discontinuing one when it has been shown to be of no benefit. Despite this, families often have great difficulty in asking for tube feedings

to be stopped once they have begun, regardless of whether they are helpful or harmful. Therefore, it is best to have this discussion in the beginning, rather than presenting it as an afterthought. Feeding tubes have been commonly used for persons with advanced dementing illnesses. There is no evidence that their use in dementias prevents aspiration pneumonia, prolongs survival, reduces the risk of pressure ulcers or infections, improves function, or provides palliation (Finucane, Christmas, & Travis, 1999). Because of their substantial risks, their use in advanced dementias should be discouraged on clinical grounds (Finucane et al., 1999). Feeding tubes are not recommended even for patients who choke on food and liquids (Hurley & Volicer, 2002). In a study of eating difficulties of persons with severe Alzheimer's, 36 of 71 (51%) residents refused food. They were all eventually fed by hand successfully, with no difference in mortality from those without eating difficulties (Volicer, Seltzer, Rheaume, et al., 1989). This alternative of giving pureed foods and sips of beverages in small amounts at a time is preferred for those with advanced dementias. The hospice team can be utilized for additional support for the patient and family. The frequent alternative is restraining patients to keep them from pulling out the tube and medicating them to treat the resulting agitation, which can lead to their developing pressure sores from the resulting immobility during the last days of life. These are common and unnecessary results from decisions for feeding tubes in terminally ill seniors.

Eating and feeding are basic to the human condition, and decisions regarding feeding tubes are often difficult for family members. By using a supportive, patient approach the care team can help the decision maker to make a choice based on facts as well as emotion. When prior counseling has taken place, it is easier for the care team to be supportive of whatever choice has been made and then work with the patient to provide the best care given that choice. Ongoing contact with the family is important as changes in status occur. After the initial discussion, patients and families have the information to modify or change their decisions if they so desire.

✦ Pneumonia in the Elderly

The prevention, diagnosis, and management of pneumonia in the geriatric population are little understood and controversial despite the proliferation of "pathways," algorithms, and a long tradition of practice and research in this disease. Pneumonia has been seen as the final common lot of the frail elderly, but efforts to reverse or ameliorate this condition have not met with success. The topics that are covered in this section include modes of infection, aspiration, diagnostic determinants of pneumonia, community-acquired versus nosocomial infection, and treatment and prevention issues.

Modes of Infection

The body's response to bacterial invasion ranges from clearance of the offending organisms to overwhelming infection. Bacterial colonization precedes infection. Colonization is the result of inadequate host defense and both immunologic and local/mechanical failures of clearance. A persistent source of bacteria is a predictor of eventual pneumonia. The source may be the nasopharynx in the young, but in the elderly it is almost

Table 20–5   Feeding Tubes: Questions to Ask

What are the underlying illnesses?
What is the prognosis?
Is the tube needed short or long term?
Is the patient's decision-making capacity intact?
Is there an advance directive or living will?
Did the patient ever express opinions on feeding tubes in the past?
Do the benefits outweigh the risks?
Are there any medical contraindications?
Would a trial of tube feeding be useful?
What are the alternatives?
Is life expectancy 6 months or less? (Hospice appropriate)

always located in the oropharynx. Progression of colonization to pneumonia requires additional events and circumstances. Prior respiratory viral infection, a history of smoking, previous antibiotic therapy, malnutrition, and serious illness combine with failure of immune response in the elderly to prepare the host for pneumonia. Immobility alone increases the rate of colonization in frail individuals. Excessive pharyngeal secretions, provoked by any kind of enteral feeding device, provide a favorable milieu for bacterial colonization.

Evidence of impaired defense against infection in the elderly includes frequent absence of fever and leukocytosis and diminished cough and expectoration. Tachypnea, tachycardia, and altered cognitive states are the more usual warning signs than fever and elevated white count. In one study, a rise in respiratory rate preceded the clinical diagnosis of pneumonia by 3 to 4 days (McFadden, Price, Eastwood, & Briggs, 1982). Physical signs are often absent in geriatric pneumonias.

Aspiration

Virtually all pneumonia at any age is aspiration pneumonia. This conceptual unity in the understanding of pneumonia has been relatively late in coming. In earlier decades, aspiration pneumonia referred to dramatic instances of large bolus delivery of gastric contents into the respiratory tract as a consequence of alcoholic stupor with vomiting, or with vomiting as a consequence of an illness associated with impaired consciousness from any cause. The offending organisms were thought to be principally *Klebsiella* and anaerobes. The locus of subsequent infection in classic large bolus aspiration pneumonia is the right lower or upper lobe. Large-volume aspiration is actually an uncommon event in seniors. The issue appears to be chronic low-volume aspiration.

Aspiration is the way that colonization of the oropharynx leads to pneumonia. Aspiration is a failure of insulation of the respiratory tract from the gastrointestinal tract. In the elderly, swallowing deficits are most often the result of neurogenic dysfunction. Misdirection of both the food bolus and secretions may occur as a product of impaired consciousness, motor dysfunction (oral and pharyngeal), deficits in sphincter function, ineffectual transport, and slowed esophageal propulsion. The problem is compounded by diminished receipt of sensory impulses and subsequent poor cough to clear the pharynx. Deep sleep favors aspiration, and the use of sedatives constitutes a pneumonia hazard.

Diagnostic Determinants of Pneumonia

Pneumonia is diagnosed during the clinical examination, by x-ray, and by laboratory results. Tubular breathing (breathing characterized by a high "whistling" sound), percussion dullness, and pulmonary rales are the exception in seniors rather than the rule. The chest x-ray radiograph, however, is often far from the gold standard that some clinicians believe it to be. The best x-ray in the evaluation of possible pneumonia is the previous one, ideally obtained at a time of relatively good health and function. Baseline chest film abnormalities abound. One seldom achieves the age of 70 or older without some previous opacity at the costophrenic angles. A proper film may confirm this possibility.

Seniors who get pneumonia have more parapneumonic effusions on the chest film than younger patients. When possible, thoracentesis should be done as an aid in diagnosis, and both chemical and bacteriologic tests performed on the aspirate to ensure precision in diagnosis. The chest tap should be followed by a repeat film with cross-table lateral views. Radiologists are most aware of the vagaries of x-ray diagnosis of pneumonia. The now current euphemism of "air space disease" is a consequence of the acknowledged eccentricities in pneumonia diagnosis. The problem is compounded by the frequent presence of coexistent congestive heart failure in seniors with pneumonia. Prior fibrotic disease and other fixed distortions of lung architecture may be present. Diaphragmatic distortion is frequently seen in seniors with infradiaphragmatic difficulties, past or present, and in those with chronic obstructive lung disease. Repeat chest films are seldom of value. It has long been known that clinical changes precede radiologic change.

The frequency of bacteremia in pneumonia, particularly in the aged, must be noted. The positive blood culture, if truly caused by the pneumonia, is the clearest guide to antibiotic therapy. What first must be established is the source of the bacteremia. In frail seniors, skin breakdown commonly provokes bacteremia. Urinary tract infection is a more common comorbidity that may produce positive blood cultures. In any of these three scenarios the antibiotic prescription will likely be the same. What is being treated is the blood culture regardless of the source of the infection (Marrie, Durant, & Yates, 1989).

Sputum culture is rarely of value as a guide to diagnosis or treatment. Gram stains are possibly more valuable, although both are fraught with collection error. As noted above, the white count may be normal and there is likely to be a paucity of immature neutrophils on the differential count. Very high white counts are more often the product of urinary sepsis than of pneumonia.

Influence of Enteral Feeding Devices

The presence of enteral feeding tubes, whether the traditional large- or small-bore nasogastric tubes or the newer percutaneous endogastric or endojejunal devices, is a risk factor for pneumonia (Galindo-Ciocon, 1993). Endogastric tubes may enhance reflux, particularly under circumstances of high gastric residuals, after PEG tube feeding. No tube prevents aspiration. The jejunostomy route may at least in theory help to prevent pneumonia. Nonetheless, these patients also demonstrate increased reflux. Acid gastric contents favor the development of gram-negative bacteria in the oropharynx and trachea, but elevation of the gastric pH by H_2-blockers or by alkaline pH feeding tube formulas increases the risk of bacterial overgrowth. If the clinical situation impels gastric mucosal protection, sucralfate, which does not affect pH, is probably the agent of choice. In any case, bleeding from the gut carries a less ominous prognosis than does pneumonia.

The value dilemma in the decision as to whether or not to institute enteral feeding is meeting the nutritional needs of the patient versus the threat of heightening susceptibility to pneumonia. This decision should not be made under circumstances of acute status change. Many patients who fail tests of swallowing may recover this function after acute systemic stress has been alleviated. The enteral tube decision is contextual in nature and should not be made reflexively after a failed swallowing challenge. Delirium, in particular, is always an acute event and its presence is not relevant to the enteral feeding decision.

Community-Acquired and Nosocomial Infection

Pneumonia is often described in terms of the location where it was acquired. "Community-acquired" pneumonia refers to infection that occurs while the patient is not institutionalized and living at home. "Nosocomial" pneumonia is contracted while the patient is hospitalized. The distinction is useful in the original choice of antibiotic therapy prior to receipt of culture data because typically each type of pneumonia tends to be caused by different organisms. But otherwise the distinction may not be important. Both are associated with the aspiration of oropharyngeal microflora, and the community in which both are operative is the oropharynx. Institutionally acquired lung infection may be more often associated with gram-negative bacteria. Community pathogens such as *Chlamydia, Haemophilus influenzae, Mycoplasma,* and *Legionella* are seldom seen in seniors admitted for pneumonia. The offending agents in hospital-acquired pneumonia are most commonly *Staphylococcus* or *Pseudomonas,* and initial treatment in this circumstance should cover these pathogens.

Issues in Treatment and Prevention

One does not have to be a historian of biologic science to appreciate the fact that recommendations for treatment of pneumonia often change. Even penicillin for *Pneumococcus* is now somewhat in disrepute. Today, treatment for pneumonia generally begins with a second-generation cephalosporin. Aminoglycosides are relatively if not absolutely problematic because of the high incidence of renal impairment in the elderly.

Mezlocillin is now active against a variety of gram-negative organisms. Vancomycin is indicated for staphylococcal disease. Clindamycin may be used when anaerobic infection is present. The frequency of antibiotic-associated diarrhea is high with this medication. Imipenem and metronidazole are now commonly employed for refractory infection. Mortality is still high in pneumonia, and treatment failure is seldom due to poor choice of antibiotics but rather to the influence of comorbidities such as other illness, hypotension, urinary incontinence, alcoholism, and absence of fever (Andrews, Chandrasekaran, & McSwiggan, 1984).

Preventive maneuvers that are clearly valid include rigorous requirement of hand washing by staff after each patient encounter. Use of H_2-blockers should be discouraged. New enteral intubation should never be instituted in the context of current treatment for pneumonia. There is as yet no solid evidence whether feeding tubes already in place should be removed with the supervention of pneumonia. The head of the bed should be elevated in patients with pneumonia and sedatives should not be given. Appropriate antibiotic therapy should be instituted without delay in accordance with the above guidelines. Blood gas determinations should be done in all cases.

Finally, to improve the outcome in pneumonia, careful management of confounding pathologies must be vigorously applied. Congestive heart failure must be kept high on the indices of suspicion. Most patients at risk of death from pneumonia have cardiac, renal, or cutaneous comorbidities. Staff members who attend geriatric patients with pneumonia must be familiar with atypical presentations, atypical host responses, and the common presence of inadequate tracheopharyngeal function.

✦ Delirium and Dementias

As the number of older individuals increases, the number of people with confusional states is also increasing. An understanding of these conditions is important for any health care professional dealing with the elderly. Though cure is usually not available for a dementia, delirium can often be reversed. As with other problems in older people, a measured and considered approach in assessment and treatment will make encounters more rewarding for clinicians and patients and their families.

Delirium is defined as a disturbance of consciousness accompanied by a change in cognition that cannot be accounted for by a preexisting or evolving dementia (American Psychiatric Association, 1994). Disturbance of consciousness is characterized by an inability to focus on or pay attention to surroundings and a fluctuating level of alertness. For example, you may introduce yourself to the patient and he or she appears to be wide awake and appropriate. Fifteen seconds later, however, the patient might be asleep or rolling the edge of the sheet and not aware of your presence. Delirium has an onset over a relatively short period of time: hours to days. Delirium is often encountered in hospitalized elderly patients. It is important to obtain a history of the patient's baseline functional and cognitive status prior to the illness and hospitalization from a family member or friend. If it was significantly better previously, it is likely that delirium is present. If the presence of delirium is missed, its cause may be overlooked, and the outcome is not likely to be as positive.

Delirium is more common in patients with dementias. For that reason, even if a senior has an established diagnosis of Alzheimer's disease, for example, one should always be aware of the possibility of a concurrent delirium. This awareness allows one to remove any possible contributing factors and help improve the patient's functional or cognitive state.

Possible contributing factors to delirium are numerous and several can be present at one time (**Table 20–6**). Illness itself can cause delirium, and a change in behavior or cognition in a frail elderly person can often be the first sign of an illness. Infections such as pneumonia can present with an onset of confused behavior, but with no fever and cough, in frail, elderly persons. Metabolic causes of delirium such as hypoglycemia, hypoxia, and hypercarbia can be assessed with laboratory tests. Dehydration and hyponatremia or hypernatremia usually result in a decreased level of consciousness. Severe hepatic or renal disease can cause delirium. Thiamine deficiency is common in alcoholics and can cause an acute Wernicke's syndrome, with confusion. Treatment with thiamine is standard in alcoholics to help prevent this. Finally, after a seizure, people commonly have a postictal state during which drowsiness and confusion are present.

Postsurgical patients can have delirium from the anesthesia, the stress of the illness or surgery itself, or from pain medications or other medications given postoperatively. A move to a new location can commonly elicit delirium. This might occur at a new home or during a hospitalization. The confusion is augmented by factors such as a different bathroom location, variation in routine, and new social contacts. When sensory cues are altered (e.g., when it becomes dark and dim), delirium can ensue. Sundowner's syndrome refers to confusion with its onset after nightfall. Typically, patients had no or fewer symptoms of delirium during the day.

Table 20–6 Causes of Delirium

Illness
Infections
Metabolic (hypoglycemia, hypoxia, hypercarbia)
Fluid or electrolyte imbalance
Hepatic or renal disease
Thiamine deficiency
Postictal
Postsurgical
Change in location
Alteration in sensory cues
"Sundowner's" syndrome
Medicines
Toxins
Withdrawal effects
Alcohol
Sedatives, hypnotics, anxiolytics

From American Psychiatric Association. (1994). *Diagnostic and Statistical Manual of Mental Disorders*, 4th ed. Washington, DC: APA.

One of the most common causes of delirium is adverse effects of medications. Any psychoactive drug should be considered a possible cause, including antidepressants, antianxiety medications, antipsychotics, opioid medications, and lithium (for use in manic-depressive illness). Drugs such as cocaine, marijuana, barbiturates, and alcohol can also cause delirium as a direct effect. Drugs including alcohol, sedatives, hypnotics, and antianxiety medications can cause delirium as a withdrawal effect (e.g., delirium tremens owing to alcohol withdrawal). Any medication with anticholinergic effects, of which there are many, can cause delirium. Antihistamines that can be obtained over the counter are in this group. Antihypertensives such as propranolol, methyldopa, hydrochlorothiazide, cimetidine (for stomach ulcer), digoxin, and anti-Parkinson's medications such as levodopa or amantadine are other frequently used medications with the potential to cause delirium. Any medication taken by an older person with delirium should be considered a possible cause, and as is always the case, only medications that are absolutely necessary should be continued.

The treatment of delirium involves removing the precipitating cause, if at all possible. Subsequent measures are likely to fail unless the cause is identified. The room should be quiet and familiar pictures and objects can help in orientation. A family member or friend can often orient the person to familiar things. If it is dark, turning a light on can often help. In rare instances, medications or restraints may be needed for safety. This should be a last resort because such measures can result in less ultimate benefit to the person.

Dementia

Dementia is characterized by the development of multiple cognitive deficits, including memory impairment. The dementia must be of sufficient severity to cause impairment in occupational or social functioning and must represent a decline from a previous higher level of functioning (Arnold & Kumar, 1993). The incidence of dementia increases dramatically with age. Dementia is estimated to affect 1% of people from age 50 to 70, and up to 50% of the very elderly (Rossor, 1994).

The diagnosis of dementia starts with the history. Usually this will be collected from the caregiver or family member because it is common for people with dementia to have no insight into their condition. Because the onset is often gradual, families may not be able to state when the problem started without specific probing questions. Inquiries about balancing the checkbook, doing income taxes, paying bills, losing things or getting lost, and forgetting important events are helpful. For a homemaker, questions about when she last prepared a full meal by herself, when she last did the housework, and if there has been any change in her social functioning are appropriate. Occupational and social history aid in developing the best questions regarding daily functioning that are specific to each person.

Many tests are available for documenting whether there is cognitive impairment. The Folstein Mini–Mental State Exam is the most commonly used screening test for dementia (Folstein, Folstein, & McHugh, 1975) (**Table 20–7**). It is a highly verbal test, and scores have been found to be affected by age, education, and cultural background, but not gender. It has been recommended that it not be used in people with less than an eighth-grade education or in people not fluent in English (Tombaugh & McIntyre, 1992). A perfect score is 30. Severity ranges for scoring are no cognitive impairment, 24 to 30; mild cognitive impairment, 18 to 23; severe cognitive impairment, 0 to 17 (Arnold & Kumar, 1993).

Alzheimer's disease is the most common cause of dementia. It is estimated to be present in 76 to 87% of cases of dementia (Morris, 1994). It is a progressive degenerative neurologic disorder that initially most noticeably affects cognition, but in its late stages affects the whole body. Because of its systemic effect, the stage of the disease can be followed by functional status as well as by cognitive status (Reisberg, 1986) (**Table 20–8**). Life expectancy is typically 7 to 10 years after diagnosis. Death most often occurs from pneumonia, urinary tract infection, or infected decubitus ulcers.

Alzheimer's disease is distinguished by a gradual onset and continuing cognitive decline (Folstein et al., 1975). A sudden onset of symptoms, focal neurologic findings such as hemiparesis or incoordination early in the course of the illness, gait disturbances, or seizures early in the course of the illness make the diagnosis of Alzheimer's disease unlikely (Stadlan, 1984).

Vascular dementia is the second most common form of dementia. It can be caused by several types of cerebrovascular lesions. These include multiple infarcts in cortical and subcortical areas, strategic single infarcts in specific areas of the brain, small vessel disease causing lacunar infarcts or white matter lesions, hypoperfusion due to cardiac arrest or other causes, and hemorrhages (Roman, Tatemichi, Erkinjuntti, et al., 1993). The *Diagnostic and Statistical Manual of Mental Disorders,* 4th edition (DSM-IV; American Psychiatric Association, 1994) criteria include focal neurologic signs and symptoms such as exaggeration of deep tendon reflexes, gait abnormalities, or weakness of an extremity, and radiologic evidence of lesions, such as multiple strokes on a computed tomography (CT) scan. These must be judged as etiologically related to the dementia. The difficulty often lies in determining whether the observed neurologic lesions or deficits are responsible for the dementia, or whether Alzheimer's or another condition is also present.

Elderly persons should be screened for "reversible" dementias. These dementias result from hypothyroidism, neurosyphilis,

Table 20–7   Mini–Mental State Examination

Maximum Score	Score	
		Orientation
5	( )	What is the (year) (season) (date) (day) (month)?
5	( )	Where are we: (state) (county) (town) (hospital) (floor)
		Registration
3	( )	Name three objects: 1 second to say each. Then ask the patient all three after you have said them. Give 1 point for each correct answer. Then repeat them until he learns all three. Count trials and record.
		Attention and Calculation
5	( )	Serials 7's. 1 point for each correct. Stop after five answers. Alternatively, spell "world" backward.
		Recall
3	( )	Ask for the three objects repeated above. Give 1 point for each correct.
		Language
9	( )	Name a pencil and watch (2 points).
		Repeat the following "No ifs, ands, or buts" (1 point).
		Follow a three-stage command: "Take a paper in your right hand, fold it in half, and put it on the floor" (3 points).
		Read and obey the following:
		Close your eyes (1 point).
		Write a sentence (1 point).
		Copy design (1 point).
30	( )	Total score
		Assess level of consciousness along a continuum:
		Alert—Drowsy—Stupor—Coma

Instructions for Administration

Orientation

1. Ask for the date. Then ask specifically for parts omitted, e.g., "Can you also tell me what season it is? One point for each correct.

2. Ask in turn "Can you tell me the name of this hospital?" (town, county, etc.). One point for each correct.

Registration

Ask the patient if you may test his memory. Then say the names of three unrelated objects, clearly and slowly, about one second for each. After you have said all three, ask him to repeat them. This first repetition determines his score (0–3) but keep saying them until he can repeat all three, up to six trials. If he does not eventually learn all three, recall cannot be meaningfully tested.

Attention and Calculation

Ask the patient to begin with 100 and count backward by 7. Stop after five subtractions (93, 86, 79, 72, 65). Score the total number of correct answers. If the patient cannot or will not perform this task, ask him to spell the word "world" backward. The score is the number of letters in correct order. (e.g., dlrow = 5, dlorw = 3).

Recall

Ask the patient if he can recall the three words you previously asked him to remember. Score 0–3.

Language

Naming: Show the patient a wrist watch and ask him what it is. Repeat for pencil. Score 0–2.

Repetition: Ask the patient to repeat the sentence after you. Allow only one trial. Score 0 or 1.

Three-stage command: Give the patient a piece of plain blank paper and repeat the command. Score 1 point for each part correctly executed.

Reading: On a blank piece of paper print the sentence "Close your eyes," in letters large enough for the patient to see clearly. Ask him to read it and do what it says. Score 1 point only if he actually closes he eyes.

Writing: Give the patient a blank piece of paper and ask him to write a sentence for you. Do not dictate a sentence; it is to be written spontaneously. It must contain a subject and a verb and be sensible. Correct grammar and punctuation are not necessary.

Copying: On a clean piece of paper, draw intersecting pentagons, each side ~1 in., and ask him to copy it exactly as it is. All 10 angles must be present and two must intersect to score 1 point. Tremor and rotation are ignored.

From Folstein, M.F., Folstein, S.E., & McHugh, P.R. (1975). "Mini-Mental State." A Practical Method for Grading the Cognitive State of Patients for the Clinician. *Journal of Psychiatric Research, 12,* 189–198, with permission.

Table 20–8 Functional Assessment Staging of Alzheimer's Disease (FAST Staging)

FAST Stage	FAST Characteristics
1	No functional decrement subjectively or objectively
2	Complains of forgetting location of objects, subjective work difficulties
3	Decreased functioning in demanding work settings evident to coworkers; difficulty traveling to new locations
4	Decreased ability to perform complex tasks (e.g., planning dinner party, shopping, personal finances)
5	Requires assistance selecting attire, may require coaxing to bathe properly
6a	Difficulty dressing properly
6b	Requires assistance bathing, fear of bathing
6c	Difficulty with the mechanics of toileting
6d	Urinary incontinence
6e	Fecal incontinence
7a	Vocabulary limited to 1 to 5 words
7b	Intelligible vocabulary lost
7c	Ambulatory ability lost
7d	Ability to sit lost
7e	Ability to smile lost
7f	Ability to hold up head lost; ultimately, stupor or coma

From Reisberg, B. (1986). Dementia: A Systematic Approach to Identifying Reversible Causes. *Geriatrics, 41*, 30–46.

B_{12} or folate deficiency, depression, and normopressure hydrocephalus. Studies have shown that about 15% of dementias are caused by reversible conditions. However, the few studies that have reported follow-up data have suggested that many of these secondary dementias are not as reversible as commonly believed (Reisberg, 1986).

Although there are many causes of dementia, including others not mentioned here, the clinical approach to these patients, as well as those with delirium, is similar. To avoid overwhelming patients, one caregiver at a time should interact with them. Any interfering noise such as television or radio should be turned off. An attempt should be made to assess hearing. Ultimately, if important information must be given, it should also be communicated to the family or caregiver. See Chapters 7 and 8 for a more detailed coverage of specific strategies for communicating with patients with dementia.

✦ Ethical Issues in Geriatric Practice

Ethics are central to geriatric practice. This centrality is not difficult to understand. Decision making in geriatrics must take into account the factors of age itself, life expectancy, frailty, and cognitive impairment. These condition the patient's and the family's sense of the worth of what is left of life. Few practitioners now regard longevity itself as a good. The pivotal issue in geriatrics, by common consensus, has become quality of life.

Quality of Life

Quality of life is difficult to define and even more difficult to measure. No formulaic approach, algorithm, or functional assessment can assign a value to quality of life. The reason is that quality of life is in the arena of subjectivity. The value of the later years, even in the face of frailty, proximity of death, and difficulty with thinking, is sometimes underestimated by practitioners. Quality of life is thus an intuitive determination, but as in other intuitive exercises, hidden issues are involved in its valuation. Some of these occult markers are purely social constructs. Is there the balm of love or the perception of love present as an antidote to pain, dysfunction, loss of mobility, and loss of control of decision making? The most reliable index of quality of life has been found to be, where ascertainable, the patient's own assessment. Quality of life is then what is important to a given individual. Improving or stabilizing quality of life is the principal goal of geriatric practice. An intuitive judgment of reduced quality of life may be presented as a reason for reducing the intensity of therapeutic interventions. Ethics provides constructs for evaluating the various decisions that are made in the care of the elderly.

What Is Ethics?

Ethics is not a determination of good versus evil. Ethics concerns itself with the relative weight of competing goods—the values dilemma (Mahowald, 1994). The overreaching good is the primacy of benevolence. The exercise of benevolence is the starting point of ethical action, regardless of the theoretical postulate offered as the structure of ethics. What ethics attempts to resolve is the conflict of goods subsumed under the umbrella of benevolence. Examples abound. Freedom and independence are goods. Protection of the patient is also a good. These may and often do become the poles of an ethical dilemma—when to sacrifice freedom (guardianship, surrogate decision making) in the interests of protection. A good is not to harm. A competing good is to preserve life and health. The value conflict here is to determine what qualities of life may be served by a given intervention when the risk of that intervention cannot be stated a priori with any degree of precision. The work of ethics then becomes the management of uncertainty. The tools of ethics are reason and communication. Ineffective reasoning may sabotage good communication, and faulty communication can undo excellent reasoning. The ethical project is to balance alternatives, each with some merit. If there are no bona fide alternatives, there is no ethical question. The everyday life of the geriatrician is spent navigating through a sea of alternatives: to tube feed or not, to remove a patient from home to an institution or not, to transfer a patient from a therapeutic mode of care to comfort care or not. These are only a few of the value dilemmas in geriatric practice.

Autonomy

In modern medical ethics, autonomy has become the overwhelmingly dominant principle. The primacy of autonomy is a relatively recent development. Autonomy is the individual's right to self-determination (Singer, 1994). It implies that decisions made are voluntary and intentional and not the result of coercion, duress, or undue influence. For the elderly, particularly the frail elderly, a tradition of reliance on others (learned helplessness) may be established. There may be a history of relying on others for shopping, transportation, physical assistance, money management, and ultimately, for vital decision making.

True autonomy implies sharing information. Careful interaction with the older patient and inclusion of the patient in the work of choice is essential. For such inclusion to be practically applicable, the patient must be deemed capable of an informed choice between alternatives.

Assessment of Decision-Making Ability

The determination of competence is a function of the courts yet physicians are qualified to evaluate a patient's decision-making ability. At the extremes of behavior, there is no difficulty in determining in geriatric practice a patient's ability to make decisions. A patient who can manipulate information, understand the relevance and weight of the choices proposed, and realize the consequences of the alternatives with ease is clearly able to make decisions about medical care. At the other end of the spectrum is the patient who is comatose, unable to communicate, whose thought is disorganized, or who is permanently disoriented. A bedside judgment of impaired decision-making ability in these circumstances is not difficult to make. The problem is in the vast intermediate zone between these poles of reasoning. Here, neuropsychiatry is consulted, and there is a resort to formal testing. However, tests of decision making can be fraught with error. It is certainly possible that an individual may recover this ability after surviving acute illness. In the final analysis, physicians make determinations about decision-making ability in borderline cases. The sensibility of ethics will guide these decisions.

Advanced Directives

The problem of how to proceed in circumstances of lost or impaired decision capacity has been addressed in contemporary practice by recourse to the advanced directive (Kapp, 1985). Advanced directives are considered to encompass the living will and durable power of attorney for health care (McCullough, Doukas, Holleman, & Reilly, 1995). An advanced directive is generally created at a time when the would-be patient is sound in mind and body, and it is a hypothetical instrument. It is intended to govern in circumstances of unspecified future incapacity and cognitive impairment at a future time of crisis. Directives only take effect when the patient is incapable of making or communicating decisions about interventions. One difficulty with advanced directives resides in their hypothetical character. They are determined at a time of detachment yet are to be executed at a time of potential crisis, pain, and fear. However, this may be the best expression of the value of autonomy.

The Living Will

The living will is a statement about specific treatment preferences in the event of terminal illness. It is assumed that the document is drawn up under conditions of competency; however,

there are usually no limitations on conditions of revoking a living will (McCullough et al., 1995). Laws regarding living wills vary from state to state and definitions of terminal illness may vary.

Durable Power of Attorney for Health Care

The durable power of attorney is a document that appoints a health care surrogate in the future event of incompetency. In theory, the surrogate is assumed to behave as an instrument of the incompetent patient's desires. At the time of creation of the durable power of attorney, few would-be patients have discussed the details of decision making with the surrogates. Directions to the surrogate are usually broadly general, such as "I don't want to be on a breathing machine." Surrogates usually wish to create a family consensus before they act in accordance with the terms of the living will.

In geriatric practice, clinicians should understand the principles of ethics and the various legislative statutes and institutional policies that govern decision making. Education and communication with seniors and their families ensure sensitivity to autonomy and adherence to standards of ethics. (For more information on ethical principles, see Chapter 2.)

✦ Case Vignettes

Case One

Mrs. Jones, 87 years old, was admitted to the hospital geriatric service with a history of increasing lethargy and a decreased mental status. Her past history was significant for multiple strokes, vascular dementia, and diabetes of 30 years duration. She had been nonambulatory for 2½ years owing to leg weakness from her strokes, and she lived with her daughter, who cared for her. She had had six admissions in the past year including a fractured tibia 7 months previous to this admission. Since that time, she had been confined to bed. She also required total assistance in her other activities of daily living including feeding, dressing, bathing, and toileting. She was incontinent of urine and stool. Her most recent admission had been 2 months earlier for pneumonia.

Physical exam was significant for a weight of 53.3 kg (a loss of 22 kg in 6 months). Her height was 160 cm. She had diffuse expiratory crackles bibasilarly. Her extremities were stiff with limited range of motion. She complained of severe pain in both heels and exam revealed a 12 × 3 cm stage 4 decubitus ulcer over her left heel with black eschar and an area of exposed Achilles' tendon. A smaller 4 × 2 cm stage 4 ulcer was on the right heel with exposed bone. She scored 9 of 30 on the Folstein Mini-Mental State Exam.

Admission laboratory studies were significant for a white cell count of 5300 with 18% lymphocytes (absolute lymphocyte count 954), hemoglobin 9.0 g/dL, glucose 153 mg/dL, erythrocyte sedimentation rate (ESR) 114 mm/hr, and an albumin of 2.3 g/dL. X-rays of her feet showed changes consistent with osteomyelitis of her left heel. Chest x-ray showed a right lower lobe infiltrate consistent with pneumonia. Computed tomography (CT) scan of the head showed multiple small lacunar infarcts of the brain stem and basal ganglia.

The dietitian recommended that the patient receive 1400 kcal/day, 70 g protein/day, and 1400 cc of fluid/day. Speech-language pathology was consulted because of difficulty in swallowing. Bedside clinical exam showed pooled secretions in the oral cavity and pharynx. When placed in the full upright position, she drooled. She was able to repeat three word phrases with a soft, strained voice. Naming was delayed but accurate for simple objects. No laryngeal elevation was felt when the patient was asked to swallow, and when 2 cc of water were placed in her mouth, it ran out with no swallow attempts. The impression was dysphagia with flaccid dysarthria and decreased cognition. It was recommended that she have nothing by mouth, and that long-term tube feeding with a percutaneous endoscopic gastrostomy or percutaneous endoscopic jejunostomy tube be considered. She was treated with intravenous fluids and antibiotics for the infected decubitus ulcer and given transdermal fentanyl and morphine sulfate for the pain. The ulcers were also debrided by a plastic surgeon. Special soft boots were given to relieve pressure and help the heel pain. A conference was scheduled with her family to discuss further care.

Her daughter attended along with her granddaughter. Care team members present were her nurse, social worker, speech–language pathologist, geriatrician, and nurse practitioner, who led the meeting. All took part, with her daughter initially describing how she had been doing over the past years. Mrs. Jones's code status had already been made "do not resuscitate" and she had been consistent in saying to her daughter as well as the care team that she didn't want a feeding tube. The nurse reported that she was more comfortable, but still had some pain when moved. The speech–language pathologist discussed her swallowing problems and high risk of aspiration when fed by mouth. The geriatrician reviewed her medical problems and indicated that no matter what treatments were given, her prognosis was poor. If her illness followed its usual course, she would die within 6 months.

Feeding tubes were discussed, including benefits and risks. The hospice approach of comfort care and focus on maximizing the quality of her remaining life was presented. Her daughter was leaning toward a hospice approach at home, but wanted to discuss it with other family members before making a final decision. The next day she called with her decision for hospice care at home for Mrs. Jones. The intravenous line was removed and antibiotics discontinued. The speech–language pathologist reviewed positions and techniques for pleasure feeding, if desired, with the daughter to minimize risk of aspiration. The patient was discharged home for hospice care. At home she took small amounts of food from a spoon, and after 1½ weeks became unable to take anything and was given ice chips and mouth care. The hospice nursing assistant came three times weekly as did the nurse to help with her care, make sure she was comfortable, and give support to her daughter. The hospice social worker and spiritual care advisor also made home visits. A small dose of antianxiety medicine was added for her comfort, but no adjustment in pain medicine was required. Two and a half weeks after her return home, Mrs. Jones died in her sleep.

Case One: Study Questions and Answers

1. What other major diagnosis, not mentioned, can be made from the history, physical, and laboratory results of the previous case?

   Answer: Protein calorie malnutrition is the diagnosis. She had a weight loss of 22 kg in 6 months, serum albumin of

2.3 g/dL, and absolute lymphocyte count of 954, all of which support the diagnosis.

2. Mrs. Jones's Folstein Mini–Mental State score of 9 is consistent with severe cognitive impairment, and she has a diagnosis of vascular dementia. Should any weight be given to her stating that she doesn't want a feeding tube?

   Answer: If she appears to understand what a feeding tube is and her answers are consistent, then her own statements are important and should be weighed heavily in the ultimate decision.

3. Would Mrs. Jones have lived longer if a feeding tube had been inserted?

   Answer: It is probable that she would have lived longer. However, such factors as violation of her autonomy by placing a tube against her will, continued risk of aspiration of oral secretions, possible need for restraint on her wrists to keep her from pulling the tube out, with associated risk of developing new pressure sores, as well as other considerations must be balanced with the possible benefits of enteral feeding.

Case Two

Ms. Wright, an 80-year-old retired travel agent, lived independently in a seniors' apartment building and enjoyed social activities with friends and neighbors. She had a dog, but no living family members. Her past medical history was significant for type 2 diabetes, a small stroke from which she had recovered with "no problems, but my memory's not as good as it used to be," asthma, and osteoarthritis of her knees. She took six different medications.

One winter day, with the temperature at a record low of −20°F, she took her dog outside, slipped on a patch of ice, and was unable to get up. Half an hour later, security personnel in the apartment noticed her dog barking at the entrance. The dog led them to Ms. Wright, who was awake, but lethargic. She was taken by ambulance to the nearest hospital emergency room.

On physical exam, she could be aroused to speak, but was confused, and fell asleep easily. Her temperature was 90°F. Physical exam was otherwise unremarkable. CT of her head showed several small cerebral lacunar infarcts. She was treated for hypothermia and discharged home after a few days.

Two days later, a visiting nurse saw Ms. Wright in her apartment. She was not correctly taking her medications, which now totaled ten. Among them were drugs for anxiety, hypertension, diabetes, asthma, allergies, "heart," and "circulation." Additionally, her nurse learned that the previous night, security personnel had found her wandering in the building hallway, unable to find her apartment. Ms. Wright denied any alcohol use. Her diet appeared adequate, helped by the fact that meals were served in the apartment building's dining room. The nurse did a Folstein Mini–Mental State Exam, and Ms. Wright scored 24 of 30. Fingerstick blood glucose was 60 mg/dL.

The visiting nurse called Ms. Wright's physician, who had not cared for her during her hospitalization because she was not on staff there. The physician decided to stop the arthritis, anxiety, allergy, and circulation medicines, as there was no clear need for them. Because her glucose was low, her diabetes pill was also stopped. The nurse arranged to have her other medicines put in a plastic cassette arranged by time of day and day of the week to help Ms. Wright remember if she had taken them or not.

On follow-up visits, Ms. Wright was feeling well and functioning similarly to before her hospitalization. She scored 28 of 30 on a repeat Folstein Mini–Mental State Exam. Her dog was given to a friend when she realized the frequent trips outdoors were becoming too much to handle. She was again able to enjoy outings with her friends.

Case Two: Study Questions and Answers

1. What caused Ms. Wright's altered mental state when she arrived at the hospital?

   Answer: She had a delirium contributed to by her illness, hypothermia. From her history, she may also have had a very mild underlying dementia, which would make her more susceptible to develop delirium.

2. What was Ms. Wright's problem after her return from the hospital?

   Answer: She had delirium with contributions by multiple factors. These would include polypharmacy, adverse effects of individual drugs, and hypoglycemia. Removing unneeded drugs allowed her to return to her baseline cognitive state.

✦ Conclusion

The assessment and management of seniors require attention to the social, psychological, emotional, and physiologic factors that combine to affect their daily functioning and quality of life. A multidisciplinary approach is often the most effective and efficient way of providing the best care. By necessity, all team members must be aware of how their discipline interfaces with others on the team. Speech–language pathologists supply input on two essential functions: communication and swallowing. The impact of the contribution of speech–language pathologists is more significant when they know the physician's approach to diagnosis and treatment, and have a strong foundation in issues in geriatric practice.

References

American Psychiatric Association. (1994). *Diagnostic and Statistical Manual of Mental Disorders,* 4th ed. Washington, DC: APA

Andrews, J., Chandrasekaran, P., & McSwiggan, D. (1984). Lower Respiratory Tract Infections in an Acute Geriatric Male Ward: A One-Year Prospective Surveillance. *Gerontology, 30,* 290–296

Arnold, S.E., & Kumar, A. (1993). Reversible Dementias. *Medical Clinics of North America, 77,* 215–230

Bald, F.C. (1954). *Michigan in Four Centuries.* New York: Harper & Brothers

Barrocas, A., Belcher, D., Champagne, C., & Jastram, C. (1995). Nutrition Assessment: Practical Approaches. *Clinics in Geriatric Medicine, 11,* 675–713

Brown, I., Renwick, R., & Raphael, D. (1995). Frailty: Constructing a Common Meaning, Definition, and Conceptual Framework. *International Journal of Rehabilitation Research, 18,* 93–102

Chernoff, R. (1995). Effects of Age on Nutrient Requirements. *Clinics in Geriatric Medicine, 11,* 641–651

Cohen, D. (1994). Dementia, Depression, and Nutritional Status. *Primary Care, 21,* 107–119

Colley, C.A., & Lucas, L.M. (1993). Polypharmacy: The Cure Becomes the Disease. *Journal of General Internal Medicine, 8,* 278–283

Drickamer, M.A., & Cooney, L.M. (1993). A Geriatrician's Guide to Enteral Feeding. *Journal of the American Geriatrics Society, 41,* 672–679

Dwyer, J. (1994). Nutritional Problems of Elderly Minorities. *Nutrition Reviews, 52,* S24–S27

Finucane, T.E., Christmas, C., & Travis, K. (1999). Tube Feeding in Patients with Advanced Dementia: A Review of the Evidence. *Journal of the American Medical Association, 282,* 1365–1370

Folstein, M.F., Folstein, S.E., & McHugh, P.R. (1975). "Mini-Mental State." A Practical Method for Grading the Cognitive State of Patients for the Clinician. *Journal of Psychiatric Research, 12,* 189–198

Galindo-Ciocon, D.J. (1993). Tube Feeding: Complications Among the Elderly. *Journal of Gerontology Nursing, 19,* 17–22

Hurley, A.C., & Volicer, L. (2002). Alzheimer Disease. "It's Okay, Mama, If You Want to Go, It's Okay." *Journal of the American Medical Association, 288,* 2324–2331

Kapp, M.B. (1985). *Legal and Ethical Aspects of Health Care for the Elderly.* Ann Arbor, MI: Health Administration Press

Katz, S., Ford, A.B., Moskowitz, R.W., et al. (1963). Studies of Illness in the Aged: The Index of ADL. *Journal of the American Medical Association, 185,* 914–919

Kerstetter, J.E., Holthausen, B.A., & Fitz, P.A. (1993). Nutrition and Nutritional Requirements for the Older Adult. *Dysphagia, 8,* 51–58

Lawton, M.P., & Brody, E.M. (1969). Assessment of Older People: Self-Maintaining and Instrumental Activities of Daily Living. *Gerontologist, 9,* 179–186

Lipschitz, D.A. (1995). Approaches to the Nutritional Support of the Older Patient. *Clinics in Geriatric Medicine, 11,* 715–724

Mahowald, M.B. (1994). So Many Ways to Think: An Overview of Approaches to Ethical Issues in Geriatrics. *Clinics in Geriatric Medicine, 10,* 403–418

Marrie, T.J., Durant, H., & Yates, L. (1989). Community-Acquired Pneumonia Requiring Hospitalization: Five-Year Prospective Study. *Reviews of Infectious Diseases, 11,* 586–599

McCullough, L.B., Doukas, D.J., Holleman, W.L., & Reilly, R.B. (1995). Advance Directives. In: W. Reichel (Ed.), *Care of the Elderly,* 4th ed. (pp. 597–608). Baltimore: Williams & Wilkins

McFadden, J.P., Price, R.C., Eastwood, H.D., & Briggs, R.S. (1982). Raised Respiratory Rate in Elderly Patients: A Valuable Physical Sign. *British Medical Journal, 284,* 626–627

Metheny, N. (1993). Minimizing Respiratory Complications of Nasoenteric Tube Feedings: State of the Science. *Heart and Lung, 22,* 213–223

Morley, J.E. (1993). Nutrition and the Older Female: A Review. *Journal of the American College of Nutrition, 12,* 337–343

Morris, J.C. (1994). Differential Diagnosis of Alzheimer's Disease. *Clinics in Geriatric Medicine, 10,* 257–276

Reisberg, B. (1986). Dementia: A Systematic Approach to Identifying Reversible Causes. *Geriatrics, 41,* 30–46

Rolandelli, R.H., & Ullrich, J.R. (1994). Nutritional Support in the Frail Elderly Surgical Patient. *Surgery Clinics of North America, 74,* 79–92

Roman, G.C., Tatemichi, T.K., Erkinjuntti, T., et al. (1993). Vascular Dementia: Diagnostic Criteria for Research Studies. Report of the NINDS-AIREN International Workshop. *Neurology, 43,* 250–260

Rossor, M.N. (1994). Management of Neurological Disorders: Dementia. *Journal of Neurology, Neurosurgery, and Psychiatry, 57,* 1451–1456

Silver, A.J. (1991). Malnutrition. In: J.C. Beck (Ed.), *Geriatrics Review Syllabus: A Core Curriculum in Geriatric Medicine* (pp. 174–175). New York: American Geriatrics Society

Singer, P. (1994). *Ethics.* Oxford: Oxford University Press

Stadlan, E.M. (1984). Clinical Diagnosis of Alzheimer's Disease. In: G. McKhann, D. Drachman, M. Folstein, et al. (Eds.), *Report of the NINCDS-ADRDA Work Group Under the Auspices of Department of Health and Human Services Task Force on Alzheimer's Disease. Neurology, 34,* 940

Stuart, B, et al. (1996). *Medical Guidelines for Determining Prognosis in Selected Non-Cancer Diseases,* 2nd ed. Arlington, VA: National Hospice Organization

Tombaugh, T.N., & McIntyre, N.J. (1992). The Mini-Mental State Examination: A Comprehensive Review. *Journal of the American Geriatrics Society, 40,* 922–935

U.S. Census Bureau. (2000). *Census 2000.* U.S. Department of Commerce, Washington, D.C.

U.S. Census Bureau. *Population Projections Program.* U.S. Department of Commerce, Washington, D.C.

Volicer, L., Seltzer, B., Rheaume, Y., et al. (1989). Eating Difficulties in Patients with Probable Dementia of the Alzheimer Type. *Journal of Geriatric Psychiatry and Neurology, 2,* 188–195

Winograd, C.H., Gerety, M.B., Chung, M., et al. (1991). Screening for Frailty: Criteria and Predictors of Outcomes. *Journal of the American Geriatrics Society, 39,* 778–784

21

Neurologic Disorders: An Orientation and Overview

Nabih Ramadan and Daniel S. Newman

✦ **Anatomic Substrates**

✦ **Neurologic Examination**

✦ **Common Neurologic Tests**

✦ **Neurologic Diseases and Their Management**

An understanding of neurology, among other disciplines in medicine, is arguably the most important for the speech–language pathologist (SLP). Indeed, the nervous system provides for the control of structures that produce and modify sound into speech, and language itself is organized and constructed solely within the brain.

This chapter provides a framework for understanding the neurologic approach to problems the SLP encounters, which revolves around anatomic (Where is the lesion?) and functional (What is the lesion?) constructs. An illustrative case: Your grandmother telephones you, and, because you are an SLP, tells you that her neighbor has begun to "talk funny." You think a moment; this could mean anything. You wonder, has the usual content of conversation changed or become inappropriately jocular or puerile? Is the person now speaking in jargon or neologisms? Has the speech become softer or monotonal? Is it more hoarse or slurred? Whether you know it or not, as you attempt to figure out what Grandma means by "talk funny," you are beginning to try to localize the lesion. Your first question is likely to be, "Is she saying funny things or are the words coming out funny?" The answer to this question could tell you whether the neighbor has dysarthria, aphasia, or a disorder of thought.

✦ Anatomic Substrates

The Motor Unit

Components of speech are organized hierarchically. Tissues that actually produce sound and modify speech are either largely muscle (e.g., the tongue) or soft tissues that change their shape through the action of attached or adjacent muscle. These skeletal muscles are innervated by lower motor neurons (LMNs), which have their cell bodies in the caudal part of the brainstem, specifically the lower pons and medulla. The neuromuscular junction (NMJ) functionally connects LMN with the muscle, and together they form the motor unit. Damage or dysfunction of the motor unit leads to variants of dysarthria, which is inevitably flaccid.

Motor Control

Pyramidal System

The motor unit is under the control of several descending pathways that originate in the cerebrum or brainstem and are known collectively as the upper motor neurons (UMN). UMNs project to the spinal (corticospinal) or lower cranial nerves (corticobulbar LMNs). The corticospinal tracts descend through the pyramids in the medulla and are also designated as the pyramidal tracts. The corticobulbar tracts provide the voluntary control over the cranial nerves that produce speech.

A lesion of the corticospinal tract causes weakness and a loss or reduction of contralateral voluntary movements in the extremities. On the other hand, unilateral lesions of the corticobulbar tract have less of an effect because most lower cranial nerves are innervated bilaterally. A notable exception is the lower part of the face, which receives primarily contralateral (corticobulbar) input. Corticobulbar tract lesions have a marked effect on speech, manifesting as spastic dysarthria.

Extrapyramidal System

Other descending pathways (e.g., the rubrospinal and reticulospinal), which are collectively called the extrapyramidal system, are primarily concerned with posture and tone of the

315

upper and lower extremities, and their roles in the production of speech are less well understood. Also, other areas of the brain (e.g., basal ganglia and cerebellum) are involved with motor control but do so by way of complex feedback loops involving cortical and subcortical structures. The pyramidal and extrapyramidal motor systems are viewed as the "voluntary" and "involuntary" systems, respectively.

For example, consider a man standing ready to catch a baseball that is thrown to the right of him. When he reaches to the right to catch it, only the abduction and extension of the arm and the opening of the fingers are "voluntary." The unconscious extension of the left arm and the requisite changes of the trunk musculature are "involuntary." These changes have been largely planned and executed by the basal ganglia using real-time sensory information to maintain balance and utilizing prelearned motor programs to support the rest of the body in a stable posture while catching the ball. The cerebellum primarily smoothes and corrects the voluntary actions of the opposing muscles (i.e., agonist and antagonist) involved in the movements of the right arm as it is directed to and acquires the target.

◆ Neurologic Examination

The neurologic examination is a structured approach to evaluating the nervous system function of the patient, and includes assessments of the mental status, cranial nerves, motor function, sensory function, reflexes, gait and station, and coordination.

Mental Status

The mental status examination is usually the first neurologic function tested, even if it is done informally. Typically, the following functions are screened: arousal, attention, memory, affect, language, and drawing.

The Cranial Nerves (CN)

Olfactory Nerve (CN I)

The first-order terminals involved in perception of odors are contained in the olfactory nerves. Patients are asked whether they are able to perceive odors through one nostril while the other is occluded. Generally, small vials containing volatile agents (e.g., oil of wintergreen or camphor) are used. An inability to detect odors is termed anosmia.

Optic Nerve (CN II)

Although the rods and cones in the retina are the sense organs that convert light to electrical impulses, the fibers of the optic nerve are extensions of the first-order neurons of sight. The fibers of the optic nerve begin in the retina, exit the globe, and travel posteriorly to the optic chiasm where a partial decussation occurs. The fibers continue and end primarily in the lateral geniculate nucleus of the thalamus. A small percentage of optic nerve fibers end in the midbrain as afferents of the pupillary light reflex. CN II is tested by checking visual acuity with an eye chart as well as the visual fields. In the clinic, visual fields are usually tested by asking the patient to count or detect the movement of fingers or small objects in the visual fields. This is done with the contralateral eye covered and with the patient fixating on the examiner's eye. The examination of the optic nerve also includes a funduscopic examination with an ophthalmoscope.

Oculomotor, Trochlear, and Abducens Nerves (CNs III, IV, and VI)

The oculomotor, trochlear, abducens nerves (CNs III, IV, and VI) provide the lower motor neuron control of eye movements. In addition, the third nerve innervates the levator of the eyelid, the constrictor muscle of the pupil, and the ciliary muscle that controls accommodation. They are tested clinically by having the patient visually follow an object to the cardinal positions of gaze.

Trigeminal Nerve (CN V)

The fifth cranial nerve has both motor and sensory components. The motor component of the trigeminal nerve provides for jaw movement. Unilateral lesions are usually well tolerated, but severe bilateral lesions leave the mouth open and unable to be closed.

The sensory portion of the trigeminal nerve supplies sensation to the face as well as the buccal and nasal mucosa. The cells arise largely in the gasserian ganglion and, like all sensory nerves, send processes distal to innervate the periphery and centrally to nuclei within the central nervous system (CNS). The fibers that course peripherally do so within the three divisions of the trigeminal nerve: the ophthalmic (V_1), maxillary (V_2), and mandibular (V_3) branches. The centrally destined processes of the trigeminal sensory neurons enter the lateral pons and course rostrally or caudally in the brainstem depending on the type of sensory information they carry. Those concerned with pain and temperature descend into the medulla and upper cervical spinal cord as the descending trigeminal tract. Those carrying tactile and proprioceptive information ascend to the main sensory nucleus. The motor fibers of CN V leave the pons and innervate the muscles of mastication (the temporalis, masseter, and pterygoids) via the mandibular branch.

Of particular interest to the SLP are the maxillary and mandibular branches. The maxillary branch carries sensation from the maxilla, maxillary teeth, the mucous membranes of the upper mouth, the anterior palate, nose and nasopharynx, the inferior portion of the internal auditory meatus, and the midface. The mandibular branch conducts sensory information from the skin of the cheek, the lower teeth and jaw, and the mucosal linings of the uvula, posterior hard palate, and nasopharynx. The mandibular branch contains the proprioceptive and other sensory information from the skin on the mandible, ipsilateral side of the tongue, and the buccal surface of the cheek. The ophthalmic division can be tested with the corneal and nasal tickle reflexes. A wisp of cotton gently stroked across the junction of the sclera and cornea should elicit bilateral blinking. Similarly, a wisp of cotton introduced very gently into one of the patient's nostrils should result in the wrinkling of the nose. In both tests, the two sides are compared. The bulk of the masseter and temporalis muscles are tested by palpation of the muscles while patients clench their teeth. Once bulk has been ascertained, the strength of the muscles is tested by an attempt to open the patient's jaw with downward pressure on the chin. The pterygoids provide for lateral movement of the jaw. The jaw will deviate to the side of the weak pterygoid and will be more easily pushed in that direction. Inside the mouth, weakness of the tensor veli palatini may manifest as tilting of the uvula away from weak side. The jaw jerk reflex tests afferent and efferent function of the mandibular division of CN V.

Facial Nerve (CN VII)

As another nerve with both motor and sensory components, the facial nerve provides LMN innervation for the muscles of facial expression and the stapedius muscle. The special sensory component allows for the innervation of the taste buds on the anterior two thirds of the tongue. Parasympathetic fibers within the facial nerve innervate the lacrimal gland as well as the submandibular and sublingual salivary glands. The facial muscles are tested first by inspection of the face for symmetry and then by examining individual muscles for strength. Patients with weak facial muscles generally have fewer facial lines and wrinkles. The face looks inordinately placid. With unilateral weakness, the palpebral fissure will be wider on the weak side. When the orbicularis oculi are contracted maximally, the patient should be able to "bury" the origins of the eyelashes. Additionally, a good deal of resistance to forced eye opening should be apparent. The nasolabial folds should be roughly symmetrical; the weak side will appear flattened. With unilateral weakness the corner of the mouth will be seen to sag. When smiling, the corners of the mouth should elevate. With bifacial weakness, the smile looks more like a snarl, and whistling or drinking through a straw becomes difficult or impossible. When facial muscle weakness is owing to lower motor neuron loss as in amyotrophic lateral sclerosis (ALS), fasciculations may be seen.

A key clinical point with respect to facial weakness is the distribution of the deficit. Lower motor neuron weakness, as in Bell's palsy, generally involves all ipsilateral muscles. In a typical upper motor neuron lesion, such as a stroke, the muscles below the eyes are generally much weaker than those of the forehead and of eye closure.

Acoustic Nerve (CN VIII)

Cranial nerve VIII provides innervation for the cochlea and the end organs of the vestibular apparatus. Thus, this nerve provides the ability to hear and sense vertical, horizontal, and rotatory accelerations. Hearing may be tested at the bedside by having a patient listen for the ticking of a watch or recognize whispered words. A tuning fork is used to test whether air conduction is greater than bone conduction, as is normal. Vestibular function may be glimpsed by observing the eyes for movements in primary gaze or during pursuit movements. Detailed vestibular function testing is beyond the scope of this chapter.

Glossopharyngeal Nerve (CN IX)

This nerve supplies somatic sensation to the middle ear and the sense of taste to the posterior third of the tongue. The stylopharyngeus is the sole muscle innervated by this nerve. This muscle raises and dilates the pharynx. Testing of the CN IX is accomplished by testing the gag reflex. A cotton-tipped applicator or tongue blade that gently touches the posterior wall of the pharynx should elicit elevation and constriction of the pharyngeal musculature, as well as retraction of the tongue. Although the afferent arc of this reflex is carried through the glossopharyngeal nerve, the efferent function is conducted through the vagus. Some people, however, do not gag, so this should be considered unequivocally abnormal only if the gag is lost unilaterally.

Vagus Nerve (CN X)

The vagus nerve is a long and complex structure. It provides motor and sensory innervation to the palate, pharynx, and larynx. Additionally, it contains visceral sensory information from, and parasympathetic innervation to, thoracic and abdominal viscera. Some of the taste receptors on the posterior tongue and pharynx are vagally innervated as well. The thoracic and abdominal aspects of vagus function not relevant to speech will not be covered further in this chapter. Functionally, the vagus nerve is extremely important for both swallowing and phonation, innervating most of the muscles involved with speech and swallowing except for the stylopharyngeus (IX) and tensor veli palatini (V). For the SLP, the three relevant branches of the vagus are the pharyngeal, the superior laryngeal, and the recurrent laryngeal nerves. After these segments have branched, the vagus nerve is concerned primarily with the viscera of the thorax and the abdomen.

Shortly after exiting the skull, CN X breaks into branches. The pharyngeal branch descends to the inferior pharyngeal constrictor where it mingles with the glossopharyngeal and external branch of the superior laryngeal nerve as the pharyngeal plexus. From this plexus, efferent fibers innervate all of the muscles of the palate and the pharynx, except those noted above.

The superior laryngeal nerve, the second important branch of CN X, divides into internal and external branches. The external laryngeal nerve supplies the inferior pharyngeal constrictor and the cricothyroid muscle. The cricothyroid muscle controls pitch by lengthening the vocal cords. The internal laryngeal nerve is a pure sensory nerve that receives mucosal sensory information from the pharynx down to the level of the epiglottis, the aryepiglottic folds, and the arytenoid cartilages. It also contains proprioceptive information from the muscle spindles of the vocal apparatus.

The third relevant branch of the vagus is the recurrent laryngeal nerve. Both the left and right recurrent branches are so named because after descending to the level of the branching great vessels in the mediastinum, they double back on themselves and ascend to the larynx. The right recurrent laryngeal loops under the right subclavian artery and the left loops beneath the arch of the aorta. Both recurrent laryngeal nerves innervate all intrinsic muscles of the larynx except for the cricothyroid.

Several functions of the vagus nerve are easily tested during the neurologic exam. Inspection of the palate reveals it to look lower and less archiform on the unilaterally weak side. When the patient says /a/, there will be deviation to the normal side. The gag reflex will be reduced or abolished on the affected side. Unless palatal weakness is bilateral, hypernasality or nasal regurgitation of liquids during swallowing may not be noticeable. In bilateral weakness of the palate, speech becomes hypernasal and there is nasal regurgitation of liquids during swallowing.

Normally the vocal folds are abducted during inspiration and adducted during phonation and coughing. With unilateral abductor weakness, the voice may be hoarse but there will not usually be dyspnea. With bilateral abductor weakness, there is often severe dyspnea and inspiratory stridor. The voice may be hoarse but because both vocal folds can still be adducted, speech will not be severely affected. In a complete unilateral LMN lesion, the vocal fold lies motionless in midabduction. The voice is low pitched and hoarse, but phonation may not be affected as much, as the normal cord may be able to cross the midline. With bilateral LMN weakness, there is inspiratory stridor, dyspnea, and loss of phonation.

Accessory Nerve (CN XI)

The 11th nerve is derived from anterior horn cells from the upper four or five cervical segments. Its fibers enter the skull through the foramen magnum, travel briefly with the vagus nerve, and ultimately innervate the sternocleidomastoid (SCM) and the upper part of the trapezius (TPZ) muscles. (The lower part of the TPZ is innervated by the third and fourth cervical roots through the cervical plexus.) To test the SCM, ask the patient to turn the head away from the muscle as it is being palpated. The shoulder will appear depressed in repose and will wing somewhat with TPZ weakness. This will be accentuated with the arm abducted. Also, TPZ is needed to elevate the arm above horizontal because the supraspinatus and deltoid can only abduct the arm to approximately horizontal. To test muscle strength of the upper part of the TPZ, patients should be asked to shrug their shoulders.

Hypoglossal Nerve (CN XII)

The hypoglossal nerve is a mixed nerve that innervates the tongue. The nucleus lies in the medulla beneath the floor of the fourth ventricle. It innervates all muscles of the tongue except the palatoglossus, which is innervated by the vagus. The sensory portion of the hypoglossal nerve is concerned chiefly with tactile information and is therefore important for chewing, swallowing, and articulation. By having patients protrude their tongue, the tongue's motor function is tested. Unilateral lesions of CN XII lead to unilateral wasting, deviation of the tongue toward the weak side, and fasciculation. To test patients' strength, have them push the tongue against the inside of their cheek, lateral to the mouth while the examiner resists the pressure. With practice, the examiner should develop an appreciation of what is within the normal range. With UMN lesions, tongue movements are slower and weaker, particularly with lateral extension. In severe bilateral UMN lesions, as in ALS, the tongue may have relatively good bulk but is essentially immobile with attempted volitional movement. When the patient gags or yawns, however, greater degrees of tongue movement may become apparent. This disassociation between volitional movement and reflex movement indicates that although substantial loss of the corticobulbar tracts may have occurred, the intrinsic bulbar reflex pathways are still relatively intact.

Motor Examination

The goal of the motor examination is an assessment of the function of the motor unit and the various direct and indirect motor pathways. For the ambulatory patient this begins with an inspection of the posture of the limbs and a visual assessment of the bulk of the musculature. For example, fixed postures across joints (contractures) may be indicative of long-standing lesions of the UMN. The presence of hammer toes generally indicates long-standing LMN loss of the extensors of the toes leading to unopposed toe flexion. In essence, one's resting posture is an unfailing indicator of the combined descending forces acting through the motor unit.

After the inspection and palpation of the limbs and muscles at rest, the tone of muscles is tested by passively stretching them. Increased muscle tone or hypertonicity can manifest as spasticity, the characteristic "clasp-knife" tone seen in corticospinal tract lesions, or "rigidity" as seen in Parkinson's disease. Reduced muscle tone, or hypotonicity, is observed with acute cerebellar lesions. It is useful to observe the outstretched arms with the hands supinated while the patient closes the eyes. A "pronator drift" (the drift of the hand to pronation) indicates a subtle corticospinal tract lesion. An upward or outward drift of the arm may be an indication of a sensory system lesion, demonstrating that with the eyes closed, the brain no longer "knows" where the limb is in space.

After the bulk and tone are assessed, the strength and speed of individual muscles are tested. Numerous grading scales are used but one of the most common is the Medical Research Council's (1946) muscle strength scale in which muscle strength is graded on a 0 to 5 scale:

0 No contraction
1 Flicker or trace of contraction
2 Active movement, with gravity eliminated
3 Active movement against gravity
4 Active movement against gravity and resistance
5 Normal power

Sensory Examination

Primary somatosensory (bodily senses) modalities include (1) *discriminative touch*, which is required for recognition of size, shape, and texture of objects; (2) *proprioception*, which gives us the sense of static and dynamic position of body parts; (3) *nociception*, which signals pain and itch; and (4) *temperature* (warmth and cold). Discriminative touch and proprioception afferents are carried in the dorsal spinal column onto the thalamus, whereas nociceptive and temperature fibers run in the anterolateral spinal system on their way to the thalamus.

Primary sensory information ascends from the periphery through the spinal cord and brainstem to the thalamus in several tracts that differ in the type of information encoded. Thalamocortical fibers relay the information to the relevant cortex. In a patient without sensory complaints, this part of the exam is often limited to the detection of light touch (with a wisp of cotton) and pain (pinprick on the face and the distal aspects of the hands and feet). Additionally, vibration sense and position sense are tested in the fingers and toes. In a patient with sensory complaints, the examination would be more detailed with an attempt made to determine the distribution, nature, and degree of anesthesia.

If the lesion involves the sensory cortex or the thalamocortical radiations, a different type of sensory defect is produced. Although the ability to detect the "primary" sensations of light touch, pinprick, and vibration may not be impaired, the ability to perform certain other sensory tasks will be. Two-point discrimination can be tested with the two points of a compass, for example. The patient is asked if the examiner has touched the skin with one or two points. Normally, we can detect two distinct points separated by several millimeters on the fingertips. For a shorter distance, the two points are experienced as one. On the back or trunk, however, a several-centimeter distance or longer is needed to make this distinction. The ability to detect letters or numbers written on the palm or fingertips is referred to as "graphesthesia." Finally, the ability to recognize objects placed in the hands by virtue of their shape and texture is called "stereognosis." These abilities are also impaired with sensory lesions at, or rostral to, the thalamus.

Reflexes

The examination of reflexes provides important objective information about the integrity of the nervous system in two ways. First, most reflexes are mediated by monosynaptic or oligosynaptic (a few synapses) pathways that have afferent arcs outside the CNS, that enter the CNS, and that have efferent arcs that mediate a motor function in the periphery. Thus, the integrity of the nervous system in a "horizontal" sense can be assessed with the tap of a tendon.

For example, tapping on the triceps tendon at the elbow produces an afferent volley in the radial nerve that enters the spinal cord through the C7 dorsal root. The large sensory nerve fibers mediating the reflex synapse directly on lower motor neurons also in the C7 spinal cord segment. These are induced to fire and an efferent volley goes down some of the LMN destined to innervate the triceps, producing the triceps contraction. If the peripheral nerve, the dorsal or ventral root, or the spinal cord segment itself is damaged, the reflex may be abolished or reduced.

The second kind of information that reflexes provide is in a vertical sense. The briskness of a reflex is determined by the descending corticospinal tract tone. An UMN lesion produces hyperreflexia below the level of the lesion. In other words, a midthoracic spinal cord lesion would produce hyperreflexia, or exaggerated reflexes, in the legs, but the reflexes in the arms and cranial innervated structures would remain normal. Similarly, a unilateral corticospinal tract lesion at the level of the frontal lobe would be expected to produce hyperreflexia in all contralateral muscles that receive its projections. This is the most common scenario following a cerebral infarct producing contralateral hemiparesis.

Gait and Station

The assessment of gait and station is an essential part of the neurologic examination, which may provide significant information about many different areas of the nervous system. Standing upright is possible only with adequate proprioceptive information concerning the location of the body and limbs in space, muscular power to maintain the erect posture, and vestibular and visual input to centers involved in "righting reflexes." Locomotion involves voluntary sequential firing of leg flexors and extensors as well as involuntary or "unconscious" input to the arms, legs, and trunk muscles from cortical structures such as the frontal lobe. A detailed discussion of the physiology of gait is beyond the scope of this chapter, but some examples of the insight provided by an examination of the gait are useful.

Hemiparetic Gait

The involved leg is slow and weaker, particularly in movements involving flexion of the hip and dorsiflexion of the foot. This results in patients' circumducting the leg in an attempt to avoid a premature strike of the toe. There is decreased arm swing on the involved side, and the arm may be held flexed and abducted.

Sensory Ataxic Gait

Sensory ataxic gait is an ataxic gait owing to polyneuropathy—damage to multiple peripheral nerves—or spinal cord disease. Without having a precise knowledge of the position of the feet and limbs, the patient needs a widened stance. The individual movements of the legs are exaggerated in force and degree. The visual system may provide a partial compensation for these deficits; that is, watching the ground may help compensate for the loss of proprioceptive information. Consequently, under these circumstances, the gait worsens in low light situations or when the eyes are closed. A similar gait is seen in disease affecting the portions of the cerebellum that normally coordinate the gait.

Parkinsonian Gait

The gait in parkinsonism is fairly stereotypic. The patient stands somewhat stooped with the head forward and the arms slightly flexed. The steps are shortened and perhaps shuffling. There is decreased arm swing and the patient may "festinate," that is, involuntarily speed up and begin to shuffle forward (propulsion) or backward (retropulsion). In severe parkinsonism, these abnormalities, as well as the loss of "righting reflexes," may make independent ambulation impossible.

Myopathic Gait

If there is sufficient weakness of the hip flexors and other muscles of the pelvic girdle, the patient manifests a waddling gait. Normally, when one is walking, the gluteal muscles on the weight-bearing leg elevate the contralateral hemipelvis slightly to allow the free forward swing of the non–weight-bearing leg. If these muscles are weak, when the patient walks, the pelvis tilts downward on the side of the free-swinging leg, producing a waddling from side to side. This same abnormality occurs in neurogenic weakness if it prominently affects the hip girdle muscles, particularly the gluteus medius.

Coordination

Coordination primarily is a function of the cerebellum. Acute cerebellar hemispheric lesions produce a constellation of signs ipsilateral to the lesion: hypotonia, ataxia, tremor, and a slight amount of weakness. These signs often improve over time. Two common tests of cerebellar function are the "finger–nose–finger" test (in which patients alternately touch the examiner's finger, their own nose, the examiner's finger, etc.), and the "heel–shin" test (in which patients carefully slide their heel along the contralateral tibia from knee to ankle). The cerebellum is vital for the motor control of coordinated movement. With cerebellar lesions, there is decomposition of the planned movement. In the "heel–shin" test, for example, one might see jerky movements that represent abnormalities in the degree, duration, and timing of the contraction of the quadriceps (as the heel slides distally), and the relaxation of the hamstrings and iliopsoas muscles.

✦ Common Neurologic Tests

Electrophysiologic Tests

Electroencephalography (EEG) and electromyography (EMG) are both diagnostic testing modalities based on the fact that nerve cells and muscle are electrically active tissues. They maintain measurable voltages (potentials) across their membranes at rest and generate changes in these potentials as a means of integrating and communicating information to and from other cells. EEG and EMG exploit these properties for diagnostic purposes.

Electroencephalography

An EEG is a record of brain electrical activity generated by electrodes positioned on the scalp. The electrodes are placed in a standardized format that uses common anatomic landmarks as points of reference. The recorded activity directly reflects the activity of the cortex below, specifically the postsynaptic potentials of the large vertically oriented pyramidal cells (**Fig. 21–1**). Indirectly, though, structural or functional abnormalities of the underlying white matter or of the thalamocortical projections may produce characteristic changes as well.

The EEG is principally used to classify and prognosticate seizure disorders. For example, some EEG patterns are highly reliable signatures of a given epileptic syndrome, and therefore highly predictive of effective treatment with one or another class of anticonvulsants. Certain EEG patterns are suggestive of heritable, though benign and self-limited, seizure disorders. In others, the pattern suggests a severe disorder of brain function and portends a dismal future for the patient.

Generally, a localized "spike and wave," "spikes," or other paroxysmal activities can be suggestive of a seizure focus. The electroencephalographer looks for either the maximal amplitude of the spike discharge or phase reversal of the spike between adjacent electrodes to localize the focus on the underlying brain (**Fig. 21–2**).

An EEG is used in the diagnostic evaluation of spells of altered consciousness, for which the cause may not be obvious on routine history and physical examination. An EEG may differentiate an epileptic from a nonepileptic spell. Factors that improve the diagnostic yield of an EEG in the evaluation of spells of altered consciousness include 24-hour sleep deprivation, sleep, hyperventilation, and photic stimulation. In epileptic patients studied repeatedly over time, at least 90% ultimately demonstrate epileptiform EEG activity (Marsan & Zivin, 1970).

EEG is used in the evaluation of brain death (i.e., the irreversible cessation of brain function). In this circumstance, a "flat" or isoelectric record is obtained (Silverman, Saunders, Schwab, & Masland, 1969). Finally, EEG is used in surgical monitoring of cerebral function, for example, during carotid endarterectomy.

Electromyography and Nerve Conduction Studies

Conventionally, EMG is a test constructed of two parts: the nerve conduction study (NCS) and the needle exam (NE), which is, strictly speaking, the electromyogram. Nerve conduction studies are capable of assessing peripheral motor and sensory nerve function, as well as that of the neuromuscular junction.

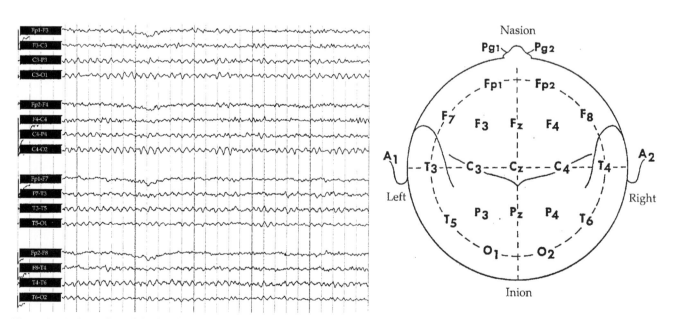

Figure 21–1 The outline of the head, seen from above, shows the standardized placement of electrodes according to the International 10–20 system. The EEG record indicates a normal 16-channel EEG recorded in an anterior to posterior bipolar montage.

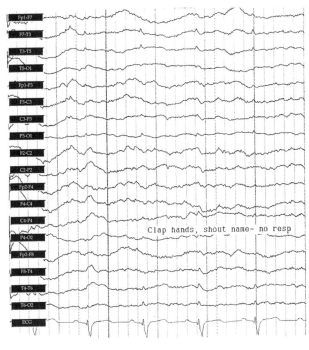

Clap hands, shout name- no resp

A

Figure 21–2 (A) Electroencephalogram (EEG) in severe diffuse encephalopathy. The bottom line is the electrocardiogram (ECG). Note that the record is characterized by slow irregular activity that is unresponsive to loud clapping and calling the patient's voice. Note also that some of the sharper waveforms are actually ECG artifact. **(B)** A focal onset secondary generalized seizure. Note that rhythmic activity begins in the right temporal area and subsequently spreads to involve the whole brain. The dark sharp lines on the right side of the record are motor/muscle artifact caused by the onset of tonic-clonic activity in the muscles of the head and face.

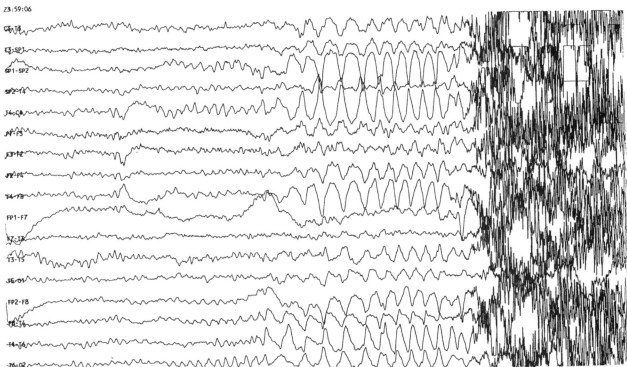

B

Although peripheral nerves are found in a wide variety of diameters, only the large myelinated (and hence rapidly conducting) fibers are measured using most conventional techniques. Essentially, the smaller fibers generate such small signals that, without special techniques, they are lost in the "noise."

To understand the NCS changes seen in pathologic conditions, it is useful to imagine a plastic-covered telephone wire as a model for a myelinated nerve fiber. The central copper wire is analogous to the axon. It carries the information encoded in the electrical current; if it is severed, the call is lost. The plastic coating, analogous to the myelin sheath synthesized by the Schwann cell, provides for isolation and insulation of the line. If the plastic sheath is damaged, there can be cross talk or "shorts" between wires. Additionally, in myelinated nerve fibers (but not phone lines), the relationship between the normal sheath and the axon it envelops is vital for normal conduction. If the myelin sheath is damaged, conduction in the axon may slow or cease altogether, something known as "conduction block."

The NCS is generally performed by percutaneously stimulating an accessible portion of peripheral nerve and simultaneously recording from a proximal or distal portion of the nerve or a muscle innervated by the nerve. In the case of

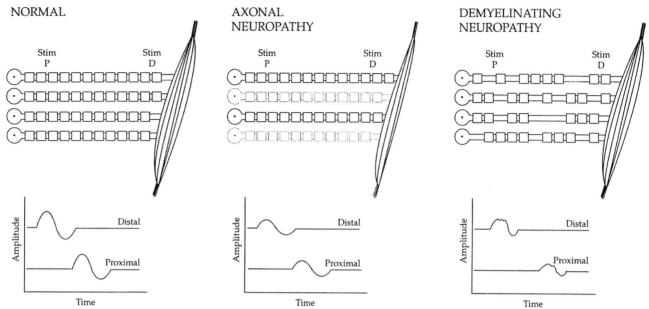

NORMAL   AXONAL
                         NEUROPATHY

DEMYELINATING
NEUROPATHY

Figure 21–3 (A) A stylized motor nerve conduction study. The four myelinated nerves are stimulated distally and proximally to yield the two traces shown below. The compound motor unit action potential (CMAP) is the summed electrical potential of the four individual motor unit action potentials. The amplitude and latencies of the responses are usually recorded. **(B)** In axonal neuropathies, or in any axon loss lesion, the loss of axons leads to a loss of muscle bulk and hence a loss of the summed individual action potentials. Note that the latencies and therefore the calculated conduction velocity are relatively spared. **(C)** In demyelinating neuropathies the random multifocal loss of internodes of myelin leads to the unpredictable slowing in individual nerve fibers. The third fiber from the top has lost too many internodes to conduct and fails to activate its muscle fibers. The resulting waveforms are therefore delayed, "dispersed," or notched because of the temporal dissynchronization of the individual motor unit action potentials, and of lower amplitude because of the complete loss of conduction of one of the nerve fibers.

sensory nerves, the recording is made with applied disk or ring electrodes directly above the nerve. When recording from motor nerves, disk electrodes are placed directly over the muscle innervated by the nerve. The resulting evoked response is actually generated by the muscle itself. Because of these differences, although sensory nerve action potentials are in the microvolt range, motor-evoked responses, representing the depolarization of many grams of electrically excitable muscle tissue, are in the millivolt range. The data obtained using these techniques include conduction velocity, terminal or distal latencies, and measurements of the sensory and motor-evoked response amplitudes.

Disorders of peripheral nerve generate a fairly limited number of abnormalities of these measures despite the limitless number of insults or diseases that can affect them. **Fig. 21–3** illustrates the characteristic abnormalities seen in common disease states.

Axonal Neuropathy In an axonal neuropathy, as individual axons are lost, the number of individual elements participating in the conduction are decreased and the resulting amplitude is diminished. Although **Fig. 21–3B** illustrates a motor fiber with its connection to the muscle, the situation is exactly analogous to a sensory conduction. Because axonal disease does not involve the Schwann cell (i.e., the myelin sheath), the distal latency and conduction velocity are relatively spared. The results are summarized in **Table 21–1**.

Demyelinating Neuropathy As can be seen from **Fig. 21–3**, in an acquired multifocal demyelinating neuropathy (e.g., the Guillain-Barré syndrome), with proximal stimulation, individual motor unit action potentials may be delayed. This has several consequences. First, the terminal latency can be

delayed, and the resulting conduction velocity will be slowed. Second, as the individual motor unit action potentials are delayed, the resulting compound motor unit action potential (CMAP) is less synchronous with respect to time. As the individual motor unit action potentials are temporally dispersed, their positive and negative phases begin to cancel electrically. This results in a CMAP that is of lower amplitude and potentially spread out with respect to time or "temporally dispersed."

A "conduction block" of that axon may take place if the process causing the demyelinating neuropathy damages a sufficient portion of the myelin sheath. In essence, while still alive and functioning in many ways, the individual motor fiber may cease to participate in voluntary contraction of the muscle. This manifests clinically as weakness.

Focal Neuropathy The NCS are very useful for detecting focal neuropathies, and the carpal tunnel syndrome (CTS) is a common and prototypical example. Carpal tunnel syndrome represents the clinical manifestations of a median nerve

Table 21–1 Nerve Conduction Findings in Peripheral Neuropathy

Type of Neuropathy	Terminal Latency	Conduction Velocity	Amplitude
Axonal	Normal or slightly decreased	Normal or slightly decreased	Reduced
Demyelinating	Increased	Decreased	Normal or slightly decreased

compression as it passes through a bony tunnel of wrist bones with nine flexor tendons. The roof of this tunnel is an unyielding sheet of connective tissue. If for any reason the space needed by the nerve is compromised (e.g., by edematous swelling of the contents of the tunnel during pregnancy), the myelin sheaths of the median nerve axons may become sufficiently distorted to cause conduction slowing, conduction block, or, when extreme, axonal loss. These three features are seen in median neuropathies at the wrist and essentially all other focal neuropathies as severity progresses.

Tests of Neuromuscular Transmission   In the previous figures illustrating the effects of demyelination and conduction block on the measured aspects of motor nerve conduction, the NMJ was omitted for simplicity. Several disorders of neuromuscular transmission are of great clinical relevance to the neurologist and SLP. The most common and prototypical disorder of neuromuscular transmission is myasthenia gravis (MG). MG is characterized by fatigable weakness of striated muscle caused by dysfunction at the NMJ. It may present as and be confined to the extraocular muscles, causing ptosis and diplopia. In more severe cases it may involve all axial and appendicular muscles including those of swallowing, speaking, and breathing. Myasthenic involvement of swallowing and respiratory function is considered a life-threatening illness.

Several tests of neuromuscular transmission are used to diagnose MG or measure the effect of therapy. Repetitive nerve stimulation (RNS), known as the Jolly test, and single-fiber EMG (SFEMG) are the most common. Before describing these tests, a brief overview of the physiology of neuromuscular transmission will be helpful. When a motor nerve is stimulated, a wave of depolarization proceeds toward the nerve terminal. Close to the terminal, the motor axon branches into many small nerve endings, each of which ends in close apposition to a single muscle fiber. When the wave of depolarization proceeds to the end of each nerve terminal, the resulting voltage change induces an influx of calcium from the extracellular space. The rise in calcium concentration at the nerve terminal causes the release of many membrane-bound packets of the neurotransmitter acetylcholine (ACh) into the synaptic cleft. The ACh quickly diffuses across the cleft and binds to postsynaptic ACh receptors (AChRs) on the muscle fiber. When a molecule of ACh binds to the AChR, a conformational change occurs in the receptor that causes a small depolarization of the muscle membrane to take place. There are many AChRs on the muscle membrane, and if enough are stimulated, the small

depolarizations of the muscle membrane summate and cause the muscle fiber to reach threshold. At threshold, a muscle fiber action potential takes place. As the muscle fiber depolarizes along its whole length, it begins to contract and generate force, a process known as "excitation-contraction coupling."

MG is an autoimmune disease characterized by the production of autoantibodies to the postsynaptic AChR. When the antibody binds to the receptor, it causes its premature destruction. Thus, in MG there is a paucity of functionally useful AChR.

One other fact must be appreciated to understand the physiology of fatigable weakness in MG. When the nerve terminal depolarizes and the waiting packets of ACh are released into the synaptic cleft, there is a normal diminution of the number of packets released with each successive stimulation. If the first stimulation induced the release of, say, 100 packets, by the fourth stimulation perhaps 50 would be released. Under normal circumstances 50 would be more than enough to produce a muscle action potential, but in MG, if a large percentage of AChRs have been destroyed or are nonfunctional because of antibody attack, the 50 packets of ACh may be inadequate to cause the depolarization of the muscle fiber. The failure to depolarize is manifested clinically as weakness.

In the technique of RNS, stimulating electrodes are placed on a motor nerve and recording electrodes on a muscle supplied by the motor nerve. Four to 10 shocks at 2 to 3 Hz (aptly named repetitive stimulation) are given, and the amplitude of the evoked motor responses is measured at the first and fourth stimulation. Amplitude decrements of greater than 10% are considered pathologic and suggestive of a defect in neuromuscular transmission (**Fig. 21–4**).

Single-fiber EMG is a more sensitive and more complex test used to detect defects of neuromuscular transmission. The patient is asked to barely activate a muscle while a special needle electrode is maneuvered until two spike potentials firing "simultaneously" are identified. With normal neuromuscular transmission, the variation in time with consecutive discharges between the firing of the first potential and the second is extremely small, on the order of 20 to 45 microseconds (**Fig. 21–5**). The measurement of this variability is called "jitter." The reduced reliability of neuromuscular transmission in MG leads to an increased variability or jitter in the firing of a given muscle fiber action potential with respect to a second fiber from the same motor unit. Sometimes the firing of the second fiber fails altogether, an event termed "blocking." SFEMG is abnormal in greater than 95% of patients with generalized MG.

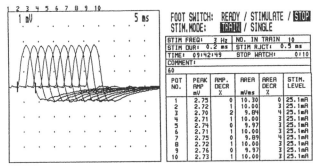

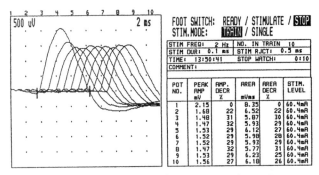

A

B

Figure 21–4 (A) A normal repetitive nerve conduction, or Jolly test. The CMAPs were recorded from the hypothenar muscle while the ulnar nerve was stimulated at 3 Hz. Note that each waveform differed in amplitude or area by less than 4%. **(B)** This Jolly test was performed on a patient with myasthenia gravis (at 2 Hz in this case). Note that with repetitive stimulation there is a marked reduction of amplitude, most prominent from the first to the second potential and reaching a nadir with the fourth stimulation. See the text for an explanation of this phenomenon.

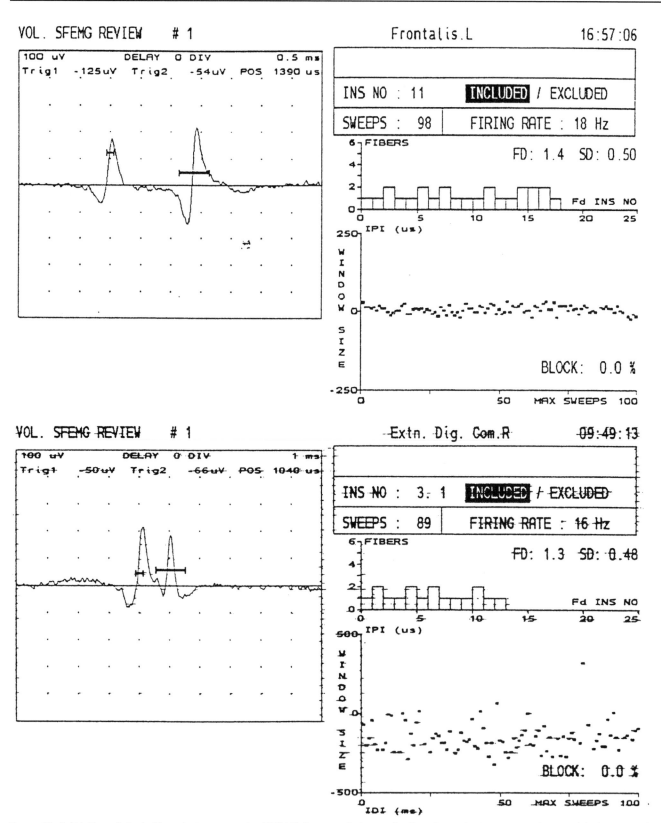

Figure 21–5 (A) Normal single-fiber electromyography (SFEMG) from the frontalis muscle. The two spikes represent the potentials from two individual muscle fibers of the same motor unit. The bold horizontal lines crossing the potentials above the baseline represent "triggers" (voltage thresholds for the computer program to recognize) for the display of the potential and the calculation of when the second spike fires relative to the first. From the interpotential interval (IPI) seen in the graph in the lower right, a calculation is made of the "jitter," or variability between the firing of the first and second muscle fibers. Most of this variability results from neuromuscular transmission. In this case the jitter was 11 μsec (normal is < 45 μsec). **(B)** This abnormal SFEMG from a patient with MG demonstrated jitter of 99 μsec.

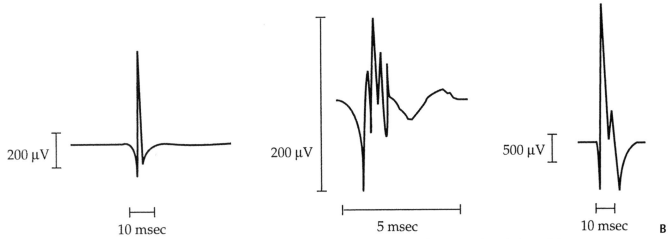

A   B

Figure 21–6 (A) Normal motor unit. **(B)** "Myopathic" motor unit. It is of low amplitude, short duration, and is polyphasic. **(C)** "Neurogenic" motor unit. It is of high amplitude, long duration, and is polyphasic. Note voltage scale.

The Role of the Needle Exam in Electromyography The needle exam (NE) is an essential part of the EMG, providing vital information on the function of the motor unit. If there is weakness from a disorder of the motor unit, the NE should be able to detect it. Even in weakness owing to disorders of the UMN, abnormalities of diagnostic significance are often apparent (e.g., changes in motor unit firing patterns or frequencies).

The NE involves the insertion of a small needle electrode into the muscle of interest. The tip of the needle acts as the recording electrode from within the muscle, and the activity is displayed on a video monitor. EMG machines assign sounds to the wave forms based on their morphologies. The question asked of the electromyographer determines which muscles will be sampled. Laryngeal EMG, both percutaneously and endoscopically performed, is becoming more common in the United States. **Fig. 21–6** illustrates characteristic findings during the needle exam.

Another method of directly obtaining information regarding the electrical activity of muscle during the EMG is by recording the surface activity of muscles (SEMG). In SEMG, the active recording electrode is placed over the belly of the muscle and the reference electrode is placed along a tendinous insertion. SEMG is insensitive to whether a muscle is denervated or whether the muscle has myopathic or neurogenic features, but it is able to provide other kinds of useful information.

SEMG is used in several clinical and research situations. It is particularly useful in "central EMG," studying the patterns and timing of muscle activation in movement disorders or other disorders of central motor control. SEMG can also be used to provide auditory or visual signals for biofeedback.

Transcranial Doppler Ultrasonography

Transcranial Doppler (TCD) ultrasonography is a noninvasive ultrasound technique that was first introduced for use in clinical practice in 1982 (Aaslid, Markwalder, & Nornes, 1982). It measures cerebral blood flow indirectly by assessing local cerebral blood flow velocity (CBF-V) in the major cerebral arteries (**Fig. 21–7**).

TCD is used primarily in the management of patients with ischemic and hemorrhagic cerebrovascular disease. Furthermore, TCD can assist in the evaluation of patients with

suspected malformations such as cerebral aneurysm or arteriovenous malformations (AVM). Also, TCD can assist in the evaluation of cerebral vasospasm, which may be posttraumatic or which follows aneurysmal subarachnoid hemorrhage (SAH). Lastly, TCD is a complementary test to the neurologic examination and EEG in assessing brain death. TCD has the advantages of being (1) noninvasive; (2) portable; (3) repeatable, providing continuous measurements; and (4) inexpensive. The disadvantages of TCD are that (1) measurements of CBF-V can be done in major arteries only; (2) the assessment is operator dependent; and (3) it is dependent on early-insonated bone windows, which are not always the case.

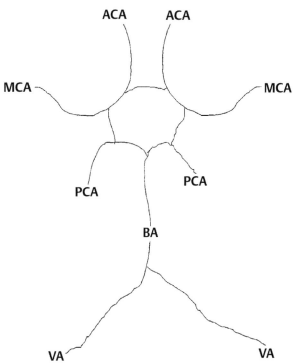

Figure 21–7 Diagrammatic representation of the circle of Willis showing the arteries that are studied by transcranial Doppler (TCD). MCA, middle cerebral artery; ACA, anterior cerebral artery; PCA, posterior cerebral artery; BA, basilar artery; VA, vertebral artery.

A recent report of the therapeutic and technology assessment subcommittee of the American Academy of Neurology (AAN) (Sloan, Alexandrov, Tegeler, Spencer, Caplan, Feldmann, Wechsler, Newell, Gomez, Babikian, Lefkowitz, Goldman, Armon, Hsu, & Goodin, 2004) indicated that TCD has an established utility in the following clinical situations:

1. Screening of children and adolescents with sickle cell disease to assess for risk of ischemic stroke.
2. Detection and monitoring of vasospasm following subarachnoid hemorrhage.

The TCD's clinical utility in the following situations remains to be determined: (1) intracranial steno-occlusive disease; (2) brain death evaluations; (3) monitoring thrombolytic therapy; (4) embolism detection; (5) monitoring during carotid endarterectomy (CEA) and coronary bypass surgery; (6) evaluation and monitoring of mass effect following middle cerebral artery infarcts; and (7) evaluation of impaired cerebral hemodynamics distal to a stenotic large cerebral vessel. The committee indicated that TCD has limited value in comparison to other methods in right-to-left cardiac shunt evaluation and in the evaluation of extracranial internal carotid artery stenosis.

Imaging Studies

The field of neuroimaging has substantially expanded in the past 25 years with the advent of computed axial tomography (CT scan) in the early 1970s and magnetic resonance imaging (MRI) in the early 1980s. In addition, cerebral angiography remains a cornerstone in the evaluation of patients with cerebrovascular disease.

Computed Tomography Scan

This technique is an x-ray computerized method used to identify abnormal structures based on (1) tissue electron density differences and contrasts; (2) displacement of normal structures; and (3) enhancement properties. Generally, structures that do not attenuate the x-ray signal are hypodense or black on CT. An example would be water or cerebrospinal fluid (CSF). On the other hand, tissues that maximally attenuate the x-ray beam are hyperdense or white on CT; a good example of a hyperdense tissue is bone. Brain and spinal cord tissue density lies between these two extremes; they appear gray on CT images. Conditions that increase the water content of brain tissue (e.g., ischemic stroke or cerebral edema) render the CT image hypodense (dark).

Alternatively, stagnant blood appears white because of its higher density than that of brain tissue or spinal cord. **Table 21–2** lists the density characteristics of normal brain tissue and some commonly seen abnormalities. Occasionally, the contents of an abnormal brain or spinal cord lesion have the same density (isodense) as that of the surrounding tissue. Thus, the CT image is not able to give us the contrast needed to identify that lesion, unless additional information is obtained. In such instances, close attention to disruption of the normal nervous system anatomy and the topographic relationship of different brain or spinal cord structures, and/or unusual enhancement following the administration of a contrast agent (usually an iodine-based compound that appears white on CT) may delineate the sought-for abnormality.

Table 21–2 Normal and Abnormal Computed Tomography (CT) Scans

CT Image	Example
Normal	Minor head injury; pseudotumor
High density	Cerebral hemorrhage; calcium-containing lesions (e.g., tuberous sclerosis)
Mixed density	Malignant brain tumors
Isodensity	Isodense subdural hematoma; benign tumors; low-grade glioma
Low density	Cerebral infarct; cysts; lipid-containing lesions; MS plaque

CT scanning is an important tool in the diagnostic evaluation of many neurologic conditions (**Table 21–3**). Most patients with one of these conditions/diseases are better evaluated with MRI than with CT for reasons described below; demonstration of fresh blood (<24 hours) and fractures may be the exceptions. CT scanning is more commonly used and more readily available than MRI because it is less expensive and quicker to perform. Also, CT scanning has the advantage over MRI in the hyperacute setting of cerebral hemorrhage. Spiral CT angiography (CTA) is a newer imaging technique that reconstructs three-dimensional (3D) images of cerebral vessels using rapid injection of intravenous contrast and helical CT scanning. CTA is useful when MR studies are contraindicated.

Magnetic Resonance Imaging

The technique of MRI depends on the mobile hydrogen concentration in tissues. Also, MRI can visualize blood vessels and fluid flow (spinal fluid or blood), and analyze tissue chemistry (magnetic resonance spectroscopy). The MRI signal is a function of deflected mobile hydrogen atoms, relaxation times referred to as T1 (longitudinal relaxation time) and T2 (transverse relaxation time), MR pulse sequences (e.g., T1-weighted and T2-weighted images), imaging protocol, and the MRI system used. The dependence on proton density, T1, and T2 allows for variable image contrast utilizing different pulse sequences. Moreover, the multiplanar capability of MR permits us to optimize the imaging plane for better anatomic

Table 21–3 Indications for CT or Magnetic Resonance Imaging (MRI) Scan in the Neurologic Workup

Condition/Disease	Examples
Cerebrovascular disease	Ischemic stroke; cerebral hemorrhage
Infections	Toxoplasmosis; brain abscess
Neoplastic disease (tumors)	
Primary benign brain tumors	Meningioma
Primary malignant brain tumors	Glioblastoma multiforme
Metastatic brain tumors	Melanoma
Spinal cord tumors	Schwannoma; metastatic breast cancer
Demyelinating disease	Multiple sclerosis
Head trauma	Contusion; fractures
Congenital malformations	Chiari; cerebral cysts

localization. Flow-sensitive pulse sequences and MR angiography provide blood flow information and reveal vascular anatomy. FLAIR (fluid-attenuated inversion recovery) imaging is T2-weighting with a suppressed CSF signal.

On T1-weighted images, CSF is hypointense and white matter is hyperintense relative to gray matter. This translates into an image where CSF is black, gray matter is dark gray, and white matter is light gray. In contrast, T2-weighted images show a white CSF signal and a gray matter signal that is lighter (more hyperintense) than that of white matter. Generally, abnormalities that increase mobile tissue water darken the T1- and lighten the T2-weighted image (e.g., ischemic stroke). On the other hand, subacute and chronic hemorrhage appears white (hyperintense) on both pulse sequences.

Contrast material is used with MRI to provide tissue contrast enhancement. The most commonly used MRI contrast agent is gadopentetate dimeglumine (gadolinium or Gd-DTPA), which does not cross the blood–brain barrier unless defective, and which shortens T1 and T2.

MRI is more sensitive than CT in detecting most brain and spinal cord abnormalities. It provides a better delineation of normal and abnormal tissues and is particularly suitable in evaluating the brainstem where CT scanning has a relatively limited value.

The indications for MRI are listed in **Table 21–3**. MRI is certainly more advantageous than CT in identifying multiple sclerosis (MS) plaques, lesions in the brainstem, early ischemic strokes (infarcts), acoustic neuromas (tumors of the eighth cranial nerve), pituitary tumors, and spinal cord cavities. MRI is very helpful in determining the age of a cerebral hemorrhage. Vascular malformations, aneurysms, and arterial occlusion are well delineated on MRI. Also, MR angiography (MRA) and the related MR venography (MRV) are noninvasive techniques that allow the visualization of arteries and veins without injecting a dye in the vessels. On MRA, arterial stenosis or occlusion, AVMs, aneurysms, and venous thrombosis are very well seen. Finally, intravenous Gd-DTPA is more sensitive than CT contrast in identifying small metastatic tumors.

Conventional Angiography

This technique was introduced in clinical medicine over 60 years ago and remains very valuable in the evaluation of patients with neurologic complaints. Cerebral and spinal angiography are performed under local anesthesia; spinal angiography is rarely performed. The procedure involves the percutaneous (across the skin) introduction of a catheter in the arterial tree (most commonly the femoral artery) and, guided by x-ray images, the injection of a dye at the desired site. The radiopaque dye highlights the injected vessel and hence permits the detection of abnormalities in the cerebral arterial or venous system. This invasive radiologic procedure carries a small risk of complications that include stroke, infection, or blood clot formation at the site of the cannulation (introduction of the catheter), or even death from a severe allergic reaction (anaphylaxis) to the dye.

Cerebral angiography is the mainstay of diagnosis of stenotic disease of the major cerebral arteries. It is also indicated in the evaluation of patients with suspected venous sinus thrombosis, although MR venography is proven equally sensitive. Angiography is also used in the diagnosis of AVMs, aneurysms, and inflammation of the blood vessels (vasculitis). Cerebral arteriography is superior to MRA in detecting intracranial arterial stenosis and small cerebral aneurysms. Arterial vasospasm can be appreciated on TCD (see above) but is best delineated on angiography.

Positron Emission Tomography

Positron emission tomography (PET) is molecular imaging test that measures metabolic activity. As such, PET is a functional imaging technique. PET imaging makes use of short-lived radiotracers to locate areas of brain activity at rest and during mental exercise. PET may detect pathology before it becomes visible with CT or MR because metabolic changes usually precede anatomic ones. PET can detect neurochemicals such as fluorine 18 (^{18}F)-DOPA and is indicated in the differential diagnosis of dementia.

✦ Neurologic Diseases and Their Management

A thorough review of neurologic diseases and their management is beyond the scope of this chapter. The following topics are meant to introduce the nonneurologist to the common and major categories of neurologic disease. For more specific information, the reader is referred to comprehensive texts in the area (Adams, Victor, & Ropper, 1997; Bradley, Daroff, Marsden, & Fenichel, 1996).

Cerebrovascular Diseases

Stroke is the third most common cause of death and the leading cause of disability in the United States (Bowler & Hachinski, 1996; Davis & Torner, 1996). The annual prevalence of stroke in the United States is over 600,000, and one third of these patients die. Stroke is subdivided into ischemic and hemorrhagic (subarachnoid hemorrhage, SAH; intracerebral hemorrhage, ICH). Patients with SAH or ICH are more likely to be severely disabled or die from stroke than those afflicted by cerebral infarction. There is some evidence that the incidence of cerebral infarction is declining partly because of better control of hypertension, but the incidences of ICH and SAH are unchanged.

Cerebral Ischemia

Cerebral ischemia is the most common cause of stroke; 75 to 85% of all strokes are ischemic. Cerebral ischemia could be permanent (i.e., cerebral infarction), or transient (i.e., transient ischemic attack, TIA). Fatality rates for cerebral infarction are less than 10% in subjects under 65 years old and about 20% in older individuals.

Risk factors for cerebral infarction are categorized as nonmodifiable (e.g., age, male gender, Black race, family history of cerebral infarction, previous stroke) or modifiable (atrial fibrillation, hypertension, myocardial infarction, diabetes mellitus, prior TIA, cigarette smoking, excessive alcohol consumption). Oral contraceptive pills, high blood lipids, obesity, and a sedentary lifestyle are risk factors for cerebral infarction in some studies but not in all (Bowler & Hachinski, 1996).

Despite major advances in the investigative studies for cerebral infarction, over 40% of ischemic strokes are of unknown cause ("cryptogenic stroke"). The most commonly identifiable causes of cerebral infarction are (1) atherosclerosis (hardening) of the large arteries supplying the brain; (2) embolism from the heart; and (3) disease of the small cerebral arteries (lacunar disease). Atherosclerosis results in cerebral infarction when a thrombus (a complex lesion that forms on the vessel wall consisting of fatty debris and blood products such as platelets and red blood cells) dislodges from one site of the diseased artery (usually at sites where shear force is maximal, such as the bifurcation of the common carotid artery into the internal and external carotid arteries) and blocks the distal portion of that vessel, preventing nutrients and oxygen from being delivered to the brain tissue. Less commonly, a clot does not dislodge, but the reduction in the large artery diameter at the site of the thrombus is severe enough to hamper flow beyond the point of constriction; this mechanism is known as hemodynamic stroke. Cerebral cardioembolism refers to ischemic strokes caused by emboli that break off from a heart chamber (e.g., left atrium) or valve. These emboli travel in the cerebral blood vessel to a point where they can't move any further and block the delivery of blood flow at that site. Lacunar disease is a condition in which the small vessels that penetrate into the brain substance are constricted or occluded; lacunar disease is caused mostly by hypertension.

Uncommon causes of cerebral infarction include blood clotting abnormalities (e.g., coagulation or platelet disorders), increased blood viscosity, sickle cell disease, migraine, dissection (tear) of the cerebral arteries, use of illicit (cocaine) or licit [oral contraceptives, phenylpropanolamine (found in cough medicines)] substances, and so on (see Tables 1, 4, 7, 8, and 9 in Ramadan & Mitsias, 1996).

Cerebral infarcts and TIAs manifest similarly with one exception: by conventional definition, TIAs last less than 24 hours (Special Report from the National Institute of Neurological Diseases and Stroke, 1990). It is important to note, however, that true TIAs (transient symptoms and signs without any evidence of brain damage) are 2 to 15 minutes in duration; symptoms that last more than 60 minutes are unlikely to reverse (Levy, 1988). The onset of symptoms with cerebral ischemia is usually abrupt. The neurologic deficits are reflections of dysfunctional or nonfunctional brain tissue supplied by the occluded artery (**Table 21–4**). The middle cerebral artery (MCA) territory

is the most common site for cerebral infarcts. Cerebral ischemia is more likely to occur in the anterior [MCA, anterior cerebral artery (ACA)] than the posterior [posterior cerebral artery (PCA), vertebral artery (VA), basilar artery (BA)] cerebral territories.

Acute Management

Optimal blood pressure control (not high but also, and equally important, not too low), control of fluid and/or electrolyte imbalance, adequate oxygenation, and maintenance of euglycemia (normal blood sugar) are some general measures used in caring for the patient with acute ischemic stroke. Patients with significant aphasia, drowsiness, obtundation, and/or brainstem stroke are best kept without food per mouth until it is determined that they are safely able to eat. This precautionary measure is intended to avoid aspiration pneumonia, a common morbidity in patients with acute stroke. Urinary tract infections are best avoided by using condom catheters in men and intermittent catheterization in women, instead of indwelling catheters. Frequent turning in bed helps prevent pressure ulcers. Venodyne boots should be worn and subcutaneous heparin should be administered (unless intravenous heparin is used) to avoid deep venous thrombosis and pulmonary embolism. Stool softeners are also recommended.

Ischemic stroke is a neurologic emergency. Every effort is exerted to evaluate and treat the patient early to avoid irreversible brain damage. Over the past 15 years, a major public awareness campaign was launched to emphasize the seriousness of cerebral ischemia and stress the need for stroke victims to seek medical attention very early. These measures allowed the evaluation of the role of thrombolytics (agents that lyse or dissolve blood clots) in the acute treatment of cerebral infarction. The efforts were fruitful as recombinant tissue plasminogen activator (rt-PA) was demonstrated to be an effective treatment in cerebral ischemia, and became the first Food and Drug Administration (FDA)-approved treatment for ischemic stroke (National Institute of Neurological Disorders and Stroke rt-PA Study Group, 1995). The role of many other drugs in stroke therapy is currently under investigation.

The patient with acute ischemic stroke is best managed in a special care unit (e.g., stroke unit) where continuous neurologic and cardiovascular monitoring is performed by skilled medical personnel. The value of close monitoring is in the early recognition and aggressive management of some of the potentially devastating sequelae of stroke such as cerebral edema or significant hemorrhagic conversion (development of blood in the area of cerebral ischemia).

Medical Prevention

Patients with acute cerebral infarction are prone to ischemic stroke recurrence, particularly in the first few weeks after the initial event and especially in patients with cerebral cardioembolism. In this high-risk group and under special circumstances, anticoagulant therapy (heparin) may be used. Other preventive medical measures include long-term use of oral anticoagulant (e.g., warfarin) or antiplatelets agents such as aspirin, ticlopidine, clopidogrel, and the combination of aspirin and dipyridamole.

In addition to the above medical therapies, patients with ischemic stroke are educated to minimize stroke risk factors (i.e., stop smoking, comply with antihypertensive and/or blood

Table 21–4 Clinical Manifestations of Cerebral Infarction

Arterial Territory	Common Symptoms and Signs
Middle cerebral artery (MCA)	Contralateral weakness and/or sensory loss (face and arm more than leg); aphasia (dominant MCA); neglect; apraxia (nondominant MCA)
Anterior cerebral artery (ACA)	Abulia; contralateral leg weakness and/or sensory loss; urinary incontinence; transcortical motor aphasia (dominant ACA); initial mutism
Posterior cerebral artery (PCA)	Contralateral hemifield loss; visual perceptual problems
Vertebral artery (VA)	Lower cranial nerve dysfunction (hoarseness, double vision, facial paralysis, swallowing difficulty, etc.); dizziness; vertigo; unsteadiness; hiccups; nausea; vomiting
Basilar artery (BA)	Locked-in-syndrome (paralysis from neck down); stupor; coma; oculomotor abnormalities (diplopia, ptosis); abnormal motor movements (chorea, hemiballismus)

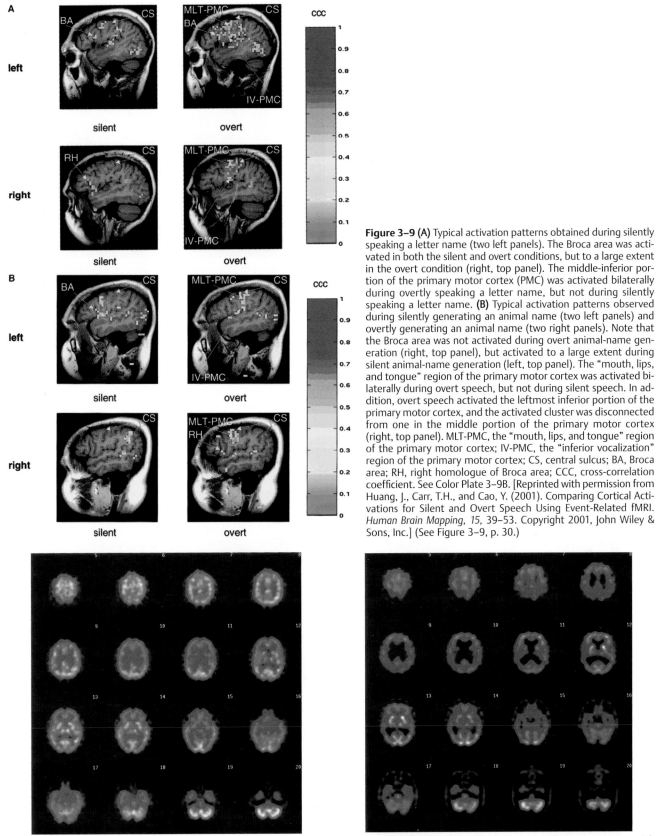

Figure 3–9 (A) Typical activation patterns obtained during silently speaking a letter name (two left panels). The Broca area was activated in both the silent and overt conditions, but to a large extent in the overt condition (right, top panel). The middle-inferior portion of the primary motor cortex (PMC) was activated bilaterally during overtly speaking a letter name, but not during silently speaking a letter name. **(B)** Typical activation patterns observed during silently generating an animal name (two left panels) and overtly generating an animal name (two right panels). Note that the Broca area was not activated during overt animal-name generation (right, top panel), but activated to a large extent during silent animal-name generation (left, top panel). The "mouth, lips, and tongue" region of the primary motor cortex was activated bilaterally during overt speech, but not during silent speech. In addition, overt speech activated the leftmost inferior portion of the primary motor cortex, and the activated cluster was disconnected from one in the middle portion of the primary motor cortex (right, top panel). MLT-PMC, the "mouth, lips, and tongue" region of the primary motor cortex; IV-PMC, the "inferior vocalization" region of the primary motor cortex; CS, central sulcus; BA, Broca area; RH, right homologue of Broca area; CCC, cross-correlation coefficient. See Color Plate 3–9B. [Reprinted with permission from Huang, J., Carr, T.H., and Cao, Y. (2001). Comparing Cortical Activations for Silent and Overt Speech Using Event-Related fMRI. *Human Brain Mapping, 15,* 39–53. Copyright 2001, John Wiley & Sons, Inc.] (See Figure 3–9, p. 30.)

Figure 3–11 Axial SPECT images of cerebral perfusion in a healthy subject obtained using the radiopharmaceutical ⁹⁹ᵐTc-ECD. Notice that perfusion levels in the parietal cortex approach those of the occipital cortex and that the distribution of tracer appears rather smooth. (Courtesy of David Wang.) (See Figure 3–11, p. 32.)

Figure 3–12 Axial SPECT images of cerebral perfusion in a patient with Alzheimer's dementia obtained using the radiopharmaceutical ⁹⁹ᵐTc-ECD. Perfusion in the parietal cortex is significantly reduced compared to that of the occipital cortex. This pattern of perfusion is typical in Alzheimer's type dementia, and is in clear contrast to that seen in healthy individuals (**Fig. 3–11**). (Courtesy of David Wang.) (See Figure 3–12, p. 32.)

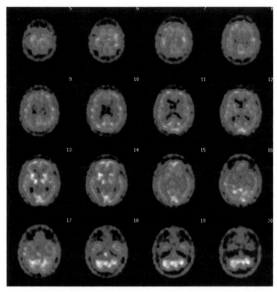

Figure 3–13 Axial SPECT images of cerebral perfusion in a patient with multiinfarct dementia (MID) obtained using the radiopharmaceutical ^{99m}Tc-ECD. Unlike the case of Alzheimer's type dementia (Fig. 3–12), perfusion levels in the parietal cortex approach those of the occipital cortex. The pattern of perfusion, however, appears mottled when compared to the healthy scan (**Fig. 3–11**), a trademark of MID. (Courtesy of David Wang.) (See Figure 3–13, p. 33.)

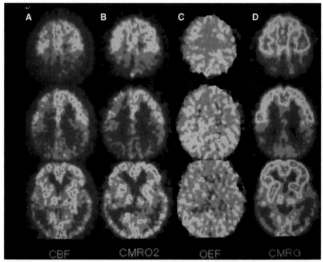

Figure 3–15 Axial PET images of (**A**) cerebral blood flow (CBF), (**B**) cerebral metabolism rate of oxygen (CMRO$_2$), (**C**) oxygen extraction fraction (OEF), and (**D**) cerebral metabolism rate of glucose (CMRG) in a patient with Alzheimer's disease. Significant reductions of CBF and CMRG and moderate reduction of CMRO$_2$ were noted in the parietotemporal region. A slight increase in OEF was observed in the same region. (See Color Plate 3–15.) [From Fukuyama, H., Ogawa, M., Yamauchi, H., Yamaguchi, S., Kimur, J., Yonekura, Y., Konishi, J. (1994). Altered Cerebral Metabolism in Alzheimer's Disease: A PET Study. *Journal of Nuclear Medicine, 35,* 1–6. Copyright 1994, Society of Nuclear Medicine, Inc., with permission.] (See Figure 3–15, p. 34.)

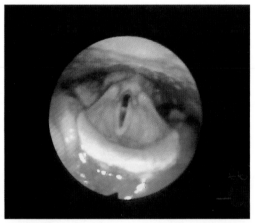

Figure 10–3 Spillage of pureed material before the swallow has begun. The material has spilled nearly to the pyriform recesses without any indication of the swallow initiation, indicating a pharyngeal delay. (See Figure 10–3, p. 153.)

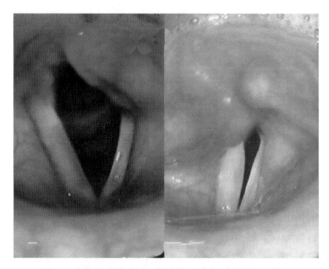

Figure 10–4 Abducted (left) and adducted (right) view of larynx with left laryngeal paralysis. Note the bowing of the affected left vocal fold visible in the abducted view. (See Figure 10–4, p. 153.)

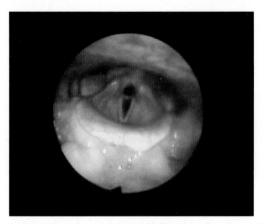

Figure 10–5 Residue of pureed material left in the valleculae and lateral channels after the swallow. (See Figure 10–4, p. 153.)

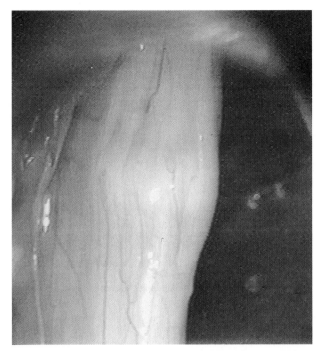

Figure 22–15 Close-up of left vocal fold cyst. (See Figure 22–15B, p. 350.)

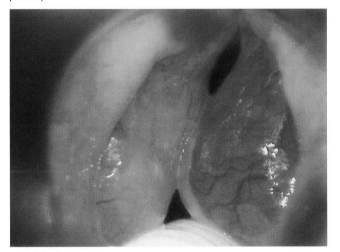

Figure 22–17 Severe polypoid degeneration of both true vocal folds in a long-time smoker. (See Figure 22–17, p. 351.)

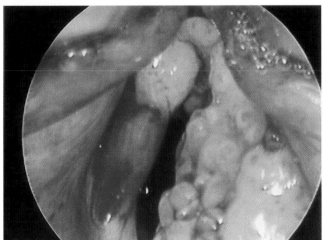

Figure 22–19 Extensive papillomatosis of the larynx in an adult. The entire right true vocal fold and the anterior left true vocal fold are involved. (See Figure 22–19, p. 352.)

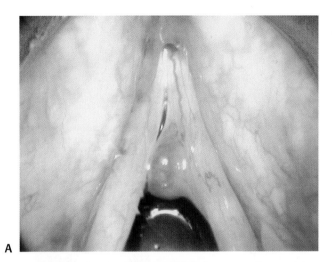

A

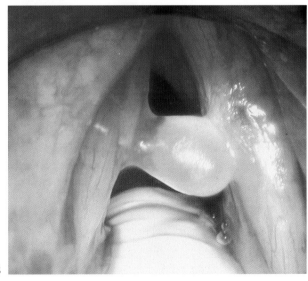

B

Figure 22–16 (A) Hemorrhagic polyp of right vocal fold with obvious enlarged feeding vessel. Also noted are polypoid changes of left anterior false vocal fold. **(B)** Pedunculated polyp of left vocal fold with reactive changes of right vocal fold (partially seen at anterior aspect of polyp on left vocal fold). (See Figure 22–16, p. 351.)

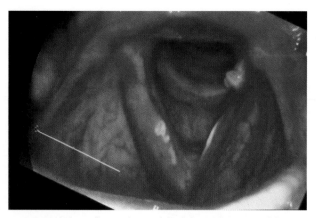

A

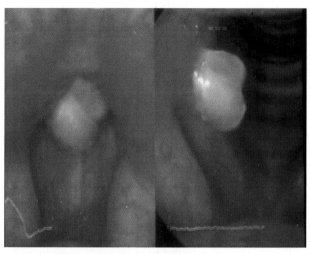

B

Figure 22–20 (A) Small granuloma of the left vocal process of the arytenoid cartilage. Also note thickening of the mucosa overlying the right vocal process and tenacious mucus on the membranous true vocal folds bilaterally. **(B)** A larger right-sided granuloma at the superior aspect of the vocal process. In this patient, the lesion does not impair glottic closure, and the voice was normal. (See Figure 22–20, p. 352.)

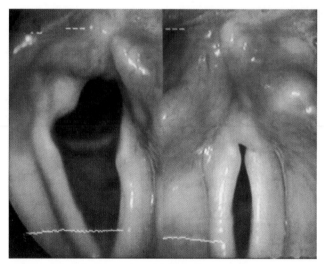

Figure 22–21 Left unilateral vocal fold paralysis: during inspiration with normal abduction of the right vocal fold (left) and during phonation with incomplete glottic closure and a resultant weak breathy voice (right). The etiology was metastatic carcinoma from the bladder to the mediastinum with involvement of the left recurrent laryngeal nerve. (See Figure 22–21, p. 353.)

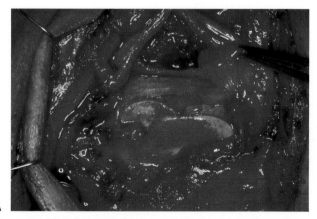

A

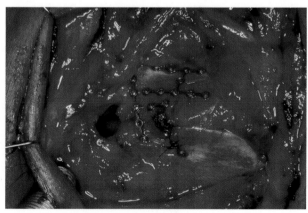

B

Figure 22–22 (A) Multiple fractures of the thyroid cartilage after a motor vehicle accident. The mucosa of the true and false vocal folds was also disrupted (not seen). **(B)** After repair of the mucosal injuries and reconstruction of the cartilaginous framework with microplates. (See Figure 22–22, p. 356.)

Table 21–5 Medical Management of Ischemic Stroke

General Measures	Acute Treatment	Medical Prevention	Risk Factor Control
Adequate oxygenation	rt-PA	Antiplatelet agents	Blood pressure
Blood pressure control	Aggressive treatment of cerebral edema (e.g., mannitol)	Anticoagulants	Diabetes
Control of blood sugar			Exercise
NPO (nothing by mouth) until judged safe			Weight loss
Frequent turning in bed			Lipids
Optimize hemodynamics			Cigarette smoking
Continual monitoring			Excess alcohol

rt-PA, recombinant tissue plasminogen activator.

sugar medications, exercise, avoid excess alcohol use, etc.) (**Table 21–5**).

Surgical Management

Patients with ischemic stroke or TIA in the territory of a severely narrowed (70 to 99%) internal carotid artery are best managed by CEA in addition to the medical therapy described above, provided the surgical risk is low (North American Symptomatic Carotid Endarterectomy Trial Collaborators, 1991). Also, it is suggested that men with asymptomatic stenosis of the internal carotid artery should undergo CEA (Executive Committee for the Asymptomatic Carotid Atherosclerosis Study, 1995). Carotid endarterectomy is a vascular surgery aimed at dissecting out the plaque (lesion composed of fat and blood products) from the diseased carotid artery. Surgical therapy in the posterior circulation is not standard care. Transluminal angioplasty (introduction of a balloon catheter in the artery and expanding the stenosis) and stenting are promising interventions.

Massive cerebral infarction and edema can result in hydrocephalus (increased size of the cerebral ventricles from blockage of CSF flow). Patients with hydrocephalus sometimes require the insertion of shunts into the ventricles to drain CSF. Also, a large infarct can cause brain herniation (displacement of the brain through rigid structures), requiring lobectomy (removal of the cerebral lobe where the infarct occurs) or hemispherectomy (removal of the diseased hemisphere) in rare instances. Finally, cerebellar ischemic strokes may be devastating unless a cerebellectomy is performed and the infarcted cerebellar hemisphere surgically removed.

Intracerebral Hemorrhage

Intracerebral hemorrhage (ICH) accounts for 5 to 10% of all strokes in the United States and 20 to 30% in Japan (Davis & Torner, 1996). The mortality rate of ICH declined dramatically from 90% in 1945–1974 to less than 50% in the 1980s (Broderick,

Table 21–6 Nonhypertensive Causes of Nontraumatic Intracerebral Hemorrhage (ICH)

Cause	Example
Blood vessels abnormality	Amyloid angiopathy; arteriovenous malformation (AVM); aneurysms; moyamoya disease
Blood abnormality	Leukemia; clotting factor deficiency; platelet dysfunction
Medications	Anticoagulants; thrombolytics; sympathomimetics (e.g., diet pills)
Illicit drugs	Cocaine; amphetamines (speed); heroin and opiates
Brain tumors	Melanoma; choriocarcinoma; lung and renal cancer; glioblastoma

Phillips, Whisnant, O'Fallon, & Bergstralh, 1989). Most ICH-related deaths occur in the first week of the event, a reflection of devastating complications such as brain herniation or massive edema. The major predictors of mortality after ICH are (1) hemorrhage size, (2) low score on the Glasgow Coma Scale (which assesses the patient's neurologic status), and (3) presence of intraventricular hemorrhage (Davis & Torner, 1996). Less than 50% of patients with ICH are functionally independent at 1 year following the hemorrhage. Similar to ischemic strokes, long-term complications following ICH include pneumonia, urinary tract infections, seizures, and deep vein thrombosis with potential pulmonary embolism.

Intracerebral hemorrhage is classified as traumatic or nontraumatic. Over 50% of nontraumatic ICH is related to hypertension. Less common causes are listed in **Table 21–6**. Cerebral amyloid angiopathy is an age-related abnormality in the cerebral blood vessels pathologically characterized by the deposition of amyloid material (an abnormal protein) in the walls of the arteries. The use of illicit drugs, particularly cocaine, led to a sharp rise in the incidence of ICH in the young. Sympathomimetics include over-the-counter drugs used for cough and weight loss; they are rarely implicated in ICH. Finally, any brain tumor can result in ICH, although metastatic lesions more commonly bleed than primary neoplasm (e.g., glioblastoma).

The neurologic symptoms and signs of ICH depend on its location (**Table 21–7**). The majority of hypertension-related ICHs occur in the deep brain structures. In decreasing frequency, the putamen, thalamus, cerebral hemispheres, and cerebellum are the most common locations of ICH. Nonhypertensive ICH is seen in the hemisphere.

Table 21–7 Clinical Manifestations of ICH by Location

Location	Symptoms and Signs
Putamen	Abrupt hemiplegia and hemisensory loss; homonymous hemianopsia; impaired consciousness; paralysis of conjugate gaze
Thalamus	Hemisensory loss; forced downward gaze; unreactive small pupils; short-term memory loss; convergence paralysis
Hemisphere	Variable depending on the lobe involved and the side
Cerebellum	Unsteadiness; dysequilibrium; vertigo; nausea and vomiting; limb incoordination
Pons	Rapid development of coma; quadriplegia; abnormal breathing; horizontal gaze paralysis; ocular bobbing

General measures of acute ICH management are similar to those used in patients with ischemic stroke (**Table 21–4**). Particular attention is paid to lower blood pressure because many patients are hypertensive and the pressure is often extremely elevated. Additional treatment strategies include (1) early endotracheal intubation of patients with depressed level of consciousness and those with large brainstem ICH (2) aggressive treatment of cerebral edema (e.g., mannitol), and (3) early recognition and treatment of the syndrome of inappropriate antidiuretic hormone (SIADH) secretion. Correction of coagulation abnormalities, when appropriate, prevents further bleeding.

The role of surgical therapy in patients with ICH is controversial (Minematsu & Yamaguchi, 1995). Cerebellar hemorrhages larger than 3 cm in maximal diameter are the exception; patients with this type of ICH are best managed by surgical evacuation of the hematoma (blood clot). Other potential candidates for surgical intervention are (1) younger patients, noncomatose, generally healthy prior to the ICH, whose hemorrhage volume is less than 50 mL; (2) patients with lobar hemorrhage, particularly in the nondominant hemisphere, whose symptoms and signs are progressing; and (3) patients who require the surgery for diagnosis (e.g., suspected tumor with unknown primary) (Kelly, 1996).

Subarachnoid Hemorrhage

Ruptured saccular aneurysms and SAH account for 6 to 10% of all strokes and up to 25% of stroke mortality (Weaver, 1995). Aneurysmal SAH occurs mostly in the fifth or sixth decade; it is more common in women in than men, and in Blacks more than Whites. Over 40% of patients with SAH either die or are severely disabled 1 year following the hemorrhage. Determinants of morbidity and mortality include age, neurologic status at presentation, the presence of hydrocephalus or intraventricular hemorrhage, thickness of the SAH layer on initial CT scan, aneurysmal location, and medical and surgical complications (Davis & Torner, 1996; Schievink, 1997).

The majority of nontraumatic cases of SAH are related to the rupture of berry aneurysms (saccular). Berry aneurysms typically form near the circle of Willis (**Fig. 21–7**); most form in the anterior circulation (anterior communicating, anterior cerebral, middle cerebral, internal carotid arteries). They are believed to develop from degenerative changes in the wall of the blood vessel secondary to hemodynamic stress (Schievink, 1997; Weaver, 1995). Risk factors for the development of berry aneurysms include hypertension, smoking, alcohol use, and systemic diseases affecting connective tissues such as polycystic kidney disease, Marfan's syndrome, sickle-cell disease, fibromuscular dysplasia, pseudoxanthoma elasticum, and coarctation of the aorta. Other types of aneurysms (mycotic or infectious; atherosclerotic), vasculitis, coagulation disorders, and licit or illicit drugs are other rare causes of SAH.

Aneurysms can expand and cause signs and symptoms related to local compression of neighboring structures. These manifestations include headache, facial pain, double vision, oculomotor nerve paralysis, weakness, and visual field defects.

Approximately 20% of aneurysmal SAHs have warning signs. These signs can be things such as a headache, dizziness, visual or ocular symptoms, nausea, or transient sensorimotor deficits (Weaver, 1995). These are believed to be the result of minor hemorrhage. When they occur, warning signs precede SAH by up to 3 months in 92% of the cases.

Table 21–8   Hunt and Hess Classification

Grade	Criteria
I	Asymptomatic or minimal headache and slight neck rigidity
II	Moderate to severe headache, neck rigidity, neurologic deficit limited to cranial nerve paralysis
III	Drowsiness, confusion, mild neurologic deficits
IV	Stupor, moderate to severe hemiparesis, early decerebrate rigidity, vegetative disturbances
V	Deep coma, decerebrate rigidity, moribund appearance

From North American Symptomatic Carotid Endarterectomy Trial Collaborators. (1991). Beneficial Effect of Carotid Endarterectomy in Symptomatic Patients with High Grade Carotid Stenosis. *New England Journal of Medicine, 325,* 445–453.

The characteristic presentation of aneurysmal rupture is explosive headache, altered consciousness, neck stiffness, and photophobia (light sensitivity). Other symptoms that may develop include diplopia, sensorimotor deficits, aphasia, vertigo, and unsteadiness of gait. Approximately 25% of patients develop seizures shortly after the aneurysmal rupture. Hunt and Hess (1968) developed a grading scale that proved important in determining the surgical risk and prognosis of patients with SAH (**Table 21–8**); patients with grade I or II have a good prognosis, whereas those with grade IV or V do not fare well.

All patients with suspected SAH should undergo an emergency head CT. If the CT is negative and the suspicion of SAH is still high, a lumbar puncture (LP) is indicated. The yield of CT in the diagnosis of SAH is 95% in the first day, 90% in the second day, and 50% a week after the aneurysmal rupture (Davis & Torner, 1996; Schievink, 1997). A spinal tap may not demonstrate hemorrhage in the first hours after SAH; it is 100% accurate between 12 hours and 2 weeks.

Once the clinical diagnosis of SAH is confirmed radiologically or by LP, cerebral angiography should be performed to look for one or several aneurysms. An initially negative angiogram should be repeated in 2 to 3 weeks to safely determine that an aneurysm is not present.

The general medical management of SAH is similar to that for ICH and ischemic stroke (Schievink, 1997; Weaver, 1995). Particular attention should be paid to keeping the room quiet to avoid agitation and having the patient's head elevated so that venous drainage is optimally maintained. Antiepileptic drugs are used to prevent seizures. Nimodipine is a standard medical therapy used to avoid the complications of vasospasm; "triple-H" therapy (hypervolemia, hypertension, hemodilution) is also employed routinely.

Surgical therapy of aneurysmal SAH consists of ligation of the aneurysm, within 48 hours of the onset of hemorrhage in patients with grades I to III and 10 to 14 days later in those with grades IV and V (Schievink, 1997; Weaver, 1995). Meshing, balloon occlusion, and stenting are used occasionally. Transluminal angioplasty is occasionally used to treat vasospasm.

Neuromuscular Diseases

Diseases of muscle can be roughly divided into those due to inherited defects (the muscular dystrophies) and those that are acquired. This distinction is admittedly arbitrary, as some myopathies may occur as hereditary disorders in some families and sporadically in others (e.g., inclusion body myositis).

The Muscular Dystrophies (MDs)

Duchenne's muscular dystrophy (DMD) is the most common muscular dystrophy in this country. As an X-linked recessive disorder, it occurs essentially only in boys. Mutations in the gene for dystrophin are associated with an absence or near absence of this protein in the muscle. Dystrophin is a membrane-associated structural protein; in its absence other glycoproteins associated with it are digested by proteases, leading to muscle fiber degeneration. The incidence is approximately 1 per 3500 male births (Emery, 1991). In a minority of cases, the disease appears to represent a new mutation. Affected boys are normal at birth but begin to manifest subtle signs of weakness when they begin to stand and walk.

Although patients do acquire walking, most are wheelchair bound by 12 years. The disease is inexorably progressive and death usually occurs from respiratory failure or pneumonia. The facial and bulbar muscles are usually spared until very late.

Treatment consists of corticosteroids, which reduce the rate at which muscle function is lost and the physical bracing of weakened limbs to allow the patient to remain mobile as long as possible (Moxley, Ashwal, Pandya, Connolly, Florence, Mathews, Baumbach, McDonald, Sussman & Wade, 2005).

Oculopharyngeal MD is a late-onset autosomal dominant disorder that is extremely rare before the age of 45. In the United States it is primarily seen in families of French-Canadian descent (Victor, Hayes, & Adams, 1962). The muscle biopsy is often characteristic. The disease usually manifests with ptosis and, later, dysphagia. Oculopharyngeal MD is progressive and currently without definitive treatment. The dysphagia may be treated with cricopharyngeal myotomy. If this does not provide sufficient relief, gastrostomy should be performed.

Myotonic dystrophy (MyoD) is the most common form of MD in the adult and is the form most likely to involve the muscles of swallowing and speaking. It is a multisystem disease that involves other tissues such as the lens of the eye, endocrine tissues, as well as smooth and cardiac muscle. The disease is caused by an expansion of an unstable region of the gene for myotonin protein kinase (Fischbeck, 1994). Clinically, the small muscles of the hands and forearm are often the first to become weak and wasted. Facial and pharyngeal muscles are invariably involved with ptosis, facial, masseter, and sternocleidomastoid wasting and weakness, giving the face a characteristic look. Pharyngeal and laryngeal weakness produces a weak hypernasal voice. There is currently no treatment for MyoD other than supportive care. Because many patients develop cardiac arrhythmia or heart failure, routine cardiac follow-up is very important.

Inflammatory Myopathies

Polymyositis (PM), dermatomyositis (DM), and inclusion body myositis (IBM) are inflammatory myopathies. They are a group of disorders characterized histologically by the presence of inflammation within muscle (Kissel, 2002; Nash & Kissel, 2001). PM is an autoimmune disorder caused by the invasion and destruction of muscle cells by mononuclear cells. DM is an immune-mediated vasculitis affecting the small blood vessels of muscle and skin. The pathophysiology of IBM is less certain. Clinically these disorders are most commonly characterized by the subacute onset of weakness of skeletal muscle. Although most of these disorders have a predilection for proximal muscles, IBM commonly causes distal weakness as well. Characteristic skin and nail changes are seen in DM. Dysphagia occurs in all inflammatory myopathies but is more common in DM and IBM. DM is the only inflammatory myopathy that occurs to any extent in children. Treatment of PM and DM consists of immunosuppression with steroids and other agents. Most patients can be controlled with these measures. IBM is notoriously difficult to treat, though some improvement may be seen with corticosteroids and intravenous immunoglobulin (IVIG) for a time. The disease is essentially progressive and ultimately quite disabling.

Disorders of Neuromuscular Transmission

Myasthenia Gravis Myasthenia gravis (MG) is an autoimmune disorder that produces fatigable weakness of skeletal muscle. It is caused by the production of autoantibodies to the post-synaptic AChR on the muscle membrane (Thanvi & Lo, 2004). These antibodies cause premature destruction of the AChR and lead to failure of neuromuscular transmission. This is manifest by decrement of the CMAP during repetitive stimulation at low rates (see above).

MG is relatively rare with a prevalence of perhaps 5 per 100,000. It has a peak incidence in women in their twenties and thirties and in men in their sixties and seventies. There is an increased incidence of thymoma in patients with MG. In some patients the disease remains confined to the extraocular muscles. In others it is generalized, involving all skeletal muscle including bulbar and respiratory muscles. Myasthenic crisis is a sudden severe decline in strength usually accompanied by respiratory failure and severe bulbar weakness. It is a life-threatening emergency requiring intubation and mechanical ventilation.

The mainstay of treatment for mild MG is anticholinesterase inhibitors such as pyridostigmine. By delaying the destruction of ACh at the NMJ, an improvement in neuromuscular transmission is achieved. More severe cases are treated by immunosuppression with corticosteroids, steroid-sparing agents such as azathioprine, or other immunosuppressant drugs like cyclosporine. For patients in crisis, plasma exchange is used to rapidly remove the offending autoantibodies. Thymectomy, even in patients without thymoma, results in an increased probability of remission in MG and is usually recommended for patients with generalized disease. The reason for this is unclear.

Lambert-Eaton Myasthenic Syndrome Lambert-Eaton myasthenic syndrome (LEMS) is another autoimmune disorder of neuromuscular transmission owing to antibodies to the voltage-sensitive calcium channel in the presynaptic motor nerve terminal (Mareska & Gutmann, 2004). Antibody-mediated loss or inactivity of these channels leads to a reduction in the calcium influx that accompanies depolarization of the nerve terminal and hence a reduction in the amount of ACh released. The failure of neuromuscular transmission by this mechanism leads to proximal weakness with relative sparing of the cranial innervated muscles. Another feature of the disease is autonomic failure manifested by xerostomia, decreased sweating, impotence, and orthostatic hypotension. Men outnumber woman by about 5:1, and in about two thirds of patients a malignancy is present, usually a small cell carcinoma of the lung (Elmqvist & Lambert, 1968). The remaining patients have LEMS on an autoimmune basis. The findings on electrophysiologic testing are distinct from those in MG. As with MG, there is decrement of the CMAP at low rates. At high rates (30–50 Hz), or immediately following maximal volitional activity, there is a profound incrementing response of the CMAP, often over 200%. Because this is an antibody-mediated disease, treatment consists of corticosteroids and steroid sparing agents (Newsom-Davis, 2003; Newsom-Davis & Murray, 1984). Additionally, 3,4-diaminopyridine is helpful for symptomatic relief. In neoplastic LEMS, tumor regression following chemotherapy and/or radiation reduces the severity of disease and may result in remission (Chalk, Murray, Newsom-Davis, Oneill, & Spiro, 1990).

Botulism   Botulism is a paralytic condition caused by the ingestion of botulinum toxin from food contaminated by *Clostridium botulinum* (Swift & Rivner, 1987). The first signs are usually xerostomia (dry mouth), abdominal cramps, and diarrhea. Generalized weakness occurs, most prominently in bulbar and ocular muscles. Diagnosis is based on the physical examination and electrophysiologic abnormalities similar to those described in LEMS. Treatment is with parenterally administered antitoxin as well as supportive care.

Disorders of Nerve

The disorders of peripheral nerve most likely to be encountered by the SLP are few but important because of their combined incidence and severity.

Guillain-Barré Syndrome   Every year at large hospitals, numerous patients are admitted with Guillain-Barré syndrome (GBS). The annual incidence is about 1 to 2 per 100,000 per year. Characteristically, the syndrome develops 1 to 3 weeks following a viral upper respiratory or gastrointestinal syndrome. The onset is often heralded by paresthesia or pain in the lower extremities. In days to weeks, an ascending progressive paralysis develops that may be complete. Severe cases develop bulbar and respiratory muscle weakness requiring mechanical ventilation and tube feeding. The dysarthria seen in this condition is flaccid.

The diagnosis of GBS is made by clinical examination, CSF exam (which demonstrates high CSF protein and few or no white blood cells), and findings consistent with multifocal demyelination on the NCS. (For a review of all aspects of this syndrome, see Ropper, Wijdicks, & Truax, 1991.)

Treatment is with either plasma exchange (McKhann, Griffen, Cornblath, Mellits, Fisher, & Quaskey, 1988) or IVIG (van der Meche, Schmitz, & Dutch Guillain-Barré Study Group, 1992). Most patients recover completely or nearly so. However, a minority are left with significant residual weakness and a few percent die in the acute phase, usually from cardiac arrest.

Amyotrophic Lateral Sclerosis   Amyotrophic lateral sclerosis (ALS) is an idiopathic degenerative disease of upper and lower motor neurons that is inevitably fatal. The annual incidence is about 2 per 100,000, and the median age of onset is in the mid- to late-fifties in most populations studied. The disease is more common in men. The mean survival from symptom onset is less than 3 years in most studies, with death usually coming from respiratory failure or pneumonia. (For a historic review, see Williams & Windebank, 1991.) Most cases (at least 90%) occur on a spontaneous basis, but a minority are inherited, almost always in an autosomal dominant manner. Approximately 20% of the familial cases in the United States result from missense mutations in the gene for Cu/Zn superoxide dismutase (*SOD1*). This enzyme functions intracellularly as a dismutase; that is, it neutralizes an extremely reactive and potentially damaging form of oxygen that is ubiquitously produced in an intermediate reaction. It has become clear that the damage of motor neurons and their subsequent death are not solely due to the *SOD1* being less efficient as a dismutase. Studies suggest that the mutant enzyme acquires new and toxic functions, a phenomenon known as "toxic gain of effect" (Gurney, Pu, Chiu, Dal Canto, Polchow, Alexander, Caliendo, Hentati, Kwon, & Deng, 1994). The pathophysiology of this disease is currently an area of active research.

The classic form of the disease is clinically characterized by both upper and lower motor neuron loss. However, individual patients are seen whose dysfunction seems to be due to either primarily UMN or primarily LMN dysfunction. Over time, most patients develop clear evidence of both UMN and LMN signs.

Approximately one third of patients experience symptomatic onset of the disease in the lower or upper extremities, and about one quarter have onset in bulbar muscles. In occasional patients, the onset is heralded by generalized weakness, respiratory failure, or fasciculation. Regardless of the site of onset, most patients ultimately experience weakness referable to bulbar musculature and are referred to the SLP.

It has been the experience of one of the authors that patients with bulbar onset disease, especially those characterized by primarily UMN features, are the group that seems to take the longest time to be referred to the neurologist. In adult patients with the insidious onset of spastic or spastic/flaccid dysarthria, ALS should always be included in the differential diagnosis. Riluzole (Rilutek®) is the only FDA-approved drug for the treatment of ALS. In two studies riluzole seemed to impart a modest survival advantage compared with placebo (Bensimon, Lacomblez, & Meininger, 1994; Lacomblez, Bensimon, Leigh, Guillet, & Meininger, 1996). Unfortunately, no statistically significant reduction in the rate of functional progression was seen.

The management of dysphagia and dysarthria are the main challenges for the SLP confronted with an ALS patient. With respect to dysphagia, a fluoroscopic swallowing study provides anatomic information that may help determine safe swallowing strategies. If aspiration is demonstrated or if bulbar function is becoming so impaired that nutritional status is beginning to suffer, percutaneous gastrostomy is offered. Surprisingly, a scientific consensus does not exist on the benefit of gastrostomy on survival in ALS. It is clear, however, that quality of life is improved by the procedure (Chio, 1999; Forbes, Colville, & Swingler, 2004; Mazzini, Corra, Zaccala, Mora, Del Piano, & Galante, 1995; Mitsumoto, Davidson, Moore, Gad, Brandis, Ringel, Rosenfeld, Shefner, Strong, Sufit, & Anderson, 2003; Strong, Rowe, & Rankin, 1999). It is recognized that ALS patients with poor respiratory function are at higher risk for morbidity and mortality following the procedure, and it is recommended that gastrostomy be performed before the forced vital capacity (FVC) falls below 50% of predicted FVC for a patient's age and sex (Miller, Rosenberg, Gelinas, Mitsumoto, Newman, Sufit, Borasio, Bradley, Bromberg, Brooks, Kasarskis, Munsat, & Oppenheimer, 1999).

Movement Disorders

Hypokinetic Movement Disorders

Parkinson's Disease Parkinson's disease (PD) is a degenerative disorder of the basal ganglia; specifically, the pigmented cells of the substantia nigra, the locus ceruleus, and the dorsal motor nucleus of the vagus are depleted. The disease affects about 1% of people over the age of 65 throughout the world. The disease is rarely familial, and essentially all cases are sporadic. Even in identical twins there is poor concordance for the disease. Environmental exposures may modify risk. For example, the disease is more common in men and nonsmokers (Morens, Grandinetti, Reed, White, & Ross, 1995). Lifelong occupational exposure to metals, particularly copper or manganese seems to be a risk factor (Gorell, Johnson, Rybicki, Peterson, Kortsha, Brown, & Richardson, 1997). Clinically, the disease is characterized by bradykinesia or akinesia, rigidity, tremor, and a loss of postural reflexes. Patients have a characteristically inexpressive or "masked" face and they blink less. When sitting, there are fewer small adjustments of posture than usual; when standing up from a chair the patient does not use the arms to push up. There may be a resting ("pill rolling") tremor of the hands. When walking, the patient is stooped, the arms flexed, and the gait short-stepped and ultimately characterized by shuffling. The loss of postural reflexes leads to falls. Given this constellation of motor signs, it is not surprising that the dysarthria of PD is hypokinetic, monotonous, and monopitched.

Rational treatment of PD is directed at reducing the pathologic effects of the loss of the dopaminergic nigrostriatal pathway. The administration of drugs containing L-dopa, a precursor of the neurotransmitter dopamine, as well as dopaminergic agonists themselves (e.g., bromocriptine, pergolide, lisuride) form the mainstay of treatment. Centrally acting anticholinergic drugs such as trihexyphenidyl are used as well, particularly in patients with prominent tremor. Selegiline is another mainstay of treatment for PD, which was shown to prevent disease progression in animals, but not in humans.

In patients with advanced disease, speech becomes progressively less understandable and the dysphagia may progress to the point where enteral feeding becomes necessary. Speech and swallowing symptoms generally are not improved by the various drug treatments.

Hyperkinetic Movement Disorders

Huntington's Disease Huntington's disease (HD), also known as Huntington's chorea, is an autosomal dominant neurodegenerative disease characterized by dementia and a choreoathetoid movement disorder. It is progressive and fatal. The disease is now known to be due to an expansion of a region on chromosome 4 leading to a gene product, or protein called "huntingtin." HD occurs in people of northern European descent with an incidence of about 5 per 100,000. The usual age of onset is in the thirties and forties, but cases are seen occasionally in the teens or after the age of 70. The disease is usually not difficult to diagnose because of family history. Patients at risk for the disease can be most reliably detected by genetic analysis for the mutation. Because there is no treatment for the disease, genetic testing under these circumstances should be performed only at specialized centers with genetic counselors familiar with the medical and ethical issues.

The disorder often begins with psychiatric manifestations such as subtle changes in personality; sometimes frank psychosis develops. Depression is common. At some point, the movement disorder begins. At first patients may seem merely fidgety, but ultimately a choreoathetoid movement disorder becomes obvious. Speech in HD is characterized by a hyperkinetic dysarthria with variable rate and loudness and imprecise consonants. Symptomatic treatment of chorea is usually accomplished with haloperidol.

Essential and Familial Tremor One of the more common hyperkinetic movement disorders is tremor; this may occur as an autosomal dominantly inherited form or it may appear sporadically, in which case it is known as essential tremor. It has an estimated incidence of over 400 per 100,000 (Haerer, Anderson, & Schoenberg, 1982). The disorder may begin in childhood but is more prevalent as a population ages. The action tremor (present when using the limb, not at rest or when supported) usually begins in the arms or as a side-to-side movement of the head. Over time, it worsens and may become quite disabling. In some patients, the cranial innervated muscles are involved and there is a wavering property to the voice. Many patients have themselves noted that the tremor abates after one or two drinks of alcohol. Treatment is with beta-blockers such as propranolol or with the anticonvulsant primidone.

Multiple Sclerosis Multiple sclerosis (MS) is a relatively common demyelinating disease of the CNS. The pathologic process causes relapsing/remitting multifocal demyelination in the brain, spinal cord, and optic nerves. The axons are relatively spared. The disease has several intriguing features. In most countries or continents studied, there is a gradient of incidence that is lowest toward the equator and rises with latitudes above or below the equator. In Blacks in the United States, at all latitudes the incidence is lower than in Whites (Kurtzke, Beebe & Norman, 1979). The same is true in Japan. In studies of migrants, the risk of the disease seems to be largely acquired by the age of 15. There is a higher incidence of MS in first-degree relatives of patients with the disease, especially identical twins. Fraternal twins have the incidence of non-twin siblings (Ebers, Bulman, & Sadovnick, 1986).

Although the lesions in MS certainly represent immune-mediated demyelination (there is evidence of antibodies directed at components of myelin and active plaques are infiltrated with certain subtypes of lymphocytes), there is no autoantibody in the classical sense.

Clinically, the disease may present with or be characterized by many different manifestations. One way to think of the possible symptoms and signs is to recall that motor, sensory, and visual, information is carried by myelinated pathways. Hence, unilateral visual loss, sensory loss or paresthesias, and varying combinations of motor weakness and spasticity can be seen. Spinal lesions may lead to complete or incomplete transverse myelitis. Although most patients have a relapsing remitting course, over time there is a tendency for the disorder to become chronic and progressive in many patients. Because of the multifocal nature of demyelination in MS, many different types of speech disorder can be seen. In some patients speech is normal, in others it is primarily ataxic, and in still others it is spastic/ataxic (Beukelman, Kraft, & Freal, 1985; Darley, Aronson & Goldstein, 1972).

Treatment involves modulation of the immune system as well as symptomatic aid. High-dose oral or parenteral glucocorticoids have been shown to reduce the period of the exacerbation, but they do not change the ultimate course of the disease. Other immunosuppressants such as azathioprine and cyclophosphamide may slow the course of decline in chronic progressive MS, but not without potentially dangerous side effects, in particular, lymphoreticular malignancies. β-Interferon is now the mainstay of treatment of relapsing remitting MS, and various forms of β-interferon are available on the market (Arnason, 1993). The recent introduction of mitoxantrone for chronic progressive MS provides hope for these patients with such course of illness.

Symptomatic treatment of spasticity may be accomplished with baclofen or tizanidine. The spasticity of the bladder may be treated with oxybutynin or tolterodine. Fatigue is sometimes effectively treated with amantadine.

Epilepsy   A seizure is a symptom of brain dysfunction characterized by disorderly electrical discharges of nerve cells. The abnormal discharge (1) may occur in a silent area of the brain causing no clinical symptoms; (2) could be limited to an island of neurons resulting in focal symptoms and signs; or (3) could spread to many areas of the brain leading to multiple symptoms and signs, and sometimes loss of consciousness. Recurrent unprovoked seizures are known as epilepsy.

It is estimated that the prevalence of epilepsy is 6 per 1000, which translates into more than 1.5 million Americans; Blacks may be more prone than Whites (Hauser & Kurland, 1975). Also, more than 200,000 epileptics have more than one seizure per month, and approximately one fourth of patients have recurrent seizures despite treatment (Hauser & Hesdorffer, 1991). Risk factors for epilepsy include mental retardation/cerebral palsy, repeated and focal febrile seizures, family history of epilepsy, central nervous system infections, moderate and severe head injury, cerebrovascular disease, brain tumors, Alzheimer's disease, excessive alcohol use and drug abuse (e.g., heroin or cocaine), and a history of asthma (Hauser & Hesdorffer, 1991).

The majority of epilepsies are idiopathic (unknown cause) (Annegers, 1993). Definite causes of seizures are multiple (**Table 21–9**). Idiopathic epilepsy is more common in children and adolescents than in adults; symptomatic epilepsy is more prevalent in adults.

Seizures are either generalized or partial (focal, local); partial seizures are further subclassified into simple partial, complex partial (indicating an impaired level, but not loss, of consciousness), and partial evolving to generalized tonic-clonic (GTC) convulsions (Commission on Classification and Terminology of the International League Against Epilepsy, 1981).

Generalized seizures are characterized by initial involvement of both hemispheres with impaired level of consciousness, bilateral motor symptoms, and widespread and bilateral neuronal discharges on electroencephalography. Grand mal and petit mal are the two main forms of generalized seizures. With grand mal, patients lose consciousness abruptly, there is tonic contraction of muscles (stridor or cry if the respiratory muscles are affected), and they fall to the ground. Soon after, convulsive movements occur for a variable period of time and are followed by a muscle-relaxation phase where the unconscious patients breathe deeply. Tongue biting, urinary and/or fecal incontinence, frothing at the mouth, and grunting occur during the GTC phase. Occasionally, patients develop a vague and ill-described feeling before they lose consciousness. When epileptic patients are awakened after a seizure, they usually feel sore and may have headache. Grand mal seizures can occur in childhood or in adulthood. They do not recur as frequently as partial seizures.

Petit mal or absence seizures are characterized by a brief (few seconds) interruption of consciousness, a blank stare, and sometimes uprolling of the eyes. Absence seizures can be isolated or could be accompanied by clonic, tonic, atonic activities, or by automatisms such as lip smacking, fumbling with clothes, and so on. Typical absence seizures occur in 4- to 12-year-old children. Simple partial seizures take the form of motor (any portion of the body may be involved in repetitive motor activities), somatosensory (manifest as numbness or tingling), special sensory (visual, auditory, gustatory, or olfactory hallucinations; vertigo, floating sensations), autonomic (pallor, perspiration, pupillary dilatation, etc.), or psychic seizures with cognitive impairment (aphasia, déjà-vu, fear, anger, etc.). Sometimes, partial seizures affect multiple body areas sequentially (jacksonian march). Complex partial seizures can evolve from simple partial or can be associated with an initial impairment of the level of consciousness. Rare types include myoclonic (single or multiple sudden and brief shock-like contractions of the face, trunk, or extremity); clonic (similar to GTC without the tonic component); tonic (GTC without clonic component); and atonic seizures (sudden loss of muscle tone).

Status epilepticus (SE) is an epileptic seizure that is "frequently repeated or so prolonged as to create a fixed and lasting condition" (Commission on Classification and Terminology of the International League Against Epilepsy, 1981). Unless attended to emergently, patients with SE are at a high risk of significant morbidity or death.

One of the most important elements in the management of patients with suspected epilepsy is to first establish the diagnosis. Many conditions can mimic seizures, including syncope (brief loss of consciousness), hyperventilation, sleep disorders, migraine, or psychiatric dissociative states. Once the diagnosis of epilepsy is made with confidence, a cause for the seizures is explored (**Table 21–9**).

Avoidance of the offending mechanism, such as alcohol, is the treatment of choice for nonrecurrent seizures. The therapy

Table 21–9   Causes of Seizures

Cause	Example
Trauma	Contusion; penetrating injury; hemorrhage
Cerebrovascular disease	Subarachnoid hemorrhage (SAH); ICH; subdural hematoma; ischemic stroke; cerebral venous thrombosis
Infections	Meningitis; encephalitis; cerebral abscess
Neoplastic disease	Primary tumors; metastatic disease
Metabolic	Hypo- and hypernatremia; hypo- and hyperglycemia; hypoxia; hypo- and hypercalcemia; kidney and liver failure
Drugs and toxins	Alcohol intoxication and withdrawal; withdrawal of antiepileptics; environmental toxins (e.g., lead)
Inherited diseases	Phenylketonuria; tuberous sclerosis; urea cycle disorders
Others	Sleep deprivation; fever in children

of epilepsy is guided by the seizure type, medication cost, and patient preference. Monotherapy (a single agent) is the recommended strategy. If an antiepileptic drug (AED) is not effective or causes significant side effects, it is preferable to change the AED rather than add another one. New AEDs have expanded the choice for patients with various forms of epilepsy (Nadkarni, LaJoie, & Devinsky, 2005). Routine blood testing (complete blood count, electrolytes, liver and kidney function tests) is performed before initiating AED therapy. When appropriate, these tests are repeated and serum blood levels of AEDs are obtained during the course of therapy.

Some patients with epilepsy fail multiple drug regimens. These patients are candidates for referral to specialized epilepsy centers that evaluate epileptics for possible surgical intervention. Localized resection of the area generating the seizures is an effective and long-term treatment in some patients with temporal lobe epilepsy (Goodman, 1996). Large resections (e.g., hemispherectomies) are occasionally performed to control intractable seizures in infants and small children.

The management of SE requires an emergent approach; the longer it takes to control SE, the worse the prognosis. The essential ABCs are protect the airway, draw blood (AED levels, glucose, sodium, calcium, gases, urea nitrogen, drug screen),

and assess and stabilize cardiac function. Rapid administration of AEDs in the first few minutes is essential. A benzodiazepine (lorazepam or diazepam) is given intermittently to stop the seizures while the AED is infusing in the vein. Sometimes patients are put into pharmacologic coma (e.g., pentobarbital) to stop the continuous electrical brain discharges that are causing SE.

✦ Conclusion

A basic understanding of functional neuroanatomy provides a useful and rational approach to the diagnosis and treatment of neurogenic communication and swallowing disorders. In general, diseases of the motor unit lead to flaccid dysarthria, and disorders of the basal ganglia and cerebellum affect the quality of movement. Degenerative, vascular, inflammatory, and neoplastic disorders of the cerebrum ultimately impact on the motor unit via central mechanisms of control. Although it is beyond the scope of this chapter to provide exhaustive coverage of all neurologic disease, we have presented the fundamental approach used by neurologists in their assessment of patients with symptoms of neurologic origin. This information complements the practice of speech–language pathology.

Study Questions

1. What are the elements of the motor unit?
2. Which tract provides the principal means of voluntary control over the cranial nerve nuclei involved in speech and swallowing?
3. Which branch of the vagus nerve is most important for controlling vocal pitch?
4. The EEG is useful in the diagnosis and prognosis of epilepsy: true or false?
5. The EMG should be abnormal in a disorder of the motor unit: true or false?
6. What are the various advantages and disadvantages of clinical imaging studies?
7. What are the most common causes of stroke?
8. How do ICH and SAH differ (other than by site)?
9. Lambert-Eaton myasthenic syndrome (LEMS) and botulism are disorders of the NMJ that largely spare the bulbar muscles: true or false?
10. Describe the various types of epilepsy.

References

Aaslid, R., Markwalder, T.M., & Nornes, H. (1982). Noninvasive Transcranial Doppler Ultrasound Recording of Flow Velocity in Basal Cerebral Arteries. *Journal of Neurosurgery, 57*, 769–774

Adams, R.D., Victor, M., & Ropper, A.H. (1997). *Principles of Neurology*, 6th ed. New York: McGraw-Hill

Annegers, J.F. (1993). The Epidemiology of Epilepsy. In: E. Wyllie (Ed.). *The treatment of Epilepsy: Principles and Practice* (pp. 157–164). Philadelphia: Lea & Febiger

Arnason, B.G. (1993). Interferon Beta in Multiple Sclerosis. *Neurology, 43*, 641–643

Bensimon, G., Lacomblez, L., & Meininger, V. (1994). A Controlled Trial of Riluzole in Amyotrophic Lateral Sclerosis. ALS/Riluzole Study Group. *New England Journal of Medicine, 330*, 585–591

Beukelman, D.R., Kraft, G.H., & Freal, J. (1985). Expressive Communication Disorders in Persons with Multiple Sclerosis: A Survey. *Archives of Physical Medicine & Rehabilitation, 66*, 675–677

Bowler, J.V., & Hachinski, V. (1996). Epidemiology of Cerebral Infarct. In: P.B. Gorelick (Ed.), *Atlas of Cerebrovascular Disease* (pp. 1.1–1.22). Philadelphia: Churchill Livingstone

Bradley, W.G., Daroff, R.B., Marsden, C.D., & Fenichel, G.M. (1996). *Neurology in Clinical Practice. The Neurological Disorders,* 2nd ed. Boston: Butterworth-Heinemann

Broderick, J.P., Phillips, S.J., Whisnant, J.P., O'Fallon, W.M., & Bergstralh, E.J. (1989). Incidence Rate of Stroke in the Eighties: The End of the Decline in Stroke. *Stroke, 20*, 577–582

Chalk, C.H., Murray, N.M.F., Newsom-Davis, J.H., Oneill, J.H., Spiro, S.G. (1990). Response of the Lambert-Eaton Myasthenic Syndrome to Treatment of Associated Small Cell Carcinoma. *Neurology, 40*, 1552–1556

Chio, A. (1999). ISIS Survey: An International Study on the Diagnostic Process and Its Implications in Amyotrophic Lateral Sclerosis. *Journal of Neurology, 246(suppl 3),* III1–5

Commission on Classification and Terminology of the International League Against Epilepsy. (1981). Proposal for Revised Clinical and Electrographic Classification of Epileptic Seizures. *Epilepsia, 22*, 489–501

Darley, F.L., Aronson, A.E., & Goldstein, N.P. (1972). Dysarthria in Multiple Sclerosis. *Journal of Speech and Hearing Research, 15*, 229–245

Davis, P.H., & Torner, J.C. (1996). Epidemiology of Subarachnoid Hemorrhage and Intraparenchymal Hemorrhage. In: P.B. Gorelick (Ed.), *Atlas of Cerebrovascular Disease* (pp. 2.1–2.15). Philadelphia: Churchill Livingstone

Ebers, G.C., Bulman, D.E., Sadovnick, A.D., et al. (1986). A Population-Based Study of Multiple Sclerosis in Twins. *New England Journal of Medicine, 315*, 1638–1642

Elmqvist, D., & Lambert, E.H. (1968). Detailed Analysis of Neuromuscular Transmission in a Patient with the Myasthenic Syndrome Sometimes Associated with Bronchogenic Carcinoma. *Mayo Clinic Proceedings, 43*, 689–713

Emery, A.E.H. (1991). Population Frequencies of Inherited Neuromuscular Diseases—A World Survey. *Neuromuscular Disorders, 1*, 19–29

Executive Committee for the Asymptomatic Carotid Atherosclerosis Study. (1995). Endarterectomy for Asymptomatic Carotid Stenosis. *Journal of the American Medical Association, 273*, 1421–1428

Fischbeck, K.H. (1994). The Mechanism of Myotonic Dystrophy. *Annals of Neurology, 35,* 255–256

Forbes, R.B., Colville, S., & Swingler, R.J. (2004). Frequency, Timing and Outcome of Gastrostomy Tubes for Amyotrophic Lateral Sclerosis/Motor Neurone Disease—A Record Linkage Study from the Scottish Motor Neurone Disease Register. *Journal of Neurology, 251,* 813–817

Goodman, R.R. (1996). Surgical Treatment of Epilepsy. In: S. Chokroverty (Ed.), *Management of Epilepsy* (pp. 309–328). Boston: Butterworth-Heinemann

Gorell, J.M., Johnson, D.D., Rybicki, B.A., Peterson, E.L., Kortsha, G.X., Brown, G.G., & Richardson, R.J. (1997). Occupational Exposures to Metals as Risk Factors for Parkinson's Disease. *Neurology, 48,* 650–658

Gurney, M.E., Pu, H., Chiu, A.Y., Dal Canto, M.C., Polchow, C.Y., Alexander, D.D., Caliendo, J., Hentati, A., Kwon, Y.W., & Deng, H.X. (1994). Motor Neuron Degeneration in Mice that Express a Human Cu,Zn Superoxide Dismutase Mutation. *Science, 264,* 1772–1775

Haerer, A.F., Anderson, D.W., & Schoenberg, B.S. (1982). Prevalence of Essential Tremor. Results from the Copiah County Study. *Archives of Neurology, 39,* 750–751

Hauser, W.A., & Hesdorffer, D.C. (1991). Epidemiology of Epilepsy. In: D.W. Anderson (Ed.), *Neuroepidemiology: A Tribute to Bruce Schoenberg* (pp. 97–119). Boca Raton: CRC Press

Hauser, W.A., & Kurland, L.T. (1975). The Epidemiology of Epilepsy in Rochester, Minnesota, 1936–1967. *Epilepsia, 16,* 1–66

Hunt, W.E., & Hess, R.M. (1968). Surgical Risk as Related to Time of Intervention in the Repair of Intracranial Aneurysms. *Journal of Neurosurgery, 28,* 14–20

Kelly, M.A. (1996). Management of Intracerebral Hemorrhage. In: P.B. Gorelick (Ed.), *Atlas of Cerebrovascular Disease* (pp. 1–20). Philadelphia: Churchill Livingstone

Kissel, J.T. (2002). Misunderstandings, Misperceptions, and Mistakes in the Management of the Inflammatory Myopathies. *Seminars in Neurology, 22,* 41–51

Kurtzke, J.F., Beebe, G.W., & Norman, J.E. Jr. (1979). Epidemiology of Multiple Sclerosis in U.S. veterans: I. Race, Sex and Geographic Distribution. *Neurology, 29,* 1228–1235

Lacomblez, L., Bensimon, G., Leigh, P., Guillet, P., & Meininger, V. (1996). Dose-Ranging Study of Riluzole in Amyotrophic Lateral Sclerosis. ALS/Riluzole Study Group II. *Lancet, 347,* 1425–1431

Levy, D.E. (1988). How Transient Are Transient Ischemic Attacks? *Neurology, 38,* 674–677

Mareska, M., & Gutmann, L. (2004). Lambert-Eaton Myasthenic Syndrome. *Seminars in Neurology, 24,* 149–153

Marsan, C.A., & Zivin, L.S. (1970). Factors Related to the Occurrence of Typical Paroxysmal Abnormalities in the EEG Records of Epileptic Patients. *Epilepsia, 11,* 361–381

Mazzini, L., Corra, T., Zaccala, M., Mora, G., Del Piano, M., & Galante, M. (1995). Percutaneous Endoscopic Gastrostomy and Enteral Nutrition in Amyotrophic Lateral Sclerosis. *Journal of Neurology, 242,* 695–698

McKhann, G.M., Griffen, J.W., Cornblath, D.R., Mellits, E.D., Fisher, R.S., & Quaskey, S.A. (1988). Plasmapheresis and Guillain-Barré Syndrome: Analysis of Prognostic Factors and the Effect of Plasmapheresis. *Annals of Neurology, 23,* 347

Medical Research Council. (1946). Aids to the Examination of the Peripheral Nervous System. Memorandum No. 45. London: Her Majesty's Stationery Office

Miller, R.G., Rosenberg, J.A., Gelinas, D.F., Mitsumoto, H., Newman, D., Sufit, R., Borasio, G.D., Bradley, W.G., Bromberg, M.B., Brooks, B.R., Kasarskis, E.J., Munsat, T.L., & Oppenheimer, E.A. (1999). Practice Parameter: The Care of the Patient with Amyotrophic Lateral Sclerosis (an Evidence-Based Review): Report of the Quality Standards Subcommittee of the American Academy of Neurology: ALS Practice Parameters Task Force. *Neurology, 52,* 1311–1323

Minematsu, K., & Yamaguchi, T. (1995). Management of Intracerebral Hemorrhage. In: M. Fisher (Ed.), *Stroke Therapy* (pp. 351–372). Boston: Butterworth-Heinemann

Mitsumoto, H., Davidson, M., Moore, D., Gad, N., Brandis, M., Ringel, S., Rosenfeld, J, Sefner, J.M., Strong, M.J., Sufit, R., & Anderson, F.A. (2003). Percutaneous Endoscopic Gastrostomy (PEG) in Patients with ALS and

Bulbar Dysfunction. *Amyotrophic Lateral Sclerosis and Other Motor Neuron Disorders, 4,* 177–185

Morens, D.M., Grandinetti, A., Reed, D., White, L.R., & Ross, G.W. (1995). Cigarette Smoking and Protection from Parkinson's Disease: False Association or Etiologic Clue? *Neurology, 45,* 1041–1051

Moxley, R.T. 3rd, Ashwal, S., Pandya, S., Connolly, A., Florence, J., Mathews, K., Baumbach, L., McDonald, C., Sussman, M., & Wade, C., et al. (2005). Practice Parameter: Corticosteroid Treatment of Duchenne Dystrophy: Report of the Quality Standards Subcommittee of the American Academy of Neurology and the Practice Committee of the Child Neurology Society. *Neurology, 11,* 13–20

Nadkarni, S., LaJoie, J., & Devinsky, O. (2005). Current Treatments of Epilepsy. *Neurology, 64 (Suppl. 3),* S2–S11

Nash, S.M., & Kissel, J.T. (2001). Inflammatory Myopathies. In: R. Pourmand (Ed.), *Neuromuscular Diseases: Expert Clinicians' Views* (pp. 199–226). Woburn, MA: Butterworth-Heinemann

National Institute of Neurological Disorders and Stroke rt-PA Study Group. (1995). Tissue Plasminogen Activator for Acute Ischemic Stroke. *New England Journal of Medicine, 333,* 1581–1587

Newsom-Davis, J. (2003). Therapy in Myasthenia Gravis and Lambert-Eaton Myasthenic Syndrome. *Seminars in Neurology, 23,* 191–198

Newsom-Davis, J., & Murray, N.M.F. (1984). Plasma Exchange and Immunosuppressive Drug Treatment in the Lambert-Eaton Myasthenic Syndrome. *Neurology, 34,* 480–485

North American Symptomatic Carotid Endarterectomy Trial Collaborators. (1991). Beneficial Effect of Carotid Endarterectomy in Symptomatic Patients with High Grade Carotid Stenosis. *New England Journal of Medicine, 325,* 445–453

Ramadan, N.M., & Mitsias, P. (1996). Nonatherosclerotic Stroke. In: P.B. Gorelick (Ed.), *Atlas of Cerebrovascular Disease* (pp. 1–7). Philadelphia: Churchill Livingstone

Ropper, A.H., Wijdicks, E.F.M., & Truax, B.T. (1991). Guillain-Barré Syndrome. Philadelphia: F.A. Davis

Schievink, W.I. (1997). Intracranial Aneurysms. *New England Journal of Medicine, 336,* 28–40

Silverman, D., Saunders, M.G., Schwab, R.S., & Masland, R.L. (1969). Cerebral Death and the Electroencephalogram. Report of the Ad Hoc Committee of the American Electroencephalographic Society on EEG Criteria for Determination of Cerebral Death. *Journal of the American Medical Association, 209,* 1505–1510

Sloan, M.A., Alexandrov, A.V., Tegeler, C.H., Spencer, M.P., Caplan, L.R., Feldmann, E., Wechsler, L.R., Newell, D.W., Gomez, C.R., Babikian, V.L., Lefkowitz, D., Goldman, R.S., Armon, C., Hsu, C.Y., & Goodin, D.S. (2004). Assessment: Transcranial Doppler Ultrasonography: Report of the Therapeutics and Technology Assessment Subcommittee of the American Academy of Neurology. *Neurology, 62,* 1468–1481

Special Report from the National Institute of Neurological Disorders and Stroke (Whisnant JP, chairman). (1990). Classification of Cerebrovascular Diseases. *Stroke, 21,* 637–676

Strong, M.J., Rowe, A., & Rankin, R.N. (1999). Percutaneous Gastrojejunostomy in Amyotrophic Lateral Sclerosis. *Journal of Neurological Science, 169,* 128–132

Swift, T., & Rivner, M. (1987). Infectious Diseases of Nerve. In: P.J. Vinken, G.W. Bruyn, & H.L. Klawan (Eds.), *Handbook of Clinical Neurology* (pp. 179–194). Amsterdam: Elsevier

Thanvi, B.R., & Lo, T.C. (2004). Update on Myasthenia Gravis. *Postgraduate Medical Journal, 80,* 690–700

van der Meche, F.G., Schmitz, P.I., & the Dutch Guillain-Barré Study Group. (1992). A Randomized Trial Comparing Intravenous Immune Globulin and Plasma Exchange in Guillain-Barré syndrome. *New England Journal of Medicine, 326,* 1123–1129

Weaver, J.P. 1995). Subarachnoid Hemorrhage. In: M. Fisher (Ed.), *Stroke Therapy* (pp. 399–435). Boston: Butterworth-Heinemann

Williams, D.B., & Windebank, A.J. (1991). Motor Neuron Disease (Amyotrophic Lateral Sclerosis). *Mayo Clinical Proceedings, 66,* 54–82

Victor, M., Hayes, R., & Adams, R.D. (1962). Oculopharyngeal Muscular Dystrophy: A Familial Disease of Late Life Characterized by Dysphagia and Progressive Ptosis of the Eyelids. *New England Journal of Medicine, 267,* 1267–1272

22

Medical and Surgical Management in Otolaryngology

Glendon M. Gardner and Michael S. Benninger

- ✦ History and Physical Examination
- ✦ Oral Cavity, Oropharynx, and Nasopharynx
- ✦ Nasal and Sinus Disorders
- ✦ Anatomy of the Larynx
- ✦ Physiology of the Larynx
- ✦ Benign Laryngeal Disorders
- ✦ Neurolaryngology
- ✦ Laryngeal Trauma
- ✦ Tracheotomy and Tracheostomy
- ✦ Professional Voice Disorders
- ✦ Gastroesophageal and Laryngopharyngeal Reflux Disease
- ✦ Acquired Immunodeficiency Syndrome and Otolaryngology
- ✦ Case Vignettes

Otolaryngologists and speech–language pathologists (SLPs) work closely together to provide comprehensive services to patients with disorders and diseases of the head and neck because of the effect of these structures on communication and swallowing. Although not all otolaryngologic patients require intervention by an SLP, knowledge of the more commonly encountered disorders and their effect on speech and swallowing functions is crucial. Medical treatment and surgical resection and repair can result in posttreatment effects that require management by an SLP.

This chapter discusses the process by which the otolaryngologist diagnoses head and neck disorders; diseases and disorders of the oral cavity, oropharynx, and nasopharynx; nasal-sinus disorders; laryngeal anatomy and physiology; laryngeal disorders, trauma, and tracheostomy; special medical issues in professional voice; laryngopharyngeal reflux disease; and head neck manifestations in AIDS.

✦ History and Physical Examination

When a patient presents to an otolaryngologist with a complaint referable to the upper airway or head and neck, the first and perhaps most critical part of the assessment is obtaining a thorough history. It is during the history that the otolaryngologist establishes a relationship with the patient and begins the mutual exchange of information in a manner that breeds trust. Traditionally, the history begins with a clarification of the chief complaint in an attempt to identify factors that are pertinent to the subsequent evaluation and treatment. The time from onset, the severity of the symptoms, whether or not the symptoms vary by time of day or exposure to certain environments or conditions, and any previous treatment for this condition should be obtained. It is important, however, not to become so focused on the main complaint that important peripheral information pertinent to the disorder or other conditions that may require assessment are ignored. A general review of other head and neck symptoms follows and then questions are asked regarding general medical health and other medical problems. A list of medications and a history of previous diseases or surgeries should be obtained. Any habits that might influence health should be considered, particularly eating habits, or whether or not the individual uses tobacco or alcohol. One cannot underestimate the power of the history, in that often the physician can come to a tentative diagnosis prior to any physical contact with the patient.

The head and neck physical examination usually begins during the history. At that time, the physician assesses speech and voice, assesses gross hearing, and notices any abnormalities of facial movement or skin conditions or masses. It is important during the head and neck exam not to focus only on the area related to the chief complaint; by doing so important physical findings may be missed. To avoid missing anything, it is reasonable to follow a sequence of evaluations despite the presenting disorder. The skin and scalp is usually evaluated first followed by an examination of the ears. The external ear and ear canal are assessed with an otoscope to identify inflammation or skin conditions. The middle ear is examined for normal landmarks and absence of infection, masses, fluid, or retraction of the ear drum. Air insufflation (pneumatic otoscopy) is particularly useful in evaluating middle ear function, negative pressure, or fluid. If any concerns are raised during otoscopy, a microscope can be used to better see any potential abnormalities. Hearing can be assessed with the use of tuning forks, although if any concerns are raised related to hearing, a formal audiogram is recommended.

A nasal examination is generally obtained with a head mirror, indirect light, and a nasal speculum. Decongesting the nose with a decongestant spray improves the view into the more posterior aspects of the nose. If concerns are raised, if visualization is difficult, or if a diagnosis needs confirmation, Benninger (1997) recommends the use of a nasal endoscope to better visualize the entire nose. The oral cavity is examined with mirror and indirect light so that two hands can be used to manipulate the tongue and other mucosal surfaces. All areas should be seen. Tongue blades depress the tongue to visualize the oropharynx, tonsils, and tongue base. Keeping the tongue blades just anterior to the junction of the anterior two thirds and posterior one third of the tongue and having the patient gently breathe minimizes the gagging sensation. With the tongue compressed, a nasopharyngeal mirror can be used to assess the nasopharynx.

The larynx typically is initially examined by indirect laryngoscopy with a laryngeal mirror. The tongue is grasped and gently pulled forward. The mirror is inserted to a point just anterior to the palate and light is directed to the mirror, which reflects onto the hypopharynx and larynx. Avoiding contacting the pharyngeal wall or base of tongue or having the patient phonate prior to placing the mirror will minimize the gag reflex. Approximately two thirds of patients can be examined well with a mirror. It is important not to focus only on the vocal folds, as other important findings related to the base of tongue, posterior pharyngeal walls, pyriform sinuses, epiglottis, and valleculae may be missed. Having the patient say different vowel sounds provides different visual angles to the larynx. Indirect laryngoscopy enables a global view of the larynx and should be performed prior to any further techniques to visualize the larynx, although it is limited in that the larynx cannot be seen during running speech or singing. To supplement the mirror view, to visualize the larynx during running speech, or if visualization is limited, a flexible laryngoscope is passed. Usually this is passed through the nose after decongestion and occasionally after application of a topical anesthetic. Not only is this instrument valuable in larynx assessment, it can be used to better visualize the nasopharynx and can be used for functional endoscopic evaluation of swallowing (FEES) or, as Bastian (1991) notes, for voice modification or biofeedback training. According to Benninger (1994), video images can be obtained for following the progress of treatment, documentation, and discussions with the patient, family or referring physician. To further augment the examination of the larynx, videostroboscopy of the larynx can be performed to assess vocal fold vibration.

The neck should be palpated for any masses, neck muscle problems, or asymmetry. The thyroid is then palpated at rest and during swallowing. Pulsating masses can be auscultated with a stethoscope listening for bruits to help identify a vascular lesion. Fine-needle aspiration is a useful tool in obtaining a pathologic diagnosis and has obviated the need in many cases for open biopsy. A neurologic assessment of the cranial nerves is part of the routine examination, whereas selective assessments of balance function should be performed if such a disorder is suggested by the preceding evaluation. A general physical examination is usually not performed on a routine basis by an otolaryngologist, although selected exams, such as of the lungs or heart, may be performed if prompted by the history and physical examination.

The need for other tests is determined by the findings of the history and physical examination. Computed tomography (CT) and magnetic resonance imaging (MRI) scanning are very useful in assessing head and neck masses or tumors and ruling out intracranial or skull base disease. CT scans are particularly useful in evaluating sinus disease. A chest x-ray is helpful in patients with head and neck tumors, cough, or hemoptysis. Swallowing and gastroesophageal reflux assessment may be considered in patients with swallowing complaints. Other medical evaluations are determined by the suspicions of disease. On occasion, an evaluation under anesthesia may be necessary to stage cancer, to obtain biopsies, or to clarify diagnosis.

✦ Oral Cavity, Oropharynx, and Nasopharynx

Anatomy

The boundaries of the oral cavity are the lips anteriorly, the buccal (cheek) mucosa laterally, the anterior tonsillar pillars posteriorly, the hard palate superiorly, and the floor of mouth inferiorly. The oral cavity contains the teeth and alveolar ridges of the mandible and maxilla, the anterior two thirds of the tongue, and the hard palate. It is also the site of the orifices of the ducts of the major salivary glands (**Fig. 22–1**).

The oropharynx begins at the anterior tonsillar pillars and extends to the hyoid bone inferiorly and to the level of the soft palate superiorly where the nasopharynx begins. The tonsils, soft palate, posterior one third of the tongue (base of tongue), and suprahyoid epiglottis are located in the oropharynx. The nasopharynx is bounded anteriorly by the choana and contains the tori tubarius and the adenoids. (The choana is the junction between the nasal cavity and nasopharynx; see **Fig. 12–1** in Chapter 12.)

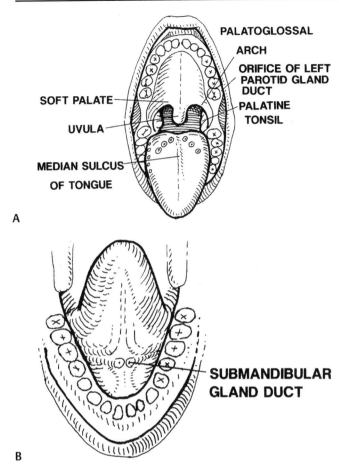

PALATOGLOSSAL
ARCH

ORIFICE OF LEFT
PAROTID GLAND
DUCT

SOFT PALATE

PALATINE
TONSIL

UVULA

MEDIAN SULCUS
OF TONGUE

A

SUBMANDIBULAR
GLAND DUCT

B

Figure 22–1 Anatomy of the oral cavity and oropharynx.

Function

The oral cavity, pharynx, and nasal cavities serve many functions. The oral cavity, oropharynx, and hypopharynx are the entrance to the digestive tract. The pharynx, nasal cavities, and oral cavity form the resonator of the voice. Abnormalities of these structures may affect speech or swallowing.

Choanal Atresia

In general, congenital problems are a result of either failure of a closed structure to open (e.g., choanal atresia) or the failure of a structure to close properly (e.g., cleft palate). The nasal placode is a thickening of the ectoderm (outer surface) of the face, which develops during the third or fourth week of gestation and invaginates, creating two nasal pits a week later (Moore, 1977). The forming nasal cavity remains separate from the pharynx at the bucconasal membrane. This membrane usually ruptures at about the eighth week of gestation. Failure to rupture leads to choanal atresia, which can be uni- or bilateral (**Fig. 22–2**).

Infants are obligate nasal breathers: they must breathe through their noses. The high position of the infant's larynx, which causes them to breathe through the nose, also enables them to eat and breathe simultaneously. Bilateral choanal atresia presents at birth with symptoms of choking, inability to nurse, and cyanosis. The diagnosis is made by unsuccessfully attempting to pass red rubber catheters through the nose to the pharynx. Various devices, the simplest of which is

a baby bottle nipple with the end cut off, are used to allow the infant to breathe through the mouth. Feeding tubes are sometimes necessary initially. Tracheotomy rarely is needed. By 2 or 3 weeks of age, the infant has often learned to breathe orally.

Surgical opening of the atresia is often done at 10 weeks of age. There are several different techniques for repairing choanal atresia including transnasal and transoral/transpalatal approaches.

Unilateral choanal atresia is less obvious and is often not diagnosed for months to years. Unilateral chronic nasal discharge is often the only symptom. Hyponasal speech is also not uncommon. Choanal atresia may be associated with other congenital anomalies.

Cleft Lip and Palate

The palate is formed by the fusion of several structures including the frontal nasal process and the palatal shelves of the maxilla, whereas the upper lip is a fusion of the lateral and medial nasal processes. This process takes place around the tenth week of gestation. Failure of proper fusion or improper breakdown of epithelial bridges may result in a variety of abnormalities of the upper lip, nose, or palate.

The least severe deformity is diastasis of the musculature of the soft palate or a submucosal cleft palate. These patients may present with velopharyngeal insufficiency with hypernasal speech and nasal regurgitation of fluids. Speech therapy often benefits patients with mild cases. For more severe cases, surgical procedures are available to reestablish the muscular integrity of the soft palate, augment the posterior pharyngeal wall, or partially close the nasopharynx with flaps.

The most severe clefting is bilateral cleft lip and complete clefting of the hard and soft palates. Various combinations of cleft lip and palate can exist, resulting in different types of feeding, speech, and cosmetic problems. Feeding difficulties in cleft palate are first due to the infant's inability to generate negative pressure to suck as air leaks through the cleft. Food in the oral cavity and oropharynx also refluxes freely into the nasopharynx and nasal cavity. Unrepaired cleft palate also results in a severely hypernasal voice, which may result in unintelligible speech. Repair of the lip is usually done when the child has fulfilled the rule of tens (i.e., 10 weeks old, 10 pounds, and hemoglobin of 10 g). The palate is repaired somewhat later, between 12 and 24 months of age (Bumsted, 1986).

Abnormalities of the musculature of the soft palate often lead to eustachian tube dysfunction due to the relationship of the tensor veli palatini and levator palatini muscles to the tori tubarius, the openings of the eustachian tubes. Middle ear effusions and sometimes more extensive ear disease are often seen in cleft palate patients. Placement of tympanostomy tubes to prevent problems from developing is advisable.

Velopharyngeal insufficiency can also be the result of lack of innervation to the soft palate via the vagus nerve. This may be seen in cerebral palsy, following poliomyelitis or in Arnold-Chiari malformation. A prosthesis that lifts the soft palate is often very effective. Bilateral lesions of the vagus nerves are extremely unlikely, whereas resection of a skull base tumor can often result in a unilateral vagal palsy with unilateral weakness of the soft palate. Surgical attachment of

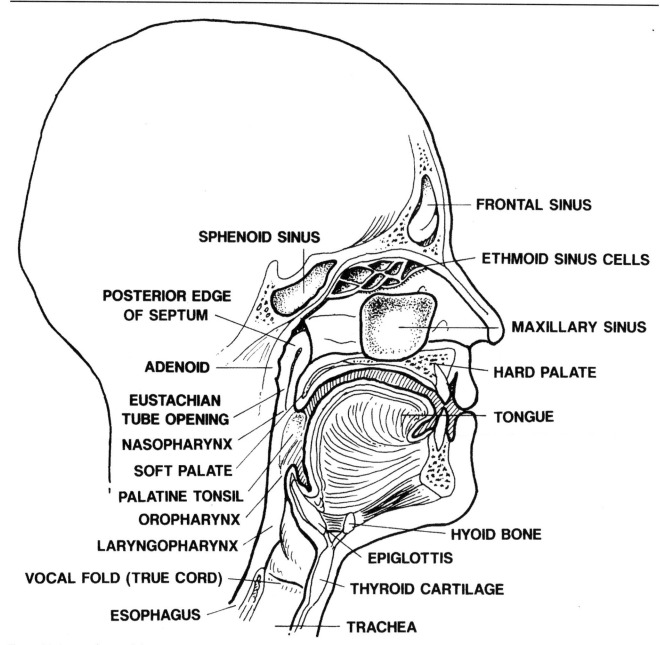

Figure 22–2 Lateral view of the upper aerodigestive tract.

the paralyzed side to the posterior nasopharyngeal wall relieves these patients of their symptoms quite well (Netterville & Vrabec, 1994).

Adenotonsillar Hypertrophy

The adenoids and palatine tonsils (commonly known just as the tonsils) are part of the ring of lymphatic tissue in the pharynx, which, with the lingual tonsils, make up Waldeyer's ring. This ring of tissue is the first part of the lymphatic system to encounter foreign substances that enter the body through the nose or mouth, and is thought to sensitize the immune system to these invaders. Problems with the tonsils and adenoids can occur when they hypertrophy and obstruct the naso- and oropharynx or they become chronically infected with bacteria, often group A, β-hemolytic streptococcus.

Hypertrophy causes hyponasal voice, nasal obstruction, snoring, chronic mouth breathing, and occasionally obstructive sleep apnea syndrome. Chronic tonsillitis causes chronic sore throat, odynophagia, and, often, halitosis. If the tonsils and adenoids do not shrink with age or remain symptomatic despite medical intervention, surgical excision of the tonsils and/or adenoids usually resolves these problems. Removal of the adenoids, however, can lead to velopharyngeal insufficiency and associated symptoms of nasal regurgitation and hypernasal voice. This usually occurs only transiently, lasting days to a few weeks, in a small number of patients (less than 5%) and is very rarely permanent (less than 1%) The permanent cases are usually seen only in children with a short palate or unrecognized submucous cleft palate. Treatment includes palatal lift prostheses or surgery to lengthen the palate or adhere it to the posterior pharyngeal wall.

Tongue Disorders

Most disorders that affect the tongue are related to changes of the mucosa, changes that can occur in any of the oral mucosa. This includes hyperkeratosis, dysplasia, and atrophy. Most mucosal abnormalities seen are very nonspecific and of little clinical significance. Many need to be biopsied to rule out carcinoma, but otherwise require no therapy.

Lack of sense of taste is usually due to a loss of sense of smell with no actual abnormality of the taste apparatus. However, various systemic illnesses and medications can diminish the overall sense of taste. Decreased taste or numbness in a specific part of the tongue should alert the clinician to the possibility of a lesion of the nerve (lingual or glossopharyngeal) supplying sensation to that portion of the tongue.

Motor function of the tongue is integral in chewing, manipulating a food bolus, swallowing, and articulating speech. Interruption of the motor innervation to the tongue is usually the result of stroke or other significant intracranial event or surgical trauma in the neck or floor of mouth. Rarely, a malignant neoplasm of the base of skull or submandibular gland presents with unilateral tongue palsy. Fortunately, the tongue is able to accommodate unilateral hypoglossal nerve palsy well, with very little long-term dysarthria or dysphagia, provided there are no other cranial nerve palsies.

Salivary Gland Disorders

The oral cavity is the site of the openings of the ducts of the major salivary glands and the site of many minor salivary glands. The three pairs of major salivary glands are the parotid glands, located anterior to the ear and superficial to the angle of the mandible; the submandibular glands, just inferior and medial to the body of the mandible; and the sublingual glands, inferior to the anterior tongue. Each gland produces saliva of slightly different composition when stimulated by the autonomic nervous system. Saliva lubricates the mouth, and enzymes within saliva initiate digestion of food. Dry mouth (xerostomia) results when the salivary glands cease to function properly. A chronically dry mouth is very uncomfortable, makes eating more difficult, and can lead to dental disease. Xerostomia can be due to simple problems, such as inadequate water intake and dehydration, or to more complex autoimmune diseases, such as Sjögren's syndrome, in which the tissue ceases to function. A common cause of xerostomia is medication that alters the autonomic input to the glands, such as antihistamines and antipsychotic and antidepressant drugs. Caffeine and alcohol have similar effects. Xerostomia is also a common side effect of radiation therapy to the oral cavity or oropharynx. Treatment first involves identifying and treating the etiology followed by the use of oral lubricants and medications that directly stimulate the salivary glands.

Infections of the Oral Cavity, Oropharynx, Nasopharynx, and Salivary Glands

Infections can occur in many different structures within and around the oral cavity and oropharynx. They can be viral, bacterial, and fungal or due to mycobacteria, some of which cause tuberculosis. The most common infection is viral pharyngitis, which causes sore throat and odynophagia (painful swallowing). The tonsils may be involved and swell enough to threaten the airway. Less common viruses, such as the herpes virus, may cause painful and infectious vesicular sores on the lips and in the mouth. Aphthous ulcers, commonly known as canker sores, are thought to be due to local trauma and possibly a nonherpetic viral infection. They are very painful and usually last about 7 days, but are not contagious. Pharyngitis and tonsillitis may also be caused by bacteria. Infection by group A β-hemolytic streptococcus (strep throat) is the most feared due to its potential systemic effects such as rheumatic fever, rheumatic heart disease, and kidney disease (acute glomerulonephritis).

The salivary glands are also prone to infection. This can be viral, as in mumps, which affects the parotid glands, or suppurative sialoadenitis, in which bacteria, usually *Staphylococcus aureus*, may infect any of the salivary glands. Stones within the ducts or glands themselves (sialolithiasis) make bacterial sialoadenitis more likely, as do dehydration and other causes of xerostomia as discussed above.

Treatment of these various infectious processes varies according to the etiology and structure involved. Hydration, analgesics, and antipyretics relieve most symptoms. Some viruses may be treated with specific antiviral agents (e.g., acyclovir is effective against herpes simplex), whereas most other viruses are not deterred by antiviral agents. Bacterial infections are treated with antibiotics. Occasionally a bacterial infection progresses into an abscess that does not respond to antibiotic therapy. Surgical drainage is then required. This can be done through either the mouth or the neck. Rather severe, life-threatening infections can develop if the abscess extends into the neck, where it can involve the great vessels or cause enough swelling to obstruct the airway. Incision and drainage of a deep neck abscess and sometimes tracheotomy are performed emergently in those cases.

Neoplasms of the Oral Cavity, Oropharynx, and Salivary Glands

The most common malignant tumor of the oral cavity and oropharynx is squamous cell carcinoma, which is usually caused by tobacco use or, to a lesser extent, alcohol abuse. This is covered in detail in Chapter 12.

Common benign tumors include papillomas, which are caused by the human papilloma virus, and fibromas, caused by trauma. Simple excision is usually curative.

Tumors may also develop within the salivary glands. If these are benign or malignant but diagnosed early, excision of the gland may effect a cure. Although relatively straightforward for the submandibular glands, it is much more complex for the parotid glands. The facial nerve leaves the skull base just inferior to the ear and courses through the substance of the parotid gland en route to the muscles of the face, which it innervates. Any surgery of the parotid gland must begin with identification and careful dissection of the facial nerve to avoid inadvertent injury, which could result in unilateral complete facial paralysis with inability to close the eye, the lips, and obvious cosmetic deformity.

Trauma of the Oral Cavity

Trauma to the oral cavity may be blunt or penetrating, with the former more common. Motor vehicle accidents and assaults are responsible for most blunt injuries that result in mandible fractures. Treating these fractures entails reestablishing normal occlusion, which may be achieved with a variety of techniques, including long-term (6 weeks) maxillomandibular fixation (MMF, wiring the jaws together) alone, MMF and wiring or plating of the fractures, or screwing and compression plating of the fractures with immediate release of MMF. The technique chosen depends on the site and direction of the fracture, as well as the surgeon's experience. When a mandible fracture is combined with other facial injuries, the repair becomes more complex and reestablishment of the normal occlusion less certain.

Penetrating injuries to the oral cavity and pharynx range from hard and soft palate lacerations, which result from children falling down on objects in their mouths, such as toy trumpets or popsicle sticks, to devastating shotgun injuries sustained in unsuccessful suicide attempts. The former warrants evaluation due to the proximity of the carotid artery to the lateral pharyngeal wall and possible damage to that structure. The latter injury requires many procedures first to salvage as much tissue as possible and then to reconstruct the face.

Sleep Disorders

Many conditions can affect sleep. Probably the most common problem with sleep is snoring, which represents turbulent airflow during sleep and affects about 50% of males and 30% of females. It is more common as people age and is more common in people who are overweight. Snoring tends to worsen after alcohol intake and when lying flat on the back. Because snoring is a sign of obstruction, it may affect one's ability to sleep.

Although snoring is often perceived as only a problem for the snorer's bed partner, it may be a sign of the more serious condition known as obstructive sleep apnea syndrome (OSAS) in which breathing stops for periods of time during sleep (apnea). Patients with OSAS commonly complain of excessive daytime sleepiness, headaches, and chronic fatigue. The condition can lead to high blood pressure, heart rhythm problems, heart failure, sudden death, and automobile accidents due to falling asleep while driving (Goode, 1986).

Apnea may be due to the central nervous system not initiating a breath, or, more commonly, a blockage developing somewhere in the throat or nasal passages, stopping the flow of air. Various abnormalities of the facial structures and throat can promote sleep apnea by blocking breathing through the nose or throat, or causing the tongue to fall back into the throat. Large tonsils, a long floppy soft palate, a large tongue, or a short mandible may promote this condition. If sleep apnea is suspected, the patient will undergo a polysomnogram, or sleep study, which involves spending a night in the sleep laboratory, or use of home-based, mobile sleep study equipment and services. While the subject sleeps, many measurements are taken of eye movements, brain wave activity (electroencephalography, EEG), heart activity, breathing activity, and oxygen saturation (level of oxygen in blood). Based on the finding of this examination the patient is diagnosed with either a snoring disorder only, or mild, moderate, or severe sleep apnea.

There are various treatments for sleep apnea. In those patients who are overweight, weight loss is extremely important and occasionally is enough to relieve the patient of these symptoms. Exercise and regimented sleep-wake cycles are also helpful.

The goal of the remainder of treatment is to keep the airway open while the patient is sleeping. This can be done with a nasal constant positive airway pressure device (nasal CPAP) in which the subject is fitted with a mask over the nose providing a constant flow of air through the nose to prevent collapse of the throat while inhaling. Although particularly effective, CPAP is sometimes poorly tolerated. Other options include oral airways, which are devices placed in the mouth that hold the tongue and jaw forward to keep the tongue from falling back and obstructing the airway. Nasal airway devices may be helpful in some patients. The oral and nasal airways are not particularly comfortable or well tolerated. Therefore, these treatments are often abandoned by the patient, who continues to suffer from the effects of sleep apnea.

Surgical procedures may permanently open the breathing passageways without the use of devices. For extremely severe sleep apnea, a tracheotomy is often done. This is the ultimate surgical procedure for this disease and works 100% of the time, but it does require long-term care of the tracheostomy tube. Most patients do not require this procedure.

Other surgical procedures are aimed at improving the airway in the nose. Several operations have been developed to open the airway at the level of the throat, the most common area that obstructs. The most popular of these is tonsillectomy and uvulopalatopharyngoplasty (UPPP). Here the surgeon removes the tonsils, which are usually contributing to the problem, and excess tissue from the soft palate (including the uvula) and pharyngeal walls. UPPP creates more room in the throat and prevents collapse of the tissues while the patient is sleeping. A staged, laser-assisted version of this procedure can now be performed as an outpatient without general anesthesia. Procedures have also been developed to pull the jaw forward, primarily to pull the tongue forward, preventing it from falling back and blocking the airway.

These procedures alter the shape and function of the pharynx and can potentially affect the voice. In most cases, if there is a change, it is a positive one, with less hyponasality in the patient who has had adenoids removed or a deviated nasal septum straightened or a less muffled voice after UPPP in one with large tonsils. A potential complication of UPPP, however, is velopharyngeal insufficiency. This occurs transiently in up to 15% of patients and permanently in less than 1% of cases.

A variety of procedures have been developed to treat primary snoring. All of these are aimed at stiffening and/or shortening the soft palate. They include injection snoreplasty (injection of a sclerosing agent into the anterior surface of the soft palate) and somnoplasty (heating the muscles of the soft palate with a radiofrequency instrument).

✦ Nasal and Sinus Disorders

Function of the Nasal Cavities and Paranasal Sinuses

The nasal cavities humidify inspired air, filter out foreign matter, provide passage of outside air to the olfactory nerves (smell), and act as a resonator for the voice. The nose is the preferred route of breathing during most activity except during strenuous exercise when the mouth is usually open. The function of the paranasal sinuses is unclear. One theory is that the sinuses serve as buffers/bumpers for trauma to the head and eyes. Another is that hollow sinuses make the head lighter (**Fig. 22–3**).

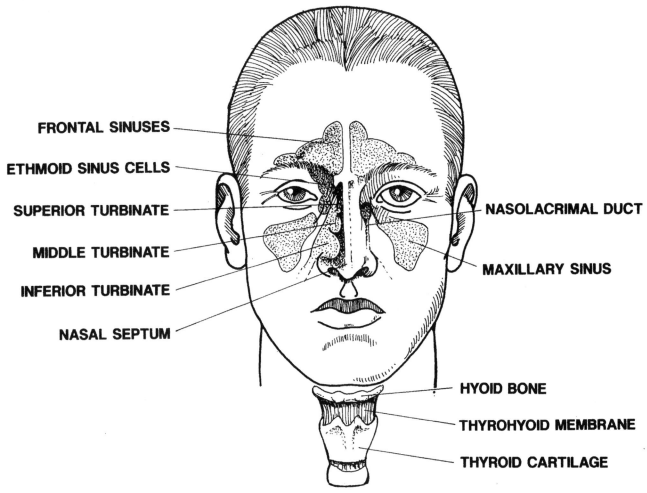

FRONTAL SINUSES

ETHMOID SINUS CELLS

SUPERIOR TURBINATE

MIDDLE TURBINATE

INFERIOR TURBINATE

NASAL SEPTUM

NASOLACRIMAL DUCT

MAXILLARY SINUS

HYOID BONE

THYROHYOID MEMBRANE

THYROID CARTILAGE

Figure 22–3 Coronal view of nasal and sinus cavities.

Disorders of the Nasal Cavities and Paranasal Sinuses

The most common nasal complaint is obstruction. Congenital problems such as choanal atresia and nasopharyngeal disease such as adenoid hypertrophy can cause obstruction, as can acquired obstructing lesions of the nasal cavities themselves. The nasal septum should be a straight, relatively thin, flat, midline structure, but it can become deviated as a person ages, obstructing (partially or completely) either one or both sides of the nose. Trauma to the nose can also cause deflection of the nasal septum or nasal bones. Benign masses, such as polyps or papillomas, and malignancies often also present with nasal obstruction, usually unilateral. Besides the obvious symptom of impaired nasal breathing, these patients often complain of decreased sense of smell, hyponasal speech, dry throat (especially in the morning), and snoring. Tumors may also cause pain and bleeding and more advanced cases can cause anesthesia of the face or eye symptoms. The inferior turbinates are responsible for providing humidity to inspired air and catching foreign substances in the mucus blanket on the mucosal surface. They can swell excessively, however, when one has allergic rhinitis or a viral upper respiratory tract infection, or they can simply grow for no apparent reason. The enlargement of the inferior turbinates also results in nasal obstruction.

Nasal obstruction may improve with medical therapy aimed at reducing swelling of the mucosal lining of the nose with oral decongestants, antihistamines (if allergy is a cause), steroid sprays, and humidification. When medical treatment fails, surgery is often curative. Straightening of the septum (septoplasty) and reconstruction of the entire nose (septorhinoplasty) are very effective procedures with few complications. Cauterizing the inferior turbinates, which leads to scarring and less ability to swell, and fracturing the turbinates and pushing them laterally also improve the airway with minimal morbidity. Sometimes a portion of the inferior turbinate is removed. Removing the entire structure can cause excessive drying and crusting in the nasal cavity and is discouraged. Removal of benign lesions such as polypectomy is also relatively straightforward, although the polyps have a tendency to recur.

Epistaxis

Bleeding from the nose (epistaxis) is another fairly common problem. Most episodes of epistaxis originate from small vessels located on the anterior septum. This results in brief relatively mild easy-to-control bleeding. Occasionally epistaxis originates from the posterior nasal cavity or nasopharynx, is much harder to control, and may possibly be life-threatening. Nasal packing or cauterizing or ligating the bleeding vessels will usually control the bleeding. Epistaxis may also be a sign of a nasal or sinus neoplasm.

Rhinitis

Allergic rhinitis is a common intermittent cause of nasal obstruction. Other symptoms include clear watery rhinorrhea, sneezing, and itchy nose and eyes. These symptoms occur in the presence of specific allergens that may be present during certain seasons (e.g., pollens, fungi) or in certain locations (e.g., dust mite, animal dander). Avoidance or elimination of the allergens provides definitive treatment, although this is frequently difficult. Few patients will part with their pets, for example. Antihistamines, steroid nasal sprays, and cromolyn nasal sprays (cromolyn prevents the mast cell from releasing histamine) may be necessary. Usually only one of these classes of medications is necessary at any one time. Antihistamines have the disadvantage of sometimes causing sedation and of excessively drying the mouth and pharynx, which can be a problem for professional voice users. Desensitization injections, commonly known as allergy shots, frequently succeed in making the person less sensitive to the allergens.

Sinusitis

Sinusitis is an infection of one or more of the eight paranasal sinus cavities. It usually follows a viral upper respiratory infection or an exacerbation of allergic rhinitis. These conditions cause swelling of the nasal mucosa including the mucosa at the naturally small openings of the sinuses. Anatomic abnormalities and polyps may also block the sinus ostia. Blockage of these openings creates a closed cavity, which is an excellent environment for the colonization and growth of bacteria, the most common pathogens in sinusitis. Symptoms of acute sinusitis include purulent nasal discharge, nasal obstruction, facial pain and pressure, fever, and occasionally headache. Treatment is aimed at opening the closed sinus cavities and eradicating the bacteria. Oral and topical nasal spray decongestants, saline nasal rinses, analgesics, rest, and antibiotics are crucial. Most acute episodes of sinusitis in immunocompetent individuals clear with one course of medical therapy.

Potential, but rare, complications of acute sinusitis include spread of the infection to the orbit, with possible injury to the eye, or intracranially, with possible meningitis, brain abscess, or cavernous sinus thrombosis. These complications usually require surgical intervention to open up and drain the affected sinus and adjacent infected area, such as the orbit.

Chronic sinusitis is quite different from the acute disease, although acute exacerbations may occur in a patient with chronic disease. The common symptoms of chronic sinusitis include chronic nasal and postnasal discharge, which is usually thick mucoid material, and varying degrees of nasal obstruction, pressure, or a heavy feeling in the face and head. Facial pain and headaches are rarely seen in chronic sinusitis and fever is also uncommon. Patients are treated in a similar manner to those with acute sinusitis, but the duration of therapy is longer. Antibiotics are prescribed for 3 weeks or longer; nasal steroid sprays and oral decongestants or antihistamines (if allergy is present) are taken indefinitely. Nasal endoscopy helps to determine whether small polyps or other lesions are obstructing the sinus ostia. A CT scan is the test of choice for assessing location and extent of disease. It often shows obstruction of the ostiomeatal complex, which is the common path of drainage for the frontal, anterior ethmoid, and maxillary sinuses. It may

also show thickening of the mucosal lining of the sinuses, a sign of chronic sinusitis. A patient who has severe enough symptoms and fails medical therapy is a candidate for surgery. A relatively new technique known as endoscopic sinus surgery (ESS) has greatly decreased the morbidity associated with sinus surgery and is the preferred technique (Redline & Young, 1993). With the increased ability to see the anatomy during surgery, more precise and more thorough removal of diseased tissue can be performed without the need for external incisions. Success rates are about 85% (Benninger, Mickelson, and Yaremchuk, 1990). Nasal polyps are often seen in patients with chronic sinusitis. They are removed during ESS and are thought to recur less often after this procedure than after a simple polypectomy.

Nasal Masses

The most common benign nasal mass is the inflammatory polyp, although it is not considered a true neoplasm (**Fig. 22–4**). As discussed above, these masses usually cause nasal obstruction and are frequently associated with allergic rhinitis or chronic sinusitis. In children, the presence of nasal polyps suggests the possibility of cystic fibrosis, which may be undiagnosed. Removal of nasal polyps involves simple polypectomy or more extensive sinus surgery, depending on symptoms and other findings. Squamous papillomas are the most common true neoplasms in the nose. They are benign and are usually cured with simple excision.

Inverted papilloma is less common and also benign. It can, however, be very aggressive and is capable of eroding through adjacent bony structures into the orbit or intracranially. Removal of these lesions requires excision of the tumor with a wide margin of normal tissue. Because these are found most commonly on the lateral nasal wall, they are usually treated with a medial maxillectomy, which removes the entire lateral nasal wall, ethmoid sinus, and medial wall of the maxilla. With a lesser operation, recurrence is common. The treatment of nasal-sinus malignancies are discussed in Chapter 12.

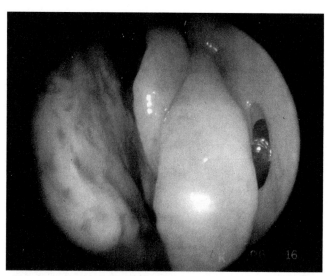

Figure 22–4 Large polyp extending from the left middle meatus into the nose. The polyps caused nasal obstruction and chronic rhinosinusitis. The patient had complete obstruction of the right nostril with polyps.

Facial Pain

Pain is a symptom that can result from many different disease processes. The most common causes of facial pain include trauma, sinusitis, and dental disease. The history suggests the diagnosis, which is usually confirmed with the physical findings. With appropriate treatment and resolution of the disease, the pain also abates. Sometimes the etiology behind the pain is not apparent or the pain does not resolve with the other symptoms.

As discussed above, acute (not chronic) sinusitis is often painful. Tenderness is elicited over the maxillary or frontal sinuses if those are involved. Inflammation of the ethmoid and sphenoid sinuses can cause pain at the top of the head and occiput, respectively. The pain, however is usually not an isolated symptom, but is associated with other signs of sinusitis.

The trigeminal nerve (cranial nerve V) supplies sensation to the face. The first division (ophthalmic) supplies the forehead, eyebrows, and eyes. The second division (infraorbital) supplies the cheek, nose, and upper lip and gums. The third division (mandibular) supplies the ear, mouth, jaw, tongue, lower lip, and submandibular region. When pain is located in a very specific nerve distribution area, lesions involving that nerve must be considered. Tumors involving the nerve usually cause other symptoms, but pain may be the only complaint, and presence of a tumor at the base of the skull or in the face must be ruled out. When the workup is negative, the diagnosis may be one of many types of neuralgia, which is a pain originating within the sensory nerve itself. Treatment is medical and in some cases surgical.

Otalgia (ear pain) can be caused by many different conditions of the ear itself, including trauma, infection, foreign body, tumor, and even cerumen impaction, or it can be a referred pain. The external ear canal and auricle receive sensory innervation from branches of four different cranial nerves: fifth (trigeminal), seventh (facial), ninth (glossopharyngeal), and tenth (vagus). These nerves also supply various other parts of the head and neck and even thorax and abdomen in the case of the tenth nerve. Inflammation of another part of these nerves, for example, the vagus nerve from a tumor of the larynx or hypopharynx, will often cause otalgia along with the local symptoms. More common conditions such as tonsillitis or an aphthous ulcer of the soft palate also commonly cause referred otalgia.

There are many craniomandibular disorders that include pain in the head and neck among many different and varied symptoms. Many of these conditions relate to the temporomandibular joint (TMJ) and surrounding structures. Internal abnormalities of the TMJ may cause local pain, otalgia, trismus, sounds within the joint during mandibular movement, and change in occlusion (Cooper, 1989). Extracapsular craniomandibular disorders are also known as myofacial pain dysfunction syndrome and are thought to be due to an abnormal relationship of the dental apparatus, the TMJs, and the neuromuscular system (Cooper, 1989). Symptoms include pains that do not seem related to the TMJ, headaches, muffled ears and other otologic symptoms, and various other vague facial, dental, and neck symptoms. The workup is first aimed at finding and correcting the underlying cause of the symptoms, such as an intracapsular lesion of the TMJ or dental malocclusion. This may require simple measures such as a bite plane to align the occlusion at night and prevent bruxism, or may require surgery of the TMJ itself. Other treatments include transcutaneous electrical neural stimulation (TENS) to control muscle spasms and relieve pain.

✦ Anatomy of the Larynx

To understand the anatomy of the larynx, it is imperative to realize that the larynx is not an anatomic site unto itself. Much of the function of the larynx is dependent on the structures that are attached and integrated with the larynx. These include the muscles and soft tissues of the neck, the trachea and the esophagus, the hyoid and mandibular bones, and the muscles of the tongue. Functionally, the larynx depends on the integration of activities with the nervous system, both afferent and efferent impulses, and coordination of activities via the central nervous system and the spinal cord. It is often simplest to think of the larynx in relationship to its four major tissue types: cartilages, muscles, nerves, and blood vessels.

There are five primary laryngeal cartilages: the thyroid cartilage, cricoid cartilage, epiglottis, and a pair of arytenoid cartilages (**Figs. 22–5, 22–6,** and **22–7**). In addition, there are smaller cartilages, the function of which is not perfectly clear. These are the paired cuneiform and corniculate cartilages, which lie in the aryepiglottic folds superior to the arytenoid cartilages. The thyroid cartilage, whose name is derived from the Greek word for shield, is the largest cartilage in the larynx and encompasses the anterior and lateral skeletal structure of the larynx. The cartilage has a greater and lesser cornua to which are attached the thyrohyoid ligament and the cricothyroid ligament, respectively, and bilateral ala. The cartilage also has an oblique line on the ala to which is attached the middle constrictor muscle. This attachment is important for the superior movement of the larynx with swallowing. The anterior thyroid cartilage extends from the thyroid notch to the anterior-inferior cartilage. The angle of the anterior cartilage tends to be more acute in men (90 degrees) than in women (120 degrees), which makes it more prominent in the neck, hence the term *Adam's apple.*

The cricoid cartilage lies just below the thyroid cartilage and is joined to the thyroid cartilage at the cricothyroid joint

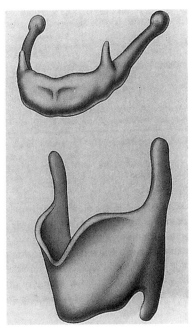

Figure 22–5 Hyoid bone and thyroid cartilage. [From Tucker, H.M. (1993). *The Larynx,* 2nd ed. New York, Thieme, with permission.]

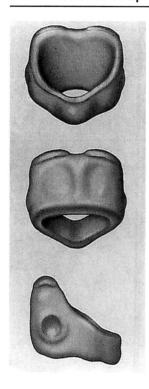

Figure 22–6 Cricoid cartilage. Top, anterior view; middle, posterior view; bottom, lateral view. [From Tucker, H.M. (1993). *The Larynx,* 2nd ed. New York, Thieme, with permission.]

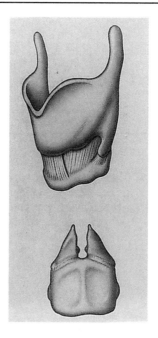

Figure 22–8 Cricothyroid joint, membrane, and ligament, above; cricoarytenoid joints, posterior view, below. [From Tucker, H.M. (1993). *The Larynx,* 2nd ed. New York, Thieme, with permission.]

between the inferior cornua of the thyroid and the lateral joint capsule of the cricoid (**Fig. 22–8**). This joint allows for rotation of the cricoid in relationship to the thyroid cartilages. The cricothyroid membrane attaches the anterior-lateral aspects of the inferior thyroid to the superior cricoid. The cricoid cartilage is the only complete ring in the upper airway with the thyroid cartilage and the tracheal rings being open posteriorly. In neonates and infants, this is the narrowest part of the upper

airway and is the most common site for upper airway obstruction. Swelling of the tissues of the subglottic region surrounded by the complete ring of fixed cricoid cartilage accounts for the airway obstruction in croup. In older children and adults, the narrowest area is the rima glottis or space between the free margins of the true vocal folds. The cricoid cartilage is shaped like a signet ring with the larger face posterior. On the upper surface of the signet portion is the cricoarytenoid joint. This joint is unique in that it allows for both rocking of the arytenoids and also anterior-posterior sliding.

The arytenoid cartilages are paired cartilages that lie on top of the cricoid cartilage at the cricoarytenoid joint. In addition to the joint, there are three main surfaces (processes) of the arytenoids: the muscular process, posterolaterally, to which is attached the posterior and lateral cricoarytenoid muscles; the vocal process, anteriorly, with the attachment of the vocalis ligament and muscle; and the posterior surface, where the interarytenoid muscle attaches.

The epiglottis is different from the other cartilages of the larynx in that it is primarily hyaline cartilage (**Fig. 22–9**). This cartilage does not ossify, whereas the other cartilages ossify with age. The epiglottis is attached to the upper, midposterior surface of the thyroid cartilage at the petiole, and laterally with the arytenoids by the aryepiglottic folds. There is an upper (lingual) and a lower (laryngeal) surface of the epiglottis. The vallecula is the area where the epiglottis meets the base of the tongue.

There are both intrinsic and extrinsic muscles of the larynx. The intrinsic muscles of the larynx are the thyroarytenoid, interarytenoid, posterior cricoarytenoid, and the lateral cricoarytenoid muscles, whereas the extrinsic muscles are the cricothyroid muscles (**Fig. 22–10**). The intrinsic muscles receive their motor innervation primarily from the recurrent laryngeal nerves (RLNs) with a small portion coming from the superior laryngeal nerve (SLN), whereas the cricothyroid receives its motor innervation from the superior laryngeal nerves (Sanders, Wu, Liancai, et al., 1993) (**Fig. 22–11**).

The lateral cricoarytenoid muscles result in rotation of the vocal process of the arytenoids toward the midline, thereby

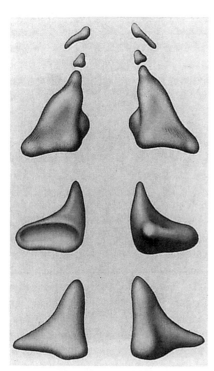

Figure 22–7 Arytenoid cartilages. Top, posterior view with cuneiform and corniculate cartilages above; middle, inferior view; bottom, anterior view. [From Tucker, H.M. (1993). *The Larynx,* 2nd ed. New York, Thieme, with permission.]

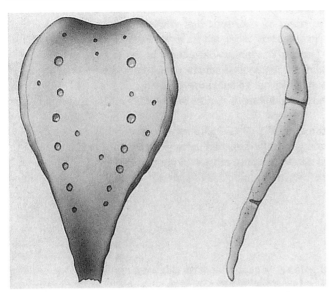

Figure 22–9 Epiglottic cartilage. Note perforations. [From Tucker, H.M. (1993). *The Larynx,* 2nd ed. New York, Thieme, with permission.]

tightening the vocal folds and slightly elongating them (**Fig. 22–12**). The thyroarytenoid (TA) muscles tense the vocal folds by shortening the arytenoids in relationship to the thyroid cartilage. The TA muscles along with the overlying vocalis ligament and mucosa are the structures that form the true vocal fold. The interarytenoids pull the muscular processes of the arytenoids together, resulting in adduction, and the cricothyroid muscles rotate the thyroid on the cricoid cartilages, thereby elongating and tensing the vocal folds. These muscles work in delicate concert to adduct the vocal folds and adjust pitch. The only pure abductor of the larynx is the posterior cricoarytenoid muscles, which rotate the vocal processes of the arytenoids laterally as they pull the muscular

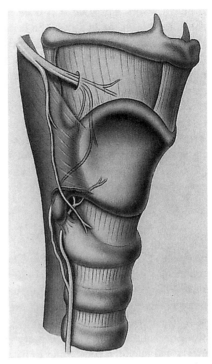

Figure 22–11 Nerve supply of the larynx. Superior laryngeal nerve course from above and recurrent laryngeal nerve approaches from below. Also note inferior constrictor muscle. [From Tucker, H.M. (1993). *The Larynx,* 2nd ed. New York, Thieme, with permission.]

processes medially. Although there is some debate, the cricothyroid muscles may also play a role in abduction with deep inspiration or with hypercapnia.

The major nerve supply to the larynx is from the superior and recurrent laryngeal nerves, which are branches of the vagus (CN X) nerve. The SLN leaves the vagus just after it exits the skull base and splits into internal and external branches. The internal branch passes through the thyrohyoid membrane to supply sensory innervation to the epiglottis and the larynx down to the level of the true vocal folds. If this sensory input is lost, there can be a significant effect on swallowing, and patients may be prone to aspiration. The external branch stays external to the larynx and supplies motor innervation to the cricothyroid muscles. The RLNs receive their names because

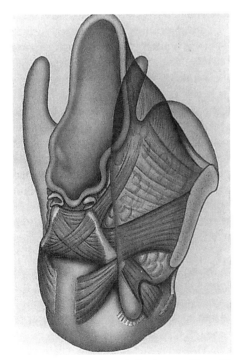

Figure 22–10 Intrinsic muscles of the larynx. [From Tucker, H.M. (1993). *The Larynx,* 2nd ed. New York, Thieme, with permission.]

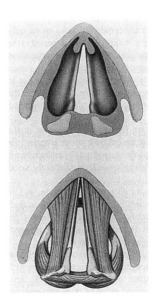

Figure 22–12 Horizontal section of larynx through the ventricles. Mucosa intact, above; mucosa removed to show intrinsic muscles of vocal folds, below. [From Tucker, H.M. (1993). *The Larynx,* 2nd ed. New York, Thieme, with permission.]

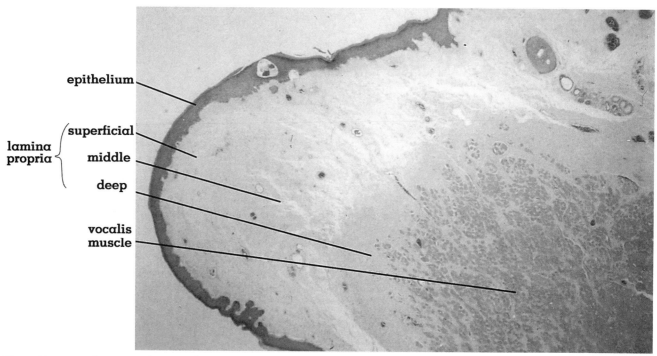

epithelium

superficial

lamina
propria

middle

deep

vocalis
muscle

Figure 22–13 Histologic coronal section of the vocal fold.

they leave the vagus nerve low in the neck and loop (recur) in the chest prior to ascending in the tracheoesophageal groove to innervate the intrinsic muscles of the larynx and provide sensation to the lower edge of the vocal folds and the subglottic region. The right RLN loops under the subclavian artery, which is at the base of the neck, higher than the left RLN, which loops under the arch of the aorta in the chest. The nerve impulses in the left RLN are slightly faster than in the right, which allows them to reach the respective muscles of the larynx at the same time (Harrison, 1981). The longer loop of the left RLN into the chest results in a higher likelihood that the left RLN will be injured by pathology in the chest (Benninger, Gardner, & Schwimmer, 2003).

The microanatomy of the vocal folds has been well described and is crucial for an understanding of the pathology and physiology of the larynx and is necessary to understand to plan treatment (Colton, 1993) (**Fig. 22–13**). The vocal folds are composed of sequential layers. The most superficial layer is the mucosa, which is stratified squamous epithelium primarily without glandular structures. Deep to the mucosa are three layers of lamina propria: a superficial layer of loose connective tissue (Reinke's space), a middle transitional layer, and a deep layer of dense connective tissue and collagen (vocal ligament). Deep to the vocal ligament is the medial belly of the vocalis (TA) muscle. It is believed that with low pitch and tension these distinct layers move independently from one another, but with elevated pitch and greater tension they tend to move more as a single unit.

◆ Physiology of the Larynx

There are three major functions of the larynx: protection, respiration, and phonation. Protection of the lungs reveals the critical role of the larynx in swallowing. Laryngeal physiology is based on a complex interaction of concerted muscular activity, sensory and motor nerve input, reflexes, and glandular

secretions. It is difficult to summarize all of these activities, although some general physiologic principles apply.

Phonation, or the production of voice, is the result of the action of the lungs, the larynx, and the resonating cavities of the upper and lower airways. As the vocal folds are brought together through the actions of the intrinsic and extrinsic muscles of the larynx, and as passive or forced-active exhalation occurs, subglottic pressure increases until it overcomes the pressure of the vocal folds held in position. The vocal folds will then part for a short period of time depending on the level of subglottic pressure and the tightness of the apposition of the vocal folds. As the vocal folds separate to allow passage of the air, two events occur that tend to bring the vocal folds back to the midline: (1) the natural tension and pressure of the vocal folds becomes greater than the decreasing subglottic pressure; and (2) the Bernoulli effect occurs, which pulls the vocal folds back to the midline. As the subglottic pressure rapidly increases, the cycle is repeated. This repetitive cycle of vocal fold closing and opening is called the myoelastic-aerodynamic theory of phonation. Factors that would allow this to occur more quickly would be associated with an increase in vocal fold frequency and an elevated pitch. These would be increasing subglottic pressure, decreasing the mass of the vocal folds, or increasing the tension on the vocal folds. Similarly, decreased subglottic pressure, increased mass, or decreased tension would result in lowering of the pitch. A mass lesion, poor pulmonary support, a thicker vocal fold (as in males), or lesser tension would all be associated with decreased pitch.

Loudness is determined by the amplitude of the vibration. Loudness can be increased or decreased without changing pitch. Other factors that are instrumental in voice production have to do with the resonating cavities of the upper airway, particularly the pharynx and oral cavity. Speech is dependent on voice production, syntax coordination, resonation, and articulation. Although subtle refinements in the normal voice are produced at the level of the larynx, the vocal folds are not necessary for voice production. Some individuals use their false vocal folds for voice production, whereas laryngectomees can produce voice through vibration of the pharynx. Quality of voice is dependent on culture, age, sex, and many other factors such as individual taste and preference.

✦ Benign Laryngeal Disorders

As described above, the larynx serves to protect the airway from aspiration, provides a valve for generating an effective cough, and is the source of the sound that is shaped by the rest of the vocal tract to produce the voice. Benign laryngeal disorders can affect any or all of these functions.

Most benign laryngeal disorders cause a change in voice quality, usually referred to as *hoarseness*. This term, among otolaryngologists and voice pathologists, is interpreted as a rough, raspy voice often with lowering of the pitch. Unfortunately, it is not quite as well defined among other physicians and the general public, and a careful history must be obtained to determine the exact nature of the voice change (Gardner & Benninger, 1996). Pain in the region of the larynx, shortness of breath, and dysphagia may also be complaints associated with benign laryngeal disorders.

Epiglottitis

Epiglottitis, also known as supraglottitis, is an acute infection of the epiglottis and aryepiglottic folds usually caused by *Haemophilus influenzae* type B (Hib). It has historically been most common in children, aged 2 to 4 years of age, but since the introduction of a Hib vaccine, the incidence in children has declined, whereas in adults it has remained stable (Frantz & Rasgon, 1993). Symptoms include rapid onset of fever, sore throat, odynophagia, and sometimes shortness of breath. Patients usually sit upright with the head extended, drooling. The severe swelling of the supraglottic structures may lead to obstruction of the airway and death by asphyxiation. Management in children involves rapidly, but calmly, controlling the airway, usually with intubation in the operating room, and then administering antibiotics. The child remains intubated until the inflammation has resolved, usually after 2 to 3 days. Adults, who are more easily examined and have a larger airway to start with, may be managed more conservatively in less severe cases. Tracheotomy is rarely needed.

Laryngomalacia

Laryngomalacia is abnormal flaccidity of the supraglottic laryngeal tissues (epiglottis and aryepiglottic folds), which collapse during inspiration, causing inspiratory stridor. This may occur shortly after birth and usually resolves spontaneously in 6 to 18 months if, as in most cases, the child is otherwise normal. The stridor fluctuates in intensity and is worse with increased inspiratory effort, such as during crying or feeding. Rarely is intervention required (Frantz, Rasgon, & Quesenberry, 1994).

Laryngitis

The most common disease of the larynx is laryngitis, which is an inflammatory condition with several different etiologies. The most common form of laryngitis is a viral infection and is usually associated with an upper respiratory tract infection. Physical findings include erythema of the vocal folds and arytenoid mucosa, excess mucus, and sometimes edema of the vocal folds. Hydration, humidification, analgesic/antiinflammatory medications, mucolytics, modified voice use, and avoidance of irritants such as cigarette smoke are the mainstays of treatment while the viral illness runs its course. In fact, these treatments help in any laryngeal disorder. Croup, which is a viral infection of the proximal trachea and subglottic region seen more commonly in young children, causes a barking cough, hoarseness, and often inspiratory stridor. Most cases respond to humidification or cool air, whereas more severe cases require systemic steroids and occasionally even intubation for airway protection.

Laryngitis is also caused by laryngopharyngeal reflux (LPR) disease and by exposure to inhaled irritants such as smoke, steam, caustic gases and other noxious substances (Koufman, Wiener, Wu, & Castell, 1988). LPR is discussed in detail later in the chapter.

Chronic cough owing to pulmonary disease may also lead to inflammation of the glottis, frequently in the region of the vocal processes of the arytenoids, which make rather violent contact with throat clearing and uncontrolled coughing fits. Some medications used to treat asthma, such as inhaled steroids, may also cause edema and erythema of the vocal folds and should not be used to treat laryngitis.

Benign Laryngeal Masses, Nodules, Polyps, and Cysts

Any lesion that changes the mass of one or both vocal folds or prevents the vocal folds from closing completely during the glottic cycle will cause dysphonia. The common benign lesions of the vocal folds include vocal fold nodules, polyps, and cysts. A less common lesion is sulcus vocalis. Each of these has a different etiology and treatment. Often, the diagnosis of a vocal fold lesion is obvious on indirect or fiberoptic laryngoscopy. According to Woo, Colton, Casper, and Brewer (1991) and Sataloff, Spiegel, and Hawkshaw (1991), videostroboscopy is of help in differentiating between the different masses in one fourth to one third of cases.

Nodules are the result of vocal abuse or phonotrauma and are usually bilateral symmetric lesions that involve the mucosa and submucosal space (**Fig. 22–14**). Repeated contact at the midportion of the membranous vocal folds causes

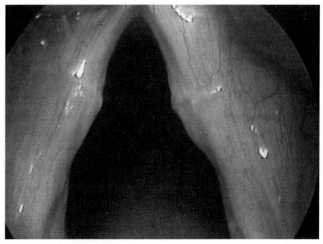

Figure 22–14 Bilateral vocal fold nodules.

thickening and often incomplete keratinization of the mucosa. The junction between the epithelium and submucosa, the basement membrane zone (BMZ), is often damaged (Loire, Bouchayer, Cornut, & Bastian, 1988). Often, what appears to be a nodule is actually transient localized edema sometimes referred to as physiologic swelling which usually resolves in 1 to 2 days following heavy voice use (Sataloff, 1991). For longer lasting lesions, voice therapy is the primary treatment. Surgery is reserved for those patients whose dysphonia persists after 3 to 6 months of intense therapy (Sataloff, 1991; Werkhaven & Ossoff, 1991). When surgery is necessary, very conservative excision of only the abnormal tissue is performed. All normal mucosa should be preserved and extreme care taken to avoid trauma to the vocal ligament, which is not typically abnormal with vocal nodules. This may be done with either very fine microsurgical instruments or with the CO_2 laser, although controversy exists regarding the use of the laser for vocal nodules (Benninger, 2000; Bouchayer & Cornut, 1992; Ford, 1994; Sataloff, 1991; Werkhaven & Ossoff, 1991; Shapshay, Rebeiz, Bohigian, & Hybels, 1990).

Intracordal cysts may be epidermoid cysts, which are most likely congenital, or mucus retention cysts resulting from obstruction of mucous gland ducts, which in turn may be due to inflammatory or traumatic processes (Milutinovic & Vasiljevic, 1992) (**Fig. 22–15**). Frequently there is no apparent predisposing cause. Only the epidermoid cyst is a true cyst and is located in the submucosa, often with surrounding fibrous reaction (Loire et al., 1988). They are usually unilateral, although a contralateral reactive nodule may be present, making the misdiagnosis of classic vocal fold nodules somewhat common. Videostroboscopy is especially helpful in differentiating between these two entities (Sataloff et al., 1991). Although voice therapy may improve the voice despite the presence of the cyst, excision is usually required to achieve the best voice result. According to Koufman and Blalock (1989), preoperative voice therapy improves the likelihood of a good result. Excision of cysts is usually performed using microdissection with cold instruments (i.e., no laser). An

incision is made through the mucosa into Reinke's space (superficial layer of the lamina propria) and the mucosa elevated off the cyst. The cyst is then dissected off of the vocal ligament (middle and deep layers of lamina propria), taking great care to avoid trauma to that structure and to avoid rupturing the cyst (Bouchayer & Cornut, 1992; Courey, Gardner, Stone, & Ossoff, 1995; Ford, 1994; Sataloff, 1991; Werkhaven & Ossoff, 1991). Excising the cyst intact is the only way of ensuring that the entire cyst has been removed, lessening the likelihood of recurrence (Bouchayer & Cornut, 1992). The often-encountered contralateral reactive nodule is assessed intraoperatively as to consistency. If it is soft, it will often resolve after excision of the cyst, but if it is hard and fibrotic the nodule should be excised as discussed above for vocal nodules.

Vocal fold polyp is a term that includes any non–neoplastic-appearing lesion that is not a nodule or granuloma (**Fig. 22–16**). Polyps may be broad-based or pedunculated, unilateral or bilateral, firm or extremely soft, very small (2 mm) or huge, appearing to obstruct the airway, although they rarely do as they flop in and out of the lumen. They may be the result of a submucosal hemorrhage, vocal abuse, or smoking. The onset of dysphonia associated with a hemorrhagic polyp is usually sudden with a history of severe coughing or screaming immediately prior to onset of the disorder not uncommon. With pedunculated polyps, the result after excision is excellent. The procedure involves making an incision at the base of the lesion, again taking care to avoid trauma to the surrounding normal mucosa and the underlying vocal ligament. Broad-based sessile polyps are excised with the same techniques, but the resulting mucosal defect is naturally larger, and the results, although still usually excellent, are less predictable. Excision may be done with microsurgical instruments or with the CO_2 laser (Sataloff, 1991; Ford, 1994; Shapshay et al., 1990).

Diffuse, chronic edema of the true vocal fold may be referred to as Reinke's edema, polypoid corditis, or polypoid degeneration (Loire et al., 1988) (**Fig. 22–17**). There is a generalized accumulation of fluid within the matrix of the superficial layer of the lamina propria, or Reinke's space (Werkhaven & Ossoff,

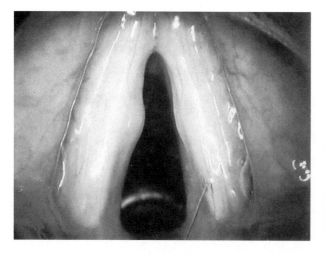

A

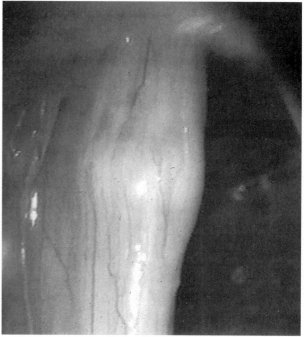

B

Figure 22–15 **(A)** Left vocal fold cyst with small reactive right vocal fold nodule. **(B)** Close-up of left vocal fold cyst (different patient than in **A**). (See Color Plate 22–15B.)

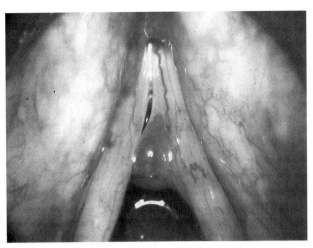

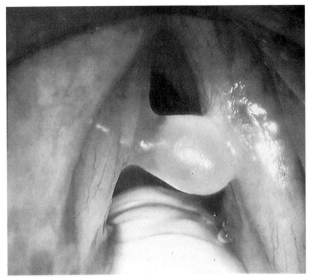

A

B

Figure 22–16 (A) Hemorrhagic polyp of right vocal fold with obvious enlarged feeding vessel. Also noted are polypoid changes of left anterior false vocal fold. **(B)** Pedunculated polyp of left vocal fold with reactive changes of right vocal fold (partially seen at anterior aspect of polyp on left vocal fold). (See Color Plates 22–16A and B.)

1991). This is usually due to smoking and other sources of chronic irritation, such as chronic coughing or throat clearing, and may be related to LPR as well. It may also represent the myxedema of hypothyroidism. With mild or early polypoid corditis, an improvement may be seen with a cessation of the inciting irritation, such as smoking. Long-standing cases will require surgical intervention for improvement of the voice. It is crucial that smokers quit prior to, or at least at, the time of surgery to avoid a recurrence of the condition (Lumpkin, Bennet, & Bishop, 1990; Hojslet, Moesgaard-Nielson, & Karlsmore, 1990). Surgery involves making an incision on the superior surface of the true vocal fold through the mucosa into Reinke's space and elevating the mucosa. The edematous matrix is then removed, taking care to avoid trauma to the vocal ligament, and the mucosa is redraped and trimmed (Courey et al., 1995). If the mucosa is relatively normal, its preservation will yield a better result than simply stripping it all away (Lumpkin, et al., 1990). If, however, there are changes, such as leukoplakia, suggestive of a neoplastic process, the abnormal mucosa must be removed for histologic examination.

Sulcus vocalis is an extremely rare condition in which there is a furrow, or sulcus, of mucosa along the rima glottis that is adherent to the underlying vocal ligament (**Fig. 22–18**). There are several types of sulcus vocalis including physiologic sulcus, type 2 sulcus (vergeture), and type 3 sulcus vocalis. There are different theories behind the etiology of each of these types, including rupture of a previously present intracordal cyst for the third type. Treatment depends first on identifying the pathology correctly. Type 2 sulcus (vergeture) is treated with microdissection and type 3 with excision (Ford, Inagi, Bless, et al., 1996).

Benign Neoplasms

The most common benign neoplasm of the vocal fold, by far, is the squamous papilloma (Jones, Myer, & Barnes, 1984) (**Fig. 22–19**). Laryngeal papillomatosis is more common in children, but can occur at any age. Dysphonia is the first symptom, but neglected or aggressive disease can progress to airway

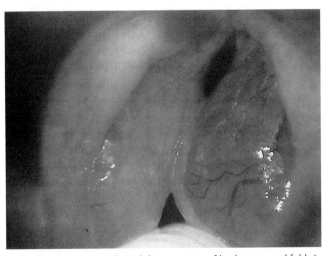

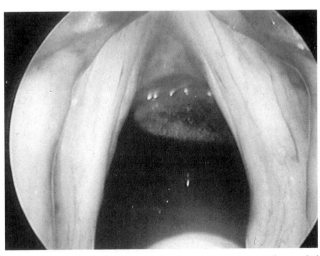

Figure 22–17 Severe polypoid degeneration of both true vocal folds in a long-time smoker. (See Color Plate 22-17.)

Figure 22–18 Bilateral sulcus vocalis. Furrows are seen on the medial aspect of both true vocal folds.

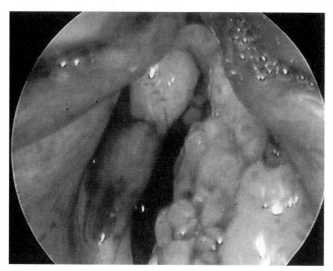

Figure 22–19 Extensive papillomatosis of the larynx in an adult. The entire right true vocal fold and the anterior left true vocal fold are involved. (See Color Plate 22–19.)

obstruction and even death. The etiology seems to be human papilloma virus (HPV) infection, but an infecting source is usually not apparent. Treatment is excision or ablation of the papillomata to restore the airway and normal contours of the vocal folds to improve voice. A variety of techniques exist for removal of the papillomas including cold instrument dissection with microinstruments, excision with the microdebrider (shaver) or ablation with the CO_2 laser or recently the pulse-dye laser (Pasquale, Wiatrak, Woolley, et al., 2003). The choice of technique generally depends on the surgeon's experience. The disease is extremely unpredictable and may recur within 1 month or disappear forever after only one treatment. Because of this uncertain prognosis, surgical excision must be conservative and preserve all normal anatomy despite often very extensive disease that obscures all normal landmarks. Overaggressive surgery can lead to scarring of the vocal folds and formation of glottic webs, which impair both voice and airway (Ossoff, Werkhaven, & Dere, 1991). When the papillomatosis goes into remission, which in children often happens at puberty, the remaining laryngeal abnormalities are often the result of the surgery and not the

disease process itself. Avoiding surgical trauma to the larynx can be difficult because these patients, especially children, commonly undergo many procedures. In more severe cases, the papillomatosis may spread down the trachea and even reach the carina and mainstem bronchi and lung parenchyma.

Medical treatment for recurrent respiratory papillomatosis (RRP) remains experimental. Systemic therapy with indole-3-carbinol (I3C) has shown some promise while injection of the lesions and surrounding tissue with the antiviral agent cidofovir seems to be the most effective addition to treatment for RRP (Pransky, Albright, & Magit, 2003; Rosen & Bryson, 2004).

Benign neoplasms of the vocal folds, other than papillomata, are extremely rare. Other tumors include oncocytic tumors, granular cell tumors, hemangiomas, adenomas, rhabdomyomas, and neurofibromas (Olson, 1991). Treatment usually involves excision with a minimal amount of normal tissue.

Granulomata are lesions that are not considered true neoplasms and consist of masses of granulation tissue. They commonly occur on the vocal process of the arytenoid cartilage as a result of some irritation such as endotracheal intubation, frequent coughing and throat clearing, and vocal abuse with a hard glottal attack or LPR (Olson, 1991) (**Fig. 22–20**). Ossification of the arytenoid cartilage as determined by CT scan suggests that perichondritis may play a role (McFerran, Abdullah, Gallimore, Pringle, & Croft, 1994). Treatment options include antireflux measures, voice therapy, steroids, surgical excision, and Botox injection (to decrease the force of arytenoid contact) (Nasri, Sercarz, McAlpin, & Berke, 1995). Granulomas have a tendency to recur after excision if the inciting etiology, such as LPR, is not eliminated, and this is best addressed before surgery (Koufman et al., 1988; McFerran et al., 1994; Sataloff, 1991; Werkhaven & Ossoff, 1991).

Functional Voice Disorders

Not all dysphonia is attributable to vocal fold masses or neurologic disorders (see below). Occasionally, a patient describes onset of a rough raspy voice, a weak breathy voice, or a whisper voice following an episode of laryngitis. With resolution of the other symptoms of laryngitis (pain, dysphagia, and cough) the dysphonia persists. The history often includes periods of

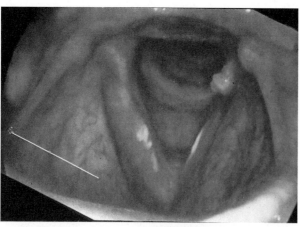

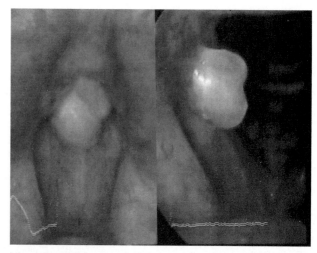

A

Figure 22–20 (A) Small granuloma of the left vocal process of the arytenoid cartilage. Also note thickening of the mucosa overlying the right vocal process and tenacious mucus on the membranous true vocal folds

B

bilaterally. **(B)** A larger right-sided granuloma at the superior aspect of the vocal process. In this patient, the lesion does not impair glottic closure, and the voice was normal. (See Color Plates 22–20A and B.)

normal voice followed by sudden unexplained onset of the dysphonic voice, although the dysphonia can be constant for long periods of time. The patient often attributes the sudden changes to some real phenomenon such as cold air, change in weather, or perceived allergies and sinus-related disease. Onset may also be slow and gradual. Laryngeal examination may reveal many different findings including an open posterior glottis with rotated arytenoids, an open glottis along the entire length of the vocal folds with normal motion, and various configurations of supraglottic hyperfunction. Although there is generally no organic disease to be found, continued abnormal laryngeal behavior may lead to the development of a secondary lesion such as vocal nodules.

The abnormal voice in patients with rapid onset of dysphonia described above is due to improper voice production technique, although it is usually done unconsciously. It is thought that during an acute laryngeal illness, when changes in the vocal folds alter the voice, some patients alter their speaking technique, sometimes in improper ways, to overcome the laryngeal pathology. When the acute inflammation resolves, most patients naturally resume their normal speaking technique, but some continue their maladaptive behavior unaware of what they are doing. Many of these patients have been told by other physicians that there is nothing wrong with them and that "it's all in your head." Many are quite frustrated by the time they meet an otolaryngologist or speech pathologist who understands their problem. Fortunately, these patients usually respond quickly to voice therapy when properly applied.

Excessive muscular tension within the larynx also causes dysphonia, with the only abnormal finding being that of various patterns of constriction of the supraglottis. This group of nonorganic voice disorders is referred to as muscle tension dysphonia, which is a subclass of functional voice disorders (Koufman & Blalock, 1991). When such a diagnosis is entertained, any suggestion of organic disease should be worked up while voice therapy is commenced. Often supraglottic hyperfunction is compensating for organic glottic insufficiency due to vocal fold immobility, a defect in the vocal fold, or a mass that impairs closure.

In some cases, a functional voice disorder is conscious, and patients are looking for gain from their problem. This gain may be in the form of increased attention or sympathy from friends and family or monetary in the form of disability claims. The clinician must be alert to this possibility as these patients are often quite resistant to therapy. Premature surgical intervention must be avoided to prevent creation of real iatrogenic laryngeal abnormalities.

Conversion aphonia or dysphonia usually has sudden onset and is associated with a predisposing event that may have nothing to do with the voice at all. This is discussed in more detail in Chapter 13.

✦ Neurolaryngology

Neuroanatomy and Reflexes

The gross neuroanatomy of the larynx was described in some detail in the preceding sections of this chapter. However, much of laryngeal function is dependent on fine coordination of proprioception, chemical and temperature receptors, and efferent muscular innervation. This fine balance can be upset

Table 22–1 Common Etiologies of Vocal Fold Immobility at Henry Ford Hospital (1985–1991)

Etiology	Number of Patients (%)
Miscellaneous (including idiopathic)	54 (34.0)
Malignancy (not including larynx)	39 (24.5)
Trauma/iatrogenic (not including thyroidectomy)	36 (22.6)
Thyroidectomy	16 (10.1)
Neurologic	14 (8.8)
Total	159 (100)

with injuries to the laryngeal nerves, mucosal injury, or neurologic disorders or diseases.

Vocal Fold Paralysis

The innervation of the laryngeal muscles can be disrupted anywhere from the nucleus ambiguus to the neuromuscular junction. If this injury is partial and some muscular activity occurs, then such an injury is called a paresis. If complete, then the injury is termed a paralysis. Vocal fold paralysis can be temporary or permanent. One of the problems with evaluating an immobile vocal fold is that when a vocal fold is immobile it can be due to loss of innervation (paralysis) or joint fixation. For the sake of this discussion, a distinction will be made when relevant but otherwise lack of movement of the vocal fold will be termed vocal fold immobility, either unilateral (UVFI) or bilateral (BVFI). The most common etiologies for VFI determined by recent review at Henry Ford Hospital (Detroit, MI) are noted in **Table 22–1**. Although iatrogenic injury, primarily during thyroid surgery has traditionally been the most common causes of both UVFI and BVFI, recently nonlaryngeal neoplasms have become the most common identifiable cause (Benninger, Crumley, Ford, et al., 1994; Terris, Arnstein, & Nguyen, 1992; Tucker, 1980) (**Fig. 22–21**). Because

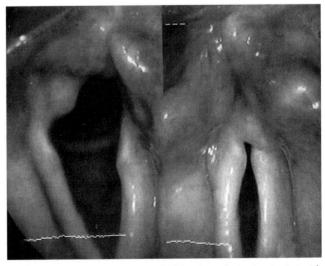

Figure 22–21 Left unilateral vocal fold paralysis: during inspiration with normal abduction of the right vocal fold (left) and during phonation with incomplete glottic closure and a resultant weak breathy voice (right). The etiology was metastatic carcinoma from the bladder to the mediastinum with involvement of the left recurrent laryngeal nerve. (See Color Plate 22–21.)

of this, unless a cause is clearly identified, some evaluation of the neck and chest is recommended to rule out a neoplasm. At present, we recommend a chest x-ray and a CT or MRI scan of the neck from the skull base to the thoracic inlet, essentially following the entire course of the superior and recurrent laryngeal nerves (Altman & Benninger, 1997). It is likely the idiopathic paralysis is the most common cause, but because many of these are felt to recover spontaneously, the temporary dysphonia may be overlooked or disregarded as anything more than laryngitis.

UVFI is most commonly caused by injury to the laryngeal nerves, although joint disruption or fixation from intubation, neck trauma or rheumatoid arthritis should be considered. Once the etiology of the immobility is determined, or once a neoplastic cause is ruled out for idiopathic immobility, then treatment is determined by the cause and the likelihood of recovery. A dislocated arytenoid should be reduced, a transected nerve reanastomosed, and rheumatoid arthritis appropriately treated. Electromyography of the larynx can be performed to clarify whether the immobility is caused by joint fixation or paralysis or to help to determine if recovery is likely in a paralyzed fold.

If a paralysis is confirmed, then the clinician has an opportunity to observe the patient or recommend a course of voice therapy. Some patients regain a satisfactory voice with voice therapy alone, obviating the need for more aggressive management (Benninger et al., 1994). Many recommend a period of observation and short course voice therapy for up to a year prior to surgical treatment to allow adequate time for accommodation or to wait for nerve recovery, which can take up to a year. With the availability of electromyography (EMG), some of the guesswork has been eliminated. Even if denervated, vocal fold function can return. However, if there is no evidence of reinnervation at 6 months, it has been our experience that it is very unlikely that function will return (Benninger et al., 1994). If by that time the voice is inadequate for the patient's social and occupational needs despite a course of voice therapy, then surgical management should be considered. Some patients may require earlier intervention, particularly if they have significant problems with aspiration or a voice that limits significantly their ability to fulfill occupational needs.

The type of surgical correction considered depends on several factors including the patient's need or desire for improvement of voice, the available techniques, the surgeon's experience, the degree of glottal insufficiency, and the urgency or need for permanency of the procedure. Many techniques are available, and combinations of techniques are occasionally needed. Vocal fold injections have been used for many years and a variety of substances have been found to be of value. If a temporary improvement is needed, then Gelfoam or Cymetra can be injected into the vocal fold. This usually lasts anywhere from 4 to 12 weeks and then reabsorbs. It is also a good technique for predicting the results of more permanent therapy or while waiting for possible recovery. Teflon paste injection is a generally reliable and predictable method of medializing the paralyzed vocal fold. In recent years, it has lost favor due to delayed granuloma formation and the irreversibility of the procedure (Gardner & Parnes, 1991). At present, we recommend Teflon in patients who have a paralyzed fold and the life expectancy is short or in patients whose general health makes them a poor operative risk. Collagen has been found to be a good method of closing small glottic

defects, but large defects have not responded well. Similarly, implantation or injection of autologous adipose has been recommended for small defects or to fine tune the results of other procedures. Both collagen and fat have the disadvantages of reabsorption and loss of effect, although some partial long-term persistence of fat has been identified. These may become more useful as more experience is gained.

The preferred method of surgically managing UVFI by most otolaryngologists at this time is by surgically medializing the immobile vocal fold. Since it was first described by Isshiki, Morita, Okamura, et al. (1974), vocal fold medialization, initially with cartilage, and now primarily with Silastic, has become the mainstay of treatment. The objective is to implant Silastic through a small window in the thyroid cartilage to push the immobile fold toward the midline to allow approximation from the opposite fold on phonation. Excellent results can be obtained particularly in young patients or those in whom the superior laryngeal nerve innervation to the cricothyroid muscle remains intact (Benninger et al., 1994; Koufman, 1986; Netterville, Stone, Tucker, et al., 1993). Other substances such as hydroxylapatite and Gore-Tex have been used in place of Silastic, although Silastic is readily available and is used by most laryngeal surgeons (Cummings, Purcell, & Flint, 1993). The advantage of Silastic medialization over vocal fold injection is that it allows for predictable results and the implant can be removed and revised if the results are suboptimal. The major disadvantage is that medialization may not adequately close a large posterior glottal chink, particularly in patients with combined SLN and RLN paralysis.

Arytenoid adduction (AA) is a procedure in which the arytenoid is rotated in a direction simulating the action of the lateral cricoarytenoid muscle, thereby adducting the vocal process to the midline. This procedure has become the preferred method of closing large posterior glottic gaps and can be performed alone or more commonly in conjunction with Silastic medialization (Tucker, 1980). The disadvantages of AA are primarily related to some technical difficulties associated with the procedure, although in experienced hands it has been an excellent addition to the capabilities in managing UVFI. Arytenoidopexy is a procedure with similar goals as AA. The arytenoids cartilage is positioned medially and then sutured to the cricoid cartilage (Zeitels, Mauri, & Dailey, 2004).

One disadvantage of the procedures described above is that they are static procedures directed at pushing or pulling the immobile vocal fold to the midline for approximation from the opposite fold, and therefore they do not return innervation to the vocal folds. Vocal fold reinnervation can potentially restore some vocal fold motion. Originally, nerve-muscle pedicle reinnervation was recommended, and although there was some evidence of clinical success and prevention of vocal fold atrophy would occur, an inability to reliably produce vocal fold motion resulted in an interest in developing other methods of reinnervation (Tucker, 1982). Subsequently, phrenic nerve and ansa cervicalis anastomosis to the recurrent laryngeal nerve or implantation directly into the laryngeal muscles has been described with some success (Crumley, 1991). The ease and predictability of Silastic medialization and AA have prevented more widespread use of reinnervation, but with ongoing investigation it is likely that this will become a more important method as time goes on.

The management of bilateral vocal fold immobility is also dependent on identification of the etiology. Unlike in UVFI, where voice and swallowing are impaired, the airway is the greatest concern with BVFI. In many cases, particularly in neonates and infants, tracheostomy may be necessary to manage the airway obstruction. Long-term management is dependent on the likelihood or timing of potential recovery. In patients whose recovery is unlikely, surgical management is usually necessary, although an occasional patient functions surprising well with no treatment. Such patients have a satisfactory voice but are usually limited in their activity levels by airway inadequacy.

When considering surgical treatment of BVFI, it is important to understand the delicate balance between good voice quality and a satisfactory airway. In general, efforts to dramatically improve the airway result in a poorer voice, and conversely attempts to retain normal voice result in some compromise in airway particularly with exercise or exertion, although a satisfactory balance is commonly attained. Several options have been advocated for lateralization of one or both vocal folds in BVFI. The first was an external direct lateralization as described by Woodman (1946). With the advent of more sophisticated endoscopic microlaryngeal techniques and particularly advances in laser technology, the Woodman procedure has been largely abandoned except in very complicated or scarred larynges. The principles of microscopic or laser surgery rely on reduction of the bulk of one or both vocal folds. This can include an arytenoidectomy, partial arytenoidectomy, or partial cordectomy, with each having distinct advantages (Dennis & Kashima, 1989; Gardner, 2000; Ossoff, Duncavage, Shapshay, Krespi, & Session, 1990). Usually, the technique used is predominantly determined by the experience of the surgeon.

Spasmodic Dysphonia

Spasmodic dysphonia (SD) is a neurologic disorder of the larynx of unknown cause that is manifested by two different characteristic voice abnormalities: adductor SD characterized by a strained or strangled voice with effortful speech, and abductor SD, which is characterized by episodes of breathiness and rapid air loss as the vocal folds spasm in an abducted position (Benninger, 1996a). Adductor SD is much more common than abductor SD. A rare patient has a combined adductor-abductor SD. Although the cause of SD is unknown, onset may occur after a traumatic event such as head trauma or a neurologic event. In some cases there may be a family history or genetic predisposition. SD is a focal dystonia of the larynx, and although it usually occurs in isolation, there is an associated tremor or other dystonia in about one fourth of patients. In most cases the onset is somewhat insidious, with gradually worsening symptoms that tend to be progressive. Many patients give a history of many years of worsening symptoms that were at first overlooked and then attributed to a functional or psychogenic cause until a diagnosis of SD is made. With better recognition of this disorder and the development of a national network of SD support groups, SD diagnosis at an early stage is becoming much more common.

The diagnosis of SD is made by the recognition of the characteristic voice and confirmed by flexible laryngoscopy where the episodes of spasm can be observed during conversational speech or when prompted by passages that precipitate spasm. At times, the diagnosis is difficult due to an associated tremor or other neurologic or neuromuscular disorder. The treatment of SD begins with a course of voice therapy. In some cases, particularly in patients with early disease, voice therapy may

be adequate alone to keep the individual functioning well and may minimize other procedures in those that require further treatment.

Unfortunately, the natural history of SD is for progression so that treatment other than voice therapy is ultimately needed. The first described successful surgical treatment for SD was unilateral recurrent laryngeal nerve section. This procedure was successful in most patients, but with long follow-up as many as 50% of patients had recurrence of their symptoms, and some had worse voices because of loss of unilateral innervation. Because of these problems, other techniques were explored. Thyroplasty with retrusion of the anterior commissure similarly had good initial results, but long-term success was achievable in only half of the patients, whereas most had significant deepening of the voice. Selective denervation has been described, but there is not enough experience to predict long-term efficacy (Berke, Blackwell, Gerratt, et al., 1999).

The treatment of choice for most laryngologists who treat patients with SD is botulinum toxin type A (Botox) injections (Benninger, 1996b; Benninger, Gardner, & Grywalski, 2001). Botox blocks the chemical interaction at the neuromuscular junction. It has been used successfully in both adductor SD, where it is almost universally effective, and in abductor SD, where results have been good but somewhat more unpredictable. Injection in adductor SD is typically into one or both of the thyroarytenoid muscles. In abductor SD, injection is into the posterior cricoarytenoid muscle. Injections are performed either intraorally or translaryngeally through the thyrocricoid space. The disadvantage of Botox is that the results are temporary and patients require repeat injections every 3 to 6 months. Overall, the high success rate and the minimal morbidity associated with the procedure have resulted in Botox becoming the treatment of choice for most cases of SD at this time. Continuation of voice therapy between injections has been found to prolong the time between injections.

Neurologic Disorders Affecting Voice

The nervous system is critical to the production of voice in coordinating the activities of the lungs larynx and resonating cavities. Kinesthetic and proprioceptive feedback are necessary for the control of phonation both through voluntary control and reflex action (Benninger, 1996b; Kirchner, 1981). Alterations in the sensory or motor function of any of the components necessary in the production of voice or speech may dramatically affect function. Although most neurologic disorders have some effect on voice, a few stand out either because of their selectivity to voice dysfunction or because of their frequency in the population. These will be discussed in more detail.

Tremor can cause significant problems in voice production. The tremor may occur because of a global disorder such as Parkinson disease or may only occur with phonation, or an essential voice tremor. At times, the tremor may worsen with stress or illness. Physical examination usually identifies the tremor, although tremor may be confused with other neurologic voice disorders such as spasmodic dysphonia. Once identified, mild tremor can usually be managed with voice therapy or with (β-adrenergic blockers, although more significant tremors may be difficult to control even with substantive pharmacologic therapy. Botox has also been used with success for essential voice tremor using the same technique as in adductor spasmodic dysphonia (Warrick, Dromey, Irish, et al., 2000).

Multiple sclerosis (MS) is a disease of undetermined cause that is characterized by demyelination of the white matter of the brainstem, spinal cord, cerebellum, and periventricular region. MS classically presents with Charcot's triad of nystagmus, dysarthric speech, and intention tremor, although this triad may not be present in many patients. MS often involves several motor and sensory functions of the head and neck including smell, vision, and facial weakness; alterations in balance; and hearing and dysarthric speech. The prevalence of MS is greater in the higher latitudes of both the Southern and Northern Hemispheres and can effect as many as 80 per 100,000 persons in some places in the United States. Most patients present between the ages of 20 and 40, with a slight male predominance (Benninger, 1996a; Garfinkle & Kimmelman, 1982). The hallmark of MS is recurring episodes of focal neurologic deficits that remit and recur, sometimes over relatively long periods of time. Over time, unfortunately, the disease does progress, with resultant permanent neurologic deficits. The diagnosis is made in an individual with suspicious symptoms by MRI scanning, which shows evidence of demyelination or by spinal tap. The treatment of MS is symptomatic. Speech, voice, swallowing, balance therapy, and hearing augmentation can be of great value in treating the patient with MS. Adrenocorticosteroids may be of value during the active phase of the disease.

Myasthenia gravis is a disease that is characterized by fatigability of muscles with gradual return of muscle strength after use. Although it can affect any striated muscle there is an increased susceptibility of the muscles innervated by cranial nerves, particularly those innervated by the facial, vagus, and oculomotor nerves. Myasthenia has a male predominance of 2:1 and occurs in about 10 per 100,000 people (Benninger, 1996a; Garfinkle & Kimmelman, 1982). The peak onset is in the sixth to seventh decades for men and in the third decade for women. Dysphonia or dysarthria occur in 6 to 25% of individuals, with the most common symptom being ptosis. Vocal fatigue with use or fatigue of the lips, tongue, and mouth while speaking or chewing are common complaints. Laryngeal dysfunction has been found to be abnormal in 60% of affected individuals. The diagnosis is made by a history of muscle fatigue with use and is confirmed by a Tensilon test. Electromyography will show fatigue on repeat electrical stimulation. The treatment of myasthenia is with acetyl cholinesterase inhibitors, steroids, and in some cases thymectomy.

✦ Laryngeal Trauma

Laryngeal trauma is often fatal and the total number of cases is difficult to measure as many victims do not reach health care facilities. Significant laryngeal injury may be the result of either blunt or penetrating trauma with motor vehicle accidents the most common cause of blunt injuries. The importance of correctly identifying an injury to the larynx or trachea is reflected in the ABCs of trauma evaluation: airway, breathing, and circulation.

If the airway is obstructed or becoming obstructed, it must be reestablished immediately. With significant laryngeal trauma, transoral endotracheal intubation is often impossible or even dangerous as it can convert a partial obstruction to a complete one (Schaefer, 1992). Therefore, a surgical airway, usually a tracheotomy, is performed to bypass the obstructed segment. Once the airway has been secured, other injuries have been assessed and the patient stabilized, the nature of the laryngeal injury is determined. If the patient is stable from the start, the larynx can be evaluated before any intervention. Preoperative evaluation includes indirect or fiberoptic laryngoscopy and CT scan of the larynx (Schaefer, 1991).

Although acute obstruction of the airway is the most dangerous aspect of laryngeal trauma, the long-term complications of laryngeal trauma can be devastating. Loss of the normal dimensions of the cartilaginous framework of the larynx and trachea or scarring within the lumen can cause chronic obstruction requiring long-term tracheotomy. Loss of innervation to the larynx can cause both airway and voice problems. Disruption and scarring of the vocal folds will cause varying degrees of voice problems. Occasionally, the larynx becomes incompetent resulting in aspiration and dysphagia.

The surgeon's goal when repairing the injured larynx is to avoid these chronic complications. This is achieved by trying to restore the original anatomy. Disrupted mucosa is sewn or grafted if there has been tissue loss. Internal laryngeal ligaments must be reattached to the cartilaginous framework, especially the anterior commissure. The laryngeal framework is restored to its original shape with use of wires, sutures, or microplates (Woo, 1990) (**Fig. 22–22**). Stents are sometimes necessary to maintain a lumen during the healing process, although the stents themselves can cause tissue reaction and scarring.

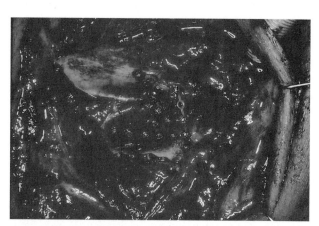

A   B

Figure 22–22 (A) Multiple fractures of the thyroid cartilage after a motor vehicle accident. The mucosa of the true and false vocal folds was also disrupted (not seen). **(B)** After repair of the mucosal injuries and reconstruction of the cartilaginous framework with microplates. See (Color Plates 22–22A and B.)

After the initial repair of the laryngeal injury, more surgery may be necessary if problems persist with airway, voice or swallowing. These revision procedures may be done either endoscopically or through an open approach, depending on the particular problem being addressed. Once healing is complete, most patients can be decannulated. Voice results are more difficult to predict, and after severe trauma a normal voice is sometimes impossible to obtain. A functional voice is sometimes the most realistic goal (Schaefer, 1992). Dysphagia is not usually a severe long-term problem following laryngeal trauma.

✦ Tracheotomy and Tracheostomy

Tracheotomy is the surgical opening of the trachea to achieve an airway directly from the anterior neck to the trachea, bypassing the oral and nasal cavities, pharynx and larynx. Tracheostomy, as opposed to tracheotomy, implies a permanent opening, although the two terms are commonly used interchangeably. Tracheotomy is performed for two basic reasons: to bypass an obstruction of the airway above the proximal trachea or to provide stable long-term easy access to the airway, usually for mechanical ventilation or pulmonary toilet.

Upper airway obstruction is caused by many different processes. Tumors of the upper aerodigestive tract may block the breathing passages. Surgery to remove these lesions can also result in enough swelling, usually short term, to obstruct breathing. Tracheotomy bypasses the region of obstruction in the pharynx in patients with severe obstructive sleep apnea. Facial trauma or deep neck abscesses may cause enough swelling to require tracheotomy until that problem has resolved. Bilateral vocal fold paralysis, laryngeal and subglottic stenosis, and tracheal stenosis often lead to tracheotomy either as a permanent treatment or to secure the airway while surgical procedures are performed on the larynx or trachea to relieve the constriction. Patients with chronic lung disease and other systemic illnesses that require long-term (greater than 7 days) mechanical ventilation will benefit from tracheotomy by removing the endotracheal tube from the larynx and subglottis, where it can cause injuries that may result in dysphonia or stenosis. The tracheotomy tube is also more comfortable, better tolerated, and easier to care for than an endotracheal tube, which passes through the nasal or oral cavities en route to the larynx (Astrachan, Kirchner, & Goodwin, 1988). The shorter tracheotomy tube also decreases ventilatory dead space, thereby easing the process of weaning from the ventilator.

Tracheotomy involves making an incision through the anterior skin of the neck, dissecting between the strap muscles, avoiding or dividing the isthmus of the thyroid gland, and entering the trachea through its anterior wall in the region of the second or third tracheal rings. Fortunately, these structures, in a thin person, are relatively close to the skin, making the procedure fairly straightforward. It is much more difficult in a person with a deep neck abscess, a neck tumor, or severe scarring of the trachea itself, or in an obese person, which is often the case in patients with severe obstructive sleep apnea.

An emergency tracheotomy, in a patient with a rapidly deteriorating airway such as a trauma patient, can be a very stressful procedure and the need for speed as well as the often altered anatomy make this somewhat more difficult than an elective procedure.

A tracheotomy done for obstruction provides an airway for the patient to breathe, but does not limit the ability to speak, providing that the obstructing lesion does not impair laryngeal function. Once air is inspired through the tube into the lungs, the air can be exhaled past the tube or through a hole in the superior aspect of the tube (fenestrated tube) by plugging the external hole of the tube to redirect the air through the larynx. This can be done with a finger or a one-way valve placed on the end of the tube such as the Passy Muir valve. If the tube is needed for long-term ventilation, a cuff around the end of the tube will prevent air from passing around the tube because all the air must flow from the ventilator to the lungs without leaking. This prevents speaking. Some devices provide an external airflow above the tracheotomy tube and through the larynx for speaking while the patient is on a ventilator.

Swallowing is sometimes affected by placement of a tracheotomy tube by limiting the elevation of the larynx and trachea during the swallow. In most cases, however, the patient will be able to eat an oral diet soon after the tracheotomy has been done, providing that other medical conditions do not preclude that. A cuffed tube may impair swallowing by compressing the esophagus.

Aspiration is sometimes cited as an indication for tracheotomy in the hopes that a cuffed tube will prevent passage of food and saliva into the distal trachea. This is not a dependable method for preventing aspiration, however, so other indications for the tracheotomy should be present. Swallowing therapy should also be undertaken before the surgical procedure is performed.

Tracheotomy is a temporary condition. The tract through which the tube is placed is skin-lined only on those rare occasions when a permanent stoma is created. In most cases, when the tube is no longer needed, it can be removed and the hole will heal within days or weeks. A temporary tracheotomy wound will rarely require surgical closure. The resulting scar is usually mild if the tube has been in place for only a short time. The longer it has been in place, the more noticeable the scar will be. Revision of the scar for a better cosmetic appearance is possible at a later date. Long-term side effects of tracheotomy, which are not common, include stenosis of the trachea at the site of the stoma, voice disorders, and, rarely, dysphagia.

✦ Professional Voice Disorders

The performing or professional vocalist may experience unique and difficult-to-manage problems related to voice. Because their lifestyle and often livelihood are dependent on the quality of their voices, even minor alterations can have significant consequences. Furthermore, the drive necessary to be successful and the personality that is necessary to be visible may result in voice overuse and at a time when voice moderation would be preferred. The lifestyle of performers is often not conducive to preferred voice behaviors. They often have an active travel or recording schedule intermixed with interviews. They usually perform at night and eat after performances, predisposing them to LPR. They have poor control over their environment and are often exposed to dryness and dust, particularly when on the road. The avocational singer frequently performs after a full day's work or family commitments that often require substantial voice use.

The most critical part of the evaluation of the singer or professional speaker is taking the history. Not only should questions be asked regarding the severity, timing, and onset of the dysphonia, but also the clinician should assess the experience, training, and lifestyle of the performer. The time of the next performance and any important career performances that are upcoming should be determined. The choir singer who does not solo and does not have to sing for 2 weeks would be approached very differently from the opera or pop star who has a key performance in 3 hours. Lifestyle behaviors that could be detrimental to voice use, such as substance abuse or eating disorders (bulimia), should be identified. Environmental factors, such as allergies, dryness, dust, or frequent travel, may all affect the voice. A list of medications should be obtained. Certain medications such as diuretics or antihistamines may be used by performers without their realizing the potential drying effect, and these and all other medications should be identified.

The physical examination should be complete and include any areas that are identified as possible problems through the history. The oral cavity and pharyngeal examinations should look for signs of inflammation or dryness and evidence of reflux or allergies. Palpation of the neck may reveal neck tightness or tenderness, and scalloping of the tongue may be a sign of tension. The larynx should first be viewed with a mirror to give a global view of the pharynx and larynx. Most diagnoses are made through the history and mirror laryngoscopy. Videostroboscopy may provide additional diagnostic information, is helpful in patient education, and is very useful in following progression of the disorder or the response to treatment. Objective voice evaluations are especially important in the evaluation of the singer in allowing for assessment of minor changes in voice or progress in treatment that might not be assessed by examining the larynx.

The treatment of dysphonia in the performer usually requires the multidisciplinary input of the otolaryngologist and SLP and often requires the aid of a trained teacher of music and singing. Simple conservative measures are helpful in most individuals regardless of the specific pathology. These would include education regarding diet and lifestyle, hydration, humidification, antireflux measures, and caution regarding excessive, prolonged, or abusive vocalization. Assessment of the singing range may identify whether or not the repertoire is right for the singer. In many cases, particularly in amateur singers, technical problems with voice production would require professional voice instruction. Voice training from an SLP will minimize the negative effects of improper speaking voice use and may carry over to the singing voice.

On occasion, acute disorders, such a virus or upper respiratory tract infection may occur at a time when performances cannot be canceled or changed. In such cases, it is critical for the voice treatment team to determine whether or not proceeding has the potential for long-term or even permanent injury to the voice. If this is likely, then the performance should be canceled. Fortunately, these are rare circumstances. Usually the singer can be managed with symptomatic treatment such as humidification, hydration, decongestants, and mucolytics. Antihistamines should be avoided, if possible, because of the potential drying side effects. Inhalant steroids are not of value and may even be contraindicated in acute laryngeal inflammation. If there is evidence of a bacterial infection, antibiotics should be started, with the type of

antibiotic being determined by the likely pathogens or by culture. On rare occasions such symptomatic treatment is not sufficient and a short course of systemic steroids may be considered.

Chronic voice disorders are not uncommon in performers. The most common significant disorders are focal edema or vocal nodules. With proper voice training and modifications along with lifestyle measures and treatment for LPR, these resolve in almost all patients. Fortunately, surgery in performers is rarely indicated. If, however, it becomes necessary, it should be performed by an experienced laryngologist utilizing microscopic surgical techniques. Postoperative care should be aggressive and multidisciplinary. The recovery should be graduated and the performer should return to singing only when there is evidence of complete recovery.

✦ Gastroesophageal and Laryngopharyngeal Reflux Disease

Gastroesophageal (GERD) and laryngopharyngeal reflux (LPR) have been recently identified as being either causative or a cofactor in many diseases and disorders of the esophagus, pharynx, larynx, and upper respiratory tract. Studies have shown that reflux is a likely cause of unexplained cough, globus sensation, hoarseness, and chronic throat clearing (Koufman, 1991). Furthermore, LPR is often confused with sinus disease in that patients complain of thick mucus sticking in the throat and attribute such symptoms to posterior nasal drainage from sinus disease, even if they have no other nasal or sinus symptoms. Throat clearing can become habitual, and the constant irritation from that activity can cause the symptoms to persist.

There are four major mechanisms for the prevention of GERD or LPR: (1) the upper esophageal sphincter (UES), which is primarily the cricopharyngeus muscle, that has resting tone and relaxes with swallowing; (2) esophageal motility; (3) the lower esophageal sphincter (LES), which is a pseudo-sphincter created by a pressure differential between the thorax and abdominal cavities; and (4) gastric motility and emptying. The three major causes of reflux disease are decreased esophageal motility, decreased LES tone, and delayed gastric emptying (Benninger, 1996b). There is some debate related to the role of the UES in reflux disease, but given that pharyngeal reflux occurs would suggest an important role. Most reflux disease is the result of lifestyle and diet. High-fat foods, alcohol, caffeine, and large meals all predispose to reflux. Furthermore, late-night eating, just prior to bedtime, prompts acid and pepsin production to digest the food, and recumbency precludes the gravitational aid in the prevention of reflux. Overweight individuals are more likely to reflux, and age can result in changes in LES tone. Finally, hiatal hernias can result in loss of LES prevention of reflux.

The typical patient with LPR often presents with a different constellation of symptoms from those with GERD. Whereas GERD patients often complain of dyspepsia and heartburn, those with LPR usually have nonspecific symptoms such as mild hoarseness that is usually worse in the morning, a foreign body or globus sensation, nocturnal cough, or the need to chronically clear the throat. The diagnosis in such patients is usually made by history suggestive of LPR, noting that 50% of patients with LPR do not get the classic symptoms of GERD such as heartburn or acid indigestion. The physical examination may reveal some thickening or edema of the posterior commissure or arytenoids mucosa, and occasionally reveals erythema or cherry-red arytenoids. With advanced or prolonged reflux, contact ulcers, granulomas, leukoplakia, evidence of chronic inflammation, or diffuse edema can be seen. Vocal fold nodules, long thought to develop only because of phonotrauma, often respond to treatment for LPR along with voice therapy. There has been some suggestion that reflux may even be a factor or cofactor in the development of laryngeal cancer. In some patients reflux may precipitate laryngospasm or exacerbate asthma. Finally, a relationship has been established between reflux and sudden infant death syndrome (SIDS) (Kelly & Shannon, 1982).

The treatment of LPR is dependent on the severity of symptoms and the certainty of the diagnosis. In most cases, diet and lifestyle are the major causes of GERD and LPR where dietary and lifestyle modifications will be adequate to alleviate the symptoms. Smaller meals; a low-fat diet; avoidance of alcohol, tobacco, and caffeine; not eating for 3 to 4 hours before bedtime; weight control; and elevation of the head of the bed will control the symptoms in most patients. With severe reflux and hiatal hernia, avoidance of heavy lifting or stooping or wearing tight clothing may be recommended. If these conservative measures are unsuccessful, a trial of antacids especially at bedtime may be suggested. If unsuccessful, a trial of a more aggressive pharmacologic treatment can be considered or objective testing if the diagnosis is uncertain.

Several tests have been advocated for the diagnosis of GERD and LPR. A barium cine swallow may make the diagnosis or identify a hiatal hernia but has a relatively high false-negative rate. Acid perfusion tests, pH probing, esophageal manometry, and endoscopy can be considered. The gold standard for evaluation of reflux, particularly LPR, is 24-hour double pH probe testing, which facilitates measurement in the lower esophagus and pharynx simultaneously. These tests may be cumbersome for the patient and are expensive. An alternative to testing is a trial of medication. A proton pump inhibitor results in acid suppression in most patients and therefore should eliminate symptoms if reflux is the cause. Occasionally, doubling of the recommended dosage is necessary. If this is successful in disease control, then a dietary-lifestyle modification should be implemented. The proton-pump inhibitor can be continued, although most patients can be converted to a less expensive medication such as an H_2 blocker.

✦ Acquired Immunodeficiency Syndrome and Otolaryngology

Acquired immunodeficiency syndrome (AIDS) is caused by the human immunodeficiency virus (HIV). This disease has had a profound impact on otolaryngology as with all areas of medicine. Many patients experience their first symptoms of AIDS in the head and neck. Otolaryngologists must be alert to the signs of AIDS and be prepared to make the diagnosis when these patients present.

Although certain infectious processes are much more common in AIDS patients, all common infections may occur in the AIDS population, including sinusitis, pharyngitis, tonsillitis, and otitis media and externa. These frequently seen conditions, however, often fail to respond to the usual course of treatment, requiring repeated courses of antibiotics and perhaps surgery when complications occur. This resistance to treatment should alert the clinician to a possible immunodeficiency.

Candida infections of the oral cavity, pharynx, larynx, and esophagus are more common in patients with AIDS. Herpes simplex and zoster infections are also more frequent and more severe in AIDS patients (Marcusen & Sooy, 1985). Giant herpetic ulcers may affect the mouth, nose, or face (Lucente, 1993). Other ulcers of the oral cavity, specifically aphthous ulcers, may also develop into giant ulcers and are extremely painful and difficult to treat. Hairy leukoplakia is a benign and painless condition that is also associated with HIV infection.

Nasopharyngeal lymphoid proliferation may present with nasal obstruction, snoring, and serous otitis media with hearing loss. The findings of apparent adenoid hypertrophy in an adult with HIV infection risk factors should prompt the appropriate tests.

Kaposi's sarcoma is a previously rare neoplasm that is the most common neoplastic process in AIDS patients (Singh, Har-El, & Lucente, 1994). These lesions may be in the skin, lymph nodes, or any mucosal surface of the head and neck. Treatment is symptomatic.

The most common neck mass in patients infected with HIV is the enlarged lymph node. If one of these enlarged nodes becomes significantly larger than the rest, a diagnosis of lymphoma, which is associated with AIDS, must be considered. Benign lymphoepithelial lesions of the parotid glands have also been noted in patients who are HIV seropositive (Tunkel, Loury, Fox, et al., 1989). These lesions are typically cystic and bilateral and can grow quite large. Diagnosis is based on the clinical presentation and fine-needle biopsy to rule out other neoplasms. Excision, which involves superficial or total parotidectomy with facial nerve dissection, is reserved for neoplasms; benign lymphoepithelial lesions of the parotid glands should be followed for repeated aspirations of fluid as needed for comfort or sudden changes in size, which may indicate the development of a lymphoma.

Fifty percent of AIDS patients present with an opportunistic pulmonary infection such as *Pneumocystis carinii* pneumonia. Cough is the most common symptom of these infectious processes.

✦ Case Vignettes

Case One

A 43-year-old woman experienced blunt trauma to the left neck secondary to a snowmobile accident. She immediately noticed a change in voice and mild dysphagia. On presentation to the emergency department, she was noted to have ecchymosis of the left neck and an immobile left vocal fold in a paramedian position with incomplete approximation from the other fold. She had no shortness of breath. She was discharged to be reevaluated in 3 to 4 weeks. On repeat evaluation, the vocal fold was still found to be in a paramedian position with improved, but incomplete, approximation from the other side. Her voice remained breathy with poor glottal coup. A videostroboscopic analysis revealed an asymmetrical vertical plane and asymmetrical vibration with a large glottic chink. The patient was referred for voice therapy. Following 6 weeks of treatment, the patient had improvement of her voice with longer maximum phonatory times and decreased air wasting. Nonetheless, her voice was inadequate for her occupational and social needs. She was in sales for a major manufacturing corporation.

Electromyography of the larynx was performed and showed fibrillation potentials from the thyroarytenoid muscle and normal innervations of the cricothyroid muscle. To temporize her voice, vocal fold injection of Gelfoam was performed with near normalization of the voice. On 6-week evaluation, the vocal fold was again found to be lateralized. However, there was good approximation from the opposite side and, although mildly dysphonic, the patient has satisfactory voice for her job. It was elected to have her follow-up with the SLP pathologist and return to the otolaryngologist in 6 months. On repeat evaluation, her voice had returned completely to normal, and physical examination revealed a normally mobile left vocal fold, good approximation to midline, and return of normal vocal fold waveform vibration on videostroboscopy.

This case has value to the SLP because it shows the somewhat elongated treatment course of patients with vocal fold paralysis. It verifies the critical role of voice therapy in the early stages of the disease, with the potential of vocal fold normalization through accommodation. It also confirms the important roles of diagnostic testing, including videostroboscopy, airflow analysis, and electromyography, in the evaluation and treatment of patient with unilateral vocal fold immobility.

Case Two

A 5-year-old boy was referred by his pediatrician to an otolaryngologist for chronic mouth breathing, snoring, hyponasal speech, periods of apnea at nighttime, and enuresis. Physical examination revealed 3+/4 tonsil hypertrophy and diffuse adenoid hypertrophy. Given the child's history of obstructive sleep apnea symptoms, enuresis, and tonsillar and adenoid hypertrophy, a tonsillectomy and adenoidectomy were performed. Although the child immediately experienced improvement in his sleep and elimination of his snoring, enuresis, and chronic mouth breathing, the parents noted that the child's voice had changed from being hyponasal to being very hypernasal with a loss of air with production of certain oral sounds, persisting for 2 weeks following the procedure. Examination of the pharynx revealed good healing in the tonsillar and adenoid sites and normal movement of the palate. The otolaryngologist recommended observation, and 6 weeks following the surgery the hypernasal speech was eliminated.

✦ Conclusion

Otolaryngologic patients can present with disorders that affect speech functions (phonation, resonance, and articulation) and swallowing. Communication between the disciplines of otolaryngology and speech–language pathology can be fostered by familiarity with the process of diagnosis and treatment in each area. This chapter provided an introduction to those areas in the field of otolaryngology that are of the most significance to the speech–language pathologist.

Study Questions

1. What are the anatomic boundaries of the oral cavity?
2. What are the symptoms of bilateral choanal atresia in a newborn infant? Why do they occur?
3. Identify the common causes of velopharyngeal insufficiency in children?
4. What are the common causes of xerostomia?
5. Describe the sensory innervation to the face.
6. How do the cricothyroid muscles act to aid in adduction of the vocal fold? What is the innervation of this muscle?
7. Explain the myoelastic aerodynamic theory of phonation.
8. Name three causes of Reinke's space edema.
9. What are the two most common causes of unilateral vocal fold paralysis?
10. How does botulinum toxin act to eliminate the symptoms of spasmodic dysphonia? Is this effect permanent? Why?
11. What is the most important part of the clinical evaluation of a voice disorder in a performer?
12. Describe three common head and neck manifestations of AIDS.

References

Altman, J., & Benninger M.S. (1997). The Evaluation of Unilateral Vocal Fold Immobility: Is Chest X-Ray Enough? *Journal of Voice, 11,* 364–367

Astrachan, D.I., Kirchner, J.C., and Goodwin, W.J. (1988). Prolonged Intubation vs. Tracheotomy: Complications, Practical and Psychological Considerations. *Laryngoscope, 98,* 1165–1169

Bastian, R.W. (1991). Videoendoscopic Evaluation of Patients with Dysphagia: An Adjunct to the Modified Barium Swallow. *Otolaryngology Head Neck Surgery, 104,* 339–350

Benninger, M.S. (1994). The Medical Examination. In M.S. Benninger, B. Jacobson, & A. Johnson (Eds.), *Performing Arts Medicine: The Care and Prevention of Professional Voice Disorders* (pp. 86–96). New York: Thieme

Benninger, M.S. (1996a). Dysphonias Secondary to Neurologic Disorders. *Journal of Singing,* May/June, 29–32

Benninger, M.S. (1996b). Treatment of Dysphonias Secondary to Gastroesophageal Reflux. In: P. Clemente (Ed.), *Voice Update.* Amsterdam: Elsevier Science

Benninger, M.S. (1997). Nasal Endoscopy: Its Role in Office Diagnosis. *American Journal of Rhinology, 11,* 177–180

Benninger, M.S. (2000). Microdissection or Microspot CO$_2$ Laser for Limited Vocal Fold Benign Lesions: A Prospective Randomized Trial. *Laryngoscope, 110(2 Pt 2 suppl 92),* 1–17

Benninger, M.S., Crumley, R.L., Ford, C.N., et al. (1994). Evaluation and Treatment of the Unilateral Paralyzed Vocal Fold. *Otolaryngology Head Neck Surgery, 111,* 497–508

Benninger, M.S., Gardner, G., & Grywalski, C. (2001). The Outcomes of Botulinum Toxin Treatment for Patients with Spasmodic Dysphonia. *Archives of Otolaryngology-Head & Neck Surgery, 127,* 1083–1085

Benninger, M.S., Gardner, G.M., & Schwimmer, C. (2003). Laryngeal Neurophysiology. In: J. Rubin, R. Sataloff, & G. Korovin (Eds.), *Diagnosis and Treatment of Voice Disorders,* 2nd ed. (pp. 107–113). Clifton Park, NY: Thomson Delmar

Benninger, M.S., Mickelson, S.A., and Yaremchuk, K. (1990). Functional Endoscopic Sinus Surgery. Morbidity and Early Results. *Henry Ford Hospital Medical Journal, 38,* 5–8

Berke, G.S., Blackwell, K.E., Gerratt, B.R., et al. (1999). Selective Laryngeal Adductor Denervation-Reinnervation: A New Surgical Treatment for Adductor Spasmodic Dysphonia. *Annals of Otology, Rhinology, and Laryngology, 108,* 227–231

Bouchayer, M., & Cornut, G. (1992). Microsurgical Treatment of Benign Vocal Fold Lesions: Indications, Technique, Results. *Folia Phoniatrica, 44,* 155–184

Bumsted, R.M. (1986). Cleft Lip and Palate. In: C.W. Cummings, J.M. Frederickson, L.A. Harker, et al. (Eds.), *Otolaryngology-Head and Neck Surgery* (pp. 1129–1168). St. Louis: CV Mosby

Colton, R.H. (1993). Physiology of Phonation. In: M.S. Benninger, B. Jacobson, & A. Johnson (Eds.), *Vocal Arts Medicine: The Care and Prevention of Professional Voice Disorders* (pp. 30–60). New York: Thieme

Cooper, B.C. (1989). Craniomandibular Disorders. In: B.C. Cooper, & F.E. Lucente (Eds.), *Management of Facial, Head and Neck Pain* (pp. 153–255). Philadelphia: W.B. Saunders

Courey, M.S., Gardner, G.M., Stone, R.E., & Ossoff, R.H. (1995). Endoscopic Vocal Fold Microflap: A Three-Year Experience. *Annals of Otology, Rhinology, and Laryngology, 104,* 267–273

Crumley, R.L. (1991). Update: Ansa Cervicalis to Recurrent Laryngeal Nerve Anastomosis for Unilateral Laryngeal Paralysis. *Laryngoscope, 101,* 384–387

Cummings, C.W., Purcell, L.L., & Flint, P.W. (1993). Hydroxylapatite Laryngeal Implants for Medialization: Preliminary Report. *Annals of Otology, Rhinology, and Laryngology, 102,* 843–851

Dennis, D.P., & Kashima, H. (1989). Carbon Dioxide Laser Posterior Cordectomy for Treatment of Bilateral Vocal Cord Paralysis. *Annals of Otology Rhinology, and Laryngology, 98,* 930–934

Ford, C.N. (1994). Phonosurgery. In: M.S. Benninger, B.H. Jacobson, & A. Johnson (Eds.). *Vocal Arts Medicine* (pp. 344–355). New York: Thieme

Ford, C.N., Inagi, K., Bless, D.M., et al. (1996). Sulcus Vocalis: A Rational Analytical Approach to Diagnosis and Management. *Annals of Otology, Rhinology, and Laryngology, 105,* 189–200

Frantz, T.D., & Rasgon, B.M. (1993). Acute Epiglottitis: Changing Epidemiologic Patterns. *Otolaryngology Head and Neck Surgery, 109,* 457–460

Frantz, T.D., Rasgon, B.M., & Quesenberry, Jr., C.P. (1994). Acute Epiglottitis in Adults. Analysis of 129 Cases. *Journal of the American Medical Association, 272,* 1358–1360

Gardner, G.M. (2000). Posterior Glottic Stenosis and Bilateral Vocal Fold Immobility: Diagnosis and Treatment. *Otolaryngolic Clinics of North America, 33,* 855–877

Gardner, G.M., & Benninger, M.S. (1996). The Definition and Measurement of Hoarseness. *Current Opinion in Otolaryngology-Head & Neck Surgery, 4,* 113–120

Gardner, G.M., & Parnes, S. (1991). Status of the Mucosal Wave Post Teflon Vocal Cord Injection vs. Thyroplasty. *Journal of Voice, 5,* 64–73

Garfinkle, T.J., & Kimmelman, C.P. (1982). Neurologic Disorders: Amyotrophic Lateral Sclerosis, Myasthenia Gravis, Multiple Sclerosis, and Poliomyelitis. *American Journal of Otolaryngology, 3,* 204–212

Goode, R.L. (1986). Sleep Disorders. In C.W. Cummings (Ed.) *Otolaryngology, Head and Neck Surgery* (pp. 1449–1457). St. Louis: Mosby-Year Book

Harrison, D.F.N. (1981). Fibre Size Frequency in the Recurrent Laryngeal Nerves of Man and Giraffe. *Acta Otolaryngologica, 91,* 383–389

Hojslet, P.E., Moesgaard-Nielson, V., & Karlsmore, M. (1990). Smoking Cessation in Chronic Reinke's Oedema. *Journal of Laryngology and Otology, 104,* 626–628

Isshiki, N., Morita, H., Okamura, H., et al. (1974). Thyroplasty as a New Phonosurgical Technique. *Acta Otolaryngologica, 78,* 451–456

Jones, S.R., Myers, E.N., & Barnes, L. (1984). Benign Neoplasms of the Larynx. *Otolaryngolic Clinics of North America, 17,* 151–178

Kelly, D.H., & Shannon, D.C. (1982). Sudden Infant Death Syndrome and Near Sudden Infant Death Syndrome: A Review of the Literature 1964–1982. *Pediatric Clinics of North America, 29,* 1241–1261

Kirchner, J.A. (1981). Laryngeal Afferent Systems in Phonatory Control. *ASHA Reports, 11,* 31–35

Koufman, J.A. (1986). Laryngoplasty for Vocal Fold Medialization: An Alternative to Teflon. *Laryngoscope, 96,* 726–731

Koufman, J.A. (1991). The Otolaryngologic Manifestations of Gastroesophageal Reflux (GERD): A Clinical Investigation of 225 Patients Using Ambulatory pH Monitoring and an Experimental Investigation of the Role of Acid and Pepsin in the Development of Laryngeal Injury. *Laryngoscope 101 (4 pt 2 suppl 53),* 1–78

Koufman, J.A., & Blalock, P.D. (1989). Is Voice Rest Never Indicated? *Journal of Voice, 3,* 87–91

Koufman, J.A., & Blalock, P.D. (1991). Functional Voice Disorders. *Otolaryngology Clinics of North America, 24,* 1059–1073

Koufman, J.A., Wiener, G.J., Wu, W.C., & Castell, D.O. (1988). Reflux Laryngitis and Its Sequelae: The Diagnostic Role of Ambulatory 24-Hour pH Monitoring. *Journal of Voice, 2,* 78–89

Loire, R., Bouchayer, M., Cornut, G., & Bastian, R.W. (1988). Pathology of Benign Vocal Fold Lesions. *Ear Nose and Throat Journal, 67,* 357–362

Lucente, F.E. (1993). Impact of the Acquired Immunodeficiency Syndrome Epidemic on the Practice of Laryngology. *Annals of Otology, Rhinology, and Laryngology, 161,* 1–24

Lumpkin, S.M.M., Bennet, S., & Bishop, S.G. (1990). Postsurgical Follow-Up Study of Patients with Severe Polypoid Degeneration. *Laryngoscope, 100,* 399–402

Marcusen, D.C., & Sooy, C.D. (1985). Otolaryngologic and Head and Neck Manifestation of Acquired Immunodeficiency Syndrome (AIDS). *Laryngoscope, 95,* 401–405

McFerran, D.J., Abdullah, V., Gallimore, A.P., Pringle, M.B., & Croft, C.B. (1994). Vocal Process Granulomata. *J Laryngol Otol, 108,* 216–220

Milutinovic, Z., & Vasiljevic, J. (1992). Contribution to the Understanding of Vocal Fold Cysts: A Functional and Histologic Study. *Laryngoscope, 102,* 568–571

Moore, K.L. (1977). *The Developing Human,* 2nd ed. Philadelphia: W.B. Saunders

Nasri, S., Sercarz, J., McAlpin, T., & Berke, G. (1995). Treatment of Vocal Fold Granuloma Using Botulinum Toxin Type A. *Laryngoscope, 105,* 585–588

Netterville, J.L., Stone, R.E., Tucker, E.S., et al. (1993). Silastic Medialization and Arytenoid Adduction: the Vanderbilt Experience. A Review of 116 Phonosurgical Procedures. *Annals of Otology, Rhinology, and Laryngology, 102,* 413–424

Netterville, J.L., & Vrabec, J.T. (1994). Unilateral Palatal Adhesion for Paralysis After High Vagal Injury. *Archives of Otolaryngology-Head and Neck Surgery, 120,* 218–221

Olson, N.R. (1991). Laryngopharyngeal Manifestations of Gastroesophageal Reflux Disease. *Otolaryngolic Clinics of North America, 24,* 1201–1213

Ossoff, R.H., Duncavage, J.A., Shapshay, S.M., Krespi, Y.P., & Session, G.A. (1990). Endoscopic Laser Arytenoidectomy Revisited. *Annals of Otology, Rhinology, and Laryngology, 99,* 764–771

Ossoff, R.H., Werkhaven, J.A., & Dere, H. (1991). Soft-Tissue Complications of Laser Surgery for Recurrent Respiratory Papillomatosis. *Laryngoscope, 101,* 1162–1166

Pasquale, K., Wiatrak, B., Woolley, A., et al. (2003). Microdebrider versus CO_2 Laser Removal of Recurrent Respiratory Papillomas: A Prospective Analysis. *Laryngoscope, 113,* 139–143

Pransky, S.M., Albright, J.T., & Magit, A.E. (2003). Long-Term Follow-Up of Pediatric Recurrent Respiratory Papillomatosis Managed with Intralesional Cidofovir. *Laryngoscope, 113,* 1583–1587

Redline, S., & Young, T. (1993). Epidemiology and Natural History of Obstructive Sleep Apnea. *Ear, Nose and Throat Journal, 72,* 20–26

Rosen, C.A., & Bryson, P.C. (2004). Indole-3-Carbinol for Recurrent Respiratory Papillomatosis: Long-Term Results. *Journal of Voice, 18,* 248–253

Sanders, I., Wu, B., Liancai, M., et al. (1993). Innervation of the Human Larynx. *Archives of Otolaryngology Head and Neck Surgery, 119,* 934–939

Sataloff, R.T. (1991). Structural and Neurological Disorders and Surgery of the Voice. In: R. Sataloff (Ed.), *Professional Voice: The Science and Art of Clinical Care* (pp. 267–299). New York: Raven Press

Sataloff, R.T., Spiegel, J.R., & Hawkshawk, M.J. (1991). Strobovideolaryngoscopy: Results and Clinical Value. *Annals of Otology, Rhinology, and Laryngology, 100,* 725–727

Schaefer, S.D. (1991). Use of CT Scanning in the Management of the Acutely Injured Larynx. *Otolaryngolic Clinics of North America, 24,* 31–36

Schaefer, S.D. (1992). The Acute Management of External Laryngeal Trauma: A 27-Year Experience. *Archives of Otolaryngologic Head and Neck Surgery, 118,* 598–604

Shapshay, S.M., Rebeiz, E.E., Bohigian, R.K., & Hybels, R.L. (1990). Benign Lesions of the Larynx: Should the Laser Be Used? *Laryngoscope, 100,* 953–957

Singh, B., Har-El, G., & Lucente, F.E. (1994). Kaposi's Sarcoma of the Head and Neck in Patients with Acquired Immunodeficiency Syndrome. *Otolaryngolic Head and Neck Surgery, 111,* 618–624

Terris, D.J., Arnstein, D.P., & Nguyen, H.H. (1992). Contemporary Evaluation of Unilateral Vocal Cord Paralysis. *Otolaryngologic Head and Neck Surgery, 107,* 84–89

Tucker, H. (1980). Vocal Cord Paralysis 1979: Etiology and Management. *Laryngoscope, 90,* 585–590

Tucker, H.M. (1982). Nerve-Muscle Pedicle Reinnervation of the Larynx: Avoiding the Pitfalls and Complications. *Annals of Otolaryngology, Rhinology, and Laryngology, 91,* 440–444

Tunkel, D.E., Loury, M.C., Fox, C.H., et al. (1989). Bilateral Parotid Enlargement in HIV-Seropositive Patients. *Laryngoscope, 99,* 590–595

Warrick, P., Dromey, C., Irish, J.C., et al. (2000). Botulinum Toxin for Essential Tremor of the Voice with Multiple Anatomical Sites of Tremor: A Crossover Design Study of Unilateral Versus Bilateral Injection. *Laryngoscope, 110,* 1366–1374

Werkhaven, J., & Ossoff, R.H. (1991). Surgery for Benign Lesions of the Glottis. *Otolaryngolic Clinics of North America, 24,* 1179–1199

Woo, P. (1990). Laryngeal Framework Reconstruction with Miniplates. *Annals of Otolaryngology, Rhinology, and Laryngology, 99,* 772–777

Woo, P., Colton, R., Casper, J., & Brewer, D. (1991). Diagnostic Value of Stroboscopic Examination in Hoarse Patients. *Journal of Voice, 5,* 231–238

Woodman, D. (1946). A Modification of the Extralaryngeal Approach to Arytenoidectomy for Bilateral Abductor Paralysis. *Archives of Otolaryngology, 43,* 63–65

Zeitels, S.M., Mauri, M., & Dailey, S.H. (2004). Adduction Arytenopexy for Vocal Fold Paralysis: Indications and Technique. *Journal of Laryngology and Otolaryngology, 118,* 508–516

23

Drug-Induced Communication and Swallowing Disorders

Tami Remington and Susan C. Fagan

- ✦ Definition of an Adverse Drug Reaction
- ✦ Evaluation of a Patient Experiencing a Drug-Induced Disease
- ✦ Drug-Induced Dysphonia
- ✦ Drug-Induced Speech and Language Impairments
- ✦ Drug-Induced Swallowing Disorders

The use of prescription and over-the-counter medications is increasing, and patients seen by speech–language pathologists (SLPs) are likely to be taking multiple medications for treatment of neurologic and other conditions (**Appendix 23–1**). With the use of any drug, the potential exists to cause unwanted effects that can result in serious morbidity or mortality. An Institute of Medicine (1999) report heightened awareness of the problems of adverse drug events. It is estimated that adverse drug events result in more than 2 million injuries each year, and the cost of drug-induced injuries and death was estimated at more than $177 billion in 2000 (Ernst & Grizzle, 2001). Health care providers across all disciplines are called on to be vigilant in their efforts to prevent, detect, and resolve drug-related problems.

✦ Definition of an Adverse Drug Reaction

An adverse drug reaction (ADR) is one type of adverse drug event and is defined as "any response to a drug which is noxious and unintended, and which occurs at doses normally used in man for prophylaxis, diagnosis, or therapy of disease, or for the modification of physiologic function" (World Health Organization, 1975). When it is an extension of the expected pharmacologic effect of the drug, it tends to be predictable and dose dependent. However, unexpected, bizarre reactions (idiosyncratic reactions) can also occur that are unrelated to the drug's pharmacologic action.

Health care professionals have an obligation to minimize the risk associated with drugs and to optimize outcomes from drug therapy. Knowledge of drug-induced communication and swallowing disorders will promote prevention, assist in early detection, and ensure prompt action once a reaction has occurred. This chapter discusses the various adverse effects of drugs that have resulted in communication and swallowing disorders as described in the literature. The classification of these effects into certain categories is at times difficult because authors may use vague descriptions or various labels for a particular communication disorder. For simplification, drug-induced effects consisting of dysarthria, apraxia, and aphasia have been gathered under speech and language effects.

✦ Evaluation of a Patient Experiencing a Drug-Induced Disease

Once an adverse event has occurred, a systematic approach to evaluating the patient promotes proper management and prevention of similar occurrences. First, the clinical status of the patient should be assessed. If the patient is experiencing life-threatening effects, such as those that interfere with airway, breathing, or circulation, then emergency medical attention is imperative. Examples of potentially life-threatening effects include stridor, angioedema, laryngospasm, wheezing, or hypotension. The investigation and action taken in response to other reactions can be prioritized by the degree of compromise the patient is experiencing.

To determine whether the reaction was drug induced, the circumstances surrounding the adverse event must be accurately and thoroughly investigated. Information should be collected directly from the patient if possible and as soon as possible to improve the accuracy and reliability of the data. Detailed information is obtained on the complaint, including its location, severity, timing, onset, duration, associated symptoms, modifying factors (what makes it better or worse), and context (under what circumstances does the complaint occur, and has it happened before). Determining the patient's

Table 23–1   Assessment of Likelihood that an Adverse Event is Drug Induced

	Yes	No	Do Not Know Score
1. Are there previous conclusive reports on this reaction?	+1	0	0
2. Did the adverse event appear after the suspected drug was administered?	+2	−1	0
3. Did the adverse reaction improve when the drug was discontinued or a specific antagonist was administered?	+1	0	0
4. Readministered?	+2	−1	0
5. Are there alternative causes (other than the drug) that could on their own have caused the reaction?	−1	+2	0
6. Did the reaction reappear when a placebo was given?	−1	+1	0
7. Was the drug detected in the blood (or other body fluids) in concentrations known to be toxic?	+1	0	0
8. Was the reaction more severe when the dose was increased, or less severe when it was decreased?	+1	0	0
9. Did the patient have a similar reaction to the same or similar drugs in any previous exposure?	+1	0	0
10. Was the adverse event confirmed by any objective evidence?	+1	0	0
Total score[a]			

[a]Association between drug and reaction: 9, definite; 5–8, probable; 1–4, possible; 0, doubtful.

current medication history will help in the investigation as well. The clinician must determine what the patient is actually taking, including prescription medications, over-the-counter and alternative therapies (including herbal remedies), and recreational drugs. The history of dosage changes, initiation of new drugs, and discontinuation of past drugs should also be collected.

Next, previous occurrences of the adverse event should be noted, particularly as they relate to any of the patient's medications. To review adverse effect profiles of drugs, sources such as package inserts (found in drug packaging and in the *Physicians' Desk Reference*), American Hospital Formulary Service (AHFS) Drug Information, or *Facts and Comparisons* can be consulted. Direct communication with drug manufacturers is often helpful. They have reports of postmarketing ADRs that are not yet in the package insert and are often able to provide written information on an ADR. Investigation into the primary literature will yield detailed descriptions of drug-induced diseases and is particularly useful for idiosyncratic reactions or reactions from new drugs.

Proving causality between the drug and the adverse event is difficult, and often a clear conclusion is not reached. In general, however, the likelihood that an adverse event is drug induced can be estimated using previously developed criteria (**Table 23–1**) (Naranjo, Busto, Sellers, et al., 1981). Also, comparing the patient's reactions to those discovered in a review of the literature is helpful. The temporal relationship of the initiation of the drug or changes in the dosage and the onset of the event, characteristics of presentation, preexisting risk factors that the patient may possess, the possibility of involvement of drug interactions, alternative causes for the reaction including symptoms of underlying disease, and other iatrogenic causes can be significant.

A plan of action should be developed and implemented in collaboration with the patient and the patient's primary health care provider based on the acuity and severity of the adverse event and recommendations reported in the literature. This plan should include supportive and direct care for the patient's problem, but could possibly include no treatment at all. The necessity of discontinuing the therapy in question should be addressed. Discontinuing therapy is often the best solution if alternative safe and effective therapy is available. But if the benefits of therapy outweigh the burden of the ADR, therapy may be continued with or without treatment for the ADR. Other drug restrictions should be identified to prevent cross-reactivity with similar drugs. Implementation of the plan requires informing the patient, the patient's primary health care provider, and the patient's pharmacist of the nature of the reaction and the proposed resolution. Written documentation will support the diagnosis and treatment plan to ensure that information is communicated accurately.

If the reaction has occurred secondary to a new drug or is very unusual or serious, it should be reported to the manufacturer and to the Med Watch program at the Food and Drug Administration (FDA) (**Fig. 23–1**). Often serious ADRs of new drugs are not recognized until they are released for general use owing to the low incidence of the event. Reporting the reaction assists the FDA and drug manufacturers in providing information to health care professionals to promote the safe use of medications.

Reporting the ADR in the medical literature is important if it has not been widely described to further improve general knowledge of the adverse effects of the drug and assist other clinicians in their investigation of the topic. Institutional adverse drug reaction forms are also available in most settings, and all ADRs should be reported by this mechanism to contribute to internal monitoring of safety of drug therapy.

✦ Drug-Induced Dysphonia

Inhaled Steroid Preparations

Although few drugs have been associated with changes in voice or dysphonia, inhaled steroid preparations used in the chronic management of lung disease are frequently

U.S. Department of Health and Human Services

MEDWATCH

The FDA Safety Information and
Adverse Event Reporting Program

For **VOLUNTARY** reporting of
adverse events and product problems

Page _____ of _____

Form Approved: OMB No. 0910-0230 Expires: 09/30/05
See OMB statement on reverse

FDA Use Only

Triage unit
sequence #

A. Patient information

1. Patient identifier	2. Age at time of event: or _____ Date of birth:	3. Sex ☐ female ☐ male	4. Weight _____ lbs or _____ kgs
In confidence			

B. Adverse event or product problem

1. ☐ Adverse event   and/or   ☐ Product problem (e.g., defects/malfunctions)

2. Outcomes attributed to adverse event (check all that apply)

☐ death _____ (mo/day/yr)
☐ life-threatening
☐ hospitalization - initial or prolonged

☐ disability
☐ congenital anomaly
☐ required intervention to prevent permanent impairment/damage
☐ other: _____

3. Date of event (mo/day/yr)	4. Date of this report (mo/day/yr)

5. Describe event or problem

6. Relevant tests/laboratory data, including dates

7. Other relevant history, including preexisting medical conditions (e.g., allergies, race, pregnancy, smoking and alcohol use, hepatic/renal dysfunction, etc.)

PLEASE TYPE OR USE BLACK INK

C. Suspect medication(s)

1. **Name** (give labeled strength & mfr/labeler, if known)

#1

#2

2. Dose, frequency & route used	3. Therapy dates (if unknown, give duration) from/to (or best estimate)
#1	#1
#2	#2

4. **Diagnosis for use** (indication)

#1

#2

5. Event abated after use stopped or dose reduced
#1 ☐ yes ☐ no ☐ doesn't apply
#2 ☐ yes ☐ no ☐ doesn't apply

6. Lot # (if known)	7. Exp. date (if known)
#1	#1
#2	#2

8. **Event reappeared after reintroduction**
#1 ☐ yes ☐ no ☐ doesn't apply
#2 ☐ yes ☐ no ☐ doesn't apply

9. NDC # (for product problems only)
- -

10. **Concomitant medical products** and therapy dates (exclude treatment of event)

D. Suspect medical device

1. Brand name

2. Type of device

3. Manufacturer name & address	4. Operator of device ☐ health professional ☐ lay user/patient ☐ other: _____

5. **Expiration date** (mo/day/yr)

6.
model # _____
catalog # _____
serial # _____
lot # _____
other #

7. **If implanted, give date** (mo/day/yr)

8. **If explanted, give date** (mo/day/yr)

9. **Device available for evaluation?** (Do not send to FDA)
☐ yes   ☐ no   ☐ returned to manufacturer on _____ (mo/day/yr)

10. **Concomitant medical products** and therapy dates (exclude treatment of event)

E. Reporter (see confidentiality section on back)

1. Name & address	phone #

2. Health professional? ☐ yes ☐ no	3. Occupation	4. Also reported to ☐ manufacturer ☐ user facility ☐ distributor

5. If you do NOT want your identity disclosed to the manufacturer, place an " X " in this box. ☐

FDA

Mail to: **MEDWATCH**
5600 Fishers Lane
Rockville, MD 20852-9787

or FAX to:
1-800-FDA-0178

FDA Form 3500 (11/02)   Submission of a report does not constitute an admission that medical personnel or the product caused or contributed to the event.

Figure 23–1 Reporting from for the Med Watch program of the Food and Drug Administration.

ADVICE ABOUT VOLUNTARY REPORTING

Report adverse experiences with:
- medications (drugs or biologics)
- medical devices (including in-vitro diagnostics)
- special nutritional products (dietary supplements, medical foods, infant formulas)
- cosmetics
- medication errors

Report product problems – quality, performance or safety concerns such as:
- suspected contamination
- questionable stability
- defective components
- poor packaging or labeling
- therapeutic failures

Report SERIOUS adverse events. An event is serious when the patient outcome is:
- death
- life-threatening (real risk of dying)
- hospitalization (initial or prolonged)
- disability (significant, persistent or permanent)
- congenital anomaly
- required intervention to prevent permanent impairment or damage

Report even if:
- you're not certain the product caused the event
- you don't have all the details

How to report:
- just fill in the sections that apply to your report
- use section C for all products except medical devices
- attach additional blank pages if needed
- use a separate form for each patient
- report either to FDA or the manufacturer (or both)

Confidentiality: The patient's identity is held in strict confidence by FDA and protected to the fullest extent of the law. FDA will not disclose the reporter's identity in response to a request from the public, pursuant to the Freedom of Information Act. The reporter's identity, including the identity of a self-reporter, may be shared with the manufacturer unless requested otherwise.

If your report involves a serious adverse event with a device and it occurred in a facility outside a doctor's office, that facility may be legally required to report to FDA and/or the manufacturer. Please notify the person in that facility who would handle such reporting.

Important numbers:
- 1-800-FDA-0178   to FAX report
- 1-800-FDA-1088   to report by phone or for more information
- 1-800-822-7967   for a VAERS form for vaccines

To Report via the Internet:
https://www.accessdata.fda.gov/scripts/medwatch/

The public reporting burden for this collection of information has been estimated to average 30 minutes per response, including the time for reviewing instructions, searching existing data sources, gathering and maintaining the data needed, and completing and reviewing the collection of information. Send comments regarding this burden estimate or any other aspect of this collection of information, including suggestions for reducing this burden to:

DHHS Reports Clearance Office
Paperwork Reduction Project (0910-0291)
Hubert H. Humphrey Building, Room 531-H
200 Independence Avenue, S.W.
Washington, DC 20201

Please DO NOT
RETURN this form
to this address.

U.S. DEPARTMENT OF HEALTH AND HUMAN SERVICES
Public Health Service • Food and Drug Administration

FDA Form 3500-back   **Please Use Address Provided Below – Just Fold In Thirds, Tape and Mail**

**Department of
Health and Human Services**
Public Health Service
Food and Drug Administration
Rockville, MD 20857

Official Business
Penalty for Private Use $300

BUSINESS REPLY MAIL
FIRST CLASS MAIL   PERMIT NO. 946   ROCKVILLE, MD

POSTAGE WILL BE PAID BY FOOD AND DRUG ADMINISTRATION

NO POSTAGE
NECESSARY
IF MAILED
IN THE
UNITED STATES
OR APO/FPO

MEDWATCH
The FDA Safety Information and Adverse Event Reporting Program
**Food and Drug Administration
5600 Fishers Lane
Rockville, MD 20852-9787**

Figure 23–1 *(Continued)*

implicated (**Table 23–2**). In patients who use inhaled steroids regularly, as many as 77% report the development of dysphonia (Lavy, Wood, Rubin, & Harries, 2000; Toogood, Jennings, Greenway, et al., 1980; Williams, Baghat, Stableforth, et al., 1983; Williamson, Matusiewicz, Brown, et al., 1995). However, in a study of children, there was no increased risk of dysphonia among those receiving inhaled steroid compared with placebo-treated subjects (Agertoft, Larsen, & Pedersen, 1998). The occurrence of dysphonia appears to be dose-related (Toogood et al., 1980; Williamson et al., 1995). Onset of symptoms is highly variable, with some patients developing symptoms early in therapy whereas others' symptoms are delayed up to 112 weeks (Williams et al., 1983). Although dysphonia can occur alone, it is often accompanied by other symptoms including oral candidiasis, throat irritation, and cough.

Visualization of the vocal folds in patients experiencing inhaled steroid-induced dysphonia yields variable findings. Bowing of the vocal cords is frequently observed. However, not all patients exhibit this finding, although it is observed in some patients without dysphonia (Lavy et al., 2000; Toogood et al., 1980; Williams et al., 1983; Williamson et al., 1995). Among patients with the abnormality, resolution of the bowing and/or dysphonia often occurs within 16 weeks after discontinuation of the steroid (Toogood et al., 1980; Williams et al., 1983; Williamson et al., 1995). Recurrence of symptoms was noted in some patients who reinstituted therapy. Mucosal changes have also been seen, including thickened mucus and evidence of fungal infection (Lavy et al., 2000). Supraglottic hyperfunction may be present (Lavy et al., 2000).

The mechanism of dysphonia associated with inhaled steroids is likely to be multifactorial and is still being investigated. Trauma to the vocal folds from the rapid discharge of propellant from metered-dose inhaler preparations may cause voice changes. Dysphonia from the administration of metered-dose inhalers without steroid occurs, although at a lower frequency (Campbell, 1984; Skinner & Williams, 1984). The incidence of dysphonia from other forms of inhaled steroids such as dry powder inhalers seems to be less, and dysphonia may improve within 4 weeks after converting to this dosage form from a metered-dose inhaler (Crompton, Sanderson, Dewar, et al., 2000; Streeton, 1984). However, the use of a spacer device with metered-dose inhalers, which eliminates vocal fold trauma from the forceful discharge of the propellant, does not significantly reduce the incidence of dysphonia (Williamson et al., 1995).

Dysphonia with the use of inhaled steroids could also be caused by local effects of the steroid. It is hypothesized that steroid deposited in the larynx may induce local myopathy of laryngeal muscles or mucosal atrophy that would affect vocal fold function and produce bowing of the vocal cords (Lavy et al., 2000; Williams et al., 1983). This would account for the failure of spacers to reduce the incidence of dysphonia because they may actually increase deposition of steroid in the larynx (Inhaled steroids and dysphonia 1984). Mouth rinsing after steroid inhaler use has been reported to be protective against dysphonia (Toogood, Jennings, Baskerville, et al., 1984; Toogood et al., 1980).

Supraglottic hyperfunction may be the cause of dysphonia in some patients (Lavy et al., 2000). This abnormality may arise as a musculoskeletal accommodation to mucosal changes or be secondary to asthma itself.

Androgenic Steroids

Virilization of the voice occurs as an extension of the pharmacologic effect with the use of androgenic steroids, particularly in women (**Table 23–1**) (Baker, 1998). Danazol is known to cause deepening of the voice, hoarseness, and vocal instability in as many as 38% of patients (Newman & Forbes, 1993). It is hypothesized that the mechanism of voice virilization is inflammation of the vocal folds or alteration of muscle tissue and coordination (Baker, 1998; Boothroyd & Lepre, 1990). Increased vocal fold rigidity has been noted and was thought to be due to a local increase in muscle tissue with a concomitant decrease in connective tissue (Gerritsma, Brocaar, Hakkesteegt, et al., 1994). Voice virilization from androgenic steroids usually occurs within the first 3 months of therapy and is often irreversible, even on discontinuation of therapy (Baker, 1998; Boothroyd & Lepre, 1990; Newman & Forbes, 1993; Wardle, Whitehead, & Mills, 1983).

Vocal Fold Paresis and Paralysis

Vinca Alkaloids

Drug-induced vocal fold paresis and paralysis are unusual but have been reported (**Table 23–2**). The most frequently implicated agents are the vinca alkaloids, namely, vincristine and vinblastine. These agents are known to be generally neurotoxic, and presenting symptoms usually include constipation, urinary retention, decreased deep tendon reflexes, paresthesia, and distal sensory loss. Vocal fold paralysis rarely occurs, and is thought to be another manifestation of neurotoxicity (Whittaker & Griffith, 1977). It has been hypothesized that the vinca alkaloids may combine with neural proteins, leading to accumulation of neurofilaments and ultimately impairing axoplasmic flow and causing neural degeneration (Delaney, 1982). Vocal fold dysfunction with vincristine and vinblastine is thought to be dose dependent, although it has been reported in patients receiving low-dose vincristine as well (Alfredsunder, Hochman, & Kaplan, 1992; Whittaker & Griffith, 1977). Other risk factors may include underlying neuropathy or autoimmune disease (Alfredsunder et al 1992).

The presentation of vinca alkaloid-induced vocal fold paralysis is somewhat variable. Hoarseness, dry cough, sore throat, neck pain, aphonia, and stridor have been reported (Alfredsunder et al., 1992; Delaney, 1982; Tobias & Bozeman, 1991; Whittaker & Griffith, 1977). These complaints can be accompanied by symptoms consistent with general neuropathy, such as hypotonia, constipation, and paresthesia (Delaney, 1982; Tobias & Bozeman, 1991). On visualization of the vocal folds by direct or indirect laryngoscopy, unilateral and bilateral vocal fold paresis and paralysis have been noted. Onset of symptoms occurs 2 weeks to 7 months after administration of the first dose of vincristine or vinblastine, and resolution of signs and symptoms usually occurs within 6 weeks after drug discontinuation (Alfredsunder et al., 1992; Delaney, 1982; Tobias & Bozeman, 1991; Whittaker & Griffith, 1977).

Neuroleptic Agents

Vocal fold dysfunction has rarely been reported with the use of neuroleptic agents (**Table 23–2**). Haloperidol and fluphenazine have induced dysphonia in a patient after 3 years of therapy. It was felt that dysphonia was associated with the development

Table 23–2 Drug-Induced Speech and Swallowing Disorders

Drug or Drug Class	Disorder(s)	Proposed Mechanism(s)	References
Alcohol	Dysarthria	Decreased cognition	(Sobell, Sobell, & Coleman, 1982)
Alendronate	Mechanical dysphagia	Local chemical irritation of the esophagus	(Maconi & Porro, 1995; De Groen, Lubbe, Hirsch, et al., 1996; Colina, Smith, Kikendall, & Wong, 1997)
Anticholinergics	Dysarthria	Reduced activity of acetylcholine	(Duvoisin & Katz, 1968)
Antidepressants	Speech blockage	Unknown	(Schatzberg, Cole, & Blumer, 1978; Sandyk, 1983)
	Stuttering	Unknown	(Garvey & Tollefson, 1987; Quader, 1977; British Medical Journal, 1977; Masand, 1992; Meghji, 1994; Guthrie & Grunhaus, 1990; McCall, 1994; Brewerton, Markowitz, Keller, & Cochrane, 1996; Christensen, Byerly, & McElroy, 1996; Friedman, Guthrie, & Grunhaus, 1990)
Antiepileptics	Dysarthria	Cerebellar damage	(Riely, 1972; Jaster & Abbas, 1986)
Neuroleptics	Dysarthria	Unknown	(Gaile & Noviasky, 1998)
	Dysphonia	Tardive dyskinesia	(Lieberman & Reife, 1989)
	Neurogenic dysphagia	Inhibition of esophageal or pharyngeal/laryngeal motility	(McCarthy & Terkelsen, 1994; Cordeiro & Arnold, 1991; Moss & Green, 1982; Woodring, Martin, & Keefer, 1993; Sliwa & Lis, 1993; Pearlman, 1994; Wardell, 1957; Farber, 1957; Feldman, 1957; Hollister & Kosek, 1965; Plachta, 1965; Hollister, 1957; Zlotlow & Paganini, 1958)
		Pharyngeal-laryngeal dystonia	(Solomon, 1977; Flaherty & Lahmeyer, 1978; Cruz, Thiagarajan, & Harney, 1983; Stones, Kennie, & Fulton, 1990; Nair, Saeed, Shahab, et al., 2001; Casteels-Van Daele, Jaeken, Van der Schueren, et al., 1970)
	Speech arrest	Tardive dyskinesia	(Weiden, & Harrigan, 1986; Gregory, Smith, & Rudge, 1992; Crane & Paulson, 1967; Crane, 1968; Yassa & Jones, 1985)
		Acute dystonia	(Marcotte, 1973)
	Stuttering	Tardive dyskinesia	(Schmidt & Jarcho, 1966; Faheem, Brightwell, Burton, & Struss, 1982; Kane & Taylor, 1963; Angrist & Gershon, 1973)
		Imbalance of dopamine, acetylcholine, norepinephrine and serotonin	(Nurnberg & Greenwald, 1981; Adler, Leong, & Delgado, 1987; Thomas, Lalaux, Vaiva, et al., 1994; Ebeling, Compton, & Albright, 1997; Supprian, Retz, & Deckert, 1999; Duggal, Jagadheesan, & Nizamie, 2002; Lee, Lee, Kim, et al., 2001; Mahr & Leith, 1990)
Benzodiazepines	Neurogenic dysphagia	Inhibition of pharyngeal/laryngeal motility	(Wyllie, Wyllie, Cruse, et al., 1986)
	Dysarthria	Impaired cognition	(Gottschalk, 1977; Ishikawa, Hato, Tauchi, & Wada, 1988; Matson & Thurlow, 1988; Wilson, Petty, Perry, & Rose, 1983)
	Stuttering	Direct benzodiazepine effect in the brain	(Elliott & Thomas, 1985)
	Aphasia		(Wilson, Petty, Perry, et al., 1983)
Botulinum toxin	Neurogenic dysphagia	Impaired laryngeal movement	(Jankovic & Schwartz, 1991; Poewe, Schelosky, Kleedorfer, et al., 1992; Comella, Tanner, DeFoor-Hill, et al., 1992; Kessler, Skutta, & Benecke, 1999; Tuite & Land, 1996; Thobois, Brousolle & Toureille, 2001; Nix, Butler, Roontga, et al., 1992)
Butorphanol	Apraxia	Unknown	(Gora-Harper, Suahara, & Gray, 1995)
Chloroquine	Dysphagia	Unknown	(Gustafsson, Walker, Alvan, et al., 1983)
Cytarabine/ methotrexate	Dysphagia	Unknown	(Marmont & Damasio, 1973)
Digoxin	Dysphagia	Unknown	(Kelton & Scullin, 1978)
Doxycycline	Mechanical dysphagia	Local chemical irritation of the esophagus	(Bokey & Hug, 1975; Palmer, Selbst, Shaffer, & Proujansky, 1999)
Hydralazine	Dysphonia	Laryngeal ulcerations from necrotizing vasculitis	(Weiser, Forouhar & White, 1984)
L-dopa	Dysphagia	Unknown	(Wodak, Gilligan, Veale, et al., 1972)
	Stuttering	Increased dopaminergic activity	(Louis, Winfield, Fahn & Ford, 2001)
Lithium carbonate	Dysarthria	Neurotoxicity	(Bond, Carvalho, & Foulks, 1982; Singh, 1982, Lewis, 1983; Solomon & Vickers, 1975)
Methylphenidate	Stuttering	Increased dopaminergic activity	(Burd & Kerbeshian, 1991)
Metoclopramide	Dysarthria	Antidopaminergic effects	(Sandyk, 1983; Walsh, 1982)
	Dysphonia	Supraglottic dystonia	(Warren, 1998)

Table 23–2 *(Continued)*

Drug or Drug Class	Disorder(s)	Proposed Mechanism(s)	References
Metrizamide (contrast agent)	Stuttering	Immune-mediated or pial vasculature vasospasm	(Masdeu, Glista, Rubino, et al., 1983)
	Aphasia		(Sarno, 1985)
Nonsteroidal antiinflammatory agents	Dysphagia	Local chemical irritation of the esophagus	(Kim, Hunter, Wo, Davis, & Waring, 1999)
Pemoline	Stuttering	Increased dopaminergic transmission	(Burd & Kerbeshian, 1991)
Potassium chloride	Mechanical dysphagia	Local chemical irritation of the esophagus	(Pemberton, 1970; Chesshyre & Baimbridge, 1971; Rosenthal, Adar, Militianu, et al., 1974; Howie & Strachan, 1975; McCall, 1975; Peters, 1976; Twplick, Twplick, Ominsky, et al., 1980)
		Obstruction of esophagus from tablet	(Ashout, Salama, Morris, et al., 1984)
Procainamide	Dysphagia	Interference with neuromuscular transmission?	(Miller, Oleshansky, Gibson, & Cantilena, 1993)
Sildenafil	Dysphagia	Local chemical irritation of the esophagus	(Higuchi, Ando, Kim, et al., 2001)
Tetrabenazine	Dysphagia	Unknown	(Snaith & Warren, 1974; Critchley, 1976; Huang, McLeod, Holland et al., 1976)
Theophylline	Stuttering	Unknown	(McCarthy, 1981)
Quinidine	Mechanical dysphagia	Local chemical irritation of the esophagus	(Twplick, Twplick, Ominsky, et al., 1980; Mason & O'Meara, 1981; Kikendall, 1999; Wong, Kikendall, & Dachman, 1986)
		Physical obstruction of esophagus from tablet	(Bohane, Perrault, & Fowler, 1978)
Steroids, epidural	Dysphonia	Vocal fold edema	(Slipman, Chow, Lenrow, et al., 2002)
Steroids, inhaled	Dysphonia	Vocal fold trauma or deformities	(Toogood, Jennings, Greenway, et al., 1980; Williams, Baghat, Stableforth, et al., 1983; Williamson, Matusiewicz, Brown, et al., 1995; Lavy, Wood, Rubin, & Harries, 2000; Streeton, 1984; Anon, 1984; Toogood, Jennings, Baskerville, et al., 1984)
Steroids, androgenic	Vocal virilization	Vocal fold inflammation	(Newman & Forbes, 1993; Boothroyd & Lepre, 1990; Gerritsma, Brocaar, Hakkesteegt, et al., 1994; Wardle, Whitehead, & Mills, 1983)
Tacrolimus	Apraxia and dysarthria	Unknown	(Boeve, Kimmel, Aronson, et al., 1996)
Topical oropharyngeal anesthesia	Dysphagia	Removal of sensory inputs	(Ertekin, Kiylioglu, Tarlaci, et al., 2000)
		Necessary for voluntary swallowing	
Vinca alkaloids	Vocal fold dysfunction	Neurotoxicity	(Whittaker & Griffith, 1977; Delaney, 1982; Alfredsunder, Hochman, & Kaplan, 1992; Tobias & Bozeman, 1991)
	Dysphagia	Unknown	(Chisholm & Curry, 1978)

of tardive dyskinesia because it improved with the administration of physostigmine and discontinuation of haloperidol. However, 4 weeks after the initiation of therapy with fluphenazine, the dysphonia recurred. Again, the patient's symptoms improved with physostigmine and discontinuation of therapy. Subsequent therapy with clozapine was successful (Lieberman &, Reife, 1989).

✦ Drug-Induced Speech and Language Impairments

Agents reported to influence speech and language do so by either direct injury to the involved tissues or, more commonly, by altering neurotransmitter function in the central and peripheral nervous systems (**Table 23–2**). A drug can alter neurotransmitter function by (1) increasing or decreasing the amount of neurotransmitter in the synapse available for interaction with the receptor; (2) preventing reuptake of the neurotransmitter, allowing it to persist in the synapse longer; (3) blocking the receptor so that the neurotransmitter cannot stimulate the receptor (an antagonist); and (4) stimulating the receptor directly (an agonist). Neurotransmitters affected by pharmacologic agents are acetylcholine, norepinephrine/epinephrine, γ-aminobutyric acid (GABA), serotonin, dopamine, and glutamate (**Table 23–3**).

Dysarthria

It is quite common for drugs active in the central nervous system to cause changes in speech as part of a symptom complex resulting from adverse cognitive effects of the drug (Fayen,

Table 23–3   Neurotransmitters and Their Interactions with Common Medications

Neurotransmitter	Actions	Drugs Inhibiting	Drugs Promoting
Acetylcholine	Excitatory; parasympathetic; memory	Anticholinergics; antidepressants; antiarrhythmics antihistamines	Donepezil; galanthamine; rivastigmine; pyridostigmine; neostigmine
Norepinephrine/ Epinephrine	Mood; anxiety; alertness autonomic nervous system	Beta-blockers; alpha-blockers	Epinephrine; stimulants; pseudoephedrine
GABA	Inhibitory; throughout nervous system		Benzodiazepines; barbiturates; some anticonvulsants
Serotonin	Sleep–wake cycles; emotion mood; vessel constriction;	Cyproheptadine; methysergide	Antidepressants; sumatriptan; ergots
Dopamine	Inhibitory; movement; psychoses; gastrointestinal function	Neuroleptics; metoclopramide	Levodopa; bromocriptine; pergolide; pramipexole; ropinirole; antidepressants
Glutamate	Excitatory; predominant throughout nervous system	Lamotrigine; riluzole; ketamine; phencyclidine (PCP)	

Goldman, Moulthrop, & Luchins, 1988; Miller, Richardson, Jyu, Lemay, Hisock, & Keegan, 1988). "Slurred speech," dysfluency, and word unintelligibility describe the dysarthria reported to be related to medication usage. More uncommon, however, are the speech disorders occurring as a solitary symptom of the adverse effects of the drug. Dysarthria, aphonia, mutism, and speech blockage have all been associated with administration of drugs, with various degrees of severity and duration.

Lithium Carbonate

Lithium carbonate is used to treat bipolar disorders and has been associated with both transient and persistent dysarthria when the drug is used alone or in combination with neuroleptic therapy (Bond, Carvalho, & Foulks, 1982; Lewis, 1983; Singh, 1982; Solomon & Vickers, 1975). Blood lithium concentrations above 2 mEq/L have been consistently associated with slurred speech, which is usually accompanied by other signs of lithium toxicity such as tremor. However, in some cases the onset of the dysarthria ranges from weeks to years after the initiation of therapy and is not always related to elevated concentrations of lithium in the blood. In all cases withdrawal of lithium was associated with improvement of symptoms, but persistent dysarthria, suggested to be due to an irreversible neurotoxicity of the drug, has been reported (Bond et al., 1982; Lewis, 1983; Singh, 1982).

Neuroleptic Agents

Neuroleptics may cause speech arrest or inability to articulate words by either of two distinct mechanisms (Faheem, Brightwell, Burton, & Struss, 1982; Gaile & Noviasky, 1998; Kane & Taylor, 1963; Marcotte, 1973; Schmidt & Jarcho, 1966). The first occurs early in treatment (hours to days after initiation) and is a result of an acute dystonic reaction. The speech difficulty may be accompanied by oculogyric (eye movement) crisis, choreoathetosis, and cervicolingual masticatory crisis, and usually responds quickly to discontinuation of the agent and administration of an anticholinergic medication. Young patients receiving phenothiazine or butyrophenone (haloperidol) derivatives by parenteral routes seem to be at particular risk of this adverse effect (Marcotte, 1973).

The second type of speech disorder associated with neuroleptic administration has been associated with tardive

dyskinesia (Angrist & Gershon, 1973; Faheem et al., 1982; Kane & Taylor, 1963; Schmidt & Jarcho, 1966). These movement disorders are delayed in onset (a minimum of months after initiation of treatment) and are thought to be related to the duration of therapy. The symptoms of tardive dyskinesia usually include purposeless movements of the arms, hands, legs, and face (akathisia), and the disorder tends to persist and worsen after discontinuation of the neuroleptic. Increasing the neuroleptic dose may alleviate the symptoms temporarily, but no benefit of anticholinergic medication can be expected. Older patients appear to be at greatest risk of tardive dyskinesia, but all patients on prolonged neuroleptic therapy are at risk.

Benzodiazepines

Benzodiazepines are known to adversely affect speech through their effects on cognition (Gottschalk, 1977). There have been reports, however, of speech disturbances occurring in the absence of, or in disproportion to, other cognitive effects of the drug. In one case, a 3-year-old girl was given high-dose intravenous diazepam (37.5 mg over 15 hours) for control of agitation after a surgical procedure (Ishikawa, Hato, Tauchi, & Wada, 1988). Four hours after the final dose of diazepam, the patient was noticed to be anarthric and subsequently dysarthric, which gradually improved and disappeared at 180 hours after the final diazepam dose. In a case involving the short-acting benzodiazepine midazolam, dysarthria accompanied by hypotension and drowsiness developed in a 67-year-old man, 5 minutes after an intramuscular injection of the drug (Matson & Thurlow, 1988). The hypotension and dysarthria dissipated after 25 minutes but the drowsiness persisted.

Antidepressants

Speech blockage has been reported to occur with many different antidepressants (Sandyk, 1983; Schatzberg, Cole, Blumer, 1978; Sholomskas, 1978). In the majority of patients, the onset of the symptom is within the first few weeks of therapy and resolution occurs within a few days of reduction in the dose or a discontinuation of the therapy. Although it is thought to be more common in older patients (Sandyk, 1983), it has been reported in the young and should be considered in this patient population (Sholomskas, 1978).

Metoclopramide

Metoclopramide is a dopamine antagonist used for its antiemetic and promotility properties. Extrapyramidal side effects such as acute dystonic reactions are not uncommon, but isolated speech disturbance is quite rare (Sandyk, 1983; Walsh, 1982). One 25-year-old woman developed dysarthria after receiving high-dose metoclopramide for 72 hours preoperatively (Walsh, 1982). The dysarthria persisted for 6 weeks after she received her last dose of metoclopramide. In an elderly patient, metoclopramide was associated with a severe dysarthria that developed after 6 weeks of chronic therapy for dyspepsia (Sandyk, 1983). The dysarthria was accompanied by a resting tremor and decreased tongue mobility. After discontinuation of the metoclopramide, the neurologic problems disappeared over several weeks. In a second elderly patient, the dysarthria developed after a single intramuscular dose and took 8 weeks to resolve (Sandyk, 1983).

Other Drugs

Other pharmacologic agents associated with speech disorders are anticholinergics (Duvoisin & Katz, 1968), intranasal butorphanol (Gora-Harper, Sunahara, & Gray, 1995), alcohol (Sobell, Sobell, & Colemen, 1982), tacrolimus (Boeve, Kimmel, Aronson, et al., 1996), and antiepileptics (Jaster & Abbas, 1986; Riley, 1972). In most cases, the symptoms resolve quickly on discontinuation of the drug. In the cases of anticholinergics and butorphanol, reversal with an acetylcholinesterase inhibitor (physostigmine) (Duvoisin & Katz, 1968) and opiate antagonist (naloxone) (Gora-Harper et al., 1995), respectively, have been used with success. In the case of hydantoin antiepileptics (phenytoin), however, chronic neurotoxicity has been reported after long-term therapy and the implication of permanent cerebellar damage has been suggested (Riley, 1972).

Aphasia

Benzodiazepines

A jargon aphasia related to clobazam, a benzodiazepine used as an antiepileptic agent, was reported in an 18-year-old man with a history of seizures and migraine with aura (Wilson, Petty, Perry, & Rose, 1983). After 3 weeks of therapy, he developed minute-long episodes of sudden-onset extended neologisms that gradually improved for the 5 days after the discontinuation of clobazam. The authors proposed an interaction between his partial seizures and the clobazam as the cause of the aphasia. In all cases of benzodiazepine-associated language disorders, onset and duration seem to be related to the pharmacokinetic characteristics of the particular agents, and no permanent neurotoxicity appears to exist.

Metrizamide

Aphasia has been reported as complication of metrizamide myelography (Masdeu, Glista, Rubino, et al., 1983; Sarno, 1985). The authors have characterized the aphasia as motor, expressive, and conduction. Onset of symptoms has ranged from 1 to 18 hours after the administration of the drug. The duration of the aphasia is typically brief, about 36 hours.

The actual mechanism for the aphasia is unknown, but was theorized to be neurotoxic rather than a phenomenon of seizure.

Drug-Induced Stuttering

Antidepressants

Although it is unusual, drugs have been reported to induce stuttering in patients with and without a previous history of stuttering (**Table 23–2**). Antidepressants are most frequently implicated, but the mechanism by which they induce stuttering is not entirely clear. Cases of tricyclic antidepressants causing stuttering were first published in the 1970s and the condition may be underreported. Although there are relatively few cases of antidepressant-induced stuttering published, four of 98 patients receiving tricyclic antidepressants in one study required discontinuation of their drug owing to stuttering (Garvey & Tollefson, 1987).

Amitriptyline and one of its analogues, dothiepin, were associated with stuttering in two cases when the drugs were utilized in relatively low doses (Quader, 1977). The onset of symptoms was 3 to 4 days and discontinuation of therapy was indicated in both cases. Spontaneous resolution of symptoms followed in 2 days in the amitriptyline patient and in an unspecified time in the dothiepin patient. Stuttering was accompanied by other symptoms that were labeled as dysarthria by the authors, but later described as a nonspecific involuntary movement that interrupted the patients' speech (Saunders, 1977). The authors hypothesized that stuttering was due to anticholinergic effects of the drugs on the cerebellar connections and striatum.

Desipramine is another tricyclic antidepressant that has been reported to cause stuttering in a patient who had previously tolerated another antidepressant, doxepin (Masand, 1992). Stuttering occurred 4 months after initiating treatment, and recurred within 1 day of rechallenge. The patient's serum desipramine level was reported to be 439 ng/mL, which is slightly higher than the therapeutic range of 150 to 300 ng/mL, but is not in the toxic range of >1000 ng/mL. The patient experienced concomitant jaw myoclonus, and the authors did not speculate as to the mechanism of the reaction.

Newer antidepressants that belong to the class of serotonin reuptake inhibitors have produced stuttering. Fluoxetine and sertraline have been associated with stuttering in five patients within 4 weeks of initiating therapy (Brewerton, Markowitz, Keller, & Cochrane, 1996; Christensen, Byerly, & McElroy, 1996; Guthrie & Grunhaus, 1990; McCall, 1994; Meghji, 1994). One patient had a past medical history of stuttering, whereas the others did not. In four of five patients, drug discontinuation produced resolution of stuttering within 2 weeks (Brewerton et al., 1996; Christensen et al., 1996; Guthrie & Grunhaus, 1990; McCall, 1994). However, the other patient had a much slower resolution of the stuttering and required speech therapy (Meghji, 1994). Proposed mechanisms for this reaction were an abnormality in serotonin function (Guthrie & Grunhaus, 1990) or a type of akathisia (motor restlessness and anxiety) due to inhibition of dopamine activity in the right hemisphere by serotonergic or noradrenergic activity of these agents (Brewerton et al., 1996; Christensen et al., 1996; Friedman, Guthrie, & Grunhaus, 1990).

Neuroleptic Agents

Many neuroleptic agents have been associated with drug-induced stuttering. The first reports consisted of two patients who were receiving therapy with fluphenazine or chlorpromazine (Nurnberg & Greenwald, 1981). Both patients had tolerated neuroleptic therapy before, but experienced stuttering 26 days after restarting therapy or 4 days after a dosage increase. In both patients, treatment with diphenhydramine, benztropine, or trihexyphenidyl was not helpful, but symptoms abated with decreasing the dosage of the offending agent. Both patients reexperienced stuttering with increased dosage of their neuroleptics. The authors speculated that this reaction could be a type of extrapyramidal symptom, but acute dystonia was ruled out because of the lack of resolution after treatment with anticholinergic agents.

Other clinicians have noted improvement in neuroleptic-induced stuttering with administration of propranolol (Adler, Leong, & Delgado, 1987). Two patients were receiving therapy with perphenazine/desipramine combination or chlorpromazine/lithium combination. The patient receiving desipramine had tolerated therapy with nortriptyline in the past. In both cases, stuttering resolved soon after administration of propranolol 10 or 20 mg three times daily. In one patient, stuttering reappeared after discontinuation of propranolol, but again resolved with resumption of therapy. This prompted the authors to propose that neuroleptic-induced stuttering has an etiology similar to akathisia (i.e., imbalance of dopaminergic, cholinergic, and noradrenergic systems in the brain) because it responded to the same treatment as akathisia.

An atypical neuroleptic agent, clozapine, has also been known to induce stuttering in a four patients (Duggal, Jagadheesan, & Nizamie, 2002; Ebeling, Compton, & Albright, 1997; Supprian, Retz, & Deckert, 1999; Thomas, Lalaux, Vaiva, et al., 1994). Occurrence of symptoms seemed to be dose dependent in that it occurred after dose increases in patients who tolerated lower doses. Changes on electroencephalography were demonstrated in three patients, and the authors hypothesized that the patients' symptoms may have been related to epileptiform activity. In three patients, stuttering remitted despite continuation of clozapine after reduction of the dose with or without initiation of effective antiepileptic therapy (Duggal et al., 2002; Ebeling et al., 1997; Supprian et al., 1999). In one case, discontinuation of therapy resulted in resolution of symptoms within 5 days, but symptoms recurred on rechallenge with the drug (Thomas et al., 1994).

Risperidone, a high-potency atypical neuroleptic, has been reported to induce stuttering in one patient (Lee, Lee, Kim, et al., 2001). Stuttering began 5 days after initiation of treatment and worsened with dosage increases. With continued therapy over the next 7 weeks, stuttering improved spontaneously, and was nearly resolved 2 months later.

Metrizamide

Metrizamide, a radiopaque contrast medium used in positive contrast myelography, was shown to induce stuttering in three patients (Bertoni, Schwartzman, Van Horn, et al., 1981; Pimental & Gorelik, 1985). In all patients, stuttering was accompanied by other symptoms originating in the central nervous system, such as confusion and asterixis (motor disturbance marked by intermittent sustained contractions of groups of muscles). Onset of symptoms was within 12 hours of completion of the imaging study, and symptom resolution was highly variable. In one patient, symptoms resolved within 7 days, but the other two patients required 3 to 5 months for symptom resolution. In all three patients, distribution of metrizamide to the central nervous system was confirmed by computed tomography scan. It has been proposed that the presence of dye in the central nervous system may induce an immune response or vasospasm of pial vasculature that could contribute to the development of symptoms (Pimental & Gorelik, 1985). Placing the patient in a supine position after the procedure may facilitate distribution of the dye to the brain (Bertoni et al., 1981), but a semi-upright position is not entirely protective (Pimental & Gorelik, 1985).

Other Drugs

Other drugs that have been associated with stuttering are theophylline (Gerard & Robience, 1998; McCarthy, 1981; Rosenfield, McCarthy, McKinney, et al., 1994), prochlorperazine (Mahr & Leith, 1990), methylphenidate and pemoline (Burd & Kerbeshian, 1991), levodopa (Louis, Winfield, Fahn, & Ford, 2001), gabapentin (Nissani & Sanchez, 1997), and alprazolam (Elliott & Thomas, 1985). Theophylline induced stuttering in four children and an elderly man, two of whom had documented theophylline levels within the therapeutic range. In all cases, stuttering resolved on discontinuation of the drug, but reappeared on rechallenge in three cases. No mechanisms for the reaction were proposed (Gerard & Robience, 1998; McCarthy, 1981; Rosenfield et al., 1994).

Prochlorperazine caused stuttering in a 39-year-old woman within 3 hours of administration of two doses, and was accompanied by tongue and laryngeal spasms. Although the dystonias resolved quickly, stuttering persisted and required speech therapy for 6 weeks. The authors felt the stuttering was initially part of the acute dystonic reaction, but persisted because of behavioral changes by the patient that caused disruption of the rhythm and coordination of her speech (Mahr & Leith, 1990).

A 3-year-old girl experienced stuttering 3 to 4 days after separate courses of methylphenidate and pemoline. Stuttering resolved spontaneously after therapy was discontinued. The authors proposed that stuttering may have been resulted from increased dopaminergic neurotransmission that is caused by both drugs (Burd & Kerbeshian, 1991).

Similarly, levodopa administered for the treatment of Parkinson's disease has produced stuttering in two patients (Louis et al., 2001). Discontinuation of the drug in one patient resulted in disappearance of the speech dysfluency, whereas improvements in speech were noted at the end of the dosing interval in the other patient.

Alprazolam caused stuttering in a 22-year-old woman who had previously tolerated other benzodiazepines. Within 2 hours of drug administration, she began to stutter. It resolved within 2 days of discontinuation of alprazolam, and recurred on a double-blind rechallenge. The authors stated that the onset and duration of stuttering paralleled the pharmacokinetic profile of the drug and therefore they felt that the stuttering was due to a direct action of the drug on the brain, and not anticholinergic side effects (Elliott & Thomas, 1985).

✦ Drug-Induced Swallowing Disorders

Dysphagia, defined as difficulty in swallowing, is associated with many neurologic disorders, head and neck cancer, and gastroenterologic diseases. However, many drugs have also been implicated as causes of dysphagia (**Table 23–2**). Normal swallowing is a complex function, and drugs impair swallowing by inducing a mechanical obstruction (mechanical dysphagia) or affecting neuromuscular control of swallowing (neurogenic dysphagia). Often drug-induced dysphagia resolves spontaneously after discontinuation of the offending agent, but complications including esophageal stricture, ulceration and bleeding, aspiration pneumonia, weight loss, and even death have been reported. Evaluation of all patients with dysphagia should include consideration of drug-induced causes to promote prompt diagnosis and treatment to prevent the occurrence of complications.

Mechanical Dysphagia

Drugs induce mechanical dysphagia most often indirectly by causing esophageal ulceration or inflammation. Doxycycline (Bokey & Hugh, 1975; Palmer, Selbst, Shaffer, & Proujansky, 1999), potassium chloride (Chesshyre & Braimbridge, 1971; Howie & Strachan, 1975; McCall, 1975; Pemberton, 1970; Peters, 1976; Rosenthal, Adar, Militianu, et al., 1974; Teplick, Teplick, Ominsky, et al., 1980), quinidine (Kikendall, 1999; Mason & O'Meara, 1981; Teplick et al., 1980; Wong, Kikendall, & Dachman, 1986), nonsteroidal antiinflammatory agents (Kim, Hunter, Wo, Davis, & Waring, 1999), and alendronate (De Groen, Lubbe, Hirsch, et al., 1996; Colina, Smith, Kikendall, & Wong, 1997; Maconi & Porro, 1995) have been reported to cause dysphagic symptoms by this mechanism. These drugs are chemical irritants to the esophageal mucosa, especially when prolonged contact occurs. Less frequently, the drug preparation itself can induce a mechanical dysphagia by lodging in the esophagus and preventing passage of a bolus. Agents associated with this mechanism of injury are potassium chloride (Ashour, Salama, Morris, et al., 1984), and quinidine (Bohane, Perrault, & Fowler, 1978).

Regardless of the mechanism of injury, patients usually present with symptoms of dysphagia, odynophagia, and substernal chest pain that is worsened with swallowing. Onset of symptoms ranges from immediately after the first dose of a drug to several years after initiation of therapy. Ingesting small volumes of liquid with orally administered medications (De Groen et al., 1996; Higuchi, Ando, Kim, et al., 2001; Kikendall, 1999; Macedo, Azevedo, & Ribeiro, 2001; Maconi & Porro, 1995; Mason & O'Meara, 1981), assuming a recumbent position immediately after taking medication (Bokey & Hugh, 1975; De Groen et al., 1996; Higuchi et al., 2001; Macedo et al., 2001; Maconi & Porro, 1995), recent esophageal injury from a nasogastric tube (Teplick et al., 1980), and an enlarged left atrium (Howie & Strachan, 1975; Maconi & Porro, 1995; McCall, 1975; Pemberton, 1970; Peters, 1976; Rosenthal et al., 1974) have been identified as risk factors for the development of drug-induced mechanical dysphagia. Although most reported cases are relatively uncomplicated, esophageal perforation with massive hemorrhage (McCall, 1975), stricture (Chesshyre & Braimbridge, 1971; De Groen et al., 1996; Howie & Strachan, 1975; Kim et al., 1999; Peters, 1976; Teplick et al., 1980; Wong et al., 1986), mediastinitis (Rosenthal et al., 1974), bronchoesophageal fistula (McAndrew & Greenway, 1999), and death (McCall, 1975; Rosenthal et al., 1974) have occurred. Management of drug-induced dysphagia should include discontinuation of therapy and supportive treatment involving limiting oral intake, administration of analgesics or acid-suppressive agents when necessary, and appropriate medical or surgical management of complications.

Esophageal injury and dysphagia from bisphosphonates has received particular attention. Although the incidence of serious or severe esophageal effects was found to be similar to placebo-treated patients in controlled clinical trials of alendronate (Bauer, Black, Ensrud, et al., 2000; Liberman & Hirsch, 1996;), the incidence with widespread use may be higher (Chesshyre & Braimbridge, 1971). It has been suggested that regular reinforcement of dosing instructions for patients in the trials may be responsible for the improved safety observed (Liberman & Hirsch, 1996). Less is known about the risk of esophageal injury from other bisphosphonates such as risedronate and etidronate. However, they are likely to be implicated as well because, like alendronate, they exist as free acids when dissolved in the stomach (Lanza, Hunt, Thomson, Provenza, & Blank, 2000; Macedo et al., 2001). Alendronate and risedronate are contraindicated in patients with preexisting esophageal pathology, such as strictures or achalasia, and in patients who are unable to comply with dosing instructions, which include remaining upright for at least 30 minutes after dosing. Newer dosing schedules that permit once weekly dosing (rather than daily) are favored to promote adherence to these instructions.

Neurogenic Dysphagia

Drug-induced neurogenic dysphagia occurs when a drug causes weakness of muscles involved in swallowing or incoordination of the swallowing process. Several drugs have been implicated in the interruption of the normal swallowing process by a variety of different mechanisms. Drugs reported to decrease esophageal motility include clozapine (McCarthy & Terkelsen, 1994), digoxin (Cordeiro & Arnold, 1991), molindone/benztropine combination (Moss & Green, 1982), and thiothixene/benztropine combination (Woodring, Martin, & Keefer, 1993). Many of these agents possess anticholinergic properties that have the potential to inhibit the activity of striated muscle of the pharynx, upper esophageal sphincter (UES), and upper esophagus. Clinical reports of the effect of these drugs on esophageal motility include increased tone of the UES (McCarthy & Terkelsen, 1994), esophageal muscle incoordination (Cordeiro & Arnold, 1991), decreased esophageal peristalsis (McCarthy & Terkelsen, 1994; Moss & Green, 1982), and marked esophageal dilation (Woodring et al., 1993). Other drugs, namely, haloperidol/benztropine/amitriptyline combination (Sliwa & Lis, 1993), clozapine (Pearlman, 1994) and nitrazepam (Wyllie, Wyllie, Cruse, et al., 1986), have demonstrated an ability to cause dysphagia through impairment of coordination of the pharyngeal and laryngeal phases of swallowing. Clinically, these effects manifest as delayed cricopharyngeal relaxation until after hypopharyngeal contraction (Wyllie et al., 1986), increased oral and pharyngeal transit times (Sliwa & Lis, 1993), and decreased pharyngeal peristalsis (Pearlman, 1994). Onset of dysphagic symptoms ranged from 2 days to 10 months after the offending agents were started. Some cases were complicated by pneumonia due to aspiration (Sliwa & Lis, 1993; Wyllie et al., 1986), but no other complications were noted. Discontinuation or dosage reduction of the offending agent(s) resulted in resolution of dysphagia in most cases.

Neuroleptic Drugs

Soon after widespread use of neuroleptic agents began in the 1950s and 1960s, several reports of sudden death appeared in the literature. Reserpine (Wardell, 1957), chlorpromazine alone (Farber, 1957; Feldman, 1957) and in combination with thioridazine and trihexyphenidyl (Hollister & Kosek, 1965), prochlorperazine and reserpine (Plachta, 1965), prochlorperazine (Hollister, 1957), and reserpine and an antiepileptic agent (Zlotlow & Paganini, 1958) were implicated. Onset of symptoms ranged from 3 weeks to 10 years after initiating therapy. Although the patients did not complain of dysphagia, they appeared to suddenly asphyxiate while eating. In several patients, food was found in the airway on autopsy (Farber, 1957; Hollister & Kosek, 1965; Zlotlow & Paganini, 1958). This prompted many clinicians to propose that perhaps the neuroleptic agents contributed to aspiration of food by impairing cough or gag reflexes (Von Brauchitsch & May, 1968). Later reports of neuroleptic agents inducing dysphagia also proposed the same mechanism (Hughes, Shone, Lindsay, et al., 1994; Shamash, Miall, Williams, et al., 1994; Solan, 1976). However, other investigators found no association between sudden death (Leestma & Koenig, 1968) or swallowing difficulty (Hussar & Bragg, 1969) and the introduction of phenothiazine neuroleptics.

Neuroleptics were more definitively associated with neurogenic dysphagia through the induction of pharyngeal-laryngeal dystonia. Antidopaminergic drugs such as fluphenazine (Solomon, 1977), haloperidol (Cruz, Thiagarajan, & Harney, 1983; Flaherty & Lahmeyer, 1978), fluspirilene (Stones, Kennie, & Fulton, 1990), risperidone (Nair, Saeed, Shahab, et al., 2001), and metoclopramide alone (Casteels-Van Daele, Jaeken, Van der Schueren, et al., 1970; Newton-John, 1988) and in combination with prochlorperazine (Casteels-Van Daele et al., 1970) have caused dysphagic symptoms. The onset of symptoms is typically acute and occurs within days of initiating therapy or increasing the dosage. Complaints of dysphagia can be accompanied by difficulty in speaking or breathing (Flaherty & Lahmeyer, 1978; Newton-John, 1988), or a choking feeling (Solomon, 1977) without visible evidence of dystonia. Treatment was delayed in some patients due to a lack of recognition of the cause of the complaints and a single case was complicated by aspiration pneumonia (Cruz, Thiagarajan, & Harney, 1983). All patients responded rapidly to treatment with anticholinergic drugs such as benztropine, glycopyrronium and diphenhydramine or drug discontinuation. Recurrence has occurred with rechallenge.

Tardive Dyskinesia   Neuroleptics also have the ability to interfere with swallowing by inducing tardive dyskinesia (Crane, 1968; Crane & Paulson, 1967; Gregory, Smith, & Rudge, 1992; Newton-John, 1988; Weiden & Harrigan, 1986; Yassa & Jones, 1985). Patients who develop tardive dyskinesia can have persistent, abnormal tongue movements that prevent normal swallowing (Yassa & Jones, 1985). This is clinically different from acute dystonia with respect to the onset of symptoms and response to treatment. Onset is typically years after initiation of neuroleptic therapy. Anticholinergic agents and discontinuation of therapy, which are uniformly beneficial in acute dystonia, have been reported to worsen dysphagia caused by tardive dyskinesia (Craig & Richardson, 1982; Gregory et al., 1992; Weiden & Harrigan, 1986). However, slow improvement in symptoms after discontinuation of neuroleptic therapy can occur (Crane, 1968; Gregory et al., 1992; Yassa & Jones, 1985).

Botulinum Toxin

Botulinum toxin produces dysphagia in many patients injected locally for torticollis and in those receiving injections in remote sites as well. The incidence of dysphagia in patients receiving injection of botulinum toxin into cervical muscles ranges from 21 to 57% (Comella, Tanner, DeFoor-Hill, et al., 1992; Jankovic & Schwartz, 1991; Poewe, Deuschl, Nebe, et al., 1998; Poewe, Schelosky, Kleedorfer, et al., 1992). Onset of symptoms generally occurs within 3 weeks and does not appear to be dose-related (Kessler, Skutta, & Benecke, 1999; Poewe et al., 1998). Symptoms are usually mild and do not require treatment other than discontinuation of injections. Occasionally, restriction to a soft food or liquid diet or nasogastric feeding is necessary (Kessler et al., 1999; Poewe et al., 1992; Thobois, Broussolle, & Toureille, 2001; Tuite & Land, 1996). On discontinuation of the injections, symptoms typically resolve within 8 weeks (Kessler et al., 1999). Although preexisting dysphagia is not a risk factor for the development of botulinum toxin-induced dysphagia, patients with preexisting dysphagia may experience slower resolution of drug-induced symptoms (Comella et al., 1992; Holzer & Ludlow, 1996). It has been suggested that patients with Macado-Joseph disease may be more likely to develop dysphagia and exhibit more severe and longer lasting symptoms than expected (Tuite & Land, 1996).

The mechanism by which botulinum toxin causes difficulty swallowing is not entirely clear. The toxin may diffuse into pharyngeal muscle from locally injected sites, or it may be transported through the bloodstream (Comella et al., 1992; Nix, Butler, Roontga, et al., 1992; Poewe et al., 1992). The toxin may also have an increased selectivity for pharyngeal muscle presynaptic terminals (Poewe et al., 1992; Sampaio & Castro-Caldas, 1992).

Other Drugs

Topical anesthestics applied to the oropharyngeal mucosa reliably produces dysphagia, which can lead to laryngeal aspiration (Ertekin, Kiylioglu, Tarlaci, et al., 2000). Other drugs, including digoxin (Kelton & Scullin, 1978), chloroquine (Gustafsson, Walker, Alvan, et al., 1983), L-dopa (Wodak, Gilligan, Veale, et al., 1972), tetrabenazine (Critchley, 1976; Huang, McLeod, Holland, et al., 1976; Snaith & Warren, 1974), cytarabine/methotrexate combination (Miller, Oleshansky, Gibson, & Cantilena, 1993), procainamide (Miller et al., 1993), and vincristine (Chisholm & Curry, 1978) have been reported to induce dysphagia rarely. Because of the low incidence of the reactions, the mechanisms of dysphagia are not well elucidated. However, most patients recovered uneventfully after discontinuation of the offending agent.

✦ Conclusion

This chapter has approached the topic of drug-induced communication and swallowing disturbances by reviewing the available literature regarding specific pharmacologic agents. The SLP in the medical setting is likely to come in contact with patients who are being treated with drugs highlighted in this chapter. In addition, patients may be referred for consultation regarding the acute onset of speech or swallowing symptoms that may be drug induced. Familiarity with some basic pharmacologic concepts and knowledge of the interaction between drugs and communication and swallowing disorders will enhance the process of differential diagnosis and appropriate treatment. We hope the information presented in this chapter also provides some basis for interaction between the pharmacist and SLP.

Study Questions

1. What information should be considered when attempting to determine causality between a drug and a potential adverse drug reaction?

2. What steps can be taken to prevent reexposure of a patient with a documented adverse drug reaction to the inciting agent(s)?

3. Describe the proposed mechanisms for inhaled steroid-induced dysphonia. What steps can be taken to prevent or treat dysphonia related to inhaled steroid use?

4. What are preventable risk factors for the development of drug-induced mechanical dysphagia?

5. Characterize the documented effects of certain drugs on esophageal motility and pharyngeal/laryngeal coordination.

6. Describe the presentation, time of onset, and treatment of botulinum toxin-induced dysphagia.

7. Differentiate the speech dysfunction that can occur with short- and long-term neuroleptic administration. How does treatment differ?

8. Which drugs induce stuttering most frequently?

References

Adler, L., Leong, S., & Delgado, R. (1987). Drug-Induced Stuttering Treated with Propranolol. *Journal of Clinical Psychopharmacology, 7*, 115–116

Agertoft, L., Larsen, F.E., & Pedersen, S. (1998). Posterior Subcapsular Cataracts, Bruises and Hoarseness in Children with Asthma Receiving Long-Term Treatment with Inhaled Budesonide. *European Respiratory Journal, 12*, 130–135

Alfredsunder, P., Hochman, M.C., & Kaplan, B.H. (1992). Low-Dose Vincristine-Associated Bilateral Vocal Cord Paralysis. *New York State Journal of Medicine, 92*, 268–269

Angrist, B., & Gershon, S. (1973). Behavioral Profile of a Potent New Psychotoxic Compound. *Psychopharmacologa, 30*, 109–116

Ashour, M., Salama, F.D., Morris, A., et al. (1984). Acute Dysphagia Induced by Bendrofluazide-K. *Practitioner, 228*, 524–525

Baker, J. (1998). A Report on Alterations to the Speaking and Singing Voices of Four Women Following Hormonal Therapy with Virilizing Agents. *Journal of Voice, 13*, 496–507

Bauer, D.C., Black, D., Ensrud, K., et al. (2000). Upper Gastrointestinal Tract Safety Profile of Alendronate. *Archives of Internal Medicine, 160*, 517–525

Bertoni, J.M., Schwartzman, R.J., Van Horn, G., et al. (1981). Asterixis and Encephalopathy Following Metrizamide Myelography: Investigations into Possible Mechanisms and Review of the Literature. *Annals of Neurology, 9*, 366–370

Boeve, B., Kimmel, D.W., Aronson, A.E., et al. (1996). Dysarthria and Apraxia of Speech Associated with FK-506 (Tacrolimus). *Mayo Clinical Proceedings, 71*, 969–972

Bohane, T.D., Perrault, J., & Fowler, R.S. (1978). Oesophagitis and Oesophageal Obstruction from T in Association with Left Atrial Enlargement: A Case Report. *Australian Paediatr Journal, 14*, 191–192

Bokey, L., & Hugh, T.B. (1975). Oesophageal Ulceration Associated with Doxycycline Therapy. *Medical Journal of Australia, 1*, 236–237

Bond, W.S., Carvalho, M., & Foulks, E.F. (1982). Persistent Dysarthria with Apraxia Associated with a Combination of Lithium Carbonate and Haloperidol. *Journal of Clinical Psychiatry, 43*, 256–257

Boothroyd, C.V., & Lepre, F. (1990). Permanent Voice Change Resulting from Danazol Therapy. *Australian and New Zealand Journal of Obstetrics and Gynaecology, 30*, 275–276

Brewerton, T.D., Markowitz, J.S., Keller, S.G., & Cochrane, C.E. (1996). Stuttering with Sertraline. *Journal of Clinical Psychiatry, 57*, 90–91

Burd, L., & Kerbeshian, J. (1991). Stuttering and Stimulants. *Journal of Clinical Psychopharmacology, 11*, 72–73

Campbell, I.A. (1984). Inhaled Steroids and Dysphonia. *Lancet, 1*, 744

Casteels-Van Daele, M., Jaeken, J., Van der Schueren, P., et al. (1970). Dystonic Reactions in Children Caused by Metoclopramide. *Archives of Diseases in Childhood, 45*, 130–133

Chesshyre, M.H., & Braimbridge, M.V. (1971). Dysphagia Due to Left Atrial Enlargement after Mitral Starr Valve Replacement. *British Heart Journal, 33*, 799–802

Chisholm, R.C., & Curry, S.B. (1978). Vincristine-Induced Dysphagia. *Southern Medical Journal, 71*, 1364–1365

Christensen, R.C., Byerly, M.J., & McElroy, R.A. (1996). A Case of Sertraline-Induced Stuttering. *Journal of Clinical Psychopharmacology, 16*, 92–93

Colina, R.E., Smith, M., Kikendall, J.W., & Wong, R.K.H. (1997). A New Probable Increasing Cause of Esophageal Ulceration: Alendronate. *American Journal of Gastroenterology, 92*, 704–705

Comella, C.L., Tanner, C.M., DeFoor-Hill, L., et al. (1992). Dysphagia After Botulinum Toxin Injections for Spasmodic Torticollis: Clinical and Radiologic Findings. *Neurology, 42*, 1307–1310

Cordeiro, M.F., & Arnold, K.G. (1991). Digoxin Toxicity Presenting as Dysphagia and Dysphonia. *British Medical Journal, 302*, 1025

Craig, T.J., & Richardson, M.A. (1982). Swallowing, Tardive Dyskinesia, and Anticholinergics. *American Journal of Psychiatry, 139*, 1083

Crane, G.E. (1968). Tardive Dyskinesia in Patients Treated with Major Neuroleptics: A Review of the Literature. *American Journal of Psychiatry, 124(suppl)*, 40–48

Crane, G.E., & Paulson, G. (1967). Involuntary Movements in a Sample of Chronic Mental Patients and Their Relation to the Treatment with Neuroleptics. *International Journal of Neuropsychiatry, 3*, 286–291

Critchley, E.M. (1976). Peak-Dose Dysphonia in Parkinsonism. *Lancet, 1*, 544

Crompton, G.K., Sanderson, R., Dewar, M.H., et al. (2000). Comparison of Pulmicort pMDI Plus Nebuhaler and Pulmicort Turbuhaler in Asthmatic Patients with Dysphonia. *Respiratory Medicine, 94*, 448–453

Cruz, F.G., Thiagarajan, D., & Harney, J.H. (1983). Neuroleptic Malignant Syndrome After Haloperidol Therapy. *Southern Medical Journal, 76*, 684–686

De Groen, P.C., Lubbe, D.F., Hirsch, L.J., et al. (1996). Esophagitis Associated with the Use of Alendronate. *New England Journal of Medicine, 335*, 1016–1021

Delaney, P. (1982). Vincristine-Induced Laryngeal Nerve Paralysis. *Neurology, 32*, 1285–1288

Duggal, H.S., Jagadheesan, K., & Nizamie, S.H. (2002). Clozapine-Induced Stuttering and Seizures. *American Journal of Psychiatry, 159*, 315

Duvoisin, R.C., & Katz, L. (1968). Reversal of Central Anticholinergic Syndrome in Man by Physostigmine. *Journal of the American Medical Association, 206*, 1963–1965

Ebeling, T.A., Compton, A.D., & Albright, D.W. (1997). Clozapine-Induced Stuttering. *American Journal of Psychiatry, 154*, 1473

Elliott, R.L., & Thomas, B.J. (1985). A Case Report of Alprazolam-Induced Stuttering. *Journal of Clinical Psychopharmacology, 5*, 159–160

Ernst, F.R., & Grizzle, A.J. (2001). Drug-Related Morbidity and Mortality: Updating the Cost-of-Illness Model. *Journal of the American Pharmacological Association (Washington), 41*, 192–199

Ertekin, C., Kiylioglu, N., Tarlaci, S., et al. (2000). Effect of Mucosal Anaesthesia on Oropharyngeal Swallowing. *Neurogastroenterology and Motility, 12*, 567–572

Faheem, A.D., Brightwell, D.R., Burton, G.C., & Struss, A. (1982). Respiratory Dyskinesia and Dysarthria from Prolonged Neuroleptic Use: Tardive Dyskinesia? *American Journal of Psychiatry, 139*, 517–518

Farber, I.J. (1957). Drug Fatalities. *American Journal of Psychiatry, 114*, 371–372

Fayen, M., Goldman, M.B., Moulthrop, M.A., & Luchins, D.J. (1988). Differential Memory Function with Dopaminergic Versus Anticholinergic Treatment of Drug-Induced Extra-Pyramidal Symptoms. *American Journal of Psychiatry, 145*, 483–486

Feldman, P.E. (1957). An Unusual Death Associated with Tranquilizer Therapy. *American Journal of Psychiatry, 113*, 1032–1033

Flaherty, J.A., & Lahmeyer, H.W. (1978). Laryngeal-Pharyngeal Dystonia as a Possible Cause of Asphyxia with Haloperidol Treatment. *American Journal of Psychiatry, 135*, 1414–1415

Friedman, E.H., Guthrie, S., & Grunhaus, L. (1990). Fluoxetine and Stuttering. *Journal of Clinical Psychiatry, 51*, 310–311

Gaile, S., & Noviasky, J.A. (1998). Speech Disturbance and Marked Decrease in Function Seen in Several Older Patients on Olanzapine. *Journal of the American Geriatrics Society, 46,* 1330–1331

Garvey, M.J., & Tollefson, G.D. (1987). Occurrence of Myoclonus in Patients Treated with Cyclic Antidepressants. *Archives General of Psychiatry, 44,* 269–272

Gerard, J.-M., & Robience, Y. (1998). Theophylline-Induced Stuttering. *Movement Disorders, 13,* 847–848

Gerritsma, E.J., Brocaar, M.P., Hakkesteegt, M.M., et al. (1994). Virilization of the Voice in Post-Menopausal Women Due to the Anabolic Steroid Nandrolone Decanoate (Decadurabolin). The Effects of Medication for One Year. *Clinical Otolaryngology and Allied Science, 19,* 79–84

Gora-Harper, M.L., Sunahara, J.F., & Gray, M.S. (1995). Intranasal Butorphanol-Induced Apraxia Reversed by Naloxone. *Pharmacotherapy, 15,* 798–800

Gottschalk, L.A. (1977). Effects of Certain Benzodiazepine Derivatives on Disorganization of Thought as Manifested in Speech. *Current Therapy Research and Clinical Experience, 21,* 192–206

Gregory, R.P., Smith, P.T., & Rudge, P. (1992). Tardive Dyskinesia Presenting as Severe Dysphagia. *Journal of Neurology and Neurosurgical Psychiatry, 55,* 1203–1204

Gustafsson, L.L., Walker, O., Alvan, G., et al. (1983). Disposition of Chloroquine in Man After Single Intravenous and Oral Doses. *British Journal of Clinical Pharmacology, 15,* 471–479

Guthrie, S., & Grunhaus, L. (1990). Fluoxetine-Induced Stuttering. *Journal of Clinical Psychiatry, 51,* 85

Higuchi, K., Ando, K., Kim, S.R., et al. (2001). Sildenafil-Induced Esophageal Ulcers. *American Journal of Gastroenterology, 96,* 2516–2518

Hollister, L.E. (1957). Unexpected Asphyxial Death and Tranquilizing Drugs. *American Journal of Psychiatry, 114,* 366–367

Hollister, L.E., & Kosek, J.C. (1965). Sudden Death During Treatment with Phenothiazine Derivatives. *Journal of the American Medical Association, 192,* 1035–1038

Holzer, S.E., & Ludlow, C.L. (1996). The Swallowing Side Effects of Botulinum Toxin Type A Injection in Spasmodic Dysphonia. *Laryngoscope, 106(1 pt 1),* 86–92

Howie, A.D., & Strachan, R.W. (1975). Slow Release Potassium Chloride Treatment. *British Medical Journal, 2,* 176

Huang, C.Y., McLeod, J.G., Holland, R.T., et al. (1976). Tetrabenazine in the Treatment of Huntington's Chorea. *Medical Journal of Australia, 1,* 583–584

Hughes, T.A.T., Shone, G., Lindsay, G., et al. (1994). Severe Dysphagia Associated with Major Tranquilizer Treatment. *Postgraduate Medical Journal, 70,* 581–583

Hussar, A.E., & Bragg, D.G. (1969). The Effect of Chlorpromazine on the Swallowing Function in Chronic Schizophrenic Patients. *American Journal of Psychiatry, 126,* 570–573

Institute of Medicine, Committee on Quality of Health Care in America. (1999). *To Err Is Human: Building a Safer Health System.* Washington, DC: National Academy Press

Ishikawa, T., Hato, M., Tauchi, A., & Wada, Y. (1988). Dysarthria After Large Doses of Intravenous Diazepam. *Japanese Journal of Psychiatry and Neurology, 42,* 759–761

Jankovic, J., & Schwartz, K. (1991). Botulinum Toxin Treatment of Tremors. *Neurology, 41,* 1185–1188

Jaster, P.J., & Abbas, D. (1986). Erythromycin-Carbamazepine Interaction. *Neurology, 36,* 594–595

Kane, F.J. Jr., & Taylor, T.W. (1963). An Unusual Reaction to Combined Imipramine-Thorazine Therapy. *American Journal of Psychiatry, 120,* 186–187

Kelton, J.G., & Scullin, D.C. (1978). Digitalis Toxicity Manifested by Dysphagia. *Journal of the American Medical Association, 239,* 613–614

Kessler, K.R., Skutta, M., & Benecke, R., for the German Dystonia Study Group. (1999). Long-Term Treatment of Cervical Dystonia with Botulinum Toxin A: Efficacy, Safety, and Antibody Frequency. *Journal of Neurology, 246,* 265–274

Kikendall, J.W. (1992). Pill Esophagitis. *Journal of Clinical Gastroenterology, 28,* 298–305

Kim, S.L., Hunter, J.G., Wo, J.M., Davis, L.P., & Waring, J.P. (1999). NSAIDs, Aspirin and Esophageal Strictures: Are Over-The-Counter Medications Harmful to the Esophagus? *Journal of Clinical Gastroenterology, 29,* 32–34

Lanza, F.L., Hunt, R.H., Thomson, A.B., Provenza, J.M., & Blank, M.A. (2000). Endoscopic Comparison of Esophageal and Gastroduodenal Effects of Risedronate and Alendronate in Postmenopausal Women. *Gastroenterology, 119,* 631–638

Lavy, J.A., Wood, G., Rubin, J.S., & Harries, M. (2000). Dysphonia Associated with Inhaled Steroids. *Journal of Voice, 14,* 581–588

Lee, H.-J., Lee, H.-S., Kim, L., et al. (2001). A Case of Risperidone-Induced Stuttering. *Journal of Clinical Psychopharmacology, 21,* 115–116

Leestma, J.E., & Koenig, K.L. (1968). Sudden Death and Phenothiazines: A current controversy. *Archives of General Psychiatry, 18,* 137–148

Lewis, D.A. (1983). Unrecognized Chronic Neurotoxic Reactions. *Journal of the American Medical Association, 250,* 2029–2030

Liberman, U.I., & Hirsch, L.J. (1996). Esophagitis and Alendronate. *New England Journal of Medicine, 335,* 1069–1070

Lieberman, J.A., & Reife, R. (1989). Spastic Dysphonia and Denervation Signs in a Young Man with Tardive Dyskinesia. *British Journal of Psychiatry, 154,* 105–109

Louis, E.D., Winfield, L., Fahn, S., & Ford, B. (2001). Speech Dysfluency Exacerbated by Levodopa in Parkinson's Disease. *Movement Disorders, 16,* 562–565

Macedo, G., Azevedo, F., & Ribeiro, T. (2001). Ulcerative Esophagitis Caused by Etidronate. *Gastrointestinal Endoscopy, 53,* 250–251

Maconi, G., & Porro, G.B. (1995). Multiple Ulcerative Esophagitis Caused by Alendronate. *American Journal of Gastroenterology, 90,* 1889–1890

Mahr, G., & Leith, W. (1990). Stuttering After a Dystonic Reaction. *Psychosomatics, 31,* 465

Marcotte, D.B. (1973). Neuroleptics and Neurologic Reactions. *Southern Medical Journal, 66,* 321–324

Marmont, A.M., & Damasio, E.E. (1973). Neurotoxicity of Intrathecal Chemotherapy for Leukaemia. *British Medical Journal, 4,* 47

Masand, P. (1992). Desipramine-Induced Oral-Pharyngeal Disturbances: Stuttering and Jaw Myoclonus. *Journal of Clinical Psychopharmacology, 12,* 444–445

Masdeu, J.C., Glista, G.G., Rubino, F.A., et al. (1983). Transient Motor Aphasia Following Metrizamide Myelography. *AJNR, American Journal of Neuroradiology, 4,* 200–202

Mason, S.J., & O'Meara, T.F. (1981). Drug-Induced Esophagitis. *Journal of Clinical Gastroenterology, 3,* 115–120

Matson, A.M., & Thurlow, A.C. (1988). Hypotension and Neurological Sequelae Following Intramuscular Midazolam. *Anaesthesia, 43,* 896

McAndrew, N.A., & Greenway, M.W. (1999). Medication-induced Oesophageal Injury Leading to Broncho-Oesophageal Fistula. *Postgrad Medical Journal, 75,* 379–381

McCall, A.J. (1975). Slow-k Ulceration of Oesophagus with Aneurysmal Left Atrium. *British Medical Journal, 3,* 230–231

McCall, W.V. (1994). Sertraline-Induced Stuttering. *Journal of Clinical Psychiatry, 55,* 316

McCarthy, M.M. (1981). Speech Effect of Theophylline. *Pediatrics, 68,* 749–750

McCarthy, R.H., & Terkelsen, K.G. (1994). Esophageal Dysfunction in Two Patients After Clozapine Treatment. *Journal of Clinical Psychopharmacology, 14,* 281–283

Meghji, C. (1994). Acquired Stuttering. *Journal of Family Practice, 39,* 325–326

Miller, C.D., Oleshansky, M.A., Gibson, K.F., & Cantilena, L.R. (1993). Procainamide-Induced Myasthenia-Like Weakness and Dysphagia. *Therapeutic Drug Monitoring, 15,* 251–254

Miller, P.S., Richardson, J.S., Jyu, C.A., Lemay, J.S., Hisock, M., & Keegan, D.L. (1988). Association of Low Serum Anticholinergic Levels and Cognitive Impairment in Elderly Presurgical Patients. *American Journal of Psychiatry, 145,* 342–345

Moss, H.B., & Green, A. (1982). Neuroleptic-Associated Dysphagia Confirmed by Esophageal Manometry. *American Journal of Psychiatry, 139,* 515–516

Nair, S., Saeed, O., Shahab, H., et al. (2001). Sudden Dysphagia with Uvular Enlargement Following the Initiation of Risperidone which Responded to Benztropine: Was This an Extrapyramidal Side Effect? *General Hospital Psychiatry, 23,* 231–232

Naranjo, C.A., Busto, U., Sellers, E.M., et al. (1981). A Method for Estimating the Probability of Adverse Drug Reactions. *Clinical Pharmacology and Therapy, 30,* 239–245

Newman, D., & Forbes, D. (1993). The Effects of Danazol on Vocal Parameters—Is an Objective Prospective Study Needed? *Medical Journal of Australia, 158,* 575

Newton-John, H. (1988). Acute Upper Airway Obstruction Due to Supraglottic Dystonia Induced by a Neuroleptic. *British Medical Journal, 297,* 964–965

Nissani, M., & Sanchez, E.A. (1997). Stuttering Caused by Gabapentin. *Annals of Internal Medicine, 126,* 410

Nix, W.A., Butler, I.J., Roontga, S., et al. (1992). Persistent Unilateral Tibialis Anterior Muscle Hypertrophy with Complex Repetitive Discharges and Myalgia: Report of Two Unique Cases and Response to Botulinum Toxin. *Neurology, 42,* 602–606

No author. (1984). Inhaled Steroids and Dysphonia. *Lancet, 1,* 375–376

Nurnberg, H.G., & Greenwald, B. (1981). Stuttering: An Unusual Side Effect of Phenothiazines. *American Journal of Psychiatry, 138,* 386–387

Palmer, K.M., Selbst, S.M., Shaffer, S., & Proujansky, R. (1999). Pediatric Chest Pain Induced by Tetracycline Ingestion. *Pediatric Emergency Care, 15,* 200–201

Pearlman, C. (1994). Clozapine, Nocturnal Sialorrhea, and Choking. *Journal of Clinical Psychopharmacology, 14,* 283

Pemberton, J. (1970). Oesophageal Obstruction and Ulceration Caused by Oral Potassium Therapy. *British Heart Journal, 32,* 267–268

Peters, J.L. (1976). Benign Oesophageal Stricture Following Oral Potassium Chloride Therapy. *British Journal of Surgery, 63*, 698–699

Pimental, P.A., & Gorelik, P.B. (1985). Aphasia, Apraxia and Neurogenic Stuttering as Complications of Metrizamide Myelography. *Acta Neurologica Scandinavica, 72*, 481–488

Plachta, A. (1965). Asphyxia Relatively Inherent to Tranquilization. Review of the Literature and Report of Seven Cases. *Archives of General Psychiatry, 12*, 152–158

Poewe, W., Deuschl, G., Nebe, A., et al. (1998). What Is the Optimal Dose of Botulinum Toxin A in the Treatment of Cervical Dystonia? Results of a Double Blind, Placebo Controlled, Dose Ranging Study Using Dysport. *Journal of Neurology, Neurosurgery, and Psychiatry, 64*, 13–17

Poewe, W., Schelosky, L., Kleedorfer, B., et al. (1992). Treatment of Spasmodic Torticollis with Local Injections of Botulinum Toxin. *Journal of Neurology, 239*, 21–25

Quader, S.E. (1977). Dysarthria: An Unusual Side Effect of the Cyclic Antidepressants. *British Medical Journal, 2*, 97

Riley, C.G. (1972). Chronic Hydantoin Intoxication: Case Report. *New Zealand Medical Journal, 76*, 425–428

Rosenfield, D.B., McCarthy, M., McKinney, K., et al. (1994). Stuttering Induced by Theophylline. *Ear, Nose, and Throat Journal, 73*, 914–920

Rosenthal, T., Adar, R., Militianu, J., et al. (1974). Esophageal Ulceration and Oral Potassium Chloride Ingestion. *Chest, 65*, 463–465

Sampaio, C., & Castro-Caldas, A. (1992). Botulinum Toxin and Dysphagia. *Neurology, 42*, 2233

Sandyk, R. (1983). Metoclopramide-Induced Dysarthria. *South African Medical Journal, 64*, 732

Sarno, J.B. (1985). Transient Expressive (Nonfluent) Dysphasia After Metrizamide Myelography. AJNR, *American Journal of Neuroradiology, 6*, 945–947

Saunders, M. (1977). Dysarthria with Tricyclic Antidepressants. *British Medical Journal, 2*, 317

Schatzberg, A.F., Cole, J.O., & Blumer, D.P. (1978). Speech Blockage: A Tricyclic Side Effect. *American Journal of Psychiatry, 135*, 600–601

Schmidt, W.R., & Jarcho, L.W. (1966). Persistent Dyskinesias Following Phenothiazine Therapy. *Archives of Neurology, 14*, 369–377

Shamash, J., Miall, L., Williams, F., et al. (1994). Dysphagia in the Neuroleptic Malignant Syndrome. *British Journal of Psychiatry, 164*, 849–850

Sholomskas, A.J. (1978). Speech Blockage in Young Patients Taking Tricyclics. *American Journal of Psychiatry, 135*, 1572–1573

Singh, S.V. (1982). Lithium Carbonate/Fluphenazine Decanoate Producing Irreversible Brain Damage. *Lancet, 2*, 278

Skinner, C., & Williams, A.J. (1984). Dysphonia Caused by Inhaled Steroids: Recognition of a Characteristic Laryngeal Abnormality. *Thorax, 39*, 686

Slipman, C.W., Chow, D.W., Lenrow, D.A., et al. (2002). Dysphonia Associated with Epidural Steroid Injection: A Case Report. *Archives of Physical Medicine and Rehabilitation, 83*, 1309–1310

Sliwa, J.A., & Lis, S. (1993). Drug-Induced Dysphagia. *Archives of Physical Medicine and Rehabilitation, 74*, 445–457

Snaith, R.P., & Warren H. de B. (1974). Treatment of Huntington's Chorea with Tetrabenazine. *Lancet, 1*, 413–414

Sobell, L.C., Sobell, M.B., & Coleman, R.F. (1982). Alcohol-Induced Dysfluency in Nonalcoholics. *Folia Phoniatrica (Basel), 34*, 316–323

Solan, G.M. (1976). Letter: Aspiration Pneumonia. *West Virginia Medical Journal, 72*, 18

Solomon, K. (1977). Phenothiazine-Induced Bulbar Palsy-Like Syndrome and Sudden Death. *American Journal of Psychiatry, 134*, 308–311

Solomon, K., & Vickers, R. (1975). Dysarthria Resulting from Lithium Carbonate. A Case Report. *Journal of the American Medical Association, 231*, 280

Stones, M., Kennie, D., & Fulton, J.D. (1990). Dystonic Dysphagia Associated with Fluspirilene. *British Medical Journal, 301*, 668–689

Streeton, J.A. (1984). Inhaled Steroids and Dysphonia. *Lancet, 1*, 963

Supprian, T., Retz, W., & Deckert, J. (1999). Clozapine-Induced Stuttering: Epileptic Brain Activity? *American Journal of Psychiatry, 156*, 1663–1664

Teplick, J.G., Teplick, S.K., Ominsky, S.H., et al. (1980). Esophagitis Caused by Oral Medication. *Radiology, 134*, 23–25

Thobois, S., Broussolle, E., & Toureille, L. (2001). Severe Dysphagia After Botulinum Toxin Injection for Cervical Dystonia in Multiple System Atrophy. *Movement Disorders, 16*, 764–765

Thomas, P., Lalaux, N., Vaiva, G., et al. (1994). Dose-Dependent Stuttering and Dystonia in a Patient Taking Clozapine. *American Journal of Psychiatry, 151*, 1096

Tobias, J.D., & Bozeman, P.M. (1991). Vincristine-Induced Recurrent Laryngeal Nerve Paralysis in Children. *Intensive Care Medicine, 17*, 304–305

Toogood, J.H., Jennings, B., Baskerville, J., et al. (1984). Dosing Regimen of Budesonide and Occurrence of Oropharyngeal Complications. *European Journal of Respiratory Diseases, 65*, 35–44

Toogood, J.H., Jennings, B., Greenway, R.W., et al. (1980). Candidiasis and Dysphonia Complicating Beclomethasone Treatment of Asthma. *Journal of Allergy and Clinical Immunology, 65*, 145–153

Tuite, P.J., & Lang, A.E. (1996). Severe and Prolonged Dysphagia Complicating Botulinum Toxin A Injections for Dystonia in Machado-Joseph Disease. *Neurology, 46*, 846

Von Brauchitsch, H., & May, W. (1968). Deaths from Aspiration and Asphyxiation in a Mental Hospital. *Archives of General Psychiatry, 18*, 129–136

Walsh, T.D. (1982). Chronic Dysarthria and Metoclopramide. *Annals of Neurology, 11*, 545

Wardell, K.W. (1957). Untoward Reactions to Tranquilizing Drugs. *American Journal of Psychiatry, 113*, 745

Wardle, P.G., Whitehead, M.I., & Mills, R.P. (1983). Non-Reversible and Wide Ranging Voice Changes After Treatment with Danazol. *British Medical Journal (Clinical Resident Edition), 287*, 946

Warren, J. (1998). Drug-Induced Supraglottic Dystonia and Spasmodic Dysphonia. *Movement Disorders, 13*, 978–979

Weiden, P., & Harrigan, M. (1986). A Clinical Guide for Diagnosing and Managing Patients with Drug-Induced Dysphagia. *Hospital and Community Psychiatry, 37*, 396–398

Weiser, G.A., Forouhar, F.A., & White, W.B. (1984). Hydralazine Hoarseness. *Archives of Internal Medicine, 144*, 2271–2272

Whittaker, J.A., & Griffith, I.P. (1977). Recurrent Laryngeal Nerve Paralysis in Patients Receiving Vincristine and Vinblastine. *British Medical Journal, 1*, 1251–1252

Williams, A.J., Baghat, M.S., Stableforth, D.E., et al. (1983). Dysphonia Caused by Inhaled Steroids: Recognition of a Characteristic Laryngeal Abnormality. *Thorax, 38*, 813–821

Williamson, I.J., Matusiewicz, S.P., Brown, P.H., et al. (1995). Frequency of Voice Problems and Cough in Patients Using Pressurized Aerosol Inhaled Steroid Preparations. *European Respiratory Journal, 8*, 590–592

Wilson, A., Petty, R., Perry, A., & Rose, F.C. (1983). Paroxysmal Language Disturbance in an Epileptic Treated with Clobazam. *Neurology, 33*, 652–654

Wodak, J., Gilligan, B.S., Veale, J.L., et al. (1972). Review of 12 Months' Treatment with L-Dopa in Parkinson's Disease, with Remarks on Unusual Side Effects. *Medical Journal of Australia, 2*, 1277–1282

Wong, R.K.H., Kikendall, J.W., & Dachman, A.H. (1986). Quinaglute-Induced Esophagitis Mimicking an Esophageal Mass. *Annals of Internal Medicine, 105*, 62–63

Woodring, J.H., Martin, C.A., & Keefer, B. (1993). Esophageal Atony and Dilatation as a Side Effect of Thiothixene and Benztropine. *Hospital and Community Psychiatry, 44*, 686–688

World Health Organization. (1975). *Requirements for Adverse Drug Reaction Reporting.* Geneva, Switzerland: World Health Organization

Wyllie, E., Wyllie, R., Cruse, R.P., et al. (1986). The Mechanism of Nitrazepam-Induced Drooling and Aspiration. *New England Journal of Medicine, 314*, 35–38

Yassa, R., & Jones, B.D. (1985). Complications of Tardive Dyskinesia: A Review. *Psychosomatics, 26*, 305–313

Zlotlow, M., & Paganini, A.E. (1958). Fatalities in Patients Receiving Chlorpromazine and Reserpine During 1956–1957 at Pilgrim State Hospital. *American Journal of Psychiatry, 115*, 154–156

Appendix 23–1   Pharmacological Treatment for Neurologic Diseases Commonly Occurring in Patients Seen by Speech–Language Pathologists

Disorder	Pharmacologic Treatment
Neurologic disorders	
Ischemic stroke	Aspirin, warfarin, clopidogrel, dipyridamole/aspirin, heparin, tissue plasminogen activator
Brain tumor	Dexamethasone, mannitol
Myasthenia gravis	Pyridostigmine, prednisone
Amyotrophic lateral sclerosis	Riluzole
Multiple sclerosis	Adrenocorticoid hormone (ACTH), methylprednisolone, cyclosporine, interferon, cyclophosphamide, azathioprine
Parkinson's disease	Levodopa/carbidopa, pramipexole, ropinirole, amantadine, benztropine, trihexyphenidyl, selegiline, pergolide, bromocriptine, entacapone
Essential tremor	Propranolol, metoprolol
Laryngeal disorders	
Head and neck cancer	Cyclophosphamide, doxorubicin, cisplatin, fluorouracil, carboplatin, vincristine, bleomycin, hydroxyurea, paclitaxel, mitomycin, methotrexate, interferon alfa-2b
Spasmodic dysphonia	Botulinum toxin
Vocal fold edema	Prednisone

Index

Page numbers followed by *f* or *t* indicate figures and tables, respectively.

A

AAC. *See* Augmentative-alternative communication (AAC)
ABCD. *See* Arizona Battery for the Communication in Dementia (ABCD)
Abducens nerve, 316
Accessory nerve, 318
Acetylcholine, 323
Acoustic measures of voice
  benefits, 161–162
  fundamental frequency, 162
  guidelines, 162
  harmonics-to-noise ratio, 162–163
  intensity, 163
  perturbation, 162
  phonetogram, 163
  protocol, 162*t*
  spectral analysis, 163
Acoustic nerve, 317
Acquired immunodeficiency syndrome (AIDS), 359
Acquired language disorders
  lesion-deficit studies
    aphasia, 36–39
    conclusions, 40
    history, 35–36
  neuroimaging
    CBF studies, 40–43
    functional brain activation, 43–44
    metabolism studies, 40–43
    neural bases of, 44–47
Acute care
  competency checklist, 296–297
  consultation
    documentation, 290–294
    effective, 289–290
    importance, 288
    report, 297–298
    service delivery, 284–285
  defined, 284
  documentation
    classifications, 290
    communicative care, 290–291
    neurocommunication, 291–294
    report body, 290
  education, 294–295
  examinations, 289–290
  key issues, 286–288
  organization, 285
  referral sources
    drugs/procedures, 288*t*
    neurology, 285–286
    otolaryngology, 286
    psychiatry, 286
    pulmonary medicine, 286
Acute respiratory distress syndrome (ARDS), 263
AD. *See* Alzheimer's disease (AD)
Adenocarcinomas, 184
Adenoids, 340
Adenotonsillar hypertrophy, 340
Advanced directives, 312
Adverse drug reaction, 363
Aerodigestive tract, 184, 340*f*
AIDS. *See* Acquired immunodeficiency syndrome (AIDS)
Alaryngeal communication
  artificial larynx, 194–195
  esophageal, 195
  tracheoesophageal, 195–196
Aleixa, with agraphia, 38*t*
Aleixa, without agraphia, 38*t*
ALS. *See* Amyotrophic lateral sclerosis (ALS)
Alzheimer's disease (AD)
  communicative impairments, 112*t*
  CVD-associated risk, 99–100
  differential diagnosis, 98*t*
  FAST staging, 311*t*
  FOCUSED program, 119
  FTD *vs.*, 102
  lexical-semantic impairments, 111
  Parkinson's *vs.*, 104
  rates of, 309
  related disorders, 97
  research on, 99
  symptoms, 97
  test for, 114
Alzheimer's quick test (AQT), 114
American Academy of Neurologic Communication Disorders and Sciences (ANCDS), 5
American–Speech–Language–Hearing Association (ASHA)
  certification, 61
  code of ethics, 8–9
  dementia treatment guidelines, 115

American–Speech–Language–Hearing Association (ASHA) *(Continued)*
  documentation standards, 248
  membership, 214
  standards setting by, 5
Amyotrophic lateral sclerosis (ALS)
  associated voice disorders, 172
  characterization, 332
  ICU care, 264
  management of, 332
Anatomic imaging, 20t
ANCDS. *See* American Academy of Neurologic Communication
       Disorders and Sciences (ANCDS)
Androgenic steroids, 367
Angiography, 20t, 327
Angular gyrus, 35
Anomia, 75
Anomic aphasia, 37t
Anosognosia, 74, 75
Anterior nares, 183
Antidepressants, 370–371
Antiepileptic drugs, 335
Aphasia. *See also specific syndromes*
  classification, 53–54
  client management hierarchy, 57t
  conceptual issues, 53–54
  diagnosis
    cognitive-linguistic issues, 55
    differential, 56, 58t
    life-span issues, 55–56
    neuroanatomic issues, 55
    neurophysiologic issues, 55
    sociocultural issues, 56
    tools, 54–55, 57t–59t
  drug-induced, 371
  functional activation studies, 44
  group types, 68t
  intervention planning, 57–58
  lesion location, 37t
  neuroanathomic correlates, 36–39
  neurophysiology, 41–42
  primary progressive, 102–103
  real-life consequences of, 68–69
  recovery
    CBF, 42–43
    functional activation studies, 45–47
    metabolism, 42–43
    neuroanatomic correlates, 39
  rehabilitation
    care continuum, 62
    classification, 61
    evidence-based practice, 62–68
    impaired semantic memory, 63
    perspectives on, 61–62
    SLPs' role, 61–62
    special technologies, 67
    stroke survivor groups, 68–69
  related syndromes, 38t
  TBI-associated, 75
  theoretical views, 53–54
  treatment correlates, 39–40
Aphonia conversion, 170–171
Apraxia, speech, 76
Apraxia, swallow, 135
ARDS. *See* Acute respiratory distress syndrome (ARDS)
Areodynamic measures
  application, 163
    flow, 164
    laryngeal resistance, 164
    phonation threshold pressure, 164
    protocol, 163t
    subglottal air pressure, 164
Arizona battery for the communication in dementia
       (ABCD), 115
Arnold-Chiari malformation, 339
Arousal, defined, 74
Arytenoid adduction, 354
Arytenoid cartilage, 345–346
ASHA. *See* American-Speech-Language-Hearing
       Association (ASHA)
Aspiration
  auscultation, 269
  FEES assessment, 279
  NG tubes and, 305
  pneumonia-associated, 277, 307
  prediction risks, 277–278
  tracheotomy and, 357
Ataxic dysarthria, 76
Atresia, choanal, 339
Atrophy, 101
Attention, defined, 74
Auditory perceptual analysis, 159–160
Augmentative-alternative communication (AAC), 67
Auscultation, 136, 269
Autonomy, 9, 311–312
Awareness deficits. *See* Anosognosia
Axonal neuropathy, 322

B
Bacterial infections, 341
Barium swallow, modified, 137–140
BCRS. *See* Brief cognitive rating scale (BCRS)
Beneficence, 9–10
Benzodiazepines, 370, 371
Billing. *See* Reimbursement
BiPAP, 262–263
Blood oxygenation level dependent method, 27, 29
Blue dye test, 136, 278–279
BOLD. *See* Blood oxygenation level dependent method
Boston naming test, 115
Botulism, 332, 374
Brain. *See also specific regions*
  blood flow, 35f, 40–43
  functional activation studies, 43–44
  imaging (*See* Neuroimaging)
  ischemia
    acute management, 328
    causes, 327–328
    characterization, 327
    clinical manifestations, 328t
    medical prevention, 328–329
    risk factors, 327
    surgical management, 329
  language comprehension areas, 39t
  left cerebral hemisphere, 36f
  metabolism, baseline studies, 40–43
  nerves, 183, 316–318
  perfusion, 32f
  traumatic injury
    cognitive disturbances, 74–75
    coma, 73–74
    defined, 71–72
    early stage, 81–82

incidence, 72
language disturbances, 75–76
modes of, 71–72
recovery, 81–89
rehabilitation, 77–79
sequelae following, 73–76
severity of, 72–73
speech disturbances, 76
Brainstem, 173
Brief cognitive rating scale (BCRS), 114
Broca's area
aphasia, 37
damage to, causes, 36
function, 35
Broca, Paul, 35

C
C-VIC. *See* Computed visual communication (C-VIC)
CADASIL. *See* Cerebral autosomal dominant arteriopathy (CADASIL)
Cancer. *See* Head and neck cancer
Candida, 359
CAPE-V. *See* Consensus auditory-perceptual evaluation of voice (CAPE-V)
Cardiopulmonary disease, 263–264
CARF. *See* Rehabilitation Accreditation Commission (CARF)
Carpal tunnel syndrome (CTS), 322
Cartilage, laryngeal, 345–346
CBF. *See* Cerebral blood flow (CBF)
Centers for Medicine and Medicaid Services (CMMS), 238–239
Central nervous system (CNS) imaging, 20t
Cerebral autosomal dominant arteriopathy (CADASIL), 100
Cerebral blood flow (CBF)
baseline studies, 40–43
PET image, 35f
Cerebral ischemia
acute management, 328
causes, 327–328
characterization, 327
clinical manifestations, 328t
medical prevention, 328–329
risk factors, 327
surgical management, 329
Cerebral perfusion, 32f
Cervical auscultation, 136
Change of condition, 259
Charge document, 250t
CHF. *See* Congestive heart failure (CHF)
Choana, 338
Choanae. *See* Posterior nares
Choanal atresia, 339
Chronic edema, 350–351
Chronic obstructive pulmonary disease (COPD), 263
CJD. *See* Creutzfeldt-Jakob disease (CJD)
Cleft lip, 339–340
Cleft palate, 339–340
Clinical dementia rating scale (CDRS), 114
Clinical practice guidelines (CPGs), 224, 225
Clinical reports. *See* Documentation
Clostridium botulinum, 332
CMMS. *See* Centers for Medicine and Medicaid Services (CMMS)
CNS. *See* Central nervous system (CNS)
Cognition
disturbances of, 74–75
impairment, dementia-associated, 110–111

post-TBJ, 73–76
psychogenic communication disorders and, 209
rehabilitation, 78–79
RLA rating, 80t
Cognitive-behavioral therapy, 210
Cognitive-linguistic tests, 115
Coma
defined, 73
duration of, 73–74
scales for, 72t, 73t
Communication. *See also* Language; Speech
acute care, 286t, 290–291
augmentative-alternative, 67
behaviors, rating of, 93
compensations, dementia-associated, 117
computed visual, 39–40
dysphagia care, 145
failures, 11
FOCUSED, 119t
impairment, dementia-associated, 110–111
neurocommunication, 292–294
post-TBJ, 73–76
psychogenic disorders
assessment, 209
classification, 205–208
epidemiology, 208
psychiatric comorbidity, 208–209
terminology, 205
treatment, 210–211
tracheotomy
nonverbal, 277
one-way speaking valves, 269–275
patient assessment, 269
suctioning for, 276–277
voicing options, 275–276
Comprehension
improved, strategies for, 74
modality-specific deficits, 63
single-word, 63–64
tasks, sample, 63t
Computed tomography (CT)
advanced techniques, 22–23
application, 20, 20t, 35t
defined, 19–20
general principles, 20–21
limitations, 21–22
MRI *vs.,* 26
neurologic examinations, 326
normal brain image, 21f
scanner, 21f
strengths, 21–22
temporal lobe infarct image, 28f
Computed visual communication (C-VIC), 39–40
Conduction aphasia, 37t
Conduction block, 321
Confidentiality
dementia patients, 122
principle of, 10–11
security and, 253
Congestive heart failure (CHF), 263
Consensus auditory-perceptual evaluation of voice (CAPE-V), 160
Consultation
acute care
documentation, 290–294
effective, 289–290
importance, 288

Contact granulomas, 169–170
Contact ulcers, 169–170
Continuous positive airway pressure (CPAP), 262
Conversion disorders
    aphonia, 170–171
    criteria, 207t
    dysphonia, 171–172, 208
    symptoms, 207–208
    types of, 206
Convulsions, 334
Coordination, 319–320
COPD. *See* Chronic obstructive pulmonary
        disease (COPD)
Corrective Coding Initiative (CCI), 251
Corticosteroids, 331
CPAP. *See* Continuous positive airway pressure (CPAP)
CPT. *See* Current procedural terminology (CPT)
Creutzfeldt-Jakob disease (CJD), 105
Cricoid cartilage, 345–346
Cricothyroid joint, 345–346
Criterion-referenced tests, 236, 237t
CT. *See* Computed tomography (CT)
CTS. *See* Carpal tunnel syndrome (CTS)
Cu/Zn superoxide dismutase *(SOD1),* 332
Cultural diversity, 216
Current procedural terminology (CPT), 220, 251

D
DAP. *See* Discourse abilities profile (DAP)
Data
    application examples
        goals/objectives, 242t
        pediatric SLD, 240–241
        performance improvement, 243–244
        pharyngeal dysphagia, 241–242
        precertification for services, 242
        research question formation, 244–245
        staffing needs, 243
    collection instruments, 238–239
    common uses for, 239–240
    diagnostic tests, 236
    efficacy, 239
    facility-specific, 238
    outcome tools, 238
    outcomes, 233
    periodic summaries, 238
    quality of life, 237
    rating scales, 236–237
    treatment plans, 237–238
Deafness, pure word, 39t
Delivery service issues, 6
Dementia. *See also* Alzheimer's disease (AD)
    associated disorders, 104–106
    characterization, 309
    classification, 95
    communicative impairment, 110–112
    defined, 94
    diagnosis
        approaches, 95–96
        caregivers role, 112–113
        cognitive-linguistic tests, 115
        common tools, 113t
        geriatric screening, 114
        language tests, 115
        neuropsychological tools, 114
        rating scales, 114

interventions
        caregivers role, 115
        challenges, 122–123
        communication compensations, 117
        direct, 116–120
        errorless learning quizzes, 117, 118t
        ethics, 120–123
        family visits, 118–119
        FOCUSED program, 119
        group treatment, 116
        indirect, 117–120
        individual, 117
        memory compensations, 117, 118t
        Montessori-based activities, 117, 118t
        reality orientations, 116
        reminiscence therapy, 117
        service delivery, 120
        spaced retrieval, 117, 118t
        validation therapy, 116–117
    language impairment, 111
    neurodegenerative, 96–97, 99
    posttraumatic (*See* Pugilistic Parkinsonism)
    research, 123
    subcortial, 104–106
    taxonomies, 94–95
    tests for, 309, 310t
    vascular, 309, 311
Demyelinating neuropathy, 322
Depression, dementia-associated, 95
Dermatomyositis, 331
Diagnosis-related groups (DRGs), 217–218
Diagnostic report, 248t
Diagnostic tests, 236
Diffusion-weighted imaging studies, 41–42
Direct attention training, 84t
Discourse abilities profile (DAP), 115
Discourse comprehension test, 115
Dissembling disorders, 207t
DMD. *See* Duchenne's muscular dystrophy (DMD)
Documentation
    acute care
        classification systems, 290
        communicative care, 290–291
        neurocommunication, 291–294
        report body, 290
    billing, 248–252
    clinical reports, sample, 258–259
    compliance, 252–253
    defined, 247
    format of
        computerized, 256–259
        cost and, 255–256
        customers' needs, 254–255
        physician preference survey, 255t
    legal evidence, 254
    Medicare guidelines, 252t
    patient care, 247–248
    purpose of, 247–254
    reimbursement, 249–252
    research, 253–254
    types of, 247
DRGs. *See* Diagnosis-related groups (DRGs)
Drug-induced disorders
    speech
        aphasia, 371
        dysarthria, 369–371

dysphonia, 364–369
  overview, 368t–369t
  patient evaluation, 363–364
swallowing
  dysphagia, 373–374
  overview, 368t–369t
  tardive dyskinesa, 374
Drugs
  antidepressants, 370–371
  antiepileptic, 335
  antipsycotic, 367–368, 370
  ICU, 288t
  radiopharmaceuticals, 31t, 33t, 34
  steroids, 361, 364, 367
Duchenne's muscular dystrophy (DMD), 331
Durable power of attorney, 312
Dysarthria, defined, 76
Dysarthria, drug-induced, 369–371
Dyslexia, deep, 66
Dyslexia, surface, 66
Dysphagia
  acute care population, 131–132
  bedside assessment
    bedside assessment, 133–136
    blue dye test, 136
    cervical auscultation, 136
    chart review, 133
    FEES, 136–137
    gag reflex, 135
    instruments for, 137–140
    laryngeal function, 135–136
    modified barium swallow, 137–140
    new procedures, 140–141
    positioning patients, 140t
    postural strategies, 138t
    prolonged phonation, 135
    respiratory support, 134–135
    swallow maneuvers, 139t
    voluntary tasks, 134t
    water use, 144
  endoscopy for
    as treatment guide, 154
    case study, 154–155
    indications, 148–149
    protocol, 149–154
    risks, 155–156
    sensory awareness, 154
  evidence-based practice, 143–144
  ICU assessments, 278–279
  laryngectomy-associated, 198
  management
    caregiver communication, 145
    charting progress, 144–145
    professional interactions, 144
  mechanical, 373
  neurogenic, 373
  oropharyngeal, 136
  pharyngeal, 136t
  shaker exercise, 142–143
  swallowing therapy, 141–142
Dysphonia
  conversion, 171–172, 208
  drug-induced, 364–369
  functional, 352–353
  musculoskeletal tension, 170
  spasmodic, 355

E
Eclectic voice therapy, 169
Edema, chronic, 350–351
Edema, pulmonary, 263
Education
  in acute care setting, 294–295
  continuing, 6
EEG. See Electroencephalography (EEG)
EGG. See Electroglottography (EGG)
Eight-point penetration-aspiration scale, 237t
Elderly. See also Geriatrics
  delirium in, 308–309
  dementias in, 309–311
  frailty, 302t
  functional status, 301–302
  nutrition
    needs, 302–303
    nonoral feeding, 304–306
    risk factors, 303
    status measurement, 304
  pneumonia in
    diagnosing, 307
    enteral feeding and, 307–308
    infection modes, 306–308
    prevention, 308
    treatment, 308
  population, 301
  treating, 301–302
Electroencephalography (EEG), 320, 321t
Electroglottography (EGG), 164–165
Electromyography (EMG)
  laryngeal function, 165
  needle's role, 325
  never conduction studies, 320–322
  single-fiber, 323, 324t
  vocal fold paralysis exam, 354
EMG. See Electromyography (EMG)
Emphysema, 263
Encephalopathy, HIV, 105t
Encephalopathy, Wernicke's, 105t
Endoscopy
  dysphagia treatment
    as treatment guide, 154
    case study, 154–155
    indications, 148–149
    protocol, 149–154
    risks, 155–156
    sensory awareness, 154
  nasopharyngeal, 279
Enteral nutrition
  complications, 305–306
  pneumonia and, 307–308
  tubing, 305
  use, deciding on, 306
Epidermoid cysts, 169
Epiglottitis, 349
Epilepsy, 334–335
Epistaxis, 343
Errorless learning quizzes, 117, 118t
Esophageal speech, 195
Ethics
  clinical, 12
  defined, 311–312
  dementia care
    confidentiality, 122
    contemporary, 121

Ethics *(Continued)*
 diagnostic testing, 121–122
 philosophical bases, 120–121
 privacy, 122
 professional, 121
 dilemmas
  case studies, 11–15
  factors contributing to, 10–11
 geriatrics, 311–312
 principles
  autonomy, 9
  beneficence, 9–10
  confidentiality, 10–11
  fidelity, 10–11
  justice, 10
  nonmaleficence, 9–10
  veracity, 10–11
 professional, 8–9
Etiologic voice therapy, 168
Evidence-based practice
 classification system, 226
 conceptual confusions, 226–227
 defined, 224
 guidelines, 225–226
 origins, 224–225
 terminology, 226–227
Executive functioning, defined, 74
Expiration, defined, 261
Extrapyramidal system, 315–316

F
Facial nerve, 317
Facial pain, 345
Fairness. *See* Justice
Falsetto, functional, 171–172
FAST. *See* Functional assessment stages test (FAST)
Fiberoptic endoscopic examination of swallowing (FEES)
 ICU patients, 279
 indications, 149
 interpretation, 152–154
 procedure, 136–137
 protocol, 149–154
 scoring, 152–154
Fidelity, 10–11
Flaccid dysarthria, 76
FLCI. *See* Functional linguistic communication inventory (FLCI)
Flow measures, 164
Fluoroscopy, 149*t*
Fluphenazine, 367–368, 370
fMRI. *See* Functional magnetic resonance imaging (fMRI)
Focal atrophy, 101
Focal brain damage, 36
Focal neuropathy, 322–323
Frailty, criteria, 302*t*
Frontotemporal lobar dementia (FTD)
 AD *vs.*, 102
 characterization, 101–102
 differential diagnosis, 98*t*
 variants, 102
FTD. *See* Frontotemporal lobar dementia
Functional activation studies
 language deficits, 44–47
 normal language processing, 43–44
 single-word production, 44*t*
 speech-language therapy, 47–48

Functional assessment stages test (FAST), 114, 311*t*
Functional falsetto, 171–172
Functional goals, 250–251
Functional independence measure, 232, 238
Functional linguistic communication inventory (FLCI), 115
Functional magnetic resonance imaging (fMRI)
 application, 27, 29
 BOLD, 29
 defined, 27
 naming ability study, *47f, 48f*
Functional residual capacity, 262
Fundamental frequency, 162

G
Gag reflex, 135
Gait and station, 319
Galveston Orientation and Amnesia Test (GOAT), 73*t*
Gastroesophageal reflux disease (GERD), 358–359
Gastrostomy tubes, 305–306
GBS. *See* Guillain-Barré syndrome (GBS)
GDS. *See* Global deterioration scale (GDS)
Generalized tonic-clonic convulsions, 334
GERD. *See* Gastroesophageal reflux disease (GERD)
Geriatrics. *See also* Elderly
 case studies, 312–314
 defined, 301
 ethical issues, 311–312
 polypharmacy, 302
Glasgow coma scale, 72*t*
Global aphasia, 37*t*
Global deterioration scale (GDS), 114
Glossectomy, 193
Glossopharyngeal nerve, 317
Goals, functional, 250–251
Goals, measurable, 251
GOAT. *See* Galveston Orientation and Amnesia Test (GOAT)
Granulomas, contact, 169–170
GRBAS, 160
Guillain-Barré syndrome (GBS), 264, 332

H
Haloperidol, 367–368, 370
Harmonics-to-noise ratio, 162–163
HD. *See* Huntington's disease (HD)
Head and neck
 anatomic regions
  internal compartments, 183*f*
  larynx, 184
  lymphatic systems, 184
  nasal cavity, 183
  neural systems, 184
  oral cavity, 183, 338–342
  pharynx, 183–184, 338–342
  surgical margins, *191f*
  vascular systems, 184
 examination, 337–338
Head and neck cancer
 case studies, 199–200
 diagnosis, 185–186
 incidents of, 182
 laryngeal, 188–189
 metastatic neck disease, 189
 most common, 183, 341
 multidisciplinary management, 189–190, 192–193
 nasal, 187

nasopharyngeal, 188
oral cavity, 187–188
oropharyngeal, 188
postsurgical speech
    changes, 193
    glossectomy-associated, 193
    prosthetics and, 193–194
SLP competencies, 202
SLP intervention
    outpatient, 193
    postsurgical, 192–193
    pretreatment, 192
    timing, 190
swallowing changes
    evaluation, 198–199
    radiation-associated, 198
    surgery-associated, 198
symptoms, 185
tissue changes, 184–185
treatment, 187–198
tumors, classification, 186–187
tumors, sites, 185
Health insurance
appeals, 251–252
care requirements, 223–224
denials, 251–252
government programs, 217–219
private programs, 219–220
regulation of, 220–221
Health insurance portability and accountability
    act (HIPAA), 220–221
Health-related quality of life (HQL), 312
Hemiparetic gait, 319
HIPAA. *See* Health insurance portability and accountability
    act (HIPAA)
HIV. *See* Human immunodeficiency virus (HIV)
Hood speaking valve, 271
HPV. *See* Human papilloma virus (HPV)
HQL. *See* Health-related quality of life (HQL)
Human immunodeficiency virus (HIV), 105*t*, 359
Human papilloma virus (HPV), 352
Huntington's disease (HD), 105, 333
Hydration, 302–303
Hyperkinetic movement disorders, 333
Hypertrophy, adenotonsillar, 340
Hypoglossal nerve, 318
Hypokinetic movement disorders, 333

I
ICU. *See* Intensive care unit (ICU)
IFC. *See* International Classification of Functioning,
    Disability, and Health (IFC)
Impairment measures, 230–231
Impairment, defined, 76
Inclusion body myositis, 331
Inflammatory myopathies, 331
Inhaled steroids, 364, 367
Insurance. *See* Health insurance
Intensive care unit (ICU)
admission to, 260
case studies, 280
mechanical ventilation, 262–263
medical conditions seen, 263–264
SLP role in, 260
swallowing issues
    aspiration, 277–278

assessments, 278–279
    dysphagia patients, 278–279
    ethical issues, 279–280
    tracheostomy tubes, 278
tracheostomy
    communication with tube, 269–271
    protocal, 264
    tube placement, 265–266
    tube size chart, 267–268
International classification of functioning
    and health, 77
International Classification of Functioning,
    Disability, and Health (IFC), 229
Intervention planning, 57–58
Intracerebral hemorrhage, 329–330
Inverse filter measure, 164

J
Jejunostomy tubes, 305
Jolly test. *See* Repetitive nerve stimulation
Justice, 10

K
Kaposi's sarcoma, 359
Klüver-Bucy syndrome, 101

L
Lacrimal system, 183
Lambert-Eaton myasthenic syndrome (LEMS), 331–332
Language. *See also* Speech
acquired disorders
    lesion-deficit studies, 36–40
    neuroimaging, 40–47
areas (*See* Broca's area; Wernicke's area)
comprehension areas, 39*t*
confused, 75
deficits, 44–47
disturbances, 75
impairment, dementia-associated, 111
normal processing, 43–44
postsurgical service, 193
tests, dementia, 115
Laryngeal cancer
management, 188–189
postsurgical rehabilitation
    alaryngeal speech, 194–197
    respiratory changes, 197–198
    timing, 194
surgery, 194
Laryngeal papillomatosis, 351–352
Laryngitis, 349
Laryngomalacia, 349
Laryngopharyngeal reflux (LPR), 358–359
Laryngovidostroboscoy (LVS), 165
Larynx
anatomy, 345–348
artificial, 194–195
benign disorders, 349–353
characterization, 184
function, 135–136, 164
injury to, 264
neurolaryngology, 353–356
physiology, 348–349
trauma, 356–357
LBD. *See* Lewy body disease (LBD)
Learned helplessness, 209

LEMS. *See* Lambert-Eaton myasthenic syndrome (LEMS)
Lesion-deficit studies
    aphasia, 36–39
    conclusions, 40
    history, 35–36
Leukoplakia, 184
Lewy body disease (LBD), 98*t*, 101
Lexical-semantic impairments, 111
Libertarian theories, 10
Lip, cleft, 339–340
Lithium carbonate, 370*t*
Living will, 312
Loudness, 348–349
LPR. *See* Laryngopharyngeal reflux (LPR)
Lung. *See* Respiration
LVS. *See* Laryngovidostroboscoy (LVS)
Lymphatic systems, 184

M
Magnetic resonance imaging (MRI)
    advanced techniques, 27
    application, 23–24, 35*t*
    axial magnetization, 23*f*
    axial-enhanced, 26*f*
    CT vs, 26
    defined, 23
    functional, 27, 29
    general principles, 24
    limitations, 26–27
    neurologic examinations, 326–327
    periventricular stroke image, 32*f*
    pulse sequences, normal brain, 25*f*
    scanner schematic, 22*f*
    silent picture naming, 47*f*
    strengths, 24, 26
    temporal lobe infarct image, 28*f*
Malnutrition
    delirium and, 308
    forms, 303
    indicators, 304*t*
    risk factors, 303*t*
    treatment, 304
Manage care organizations (MCOs), 219
Mattis dementia rating scale, 114
Maxillomandibular fixation (MMF), 342
MCI. *See* Mild cognitive impairment (MCI)
MCOs. *See* Manage care organizations (MCOs)
Measurable goals, 251
Mechanical dysphagia, 373
Mechanical ventilation
    competencies, 282–283
    inhalation phase, 275–276
    patient profile, 262
    types, 262–263
Med Watch Program, 365*f*–366*f*
Medial subcallosal fasiculus (MSF), 39
Medical ethics. *See* Ethics
Medical necessity, 249–250
Medicare
    administration, 217
    creation, 217
    documentation guidelines, 252*t*
    fee schedule, 219
    payment system, 217–219
Medications. *See* Drugs
Melodic intonation therapy (MIT), 39, 48

Memory
    compensations, 117, 118*t*
    defined, 74
    impaired semantic, 63
Metastatic neck disease, 189
Metoclopramide, 371
Metrizamide, 371, 372
MG. *See* Myasthenia gravis (MG)
MID. *See* Multinfarct dementia
Mild cognitive impairment (MCI), 103–104
Mini-mental status examination (MMSE), 114, 310*t*
MIT. *See* Melodic intonation therapy (MIT)
MMF. *See* Maxillomandibular fixation (MMF)
Modern spiral CT, 21
Montessori-based activities, 117, 118*t*
Montgomery tracheostomy speaking valve, 271, 272*f*
Motor neuron disorders, 172–173
Motor unit
    characterization, 315
    control, 315–316
    examinations, 318
Movement disorders. *See* specific disorder
MRI. *See* Magnetic resonance imaging (MRI)
MS. *See* Multiple sclerosis (MS)
MSF. *See* Medial subcallosal fasiculus (MSF)
MTD. *See* Musculoskeletal tension dysphonia (MTD)
Mucous retention cysts, 169
Multinfarct dementia, 33*f*
Multiple sclerosis (MS)
    associated voice disorders, 172
    characterization, 333
    management, 334
    voice effects, 356
Multislice spiral CT, 21
Muscle tension disorders, 206–207
Muscular dystrophies (MDs), 331
Musculoskeletal tension dysphonia (MTD), 170
Mutism, 38*t*, 76
Myasthenia gravis (MG)
    characterization, 331
    single fiber, 323
    voice effects, 356
MyoD. *See* Myotonic dystrophy (MyoD)
Myopathic gait, 319
Myopathies, inflammatory, 331
Myotonic dystrophy (MyoD), 331

N
Naming, impaired, 64–65
Narrative story analyses, 86–87
Nasal cancer, 187
Nasal cavity
    characterization, 183
    coronal view, 343*f*
    diseases, 343–344
    function, 339, 342
    tumors, 344
Nasogastric tubes, 305
Nasopharyngeal cancer, 188
Nasopharyngeal endoscope, 279
Nasopharynx, 338, 341
National Center for Voice and Speech, 162*t*
Neoplastic lesions, 174–175
Nerves
    conduction study, 320–321
    cranial, 183, 316–318

disorders of, 332
systems, 184
Neurobehavioral cognitive status examination, 115
Neurocognitive communication disorders
  CBF, baseline studies, 40–43
  imaging technique comparisons, 22*t*
  lesion-deficit studies
    conclusions, 40
    history, 35–36
  metabolism, baseline studies, 40–43
Neurocommunication monitoring
  clinical observations, 292–293
  result communication, 294
  result utilization, 293–294
  tool selection, 291–292
Neurodegenerative dementias
  AD *vs.*, 97, 99
  classification, 96
  diagnostic criteria, 97*t*
Neurogenic dysphagia, 373
Neuroimaging
  acquired language disorders
    CBF studies, 40–43
    functional brain activation, 43–44
    lesion-deficit studies, 35–40
    metabolism studies, 40–43
    neural bases of, 44–47
  dementia diagnosis, 95–96
  techniques
    CT, 19–23
    diffusion-weighted, 41–42
    MRI, 23–27
    perfusion-weighted, 41–42
    PET, 32–35
    SPECT, 29–32
Neurolaryngology
  neuroanatomy, 353
  reflexes, 353
  spasmodic dysphonia, 355
  vocal fold paralysis, 353–355
Neuroleptic agents
  dysphagia and, 373–374
  speech arrest and, 370
  stuttering and, 370
  vocal fold disorders and, 367–368
Neurologic disorders
  cerebrovascular, 327–335
  examinations
    angiography, 327
    coordination, 319–320
    cranial nerves, 316–318
    EEG, 320
    EMG, 320–322
    gait, 319
    imaging studies, 326–327
    mental status, 316
    motor, 318
    neuromuscular transmission, 323–325
    neuropathy, 322–323
    reflexes, 319
    sensory, 318–319
    TCD, 325–326
  neuromuscular, 330–335
Neurological diseases, 264
Neuromuscular diseases
  distinctions, 330

inflammatory myopathies, 331
  movement disorders, 331, 333–335
  nerve-associated, 332
  neuromuscular transmission-associated, 331–332
Neuromuscular transmission, 323–325, 331–332
Neuropathy, types, 322–323
Neurotransmitters, 370*t*
Nodules, 169, 349–350
Nonmaleficence, 9–10
Nonoral feeding, 304–306
Nostrils. *See* Anterior nares
Nursing Home Reform Act, 239
Nutrition. *See also* Malnutrition
  enteral, 305–308
  needs, 302–303
  parenteral, 304–305
  risk factors, 303
  status measurement, 304

O
OASIS. *See* Outcome and Assessment Information
    Set (OASIS)
Obstructive sleep apnea syndrome, 342
OCCHTA. *See* Ongoing, contextualized, collaborative
    hypothesis-testing assessment (OCCHTA)
Oculomotor nerve, 316
Oculopharyngeal MD, 331
One-way speaking valves
  contraindications, 275
  description, 269–270
  indications, 275*t*
  placement protocol, 271–273
  types of, 270–271
Ongoing, contextualized, collaborative hypothesis-testing
    assessment (OCCHTA), 86*t*
Optic nerve, 316
Oral cavity
  boundaries of, 338
  cancer, 187–188
  characterization, 183
  function, 338
  infections, 341
  trauma, 341–342
  tumors, 341
Oral reading, impaired, 65*t*
Orientation, defined, 74
Oropharyngeal cancer, 188
Oropharynx, 338, 341
OSAS. *See* Obstructive sleep apnea syndrome
Otalgia nerve, 345
Otolaryngology. *See also* specific disorders
  AIDS and, 359
  case studies, 359–360
  characterization, 286
  examinations, 337–338
Outcome and Assessment Information Set (OASIS), 239
Outcome tools, 238
Outcome-oriented practice
  complexity of, 227–228
  conceptual framework, 229
  decision making, 233
  definition of terms, 228
  measures
    costs, 231–232
    impairment, 230–231
    models, 229–230

Outcome-oriented practice *(Continued)*
    participation, 231
    satisfaction, 232
    test selection checklist, 230
  methods, 232
  program evaluation, 232–233
  time factors, 228

P
Pain
  ear, 345
  facial, 345
  management, 192
  swallowing-associated, 341
Palate, cleft, 339–340
Palatine tonsils, 340
Papilloma, 175
Papillomatosis, laryngeal, 351–352
Paradoxical vocal fold movement
  case study, 177–178
  characterization, 175
  diagnosing, 175–176
  medical descriptors, 175t
  therapeutic interventions, 177t
  treatment, 176–177
Paranasal sinuses
  disorders
    common, 343
    epistaxis, 343
    nasal massess, 344
    rhinitis, 344
    sinusitis, 344
  function of, 342
Parenteral nutrition, 304–305
Parkinson's disease
  AD *vs.*, 104
  characterization, 333
  gait in, 319
  management, 333
  mood disorders and, 104
Participation, defined, 76
Passy-Muir Ventilator (PMV)
  description, 270
  guidelines, 273t–274t
  models, 270–271
  placement, 271–273
  removal indications, 275t
  troubleshooting, 275t
Paternalism, defined, 10
Pathophysiology, defined, 76
Patient care
  confidentiality, 10–11, 122, 253
  documentation, 247–248
  security, 253
  standards for, 252–253
PDT. *See* Photodynamic therapy (PDT)
Perfusion-weighted imaging studies, 20t, 41–42
Periodic summaries, 238
Peripheral nervous system, 173
Persistent vegetative state, 73
Perturbation measures, 162
PET. *See* Positron emission tomography (PET)
Pharynx. *See also* Nasopharynx; Oropharynx
  characterization, 183–184
  function, 339
  infections, 341

Phonation
  characterization, 348
  prolonged, 135
  threshold pressure, 164
Phonetogram, 163
Phonologic impairments, 112
Photodynamic therapy (PDT), 175
Physiologic frequency range phonation.
    See Phonetogram
Physiologic voice therapy, 169
PMV. *See* Passy-Muir Ventilator (PMV)
Pneumonia
  aspiration-associated, 277, 307
  diagnosing, 307
  enteral feeding and, 307–308
  infection modes, 306–308
  prevention, 308
  treatment, 308
Polymyositis, 331
Polypharmacy, 302
Polyps, vocal, 169
Positron emission tomography (PET)
  aphasia neurophysiology, 41–42
  application, 32–33, 35t
  CBF, 35f
  defined, 32
  general principles, 33–34
  limitations, 34–35
  neurologic examinations, 327
  radiopharmaceuticals, 31t, 33t, 34
  scanner schematic, 34f
  strengths, 34
Posterior nares, 183
Posttraumatic amnesia (PTA), 72
PPA. *See* Primary progressive aphasia (PPA)
Practice. *See also* Speech-language pathologist
  acute care
    competency checklist, 296–297
    consultation, 284–285, 288–294, 297–298
    defined, 284
    education, 294–295
    key issues, 286–288
    organization, 285
    referral sources, 285–287
  consultative, 5
  evidence-based
    classification system, 226
    conceptual confusions, 226–227
    defined, 224
    guidelines, 225–226
    origins, 224–225
    terminology, 226–227
  ICU
    admissions, 260
    case studies, 280
    mechanical ventilation, 262–263
    medical conditions seen, 263–264
    swallowing issues, 277–280
    tracheotomies, 269–271
  outcome-oriented
    complexity of, 227–228
    conceptual framework, 229
    decision making, 233
    definition of terms, 228
    measures, 229–232
    methods, 232

program evaluation, 232–233
time factors, 228
scope of
cultural aspects, 216
expansion of, 215t
telepractice, 216–217
standards, 6
Pragmatics
dementia, 111
protocol, 92
rating scale, 91
TBI, 75–76
Pressure support ventilation, 262
Previous level of functioning, 250
Primary progressive aphasia (PPA), 102–103
Privacy. See Confidentiality
Procedures, ASHA guidelines, 5
Professional voice disorders, 357–358
Prosthese, 193–194, 196f
Psychiatry, 286
Psychogenic communication disorders
assessment, 209
classification, 205–208
epidemiology, 208
psychiatric comorbidity, 208–209
terminology, 205
treatment, 210–211
Psychogenic voice therapy, 168
PTA. See Posttraumatic amnesia (PTA)
Pugilistic parkinsonism, 105t
Pure word deafness, 39t
PVS. See Persistent vegetative state

Q
Quality improvement method, 233
Quality of life, 237, 311

R
Radiation, 198
Radiopharmaceuticals, 31t
RAI. See Resident assessment instrument (RAI)
Ranchos Los Ameigos rating, 80t–83t, 291t
Rating scales, 236–237
Reading, impaired, 66t
Reading, oral, 65t
Reasonable and necessary, 250
Reflexes, 319, 353
Rehabilitation
aphasia
care continuum, 62
classification, 61
evidence-based practice, 62–68
perspectives on, 61–62
SLPs' role, 61–62
special technologies, 67
stroke survivor groups, 68–69
TBI
assumptions, 79t
cognitive, 78–79
continuum, 77–78
defined, 76–77
direct attention training, 84t
Rehabilitation Accreditation Commission (CARF),
232–233, 252–253
Reimbursement
charge document, 250t

coding, 220
documentation, 248–252
Medicaid, 219
Medicare, 217–219
private heath plans, 219–220
Reminiscence therapy, 117
Repetitive nerve stimulation, 323
Research
AD, 99
dementia, 123
documentation, 253–254
ethics, 123
question formation, 244–245
Resident assessment instrument (RAI), 239
Resource utilization groups (RUGs), 218
Respiration
aiding
dysphagic patients, 134–135
mechanical ventilation, 262–263
tracheostomy, 264–277
diseases of, 263–264
ICU treatment, 262–263
medical specialists, 286
normal, 260–262
post-TE puncture, 197–198
Rhinitis, 344
Riluzole, 332
RIPA-G. See Ross information processing assessment (RIPA-G)
RLA. See Ranchos Los Ameigos
Ross information processing assessment (RIPA-G), 115
RUG. See Resource utilization groups (RUGs)
Rules of conduct, 8–9

S
Salivary gland, 341
SD. See Spasmodic dysphonia (SD)
Security, 253
Seizures, 334
Sensory ataxic gait, 319
Sensory awareness, 154, 318–319
Sentence processing, 66–67
Service delivery, 236–239
SFEMG. See Single-fiber electromyography (SFEMG)
Shaker, Reza, 142
Shiley phonate speaking valve, 271, 272f
Silent picture naming, 47f
Single photon emission computed tomography (SPECT)
application, 29–30, 31t, 35t
applications, 31t
Broca area image, 30f
cerebral perfusion images, 32f
defined, 29
gamma camera system schematic, 32f
general principles, 30–31
MID image, 33f
radiopharmaceuticals, 31t
strengths, 31–32
weaknesses, 31–32
Single-fiber electromyography (SFEMG), 176f
Single-word comprehension, 63–64
Single-word expression
cognitive process, 64f
functional activation studies, 44t
rehabilitation, 64–65
Sinuses. See Paranasal sinuses
Sinustitis, 344

Sleep apnea. *See* Obstructive sleep apnea syndrome
Sleep disorders, 342
SLPs. *See* Speech-language pathologists
Snoring, 342
*SOD*1. *See* Cu/Zn superoxide dismutase *(SOD1)*
Somatoform disorders, 209
Spaced retrieval, 117, 118*t*
Spasmodic dysphonia (SD), 173, 355
Speaking valves. *See* One-way speaking valves
SPECT. *See* Single photon emission computed tomography (SPECT)
Speech. *See also* Language
  alaryngeal
    artificial, 194–195
    esophageal, 195
    tracheoesophageal, 195–196
  anatomic substrates, 315–316
  disturbances, 76
  drug-induced disorders
    aphasia, 371
    dysarthria, 369–371
    overview, 368*t*–369*t*
    stuttering, 371–372
  esophageal, 195
  postsurgical
    alaryngeal, 194–197
    changes, 193
    glossectomy-associated, 193
    larynages-associated, 194–197
    prosthetics and, 193–194
Speech–language pathologists. *See also* Practice
  aphasia rehabilitation role, 61–62
  cancer treatment role, 182–183
  certification, 214–215
  clinical environment, 214, 215*t*
  consultative practice, 5
  continuing education, 6
  continuum of care, 4
  delivery service, 6
  dementia
    diagnosis, 112–113
    interventions, 115
    training programs, 118
  differentiating, 3–4
  endoscopy use by, 148
  ethical issues, 5–6
  evidence-based (*See* Evidence-based practice)
  funding issues, 213
  head/neck cancer intervention
    outpatient, 193
    postsurgical, 192–193
    pretreatment, 192
    timing, 190
  ICU role, 260
  interprofessional issues, 6
  issues in, 5–6
  outcome-oriented practice (*See* Outcome-oriented practice)
  practices trends, 5
  procedures, 5
  reimbursement
    coding, 220
    Medicaid, 219
    Medicare, 217–219
    private heath plans, 219–220
  skills requirements, 214–215
  subspecialization, 4–5
  technological developments, 5

Spelling, impaired, 66
Spinal cord injury, 264
Spontaneous speech recovery, 40*f*
Squamous cell carcinoma, 183, 184
Squamous papilloma, 351–352
Standardized Mini-mental state examination
    (SMMSE), 114
Steroids, androgenic, 367
Steroids, inhaled, 331, 364, 367
Stroke
  cerebral ischemia, 327–329
  dementia-associated, 99–101
  ICU care, 264
  intracerebral hemorrhage, 329–330
  periventrical, MRI image, 32*f*
  prevalence, 327
  subarachnoid hemorrhage, 330
  survivor groups, 68–69
Stuttering, 371–372
Subarachnoid hemorrhage, 330
Subcortial dementia, 104–106
Subglottal air pressure, 164
Suctioning, 276–277
Sulcus vocalis, 351
Supraglottic hyperfunction, 367
Swallowing. *See also* specific disorders
  acute care documentation, 290–291
  apraxia, 135
  aspiration, 277–278
  cancer effects on, 198–199
  drug-induced disorders, 368*t*–369*t*, 372–374
  efficacy studies, 242*t*
  FEES exam, 136–137, 279
  maneuvers, 139*t*
  modified barium, 137–140, 149
  painful, 341
  therapy
    case study, 142
    direct, 142
    ethical issues, 279–280
    indirect, 141–142
    measures, 143*t*
  tracheostomy and, 278–279, 357
Symptomatic voice therapy, 168
Syntax impairments, 112

T
Tardive dyskinesia, 374
TBI. *See* Traumatic brain injury (TBI)
TCD. *See* Transcranial doppler (TCD)
TE. *See* Tracheoesophageal puncture (TE)
Tear system. *See* Lacrimal system
Technology developments, 5
Telepractice, 216–217
Temporal lobe infarct, 28*f*
Temporomandibular joint (TMJ), 345
Test design, 230–231
Test of neuromuscular transmission, 323–325
Thiamin deficiency, 308
Thyroarytenoid muscles, 347
Thyroid cartilage, 345
Time frames, 253
TMJ. *See* Temporomandibular joint (TMJ)
Tongue disorders, 341
Tonsillectomy, 342
Tonsils, 340

Tracheoesophageal puncture (TE)
  development of, 195
  modification, 195–196
  patient candidacy for, 196–197
  respiration following, 197–198
  speech-associated with, 196
Tracheoesophageal speech, 195–196
Tracheostomy
  communications
    nonverbal, 277
    one-way speaking valves, 269–275
    patient assessment, 269
    suctioning for, 276–277
    voicing options, 275–276
  competencies, 282–283
  controversies, 264
  description, 357
  emergency, 357
  swallowing and, 357
  tubes
    controversies, 264
    placement, 265–266, 269
    selection, 267–268
    talking, 276
Tracheotomy
  defined, 357
  protocol, 264
Transcortical motor aphasia, 37t
Transcortical sensory aphasia, 37t
Transcranial doppler (TCD), 325–326
Traumatic brain injury (TBI)
  cognitive disturbances, 74–75
  coma, 73–74
  defined, 71–72
  incidence, 72
  language disturbances, 75–76
  modes of, 71–72
  recovery
    early stage, 81–82
    intermediate stage, 82–85
    late stage, 85–89
    narrative story analyses, 86–87
    OCCHTA, 86t
    RLA rating, 80t–83t
    usual course, 79, 81
  rehabilitation
    assumptions, 79t
    cognitive, 78–79
    continuum, 77–78
    defined, 76–77
    direct attention training, 84t
  sequelae following, 73–76
  severity of, 72–73
  speech disturbances, 76
Treatment. See also specific conditions
  effective, 250
  goals, 250–251
  plan, 237–238, 248t
  skilled, 250
  specificity, 250
Tremor, 333, 355
Trigeminal nerve, 316–317, 345
Trochlear nerve, 316
Tubes
  feeding, 305–308
  tracheostomy

controversies, 264
placement, 265–266, 269
selection, 267–268
talking, 276

U
Ulcers, 169–170
Upper motor neurons, 315
UPPP. See Uvulopalatopharyngoplasty (UPPP)
Utilitarian theories, 10
Uvulopalatopharyngoplasty (UPPP), 342

V
VaD. See Vascular disease (VaD)
Vagus nerve, 317–318, 347
Validation therapy, 116–117
Vascular dementia, 309, 311
Vascular disease (VaD), 98t, 99–101
Vascular system, 184
Ventilation
  defined, 261
  mechanical
    competencies, 282–283
    inhalation phase, 275–276
    patient profile, 262
    types, 262–263
  pressure support, 262
Veracity, 10–11
VHI. See Voice handicap index (VHI)
Videoendoscopy, 155–156
Vitamins, 303
Vocal fold movement
  characterization, 348
  paradoxical
    case study, 177–178, 177t
    characterization, 175
    diagnosing, 175–176
    medical descriptors, 175t
    therapeutic interventions, 177t
    treatment, 176–177
Vocal folds
  cysts, 169, 349–350
  lesions
    benign, 349–352
    brainstem-associated, 173t
    categorization, 174–175
    peripheral nerve-associated, 173t
  nodules, 349–350
  paralysis, 353–355, 367–368
  paresis, 367–368
  polyp, 350
Vocal nodules, 169
Vocal polyps, 169
Voice disorders
  cerebellar, 173
  classification, 207t
  conversion, 170–172
  diagnosis
    acoustic measures, 161–163
    aims of, 158
    areodynamic measures, 163–164
    auditory perceptual analysis, 159–160
    clinical laboratory, 161
    EGG, 164–165
    EMG, 165
    history taking, 159

Voice disorders *(Continued)*
  imaging, 165–166
  instrumental measures, 160*t*
  inverse filter measure, 164
  severity assessment, 160–161
  tools, 158–159
 etiologies, 159*t*
 extrapyramidal, 173
 functional, 169–171, 352–353
 muscular, 173–174
 myoneural junction, 173–174
 neoplastic lesions, 174–175
 neurogenic, 172–173
 neurologic, 355–356
 paradoxical vocal fold movement
  case study, 177–178
  characterization, 175
  diagnosing, 175–176
  medical descriptors, 175*t*
  treatment, 176–177
 professional, 357–358
 SD, 173
 treatment
  case study, 167–168
  options, 168–169
  principles, 166–167
Voice handicap index (VHI), 161

Voice range profile. *See* Phonetogram
Voice therapy, 210*t*
Voluntary tasks, 134*t*

W
Waldeyer's ring, 340
Wernicke's area
 aphasia, 37
 damage to, 36
 function, 35
Wernicke's encephalopathy, 105*t*
Wernicke, Carl, 35
WHO. *See* World Health Organization (WHO)
Wilson's disease, 105*t*
Word
 fluency measure, 115
 single, comprehension, 63–64
 single, expression
  cognitive process, 64*f*
  functional activation studies, 44*t*
  rehabilitation, 64–65
Word retrieval, 65*t*
World Health Organization (WHO), 77*t*, 229
Writing, impaired, 66

X
X-ray, 20